CONGENITAL HEART DISEASE – SELECTED ASPECTS

Edited by **P. Syamasundar Rao**

Congenital Heart Disease – Selected Aspects
Edited by P. Syamasundar Rao

Published by InTech
Janeza Trdine 9, 51000 Rijeka, Croatia

Notice
Statements and opinions expressed in the chapters are these of the individual contributors and not necessarily those of the editors or publisher. No responsibility is accepted for the accuracy of information contained in the published chapters. The publisher assumes no responsibility for any damage or injury to persons or property arising out of the use of any materials, instructions, methods or ideas contained in the book.

Publishing Process Manager Marina Jozipovic

Technical Editor Teodora Smiljanic

Cover Designer InTech Design Team

Additional hard copies can be obtained from orders@intechopen.com

Congenital Heart Disease – Selected Aspects, Edited by P. Syamasundar Rao
p. cm.
ISBN 978-953-307-472-6

For EU product safety concerns:
IN TECH d.o.o., Prolaz Marije Krucifikse Kozulić 3, 51000 Rijeka, Croatia,
info@intechopen.com or visit our website at intechopen.com.

Meet the editor

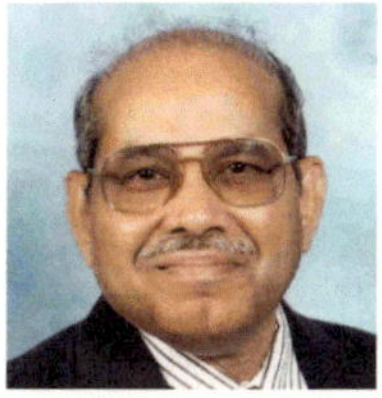

Dr. P. Syamasundar Rao is a Professor of Pediatrics and Medicine and Emeritus Chief of Pediatric Cardiology at the University of Texas-Houston Medical School and Professor of Pediatrics at the University of Texas M.D. Anderson Cancer Center in Houston, Texas, USA. Dr. Rao received his medical degree from Andhra Medical College/University in Visakhapatnam, India. He received training in Pediatric Cardiology at Stanford University, Case-Western Reserve University, and University of California in Los Angeles. After training, he joined the faculty at the Medical College of Georgia in Augusta, Georgia, USA, and became the Associate Director of Pediatric Cardiology. His subsequent positions were as follows: Consultant Pediatric Cardiologist and Chairman, Department of Pediatrics, King Faisal Specialist Hospital and Research Center in Riyadh, Saudi Arabia, Professor and Director of Division of Pediatric Cardiology at the University of Wisconsin in Madison, Wisconsin, and Professor/Director of the Division of Pediatric Cardiology at Saint Louis University School of Medicine/Cardinal Glennon Children's Hospital, St. Louis, Missouri. Dr. Rao authored 350 papers, eight monographs/books, and 55 book chapters. He lectured and made catheter intervention demonstrations in a number of countries including India, USA, Australia, Finland, Sweden, Germany, New Zealand, Brazil, and Japan.

Contents

Preface

Congenital heart defect (CHD) may be defined as an anatomic malformation of the heart or great vessels which occurs during intrauterine development, irrespective of the age at presentation. Ventricular septal defect and coarctation of the aorta are typical examples of CHDs. The reported incidence of congenital cardiac defects varies between 0.6% and 0.8% of live births. This would result in the birth of 30 to 35,000 infants with CHD each year in the United States alone. Congenital heart defects are more common than well-known congenital anomalies such as congenital pyloric stenosis, cleft lip, Down syndrome, and congenital dislocation of the hip. Nearly 50% of these babies can be managed with simple medications, observation, and follow-up without any major therapeutic intervention. However, the remaining 50%, in the past, required surgical intervention, some under cardiopulmonary bypass. Since the advent of transcatheter techniques, 50% of these babies (i.e., 25% of the total) can be managed with less invasive, percutaneous, transcatheter techniques.

Developments such as early detection of the neonates with serious heart disease and their rapid transport to tertiary care centers, availability of highly sensitive noninvasive diagnostic tools, advances in neonatal care and anesthesia, progress in transcatheter interventional procedures, and extension of complicated surgical procedures to the neonate and infant have advanced to such a degree that almost all congenital cardiac defects can be diagnosed and "corrected". The defects that could not be corrected could be effectively palliated. For achieving excellence in cardiac care, however, close interaction and collaboration of the pediatric cardiologists with neonatologists, pediatricians, general/family practitioners (who care for children with CHD), internists (who care for adults with CHD), anesthesiologists, and cardiac surgeons is mandatory. Education of physicians caring for children and adults with CHD continues to be important in achieving optimal care for the patients with heart disease.

Because of vastness of the subject, all issues related to congenital heart defects cannot be discussed in their entirety and therefore, only selected aspects will be included in this book. The book is divided into several sections, which include an overview of congenital heart defects, prevalence and etiology, some individual heart defects, management of some of the congenital heart defects, international issues, and miscellaneous issues. While there are significant advances in the understanding molecular mechanisms of cardiac development and of the etiology of CHD, these have not progressed to such a degree so as to be useful in preventing CHD at this time. Consequently, several chapters were devoted to this subject.

In the first section on the overview of congenital heart defects, I present a brief review of incidence, etiology and classification of CHD, and an overview of the nine most common congenital cardiac anomalies and their management. The exact etiology of CHD is not known, and the majority of cardiac defects can be explained by multifactorial inheritance hypothesis. The CHD may be classified as acyanotic and cyanotic defects, the former being further divided into obstructive and left-to-right shunt lesions. Pathologic, physiologic, clinical, and laboratory features of the nine most common CHD were distinctively described. Methods of management for each of these defects include transcatheter techniques for most of the acyanotic defects and by and large surgery for the cyanotic defects. Based on this review, it appears that while the etiology of CHD is not clearly identified, their recognition by clinical evaluation and non-invasive laboratory tests is possible, and their treatment with currently available transcatheter and surgical methods is feasible, effective, and safe.

In the next section on prevalence and etiology, Sayasathid and Associates from Naresuan University, Thailand, discuss epidemiology and etiology of CHD including preventative guidelines for pregnant mothers. They suggest that the number of patients with CHD continues to increase, and that epidemiology studies reveal that cases of CHD are underestimated. Huang and Liang of Guangxi Traditional Chinese Medical College in Nanning, China explore molecular mechanisms of congenital heart disease. The authors review normal cardiac development and recent discoveries of the genetic causes of CHD. They provide possible strategies for exploring these new developments to improve understanding of the genetic basis of CHD. They support the use of animal biomedical models to understand normal and abnormal function from gene to phenotype, and to provide a basis for preventive or therapeutic intervention in human diseases. In the next chapter, Minamisawa and Yokoyama from Waseda University, Japan, present recent advances in the molecular mechanism of patent ductus arteriosus (PDA). The authors describe acute and functional closure of the ductus, and discuss complex molecular mechanisms involved in ductal closure. The remodelling is reviewed, which includes the differentiation of vascular smooth muscle cells (SMCs) and endothelial cells, accumulation of extracellular matrix, vascular SMC migration into the sub endothelial region, impaired elastogenesis, and eventually fibrotic changes due to apoptosis and necrosis. The role of PGE2-EP4-cAMP signal pathway, oxygen, and calcium channels. Multiple vasoreactive stimulations in the modulator of vascular remodelling of the ductus arteriosus is also discussed. The authors conclude that this knowledge may help develop novel therapeutic strategies for patients with PDA and ductal dependent cardiac anomalies. Harmelink and Jiao of the University of Alabama in Birmingham, USA, describe bone morphogenetic protein (BMP) signaling pathways in heart development and disease. They review evidence from multiple experimental models that demonstrates the role of BMP signaling pathways in the heart development. Initially, they describe normal heart development in the mice model. Then, they describe the BMP signaling pathways in general and specific to heart development, including that of the mesoderm, myocardial wall formation, valve development, chamber septation, and outflow tract morphogenesis. The authors conclude that BMP signaling pathways are critical regulators of heart development in several species, including humans, and that mutations in the BMP pathway have been identified in humans with CHD. This insight may help develop diagnostic tests and therapeutic options for CHD in the future. Vogler et al of Sanford-Burnham Medical Research Institute in La Jolla, California, describe recent advances and findings gained from a Drosophila model for CHD. They begin with comparing Drosophila to vertebrate cardiogenesis and point out their similarities. They then allude to the lessons learned from studying Drosophila heart morphogenesis. This is followed by a discussion of manipulating the heart and genome of a fly. They also suggest that the Drosophila model is useful in elucidating the molecular mechanisms of CHD and cardiomyopathy. They conclude that development of technologies such as time-lapse analysis of heart formation, and optical techniques to study function suggest that further studies using this system will provide insights into fundamental cellular mechanisms underlying heart function and disease.

In the next section, three individual cardiac defects are reviewed. Flack and Graham from Vanderbilt University, Nashville, Tennessee, USA, describe incidence, natural history, clinical and laboratory features, and management of congenitally corrected transposition of the great arteries (CCTGA). The authors allude to the problems associated with dysfunction of left-sided, morphologic right ventricle with or without Ebstein's type of malformation of the morphologic tricuspid valve. Conventional medical management and cardiac resynchronization are discussed. Role of conventional surgical therapy and double-switch operation are also detailed. Follow-up recommendations and pregnancy outcomes are also discussed. They conclude that outcomes, based on long-term follow-up of physiologic vs. anatomic repair for CCTGA, favor anatomic correction. Ríos-Méndez of "El Cruce" Hospital in Buenos Aires, Argentina, present four cases of a double-chambered right ventricle from their institution, discuss the significance of these findings and present a literature review. The author concludes that the double-chambered right ventricle is a rare cardiac anomaly, ventricular septal defect is the most commonly-associated defect. Echocardiography (transthoracic or transesophageal), performed by a cardiologist familiar with congenital heart disease, is the method of choice for diagnosing this condition, and surgical treatment is effective with low morbidity. Pierre et al of Bichat Hospital in Paris, France, reviews features of anomalous connections of coronary arteries (ANOCOR), presents a simple classification, points out low prevalence of about 1% in the general population, discusses anatomical patterns associated with a risk of sudden death, and explores prevention of sport-related fatalities and modalities of cost-effective screening. Additionally, Pierre et al advocates multidetector CT angiography with three-dimensional reconstruction as an accurate diagnostic tool, supports surgery by the unroofing technique in ANOCOR arising from the aorta (and direct aortic implantation for ANOCOR connected with the pulmonary artery), deplores lack of long-term follow-up evaluation after surgery and support setting up of registries to determine the outcome of children and young adults (≤ 30-year old) with high-risk ANOCOR.

Management of congenital heart disease was discussed in the next section. Hadzimuratovic discusses evaluation and emergency treatment of critically ill neonates with cyanosis and respiratory distress. The author reviews some important aspects of normal and abnormal findings in physical examination, ECG, and chest x-ray films of the neonate, and suggested approaches to diagnose and treat neonates with central cyanosis. The author then discusses management of several neonatal issues, namely, heart failure in the newborn infant, hypoplastic left heart syndrome, premature neonates with a large PDA, persistent pulmonary hypertension of the newborn, and transient myocardial ischemia. Guzman et al from Cardiovascular Clinic Santa Maria in Medellin, Colombia present the results of Fontan Surgery performed at their institution. They state that management strategies for functional single ventricles have evolved into staged procedures with a goal to obtain normal ventricular pressures, volumes, and normal systemic arterial saturation. They examined the results of total cavo-pulmonary connection (Fontan operation) and conclude that the Fontan operation performed at their institution is safe with a mortality rate of 14.3%, comparable to a previously published large series.

In the next section on international issues, Bode-Thomas at the University of Jos in Nigeria reviews practical problems encountered in the diagnosis, treatment, and prevention of congenital heart diseases in the developing countries. The author initially points out that there is a paucity of data on the incidence or birth prevalence of congenital heart disease in most developing countries. This under-estimates the burden of congenital heart disease, undermining arguments for more resource allocation in the face of the many other competing health care needs. A discussion of peculiarities and challenges of CHD diagnosis and treatment in developing regions follows with a suggestion for establishing treatment centers in developing countries.

The final section includes several miscellaneous issues. Chalajour et al of Stanford University in Stanford, California, USA, discusses dynamics of myocardial cell populations following birth, and the role of cardiac progenitor cells (CPC) in neonatal myocardial tissue expansion and heart growth, as well as therapeutic strategies for congenital heart defects. The authors conclude that the presence of resident CPC in myocardium is well supported. However, controversies continue regarding the origin of CPC. Methods for activating resident CPC are still in the early discovery phase, and the potential applications of CPC-focused therapies in congenital heart disease treatment are likely in the future. Li from the University of Alberta, Canada, in a chapter on "Accurate measurement of systemic oxygen consumption in ventilated children with congenital heart disease" points out inaccuracies of using estimated oxygen consumption values (calculated by predictive equations developed by several workers in the past) in the Fick principle. These inaccuracies were found particularly in children younger than 3 years of age, whether it be in the Catheterization Laboratory or in the ICU postoperatively. The author describes the use of respiratory mass spectrometry to accurately measure oxygen consumption, and discuss the post-operative physiology following Norwood operation and its management. Itoi from Kyoto Prefectural University of Medicine in Kyoto, Japan, discusses myocardial use of energy substrates in young patients with atrial (ASD) and ventricular septal defects (VSD) and patent ductus arteriosus, (PDA) and presents their data. They conclude that myocardial energy metabolism in acyanotic CHD was sustained by fatty acid oxidation irrespective of workload. There was accelerated glucose use with overload. Lactate seemed to play an important role in maintain lactate-pyruvate redox potential. When mild myocardial workload (as in ASD), the NADH demand was complemented by lactate oxidation, while with higher workload (as in pulmonary hypertension) lactate production was accelerated to maintain the cellular redox state. Okuneva et al from E.N. Meshalkin Research Institute of Circulation Pathology and A.V. Nikolayev Institute of Inorganic Chemistry in Russia describes the results of their study to investigate the structure of cardiomyocytes, and the content of chemical elements (CE) in infants with transposition of the great arteries (TGA). They found that pathologic hypertrophy of myocardium in TGA is reflected by the decreased Zn, Br, Cr, Cl and Se content in myocardium (also Ca) and excess of Copper. They recommend that pregnant women and nursing mothers should get the optimum quantity of microelements Cr, Zn, Sr, Ni, Rb, Br, and most impotently Se (to protect the myocardium from lipid peroxidation). Se also prevents development of congenital heart diseases, including TGA, although no data to support this recommendation was presented.

There are significant advances in the understanding of the molecular mechanisms of cardiac development and of the etiology of CHD. However, these have not evolved to such a degree so as to be useful in preventing CHD at this time. Treatment of the majority of acyanotic and simpler cyanotic heart defects with currently available transcatheter and surgical techniques is feasible, effective and safe. Recent advances in medical and surgical therapy, particularly the application of staged total cavo-pulmonary connection (Fontan) have markedly improved the long-term outlook of children who have one functioning ventricle. There are a number of other developments, some of which were reviewed in this book. It is my hope that these discussions will give a fund of information to the practicing physician caring for infants, children and adults with congenital heart defects, helping them provide optimal care for their patients.

P. Syamasundar Rao, MD, FAAP, FACC, FSCAI
University of Texas at Houston Medical School
Houston, Texas,
USA

Part 1

Overview of Congenital Hear Defects

1

Congenital Heart Defects – A Review

P. Syamasundar Rao
University of Texas at Houston Medical School, Houston
USA

1. Introduction

Congenital heart defect (CHD) may be defined as an anatomic malformation of the heart or great vessels which occurs during intrauterine development, irrespective of the age at presentation. Ventricular septal defect and coarctation of the aorta are typical examples of CHDs. In this chapter, a brief review of incidence, etiology and classification of CHD, and an overview of the most common congenital cardiac anomalies and their management will be presented. Cardiac abnormalities, generally considered not congenital in origin but important cardiac problems in children, namely rheumatic heart disease, Kawasaki syndrome and cardiomyopathy will not be discussed in this review. Also, discussion of important symptoms/findings/issues with which the children are referred to pediatric cardiologists such as cardiac murmur, chest pain, syncope/dizziness, palpitation, arrhythmia, hypertension, clearance for participation in sports, coronary risk factors, bacterial endocarditis prophylaxis, ADHD medication use, clearance for non-cardiac surgery and others will not be included in the this chapter.

Incidence of congenital heart defects

The reported incidence of congenital cardiac defects varies between 0.47 to 1.17% of live births, but 0.6% to 0.8% of live births is considered typical. This would result in birth of 25,000 to 35,000 infants with CHD each year in the United States alone. Congenital heart defects are more common than well-known congenital anomalies such as congenital pyloric stenosis, cleft lip, Down syndrome and congenital dislocation of the hip.

2. Etiology

The exact cause of all congenital cardiac defects is not known. The majority of the defects can be explained by multifactorial inheritance hypothesis (Nora 1968) which states that a predisposed fetus, when exposed to a given environmental trigger (to which the fetus is sensitive) during the critical period of cardiac morphogenesis will develop the disease. This genetic and environmental interaction is most likely to be pathogenetic mechanism of congenital heart defects. Calculations based on this hypothesis predict the frequency of occurrence of the disease in first degree relatives to be square root of its frequency in the population; this fits the congenital heart disease figures (Nora 1968).

A variety of factors have statistical association with certain heart defects and these may be termed risk factors. Maternal rubella appears to have causative association with heart defects. Significantly higher incidence of serologic evidence for Coxsackie B virus infection during pregnancy in mothers of infants with congenital heart defects than in matched-control women suggested causative relationship between Coxsackie B infection and congenital heart defects, but this evidence is neither conclusive nor confirmed. Among drugs, maternal ingestion of thalidomide during pregnancy is associated with high incidence heart defects in the offspring. Similar association has been reported for some anticonvulsant drugs (particularly dilantin and trimethadione), alcohol (excessive), Lithium, sex hormones, diazepam, carticosteroids, phenolhiazine, folic acid antagonists, cocaine and dextromethamphetamines. A higher incidence of cardiac abnormalities with maternal diabetes is well known. Gross chromosomal anomalies such as trisomy 21 (Down syndrome), trisomy D and E syndromes, Turner's syndrome (XO), partial deletion of chromosome 22 and cri-du-chat (partial dilation of the short arm of chromosome 5) are associated with a higher incidence of heart defects than normal population and are likely be responsible for the congenital heart defects. Some generalized syndromes, secondary to a single mutant gene (for example, Marfan) involving multiple organ systems are associated with cardiovascular defects peculiar to that particular syndrome (Rao 1977a). Both autosomal (dominant and recessive) and sex-linked (dominant and recessive) single mutant gene syndromes have been reported with CHD. Finally, less than 1% of congenital heart defects can be explained by simple Mendelian inheritance. Autosomal dominant transmission other than single mutant gene syndrome has been reported with atrial septal defect, patent ductus arteriosus, aortic stenosis, pulmonary stenosis, tetralogy of Fallot and hypertrophic cardiomyopathy. Autosomal recessive inheritance may be present in some forms of endocardial fibroelastosis. To the best of my knowledge, sex-linked transmission has not been reported with CHD. However, recently questions have been raised as to the mitochondrial inheritance in which maternal transmission to almost all offspring occurs. In the presence of family history of congenital heart defect (parent or sibling) the probability of CHD in the offspring is higher than that seen in general population.

In summary, the cause of congenital heart defects is largely unknown and the majority of them may be explained by multifactorial inheritance hypothesis. Extensive research on gene mapping that is currently in progress may unravel previously unknown genetic mechanisms for CHD. Also, several chapters to follow address the issues related to causation of CHD.

3. Classification

Congenital heart defects may be classified into acyanotic and cyanotic depending upon whether the patients clinically exhibit cyanosis. The acyanotic defects may further be subdivided into obstructive lesions and left-to-right shunt lesions. The cyanotic defects, by definition, have right-to-left shunt. The relative incidence of these groups of defects and most common defects in each group are listed in table I. The total percent is not 100 because some of the heart defects cannot be classified into the categories listed.

4. Ayanotic heart defects: Obstructive lesions

When there is a significant narrowing of a valve or a blood vessel, there is a higher pressure proximal to the obstruction compared to the distal pressure; this pressure gradient is necessary to maintain flow across the stenotic site. Hypertrophy of the cardiac chamber proximal to the obstruction and flow disturbance across the site of obstruction and their effects will determine the clinical features.

Type of Defect	% incidence
Acyanotic	65%
Obstructive Lesions Pulmonary stenosis Aortic stenosis Coarctation of the aorta	25%
Left-to-right shunt lesions Atrial septal defect Ventricular septal defect Patent ductus arteriosus	40%
Cyanotic Tetralogy of Fallot Transposition of the great arteries Tricuspid atresia	20%

Table 1. Classification of Congenital Heart Defects

4.1 Pulmonary stenosis

The obstruction can be at valvar, subvalvar or supravalvar sites or in the branch pulmonary arteries (Rao 2000a). Valvar stenosis is the most common type and will be discussed in this section. Valvar pulmonary stenosis (PS) constitutes 7.5% to 9.0% of all CHDs. The pathologic features of valvar stenosis vary, but the most commonly found pathology is what is described as "dome shaped" pulmonary valve with fusion of the thickened pulmonary valve leaflets. Hypertrophy of the right ventricle (proportional to the degree of obstruction) and dilatation of main pulmonary artery (not related to the severity of obstruction) are also seen.

4.1.1 Symptoms

Children with PS usually present with asymptomatic murmurs, although they can present with signs of systemic venous congestion (usually interpreted as congestive heart failure) due to severe right ventricular dysfunction or cyanosis because of right-to-left shunt across the atrial septum.

4.1.2 Physical findings

The right ventricular and the right ventricular outflow tract impulses are increased and a heave may be felt at the left lower and upper sternal borders. A thrill may be felt at the left upper sternal border and/or in the suprasternal notch. The first heart sound may be normal or loud. The second heart sound is variable, depending upon the degree of obstruction and will be detailed later in this section. An ejection systolic click is heard in most cases of valvar stenosis. The click is heard best at the left lower, mid and upper sternal borders and varies with respiration (decreases or disappears with inspiration). An ejection systolic murmur (Figure 1, top) is heard best at the left upper sternal border and it radiates into infraclavicular regions, axillae and back. The intensity of the murmur may vary between grades II-V/VI; the intensity is not necessarily related to the severity of the stenosis.

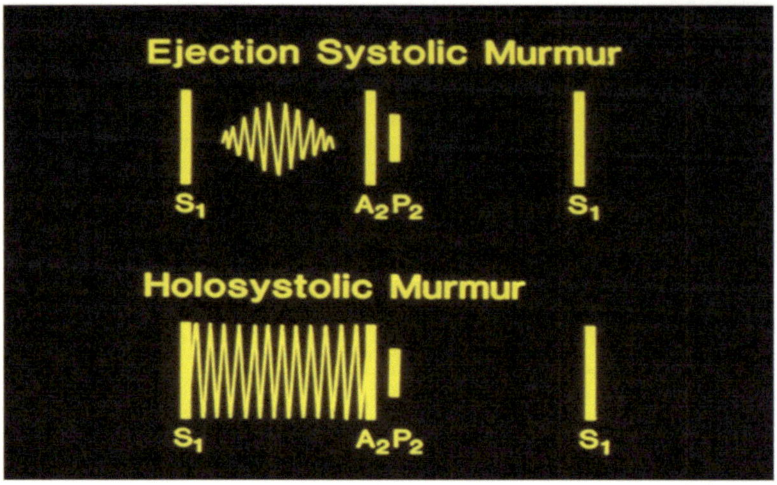

Fig. 1. Auscultatory diagrams of systolic murmurs. Ejection systolic murmur (top) begins shortly after the first heart sound (S_1) and ends shortly before the second heart sound (A_2, aortic component and P_2, pulmonary component) whereas a holosystolic murmur (bottom) begins with and obscures the S_1 and may last throughout the systole (as in the diagram) or may stop short of A_2.

4.1.3 Clinical assessment of severity

The timing of the click, the extent of splitting of the second sound, the intensity of the pulmonary component of the second sound, the length (duration) of the murmur, and timing of peaking of the systolic murmur are usually suggestive of the severity of pulmonary valve obstruction (Figure 2) (Rao 1991b, Vogelpoel & Schriere 1960).

The loudness of the ejection systolic murmur does not indicate the severity of obstruction but rather its duration and time of peaking; the longer the murmur and the later it peaks, the more severe is the PS. Similarly, the shorter the time interval between the first heart sound and ejection click, the wider the splitting of the second heart sound, and softer the pulmonary component, the more severe is the degree of pulmonary valve obstruction (Rao 2000).

4.1.4 Noninvasive evaluation

4.1.4.1 Chest x-ray

In most cases, the chest film shows no cardiomegaly, but a characteristically dilated main pulmonary artery segment (post-stenotic dilatation) is visualized. The magnitude of pulmonary artery dilatation has no bearing on the severity of pulmonary valve stenosis.

4.1.4.2 Electrocardiogram (ECG)

The ECG shows right ventricular hypertrophy; the degree of right ventricular hypertrophy is proportional to the severity of stenosis. Right atrial enlargement may be present.

4.1.4.3 Echocardiogram

The echo may show right ventricular enlargement without paradoxical septal motion and thickened and domed pulmonary valve leaflets. The Doppler flow velocity across the site of obstruction is increased and the magnitude of this increase reflects the severity of pulmonary valve stenosis. The peak instantaneous pressure gradient can be calculated by the use of a modified Bernoulli equation:

$$\Delta P = 4 V^2$$

Where, ΔP is peak instantaneous pressure gradient in mmHg and V is the peak velocity across the valve in meters/sec.

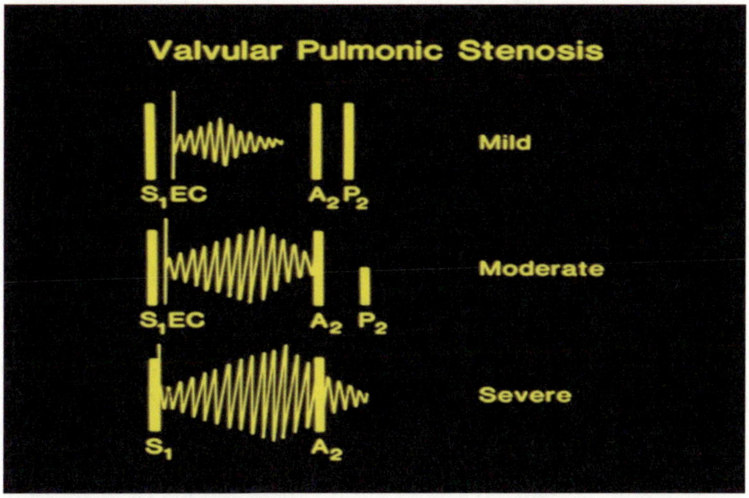

Fig. 2. In valvar pulmonary stenosis, severity of obstruction may be judged by auscultatory findings. In mild cases of pulmonary valve stenosis, the click (EC) is clearly separated from the first heart sound, almost normal splitting of the second heart sound with normal or slightly increased pulmonary component (P_2) of the second sound is heard, and an ejection systolic, diamond-shaped murmur that peaks early in systole and ends way before the aortic closure of the second heart sound is appreciated. The findings in moderate PS include an ejection systolic click that is much closer to the first heart sound than in milder forms, widely split second sound with diminished pulmonary component of the second sound and an ejection systolic murmur that peaks in mid to late systole and ends just below the aortic component (A_2) of the second sound. The features of severe valvar PS are an ejection systolic click which is either not present or falls so close to the first heart sound that it becomes inseparable from it, markedly increased splitting with a soft or inaudible pulmonary component of the second heart sound, and a long ejection systolic murmur that peaks late in systole and extends beyond the aortic component of the second sound so that the latter cannot be heard.

4.1.5 Cardiac catheterization and selective cineangiography

Though this procedure is not required for diagnosing valvar PS, it is usually required prior to therapeutic intervention, to be discussed below. The oxygen saturation data usually do not show evidence for left-to-right shunts. A right-to-left shunt across the patent foramen ovale (or an atrial defect) may be present in moderate to severe pulmonary valve obstruction. Right atrial pressure (particularly 'a' wave) may be increased. The right ventricular peak systolic pressure is increased. Trans-pulmonary valve peak-to-peak gradient is indicative of severity of obstruction. A peak-to-peak gradient in excess of 50 mmHg is usually considered an indication for therapeutic intervention. Angiocardiography usually reveals thickened and domed pulmonary valve leaflets with a thin jet of passage of contrast across the pulmonary valve. Enlargement of the right ventricle and dilated main pulmonary artery segment are also seen. In patients with severe or long-standing pulmonary valve obstruction, infundibular constriction may be seen.

4.1.6 Natural history

The natural history studies (Nugent et al 1977) have classified the degree of pulmonary valve obstruction based on peak-to-peak catheter-measured pulmonary valvar gradient: trivial = gradient < 25 mmHg; mild = gradient 25-49 mmHg; moderate = gradient 50 to 79 mmHg and severe = gradient > 80 mmHg. Patients with trivial and mild (gradients < 50 mmHg) pulmonary stenosis generally remain mild at follow-up. Patients with moderate stenosis (gradients of 50 to 79 mmHg) in contradistinction to trivial and mild stenosis, progressively increase their gradient

4.1.7 Management

Until early 1980s, surgical pulmonary valvotomy was the only treatment available, but at the present time relief of pulmonary valve obstruction can be accomplished by balloon pulmonary valvuloplasty. Indeed, at the present time balloon pulmonary valvuloplasty is treatment of choice. The indications for intervention are similar to those prescribed for surgery: a peak-to-peak systolic pressure gradient > 50 mmHg across the pulmonary valve with a normal cardiac index (Rao 1988, Rao 1989b, Rao 1998). Detailed description of the procedure of balloon valvuloplasty and the results of such a procedure are beyond the scope of this chapter; the reader is referred elsewhere for these details (Rao 2007a, Rao 2007b). In brief, a balloon catheter (with a deflated balloon) is positioned across the pulmonary valve and the balloon inflated (Figure 3); the radial forces of balloon inflation produce valve leaflet commissural disruption and thus relief of pulmonary valve obstruction (Rao 1993).

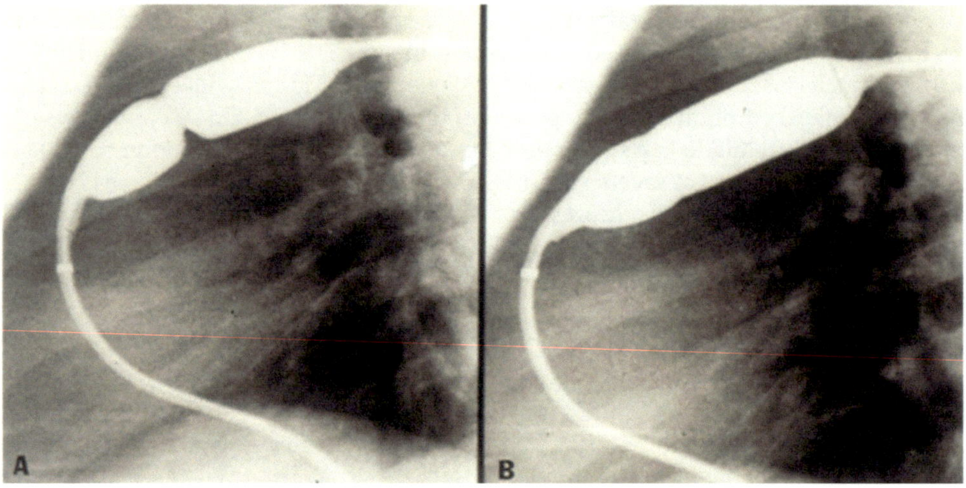

Fig. 3. Selected cineradiographic frames of a balloon dilatation catheter placed across the pulmonary valve. Note "waisting" of the balloon during the initial phases of balloon inflation (A), which is almost completely abolished during the later phases of balloon inflation (B). Reproduced with permission of the author and publisher, Rao PS: Transcatheter Therapy in Pediatric Cardiology, Wiley-Liss, Inc, New York, 1993, p. 62.

Previous recommendations are to use a balloon that is 1.2 to 1.4 times the size of the pulmonary valve annulus; however, more recent recommendations are to limit the balloon/annulus ratio to 1.2 to 1.25 (Rao 2000b, Rao 2007a, Rao 2007b). When the pulmonary valve annulus is too large to dilate with a single balloon, valvuloplasty with simultaneous inflation of two balloons across the pulmonary valve annulus is recommended. Immediate, short-term and long-term results (Figure 4) are good; although long-term results are limited (Rao et al 1998).

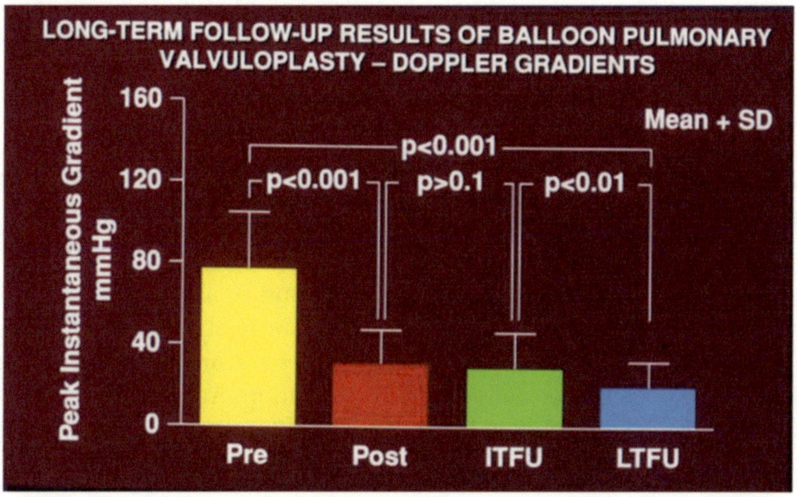

Fig. 4. Bar graph showing maximum peak instantaneous Doppler gradients, indicative of severity of pulmonary stenosis, prior to (Pre), one day following (Post) balloon pulmonary valvuloplasty and at intermediate-term (ITFU) and late (LTFU) follow-up. Note significant reduction ($p < 0.001$) after valvuloplasty, which remains unchanged ($p > 0.1$) at ITFU. However, at LTFU there was further fall ($p < 0.01$) in the Doppler gradients.

Given the success with balloon pulmonary valvuloplasty, surgery is reserved for unsuccessful balloon cases, mostly for cases with supravalvar PS, severe valve annular hypoplasia and dysplastic pulmonary valves.

In patients with mild pulmonary valve stenosis, periodic clinical follow-up, antibiotic prophylaxis prior to any bacteremia-producing procedures to prevent subacute bacterial endocarditis and no exercise restriction are recommended.

4.2 Aortic stenosis

Left ventricular outflow tract obstruction may occur at valvar, subvalvar (fixed subaortic stenosis and idiopathic hypertrophic subaortic stenosis) and supravalvar locations (Singh and Rao 2009). Valvar stenosis is the most common form and will be discussed in this section. The prevalence of congenital valvar aortic stenosis (AS) is 5% to 6% of patients with CHD. The pathology of the stenotic aortic valve is variable, most commonly it is a bicuspid valve with varying degrees of commissural fusion of thickened, domed, nonpliable valve leaflets. Tricuspid and rarely unicuspid aortic valve leaflets can also cause aortic valve obstruction. Dysplasia of the aortic valve leaflets with or without hypoplasia of the valve ring may be found in neonates and young infants. Calcification of the aortic valve leaflets so frequent in the elderly is uncommon during childhood. Dilatation of ascending aorta, post-stenotic dilatation, is seen in most cases, and the extent of aortic dilatation is independent of the severity of aortic obstruction. Hypertrophy of the left ventricular muscle is concentric in nature and is largely proportional to the degree of obstruction.

4.2.1 Symptoms

The majority of children with valvar AS are asymptomatic and the AS is detected because of a cardiac murmur heard on routine auscultation. When symptoms are exhibited, dyspnea, easy fatigability or chest pain is presenting complaint. Syncope may be a presenting complaint in some children with severe AS. In contradistinction to children, neonates and young infants usually present with dyspnea and signs of heart failure.

4.2.2 Physical findings

The left ventricular impulse is increased (left ventricular heave) in all but mild cases. A thrill may be felt at the right upper sternal border and/or in the supra-sternal notch. The first heart sound is usually normal. The second heart sound is also normal unless the aortic stenosis is extremely severe when there may be a paradoxical splitting of the second heart sound. An ejection systolic click is heard best at the apex and left mid and right upper sternal borders and the click does not vary with respiration. An ejection systolic murmur of grade II-V/VI intensity is usually heard best at the right upper sternal border with radiation into both carotid arteries. The arterial pulses are usually normal.

4.2.3 Noninvasive evaluation

4.2.3.1 Chest roentgenogram

In most cases, the chest X-ray shows a normal sized heart and a dilated ascending aorta; the latter is a sign of post-stenotic dilatation. In neonates and those with very severe heart failure cardiomegaly is seen.

4.2.3.2 Electrocardiogram

The ECG may be normal or may show varying degrees of left ventricular hypertrophy. Inverted T waves in the left chest leads indicate that aortic valve obstruction is severe. However, not all severe AS patients show T wave inversion.

None of the above described clinical and laboratory data have any predictive value in determining the severity of aortic valve obstruction.

4.2.3.3 Echocardiogram

The echocardiogram may show thickened and domed aortic valve leaflets. The aortic valve is usually bicuspid (Figure 5), with eccentric opening.

The left ventricular muscle may be thickened and its shortening fraction may be increased, depending upon the severity of AS. Doppler flow velocity across the aortic valve is increased and can be used to quantitate peak instantaneous gradient across the aortic valve in a manner similar to that described for the pulmonary valve. However, Doppler-derived mean systolic gradient appears to reflect peak-to-peak catheter gradient (see below) more accurately than peak instantaneous Doppler gradient. Mild degree of aortic insufficiency may be seen by color Doppler, even in patients without auscultatory evidence for aortic regurgitation.

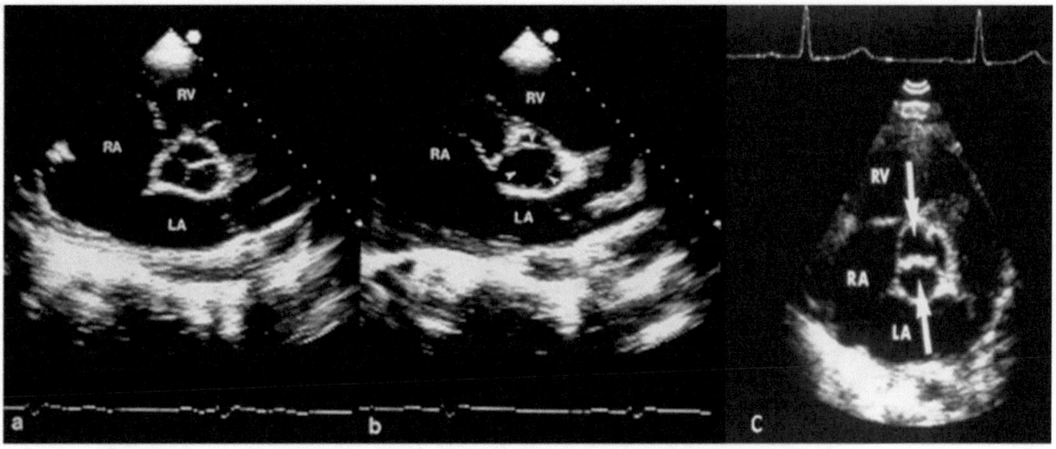

Fig. 5. Short axis views of the aorta showing aortic valve leaflets in closed (a) and open position (b) in children with tricuspid aortic valves (a and b). Bicuspid aortic valve (large arrows) is shown in c, which is commonly associated with aortic stenosis. Three aortic valve cusps and commissures (in a) are clearly seen and contrast with two valve cusps and single horizontal commissure (in c). Arrow heads in b point to open aortic valve leaflets. Neither of the children showed clinical or echo-Doppler evidence for aortic stenosis and are shown here only to demonstrate the bicuspid and tricuspid valve leaflets. LA, left atrium; RA, right atrium; RV, right ventricle.

4.2.4 Cardiac catheterization and angiography

The data show elevated left ventricular peak systolic pressure with a peak-to-peak pressure gradient across the aortic valve indicative of the severity of obstruction. Angiography will confirm thickened domed aortic valve leaflets and exclude any other abnormalities.

4.2.5 Management

The indications for intervention in valvar AS is a peak-to-peak gradient >50 mmHg with either symptoms or electrocardiographic ST-T wave changes or a peak gradient >70 mmHg irrespective of symptoms or ECG changes (Rao 1989b, Rao 1990). When pressure gradients are used as criteria for intervention (instead of valve area), it must be assured that the cardiac index is normal during pressure measurement. Until recently, surgical commissurotomy was the treatment of choice. Since the introduction of balloon valvuloplasty for valvar AS in 1983, increasing number of pediatric cardiologists, including the author of this chapter have been using balloon aortic valvuloplasty as a first therapeutic procedure for relief of aortic valve obstruction although, at this time, there is no consensus with regard to the choice of treatment mode. When surgical commissurotomy is chosen it is usually performed on cardiopulmonary bypass. When balloon valvuloplasty is performed, a balloon diameter size 80% to 100% of the size of the aortic valve annulus is chosen for valvuloplasty (Rao 1990). Immediate, short-term and long-term results following balloon aortic valvuloplasty (Figure 6) are encouraging. Only limited long-term results are available to-date (Galal et al 1997, Rao 1999).

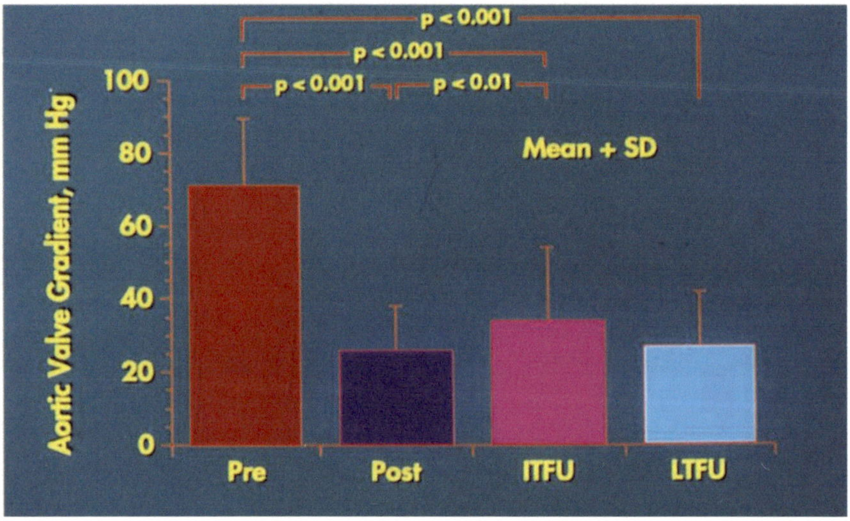

Fig. 6. Bar graph showing maximum peak instantaneous Doppler gradients, indicative of severity of aortic stenosis, prior to (Pre), one day following (Post) balloon aortic valvuloplasty and at intermediate-term (ITFU) and late (LTFU) follow-up. Note significant reduction ($p < 0.001$) after valvuloplasty, which continues to be lower ($p < 0.001$) at ITFU and LTFU.

For milder forms of AS, subacute bacterial endocarditis prophylaxis and periodic follow-up are necessary. Restriction from participation in competitive sports is recommended for all but mildest form of AS.

4.3 Coarctation of the aorta

The prevalence of coarctation of the aorta (CoA) was found to vary between 5% and 8% of CHDs; however, coarctation may be found more frequently in infants presenting with symptoms prior to one year of age. In the past, CoA was designated as preductal (or infantile) or postductal (or adult) type, depending on whether the coarctation segment was proximal or distal to the ductus arteriosus, respectively. However, a closer examination of the anatomy suggests that all coarctations are juxtaductal. The coarctation may be discrete, or a long segment of the aorta may be narrowed; the former is more common. Classic CoA is located in the thoracic aorta distal to the origin of the left subclavian artery, at about the level of the ductal structure. However, rarely, a coarcted segment may be present in the abdominal aorta. Varying degrees of hypoplasia of the isthmus of the aorta (the portion of the aorta between the origin of the left subclavian artery and the ductus arteriosus) and transverse aortic arch (the arch between the origin of the innominate artery and the left subclavian artery) are present in the majority of patients with CoA; this hypoplasia may be significant in symptomatic CoA of the neonate and infant, whereas in older children there may be only a mild degree of narrowing. The most commonly associated defects are patent ductus arteriosus, ventricular septal defect and AS. The younger the infant presents, the more likely that there is a significant associated defect. Bicuspid aortic valve and abnormal mitral valve are also seen. Sometimes, CoA is a complicating feature of a more complex, cyanotic heart defects, such as transposition of the great arteries, Taussig-Bing anomaly, double-inlet left ventricle, tricuspid atresia with transposition of the great arteries, and hypoplastic left heart syndrome. In this section, I will discuss CoA in children older than 1 year of age.

4.3.1 Symptoms

Children beyond infancy usually are asymptomatic; an occasional child will complain of pain or weakness in the legs. Most often, the coarctation is detected because of a murmur or hypertension which is detected on a routine examination (Rao 1995).

4.3.2 Physical findings

A clinical diagnosis of CoA is best made by simultaneous palpation of femoral and brachial pulses. The left ventricular impulse may be increased. A thrill is usually felt in the supra-sternal notch. The first and second heart sounds are usually normal in isolated aortic coarctation. Since a large percentage (up to 60%) of patients with CoA have associated bicuspid aortic valves, an ejection systolic click may be heard at right upper and left mid sternal borders and apex; this click does not change with respiration. An ejection systolic murmur may be heard at left or right upper sternal borders, but is usually heard best over the back in the inter-scapular regions. Sometimes a continuous murmur may be heard in the left inter-scapular region secondary to continuous flow in the coarcted segment or on the back (secondary to flow in the collateral vessels). Palpation of the brachial and femoral artery pulses simultaneously will reveal delayed and decreased or absent femoral pulses. Blood pressure in both arms and one leg must be determined: a peak systolic pressure difference of more than 20 mmHg in favor of arms may be considered as evidence for coarctation of the aorta (Rao 1995). Involvement of the left subclavian artery in the coarctation or anomalous origin of the right subclavian artery (below the level of coarctation) may produce decreased or absent left or right brachial pulses, respectively, and therefore palpation of both brachial pulses and measurement of blood pressure in both arms are important.

4.3.3 Noninvasive evaluation

4.3.3.1 Chest x-ray

Chest roentgenogram may show a normal sized heart or the heart may be mildly enlarged. Other roentgenographic features include a "3" sign on a highly penetrated chest x-ray, inverted "3" sign of the barium filled esophagus and rib-notching (secondary to collateral vessels).

4.3.3.2 Electrocardiogram

The ECG may be normal or may show left ventricular hypertrophy.

4.3.3.3 Echocardiogram

Echocardiographic studies usually reveal the coarctation in the supra-sternal notch, two-dimensional echo views of the aortic arch. Increased Doppler flow velocity in the descending aorta by continuous-wave Doppler and demonstrable jump in velocity at the coarcted segment by pulsed-Doppler technique are usually present. Extension of the Doppler flow signal into the diastole is indicative of significant obstruction. Instantaneous peak pressure gradients across the aortic coarctation can be calculated by employing modified Bernoulli equation in manner similar to that described for PS and AS. Because of higher proximal velocity, coarctation gradients may be more accurately estimated by:

$$\Delta P = 4 (V_2^2 - V_1^2)$$

Where, ΔP is peak instantaneous gradient and V_2 and V_1 are peak Doppler velocities in the descending aorta distal to the coarctation (continuous wave Doppler) and proximal to the coarctation (pulsed Doppler), respectively.
But the calculated gradient is usually an over-estimation, especially if there is no diastolic extension of the Doppler velocity (Rao and Carey 1989).

4.3.4 Catheterization and angiography

In isolated aortic coarctation, elevation of left ventricular and ascending aortic peak systolic pressure with significant peak-to-peak systolic pressure gradient across the coarctation is found. Selective aortic root or aortic arch angiography is necessary to clearly demonstrate the aortic narrowing.

4.3.5 Management

Significant hypertension and/or congestive heart failure are indications for intervention. In the presence of congestive heart failure, conventional anti-congestive measures including digitalis and diuretics should be promptly instituted. In the presence of hypertension, it is better to relieve the obstruction promptly rather than attempting to "treat" hypertension with antihypertensive drugs. Aortic coarctation may be relieved either by surgery or by balloon angioplasty. Symptomatic children should undergo relief of coarctation soon after the child is stabilized. Asymptomatic children should undergo the procedure electively. If neither hypertension nor heart failure is present, elective relief of the obstruction between the ages of 2 and 5 years is suggested. Waiting beyond 5 years is not advisable because of evidence for residual hypertension if the aortic obstruction is not relieved by the age of 5 years.
Surgical relief of aortic coarctation is the conventional treatment option. Since the description balloon angioplasty in 1983, increasing number of cardiologists, including our group, have used this technique for relief of aortic coarctation (Rao 1989c; Rao et al 1996). While I believe that balloon angioplasty is the treatment option of choice for relief of native aortic coarctation, because of concern for development of aneurysms, some cardiologists prefer surgery. Balloon angioplasty may be an effective alternative to surgery for the relief of aortic coarctation. Children older than 1 year and adults with discrete native coarctation are candidates for balloon dilatation. Long-segment coarctations or those associated with significant isthmic hypoplasia may be candidates for stent placement, especially in adolescents and adults (Figure 7).

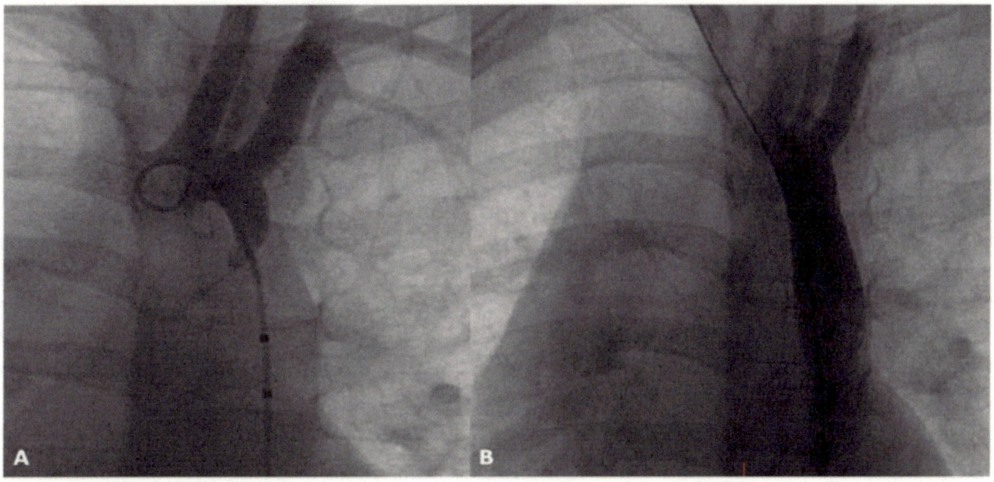

Fig. 7. Selected cine frames from aortic arch angiogram in 20-degree left anterior oblique projection demonstrating aortic coarctation with isthmic hypoplasia in an adolescent prior to (A) and immediately following (B) stent implantation.

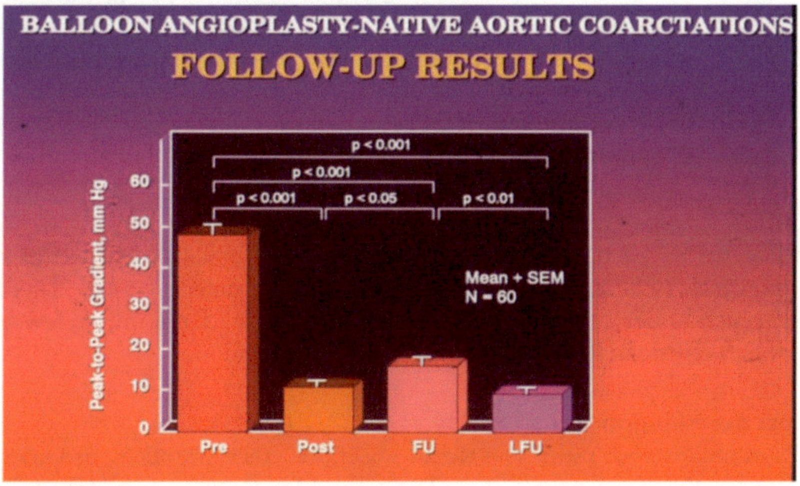

Fig. 8. Bar graph showing immediate and follow-up results after balloon angioplasty of native aortic coarctation. Peak-to-peak systolic pressure gradients across the coarctation in mmHg (mean + SEM) are shown. Note significant ($p < 0.001$) drop in the gradient following angioplasty (Pre, prior to vs. Post). The gradient increases ($p < 0.05$) slightly at a mean follow-up of 14 mo. However, these values are lower ($p < 0.001$) than those prior to angioplasty. At late follow-up (LFU), (median 5 years) following balloon angioplasty, blood pressure-measured arm-leg peak pressure difference is lower than catheterization measured peak gradients prior to ($p < 0.001$) balloon angioplasty and those obtained at intermediate-term follow-up ($p < 0.01$).

When surgical option is chosen, resection and end-to-end anastomosis, subclavian flap angioplasty or prosthetic patch angioplasty may be used depending upon anatomy of the aortic arch and coarctation and surgeon's preference. When balloon angioplasty is contemplated, the balloon size should be carefully chosen: the diameter of the balloon should be two or more times the size of the coarcted segment, but no larger than the diameter of the descending aorta at the level of diaphragm. The immediate (Figures 8) and intermediate-term results of balloon coarctation angioplasty have been good although long-term follow-up is limited (Rao 1999).

5. Ayanotic heart defects: Left-to-right shunts

When there is a defect in the partition between left and right heart structures, the oxygenated blood is shunted from left-to-right because of generally lower pressure and/or resistance in the right heart than in the left. The physical findings are either a manifestation of flow across the defects or due to effects of excessive flow across the cardiac chambers (volume overload) and valves. The magnitude of the shunt determines the clinical presentation and symptoms.

5.1 Atrial septal defect

There are three major types of atrial septal defects (ASDs) and these include ostium secundum, ostium primum and sinus venosus defects. The clinical features are essentially similar but I will mainly concentrate on ostium secundum ASDs. Atrial septal defects constitute 8% to 13% of all CHDs. Pathologically, there is deficiency of the septal tissue in the region of fossa ovalis. These may be small to large. Most of the time, these are single defects, although, occasionally multiple defects and fenestrated defects can also be seen. Because of left-to-right shunting across the defects, the right atrium and right ventricle are dilated and somewhat hypertrophied. Similarly, main and branch pulmonary arteries are also dilated. Pulmonary vascular obstructive changes are not usually seen until adulthood.

5.1.1 Symptoms

Isolated ASD patients are usually asymptomatic and are usually detected at the time of preschool physical examination. Sometimes these defects are detected when echocardiographic studies are performed for some unrelated reason. A few patients do present with heart failure in infancy, although this is uncommon.

5.1.2 Physical examination

The right ventricular and right ventricular outflow tract impulses are increased and hyperdynamic. No thrills are usually felt. The second heart sound is widely split and fixed (splitting does not vary with respiration) and is the most characteristic sign of ASD. Ejection systolic clicks are rare with ASDs. The ejection systolic murmur of ASD is soft and is of grade I-II/VI intensity and rarely, if ever, louder. The murmur is secondary to increased flow across the pulmonary valve and is heard best at the left upper sternal border. A grade I-II/VI mid-diastolic flow rumble is heard (with the bell of the stethoscope) best at the left lower sternal border. This is due to large volume flow across the tricuspid valve. There is no audible murmur because of flow across the ASD.

5.1.3 Noninvasive evaluation

5.1.3.1 Chest x-ray

Chest film usually reveals mild to moderate cardiomegaly, prominent main pulmonary artery segment and increased pulmonary vascular markings.

5.1.3.2 Electrocardiogram

The ECG shows mild right ventricular hypertrophy; the so-called diastolic volume overload pattern with rSR' pattern in the right chest leads.

5.1.3.3 Echocardiogram

Echocardiographic studies reveal enlarged right ventricle with paradoxical septal motion, particularly well-demonstrable on M-mode echocardiograms. By two-dimensional echocardiogram, the defect can be clearly visualized (Figure 9A). The type of ASD, secundum versus primum can also be delineated by the echocardiographic study. Apical and precordial views may show "septal drop-outs" without an ASD because of thinness of the septum in the region of fossa ovalis. Therefore, only subcostal views should be scrutinized for evidence of ASD. In addition, demonstration of flow across the defect with pulsed Doppler (not shown) and color Doppler (Figure 9B) echocardiography is necessary to avid false positive studied. In adolescents and adults transesophageal echo is needed to make definitive diagnosis of ASD.

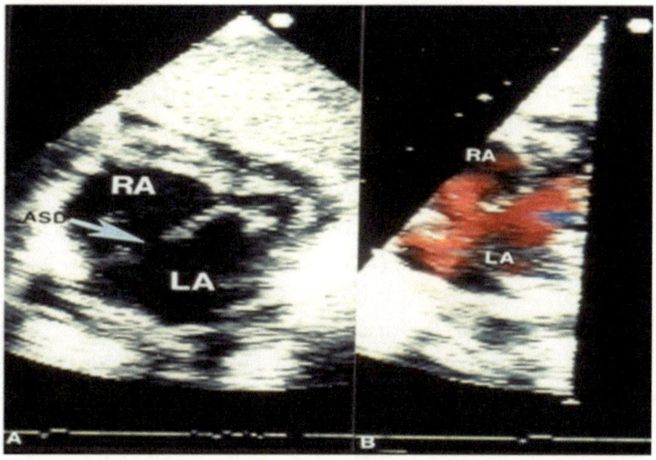

Fig. 9. Two dimensional subcostal echocardiographic view of the atrial septum (A) demonstrating a secundum atrial septal defect (ASD) in the mid septum (arrow). Color Doppler imaging shows left-to-right shunt. LA, left atrium; RA, right atrium.

5.1.4 Catheterization and angiography

Clinical and echocardiographic features are sufficiently characteristic so that cardiac catheterization is not necessary for the diagnosis. However, cardiac catheterization is an integral part of transcatheter occlusion of the ASD.

When catheterization is performed, one will observe step-up in oxygen saturation at the right atrial level. The pulmonary venous, left atrial, left ventricular and aortic saturations are within normal range. In large defects, the pressures in both atria are equal while in small defects, an inter-atrial pressure difference is noted. The right ventricular and pulmonary arterial pressures are usually normal. Calculated pulmonary-to-systemic flow ratio (Qp:Qs) is used to quantitate the degree of shunting and a Qp:Qs in excess of 1.5:1 is considered an indication for closure of ASD.

Selective angiography in the right upper pulmonary vein at its junction with the left atrium in a left axial oblique view will reveal location and the size of the ASD. When anomalous pulmonary venous connection is suspected, selective left or right pulmonary arterial angiography should be performed and the levophase of angiogram should be scrutinized for anomalous connections.

5.1.5 Management

Despite lack of symptoms at presentation, closure of the ASD is recommended so as to 1) prevent development of pulmonary vascular obstructive disease later in life, 2) reduce chances for supra-ventricular arrhythmias and 3) prevent development of symptoms during adolescence and adulthood. Elective closure around age 4 to 5 years is recommended. Closure during infancy is not undertaken unless the infant is symptomatic. Right ventricular volume overloading by echocardiogram and a Qp:Qs >1.5 (if the child had cardiac catheterization) are indications for closure.

The conventional treatment of choice is surgical correction. While the secundum ASDs can be successfully repaired by open-heart surgical techniques with a low (<1%) mortality, the morbidity with cardiac surgery is universal, and residual scar is present in all. Because of this reason several transcatheter methods have been developed. Clinical trials have been undertaken in a large number of patients with Bard clamshell septal occluder and buttoned device and feasibility and effectiveness of these devices in occluding the ASD have been demonstrated. Fractures of one or more arms of the clamshell device with occasional embolization, has prompted the investigators and the FDA to withdraw the device from clinical trials. The buttoned device has undergone clinical trials and, immediate and short-term follow-up results are encouraging (Rao et al 1994). Recently, a large number of other devices (Das Angel-Wing, ASDOS, Amplatzer, CardioSeal, Helex and others) have been introduced and clinical trials began (Chopra and Rao 2000). However, Amplatzer and Helex are the only devices that are approved by FDA for general clinical use. The experience with Amplatzer for most defects has been encouraging. Helex device is only useful in small to medium-sized defects.

Ostium primum and sinus venosus defects are not amenable to transcatheter closure and surgical correction is the treatment of choice. In the ostium primum defect, apart from closing the ASD, the mitral valve should be repaired in such a manner as to preserve its function. In the sinus venosus defect, diversion of the anomalously connected pulmonary veins into the left atrium along with the closure of the ASD should be undertaken.

5.2 Ventricular septal defect

Ventricular septal defect (VSD) is the most common CHD and constitutes 20% to 25% of all CHDs. The defect may be small, medium or large and is classified based on its location in the inter-ventricular septum (Fyler 1992). The defect is most commonly (80%) located in the membranous septum, in the subaortic region and is commonly referred to as perimembranous defect. The defect may also be located in the conal septum in the subpulmonary region and is called supracristal defect and constitutes 5% to 7% of VSDs. This type of defect is more commonly encountered in the Far East including Japan and may constitute up to 29% of VSDs. The third type, in the posterior septum, is commonly referred to as atrioventricular canal defect and approximately 8% of the VSDs are of this type.

Finally, the defect may be located in the muscular and apical portion of the ventricular septum and may make-up 5% to 20% of all VSDs, depending on the study selected. When multiple muscular defects are seen, it is often referred to as "Swiss-cheese" type of VSD.

5.2.1 Symptoms

The clinical symptomatology is largely dependent upon the size of the VSD. In small defects, the patients are usually asymptomatic and are detected because a cardiac murmur heard on routine examination. Patients with medium and large defects may present with symptoms of congestive heart failure (dyspnea, tachypnea, sweating and failure to gain weight) or with symptoms related to bronchial obstruction and/or respiratory infection.

5.2.2 Physical findings

These, again, depend upon the size of the defect. In small defects the only abnormality is a loud holosystolic murmur (Figure 1 bottom) heard best at the left lower sternal border and is sometimes referred to as "maladie de Roger". Sometimes, the holosystolic murmur may be heard best at left mid and left upper sternal borders, depending upon the direction of the VSD jet. In very small defects, murmur, though begins with first heart sound, may not last through the entire systole; the shorter the murmur, the smaller is the defect.

In medium and large defects, the right and left ventricular impulses are increased and somewhat hyperdynamic. A thrill may be felt at the left lower sternal border. The second heart sound is split unless there is pulmonary vascular obstructive disease, in which case a loud single second heart sound is heard. The pulmonary component of the second sound may be normal or increased, depending upon the degree of elevation pulmonary artery pressure. Clicks are unusual for VSD patients although they can be heard in patients whose VSDs are undergoing spontaneous closure by aneurysmal formation of the membranous ventricular septum. A holosystolic murmur is best heard at the left lower sternal border and does not usually radiate although it may be heard widely over the precordium. The intensity of the murmur may vary between grades II-V/VI. There is no significant variation of this murmur with respiration. This murmur is produced by flow across the VSD. The intensity of the murmur does not bear any consistent relationship with the size of the defect. A grade I-II/VI mid-diastolic flow rumble may be heard at the apex in patients with medium to large-sized defects and large left-to-right shunts; this murmur is heard best with the bell of the stethoscope. The mid diastolic murmur is due to increased flow across the mitral valve and usually indicates a Qp:Qs greater than 2:1.

5.2.3 Noninvasive evaluation

5.2.3.1 Chest x-ray

The x-ray shows cardiomegaly and increased pulmonary vascular markings if the shunt is large. Left atrial enlargement may be noted.

5.2.3.2 Electrocardiogram

The ECG may be normal in very small defects or may show evidence for left ventricular hypertrophy in small to moderate defects while it may show biventricular or right ventricular hypertrophy in moderate to large defects. Electrocardiographic signs of left atrial enlargement may also be seen.

5.2.3.3 Echocardiogram

Echo shows increase in left atrial and left ventricular size, which is again dependent upon the size of the VSD. The location and size of the VSD can be imaged by 2-dimensional echocardiography. Left-to-right shunting across the VSD can be demonstrated by Doppler echocardiography and color mapping (Figure 10).

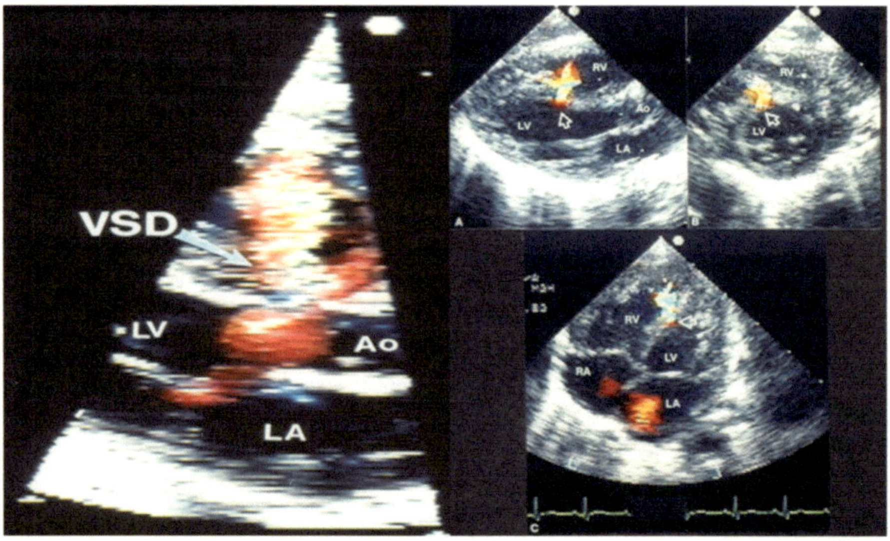

Fig. 10. Two dimensional echocardiographic views of the ventricular septum in long axis with color flow imaging (left panel) demonstrating a perimembraneous ventricular septal defect (VSD) and of the ventricular septum (arrows) in multiple views (Right panel A, B and C) with left-to-right shunt. Ao, Aorta; LA, left atrium; LV, Left ventricle; RA, right atrium; RV, Right ventricle

Peak Doppler flow velocity magnitude is inversely proportional to the size of defect. Indeed the right ventricular/pulmonary arterial pressures may be estimated by determining to peak Doppler flow velocity across the VSD.

$$\text{RV/PA peak pressure} = \text{peak arm blood pressure} - 4\,V_{VSD}^2$$

Where, RV and PA are right ventricle and pulmonary artery and V_{VSD} is the peak Doppler velocity across the VSD.

The right ventricular peak pressure may also be estimated by tricuspid back flow (regurgitant) velocity:

$$\text{RV peak pressure} = 4\,V_{TR}^2 + \text{RAP}$$

Where, V_{TR} is peak tricuspid regurgitant velocity and RAP is estimated right atrial pressure (5 mmHg).

Both formulas may help to verify internal consistency of the Doppler methodology in estimating the size of the VSD. The higher the estimated RV pressure, larger is the size of the VSD.

5.2.4 Cardiac catheterization & cineangiography

Many of the issues that require definition by catheterization in the past can be resolved by good quality echo-Doppler studies and catheterization is not routinely required. When questions cannot be satisfactorily answered, cardiac catheterization may be useful.
Step-up in oxygen saturation is observed in the right ventricle. The saturations in the left-side of the heart are usually normal. The right ventricular and pulmonary arterial pressures are normal in small VSDs and are elevated in moderate to large defects; the magnitude of elevation is proportional to the size of the VSD. Calculated Qp:Qs gives an estimate of degree of left-to-right shunting. A Qp:Qs greater than 2:1 is generally considered an indication for intervention. Pulmonary vascular resistance may be calculated:

$$PVR = (\text{Mean PA presence} - \text{Mean LA pressure})/\text{Pulmonary blood flow index}$$

Where, PVR is pulmonary vascular resistance, PA and LA are pulmonary artery and left atrium respectively.
The calculated resistance is usually 1 to 2 units and a resistance in excess of 3.0 units is considered elevated. Marked elevation of the resistance (>8.0 units) contraindicates surgical repair. When the resistance is elevated, oxygen and other vasodilating agents (Nitric oxide[NO]) should be administered to demonstrate the reversibility.
Selective left ventricular angiography in a left axial oblique view is usually required to demonstrate size and location of the VSD.

Natural history of VSDs

Knowledge of the natural history of these defects is interesting and such understanding is important in the management of children with these defects.

5.2.4.1 Spontaneous closure

Approximately 40% of VSDs spontaneously and completely close. Additional 25% to 30% of defects may become small enough not to require surgical intervention. Muscular VSDs tend to close more frequently than membraneous defects. While small defects tend to close more frequently than large defects (60% vs. 20%), even defects large enough to produce congestive heart failure or require pulmonary artery banding in infancy go on to close spontaneously. The majority of the defects close by age 2 years, most close by age 5 to 7 years, but the process of spontaneous closure continues through adolescence and adulthood. Most commonly the defect closes by apposition of leaflets of the tricuspid valve against it or by aneurysmal formation of the membranous ventricular septum.

5.2.4.2 Pulmonary vascular obstructive disease

Pulmonary vascular obstructive disease may develop in 10% of VSDs. This is probably related to the exposure of the pulmonary vascular bed to high pressure and high flow. Prompt diagnosis and closure of the defect at least prior to 18 months of age is likely to reduce the incidence of development of pulmonary vascular disease.

5.2.4.3 Development of infundibular stenosis.

Development of infundibular stenosis, the so called Gasul's transformation of the VSD may occur in 8% of the defects. There may be specific markers such as right aortic arch and increased angle of the right ventricular outflow tract that may predispose a VSD to undergo Gasul's transformation. While development of infundibular stenosis eventually requires the patient to have surgery, it indeed protects the pulmonary vascular bed and prevents development of pulmonary vascular obstruction disease.

5.2.4.4 Aortic insufficiency

Aortic insufficiency develops in approximately 5% of patients. This may either be related to prolapse of an aortic valve cusp into the VSD or lack of support to the aortic root. This complication appears to occur more commonly with supracristal VSDs than with other types. Surgical correction is indicated if moderate to severe aortic insufficiency is present.

5.2.5 Management

The management strategies depend, to a large degree, on the size of the VSD. In small VSDs, reassurance of the parents, subacute bacterial endocarditis prophylaxis and periodic clinical follow-up are all that are necessary.

In moderate-sized defects, treatment of heart failure, if present, should be undertaken. Failure to thrive and markedly enlarged left ventricle are probably indications for surgical closure. In very large defects the heart failure should be treated aggressively. If the congestive heart failure is difficult to control with the usual anti-congestive measures or if failure to thrive is present, surgical closure should be undertaken.

In large defects with near systemic pressures in the right ventricle and pulmonary artery, surgical closure should be performed prior to 18 to 24 months of age even if heart failure control and adequate weight gain are present. Total surgical correction is currently recommended. The previously used approach of initial pulmonary artery banding in small and young babies followed by surgical closure of the VSD later is no longer recommended. However, in muscular, Swiss-cheese variety of defects, initial pulmonary artery banding may be appropriate.

When the pulmonary vascular resistance is elevated, its response to oxygen and other vasodilator agents (NO), pulmonary arterial wedge angiography and sometimes, even lung biopsy may be necessary to determine the suitability for surgical closure. Patients with calculated pulmonary vascular resistance less than 8 wood units with a Qp:Qs >1.5 are generally considered suitable candidates for surgery. If the resistance drops to levels below 8 units after administering oxygen or other vasodilator agents, the patient becomes a candidate for surgery.

Large VSDs with severe elevation of pulmonary resistance (irreversible pulmonary vascular obstructive disease) are not candidates for surgery. Symptomatic treatment and erythropheresis for symptoms of polycthemia should be undertaken. These patients may eventually become candidates for lung transplantation.

When surgery is indicated, open heart surgical technique is the treatment of choice. Several investigators have attempted transcatheter occlusion of VSD in a manner similar to ASD closure. Such methods may be feasible in muscular defects (Thanopoulos et al 1999) and membranous defects with sufficient septum in the subaortic region so that the device can be implanted without interfering with aortic valve function. Specially designed Amplatzer perimembranous VSD occluders were used to close the perimembranous VSDs in clinical trials (Fu et al 2006, Holzer et al 2006), but with significant incidence of heart block (Rao 2008). At the present, FDA has only approved Amplatzer muscular VSD occluder for transcatheter closure of muscular VSDs. Some large muscular VSDs in small babies may be closed by hybrid procedures via sternotomy and a purse-string suture in the right ventricle under transesophageal echo guidance (Amin et al 2008). No device is yet approved for closure of perimembranous VSD, presumably because of concern for development of heart block (Rao 2008).

5.3 Patent ductus arteriosus

Ductus arteriosus, one of the fetal circulatory pathways, diverts the desaturated blood from the pulmonary artery into the descending aorta and placenta for oxygenation (Rao 1991a). After the infant is born, the ductus arteriosus constricts and closes spontaneously, presumably secondary to increased PO_2. But in some children, such spontaneous closure does not occur. This is more frequent in prematurely born infants. Patent ductus arteriosus (PDA) may be an isolated lesion and may be present in association with other defects. Isolated PDA constitutes 6 to 11% of all CHDs. In this section, isolated PDA beyond neonatal (and premature) period will be discussed. PDA is a muscular structure connecting the main pulmonary artery (at its junction with the left pulmonary artery) with the descending aorta at the level of left subclavian artery. The configuration of PDA varies considerably but most often it has a conical or funnel shape. The aortic end is wide and gradually narrows (ampulla) towards the pulmonary end. The narrowest segment is most often at the pulmonary end. Other types which are short and tubular and those with multiple constrictions and bizarre configuration can also be seen. Because of usually higher pressure and resistance in the systemic circuit than in the pulmonary circuit, left-to-right shunt takes place across the PDA. The degree of left-to-right shunting depends upon the minimal diameter of the ductus and ratio of pulmonary to systemic vascular resistance.

5.3.1 Symptoms

Clinical presentation depends upon the size of the ductus. If the PDA is small, there are no symptoms and it is usually detected because of a murmur detected on a routine examination. Moderate to large ducti with large shunt may either present with symptoms of easy fatigability, symptoms associated congestive heart failure or respiratory symptoms suggestive of lung collapse (very large ductus in small babies).

5.3.2 Physical findings

Left ventricular impulse is normal in small ducti and may be hyperdynamic with large shunts. A thrill may be felt at the left upper sternal border and in the suprasternal notch. The first heart sound is usually normal and the second heart sound may be buried within the murmur. In the majority of cases, a continuous murmur (Figure 11, top) is heard best at the left upper sternal border. The murmur begins in systole and continues through the second heart sound into the diastole. The systolic component of the murmur crescendos up to the second heart sound while the diastolic part descrescendos to a varying distance (time) into the diastole. The continuous murmur must be distinguished from the to-and-fro murmur; the latter is a combination of an ejection systolic murmur and an early diastolic descrescendo murmur (for example aortic stenosis and insufficiency) (Figure 11, bottom) (Rao 1991b).

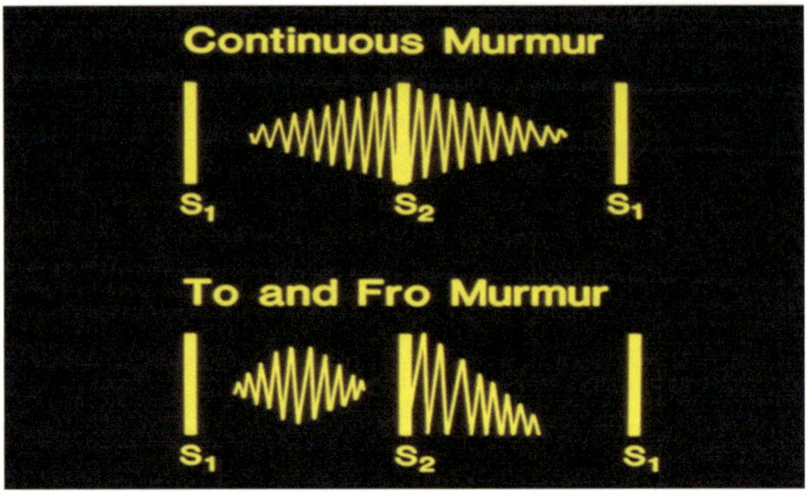

Fig. 11. Graphic representation of continuous and to-and-fro murmurs. The continuous murmur (top) begins in systole shortly after the first heart sound (S_1), crescendos up to the second heart sound (S_2) and decrescendos to a varying distance (time) into the diastole. In contradistinction to this murmur, the to-and-fro murmur (bottom) consists of an ejection systolic murmur with a separate early diastolic decrescendo murmur; note that there is a definite gap between the end of the ejection murmur and S_2.

The continuous murmur of PDA may be of grade I-V/VI in intensity. There is some beat-to-beat variation in the intensity of the murmur and for this reason it is described as machinery murmur. Multiple ejection clicks are usually heard within the murmur and this is rather characteristic of the PDA. The majority of the time, the murmur does not change with the position of the body, although the diastolic component of the murmur is heard better in a supine than in an upright position. However, in patients with very small PDA, the continuous murmur of the PDA either completely disappears or becomes only systolic in timing when the patient sits up and returns to continuous quality when the patient assumes supine position. The postulated cause of this is "kinking" of the ductus in the upright position (Thapar et al 1978). When the ductus is moderate to large in size, a mid-diastolic murmur may be heard at the apex because of increased flow across the mitral valve, such a mid-diastolic murmur suggests a Qp:Qs greater than 2:1. Arterial pulses are bounding in all but patients with very small ductus.

5.3.3 Noninvasive evaluation

5.3.3.1 Chest x-ray

Chest film may show a normal-sized heart with normal pulmonary vascular markings with small ductus while cardiomegaly, increased pulmonary blood flow and left atrial enlargement may be seen with moderate to large ductus. Collapse with secondary inflammatory process may be observed in the lung fields of small children with large ducti.

5.3.3.2 Electrocardiogram

The ECG may be normal or may show left atrial and left ventricular enlargement, depending upon the size of the ductus.

5.3.3.3 Echocardiogram

The echo may reveal varying degrees of left atrial and left ventricular enlargement, again depending upon the size of the ductus. The left ventricular contraction indices are normal unless severe myocardial dysfunction set in. Doppler echocardiography shows characteristic diastolic flow pattern in the pulmonary artery, indicative of PDA. Characteristic color flow mapping distribution is also present (Figure 12).

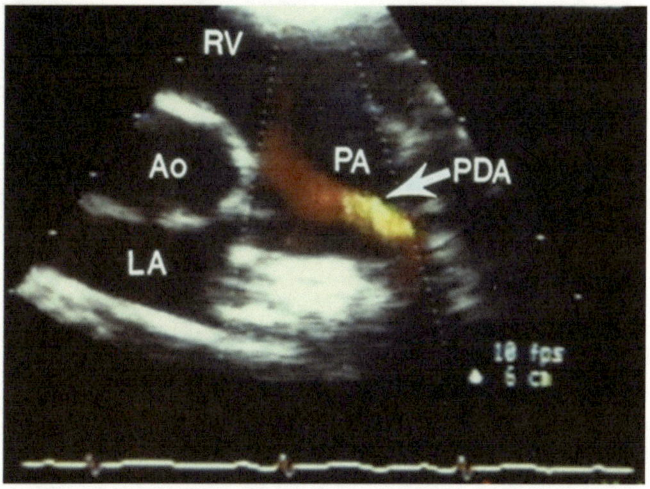

Fig. 12. Color Doppler flow mapping of the main pulmonary artery (PA) in a parasternal short axis view demonstrating the flow of the patent ductus arteriosus (PDA). Ao, Aorta; LA, Left atrium; RV, Right ventricel

5.3.4 Cardiac catheterization and selective cine angiography

These invasive studies are not necessary in the usual cases of PDA, although these procedures are integral parts of transcatheter closure.

Oxygen saturation data show a step up in oxygen saturation at the pulmonary artery level. The left heart saturations are usually normal. Calculated Qp:Qs, though usually indicates degree of shunting, it may not be accurate because of the difficulty in obtaining reliable mixed pulmonary arterial saturations. The right ventricular and pulmonary arterial pressures are normal in patients with small PDA but may be elevated if the PDA is moderate or large. Wide pulse pressure is observed in the aorta. Selective aortic arch injection demonstrates the size, shape and location of the ductus.

5.3.5 Management

It is generally believed that the presence of an isolated ductus is an indication for closure, mainly to prevent bacterial endocarditis. This can be performed at anytime, especially if associated with heart failure or pulmonary compromise. If the patient is asymptomatic, waiting until 6 to 12 months of age is generally recommended.

Until recently, surgical closure was the treatment of choice. While the risk of surgical closure is low, morbidity associated with it, namely anesthesia, endotrachial intubation and thoracotomy is universal. Because of this reason, less invasive, transcatheter closure techniques have been developed. These transcatheter methods are increasingly being used in closing PDAs. Gianturco coil occlusion of the PDA can be performed with small caliber catheters (#4F) and is the currently preferred method of occlusion for small to medium sized ducti.

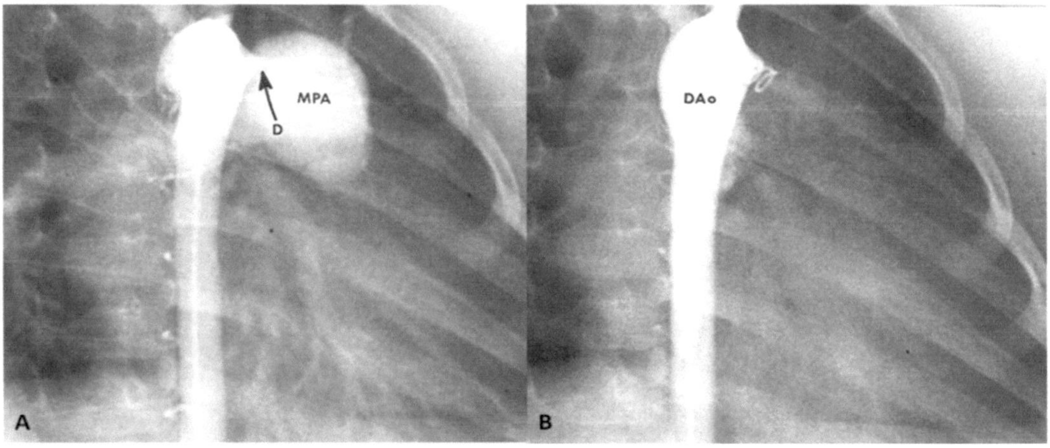

Fig. 13. Selected cine frames demonstrating a small to medium-sized patent ductus arteriosus (D) in a right anterior oblique view (A) which was occluded with a Gianturco coil (B). Dense opacification of the main pulmonary artery (MPA) prior to occlusion and no opacification following occlusion (B) are shown. DAo, descending aorta.

For large-sized PDA, surgical, video-thoracoscopic and transcatheter device closure are the available options, but most cardiologist prefer transcatheter occlusion (Rao and Sideris 1996). Amplatzer duct occluder is preferred for moderate to large PDA.

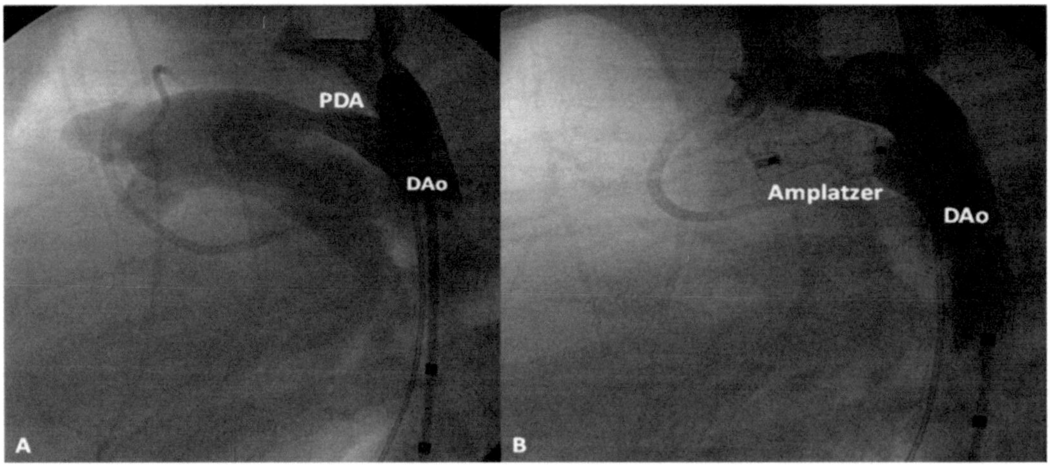

Fig. 14. Selected cine frames demonstrating a medium to large-sized patent ductus arteriosus (PDA) in a lateral view (A) which was occluded with an Amplatzer Duct Occluder (Amplatzer). Dense opacification PDA and the main pulmonary artery prior to occlusion and no opacification following occlusion (B) are shown. DAo, Descending aorta.

With wide spread use of color-Doppler echocardiography, a group of patients with color-Doppler evidence for small PDA, but without clinical features of PDA (no continuous murmur on auscultation), the so called "silent ductus" has emerged. There is no unanimity of opinion with regard to management of these patients.
Subacute bacterial endocarditis prophylaxis is recommended for all ducti prior to closure. There may not be any need for this prophylaxis three months following surgical or transcatheter closure, provided there is no residual shunt. Considerations with regard to elevated pulmonary vascular resistance with PDA are similar to those discussed under VSD section.

6. Right-to-left shunts (cyanotic heart defects)

In cyanotic congenital heart defects systemic venous blood bypasses the pulmonary circulation and gets shunted across into the left side of the heart. Thus, there is systemic arterial desaturation. By definition, cyanotic congenital heart disease does not include cyanosis due to intrapulmonary right-to-left shunting and pulmonary venous desaturation secondary to congestive heart failure. There are usually multiple defects of the heart causing right-to-left shunt. Obstruction to pulmonary blood flow (for example tetralogy of Fallot), complete admixture of pulmonary and systemic venous returns (for example, total anomalous pulmonary venous return and double-inlet left ventricle) and parallel rather than in-series circulation (transposition of the great arteries) are the causes of right-to-left shunts and cyanosis. The most important of the cyanotic CHDs are what are called "5 Ts" and are listed in table 2.

1. Tetralogy of Fallot
2. Transposition of the great arteries
3. Tricuspid atresia
4. Total anomalous pulmonary venous connection
5. Truncus arteriosus

Table 2. Common Cyanotic Congenital Heart Defects (5 Ts)

Three of these defects, namely tetralogy of Fallot, transposition of the great arteries and tricuspid atresia will be reviewed in this chapter.

6.1 Tetralogy of Fallot

Tetralogy of Fallot (TOF) is the most common cause of cyanosis beyond one year of age and constitutes 10% of all congenital heart defects. Fallot defined it as a constellation of four abnormalities to include a VSD, PS, right ventricular hypertrophy and dextroposition of the aorta. The ventricular defect is always large and non-restrictive and is located in the membranous septum in the subaortic region. Pulmonary stenosis is variable in severity and nature of obstruction. The right ventricular outflow obstruction may be mild resulting in initial left-to-right shunt at ventricular level or it may be severe causing severe cyanosis even in the neonatal period. It may be completely obstructed (pulmonary atresia) so that there is no forward flow from the right ventricle into the pulmonary artery, thus ductal dependent. The obstruction may be infundibular, valvar or supravalvar in nature or may involve branch pulmonary arteries. The stenotic component may be at a single site or may involve multiple sites. Infundibular obstruction is the most common obstruction in TOF and is due to malposition of the crista supraventricularis. The valvar stenosis may be due to valve leaflet fusion or due to valve ring hypoplasia. Right ventricular hypertrophy of severe degree is present in all cases. Dextroposition or over-riding of aorta over the ventricular septum is a variable phenomenon. The aorta is large and is thought to be due to a developmental anomaly rather than the result of physiologic abnormality of TOF. Right aortic arch is present in 25% of TOF cases.

Atrial septal defects may be present in 15% of patients with TOF in which case it may be called pentology of Fallot. Coronary artery anomalies are present in a small but significant number of cases. Origin of the left anterior descending coronary artery from the right coronary artery is the most common coronary anomaly in TOF and sometime the course of the coronary artery may be intra-myocardial.

Because the VSD is large, the systolic pressures in both ventricles are equal and for practical purposes both ventricles act as one functional chamber. The quantity of blood flow into to the systemic and pulmonary circuits depends upon their respective resistances. The level of systemic vascular resistance and the resistance offered by the right ventricular outflow tract stenosis determine the flows. The more severe the PS, the less is the pulmonary flow. In the average case of tetralogy of Fallot, the resistance offered by PS is more than that of the systemic vascular tone with consequent right-to-left shunt across the VSD. The consequent cyanosis and hypoxemia stimulate bone marrow (via kidney and erythropoitin) and produce polycythemia. While the polycythemia is helpful in increasing oxygen carrying capacity, it becomes counter-productive when the hematocrit is excessive (60 to 70%).

6.1.1 Symptoms

The clinical presentation depends upon the degree of PS. With milder degrees of PS, symptoms may not be present until late childhood while with severe PS the presentation may be in the early infancy. Typically the infant may be pink (not cyanotic) as a neonate and develops cyanosis between 2 to 6 months of age. Most usual modes of presentation are asymptomatic murmur discovered on routine auscultation, bluish color (cyanosis) observed by the parent or primary physician, hypercyanotic spells, and decreased exercise tolerance.

Hypercyanotic spells are variously described as anoxic spells, hypoxic spells, blue spells, paroxysmal dyspnea, paroxysmal hyperpnea and so no. The spells characteristically occur in tetralogy although they can be present in other lesions with similar physiology. They can occur any time between 1 month and 12 years of age but the peak incidence is 2 to 3 months. They can occur at any time of the day but most commonly seen after awakening from sleep; crying, defecation and feeding are the common precipitating factors. Spells are characterized by increasing rate and depth of respiration (hyperpnea) with increasing cyanosis, progressing to limpness and syncope, occasionally terminating in convolutions, cerebrovascular accident or death. Spells may occur in tetralogy with mild arterial desaturation and conversely may not be present in patients with severe cyanosis.

The cause or mechanism of onset of spells is not clear. Right ventricular infundibular spasm, precipitated by acute increase in endogenous catacholamines has been proposed as a mechanism. Prevention of these spells by beta-adrenergic blockade may further support this hypothesis. Since the spells have also been observed in patients with VSD and pulmonary atresia in whom infundibular spasm is singularly irrelevant, it is unlikely that the infundibular spasm is the cause in all cases. Another mechanism proposed is paroxysmal hyperpnea. During sleep oxygen consumption is reduced and there is a normal acid base balance. When the infant awakens the O_2 consumption increases and there is a slight acid base imbalance. There are adjustments made by the respiratory center to bring the imbalance back to normal. But, if there is a sudden increase in activity and consequent increase in oxygen consumption before the adjustments occur, decrease in PO_2 and pH and increase in PCO_2 take place triggering a hyperpnea response from the respiratory center and enter a vicious cycle. Hyperpnea reduces mean intrathoracic pressure, which decreases systemic and pulmonary resistances. Decreased systemic resistance is not matched with increased pulmonary flow because of dominant right ventricular outflow tract obstruction. Thus, there is even greater right-to-left shunt, further decreasing the PO_2 and pH and thus a vicious cycle (Guntheroth et al 1965, Rao 1983). Most workers believe that this is the most likely mechanism for the development of spells.

6.1.2 Physical examination

Central cyanosis is observed in most cases of' tetralogy of Fallot. However, it should be noted that mild arterial desaturation may not cause clinically detectable cyanosis. Clubbing of fingers and toes is observed beyond the first few months of life. There are usually no signs of congestive heart failure. Prominent right ventricular impulse or heave may be present. A systolic thrill may be present at the left upper sternal border. The first heart sound may be normal or slightly increased. The second heart sound is single without an audible pulmonary component. A grade III-IV/Vl long ejection systolic murmur, caused by blood flow through the right ventricular outflow tract, is usually heard at the left upper sternal border. In contrast to PS with intact ventricular septum, the murmur of tetralogy becomes shorter and less intense with increasing severity of PS. During hypercyanotic spell the murmur disappears or becomes very soft. A holosystolic murmur of VSD may be heard at the left lower sternal border in some children especially in less severe and acyanotic forms of tetralogy of Fallot. Early diastolic murmurs do not occur with TOF; the exception is TOF with syndrome of absent pulmonary valve. Continuous murmur of associated PDA is rarely heard. Older children may have an audible continuous murmur of bronchial collateral flow into the lungs.

6.1.3 Noninvasive evaluation

6.1.3.1 Chest roentgenogram

On a chest roentgenogram the heart size is usually normal to minimally increased. An uplifted apex, thought to indicate right ventricular hypertrophy may be present and is described by some as "boot-shaped" heart. Concavity in the region of pulmonary conus, reflecting hypoplasia of the pulmonary outflow tract may be present. Pulmonary vascular markings are usually diminished. A right sided aortic arch may be present. While a right aortic arch is expected to be present in 25% of TOF patients, the presence of a right aortic arch along with concave pulmonary conus and decreased pulmonary vascular markings in a chest x-ray makes the diagnosis of TOF virtually certain.

6.1.3.2 Electrocardiogram

The ECG shows signs of right ventricular hypertrophy. Right atrial enlargement is less commonly seen.

6.1.3.3 Blood work

Hemoglobin and hematocrit along with red blood cell indices should be monitored periodically in all children with cyanotic congenital heart defects including TOF. The degree and duration of hypoxemia determine the level of hemoglobin. In the absence of adequate iron intake, relative anemia with hypochromia and microcytosis may develop. Because this is a risk factor for developing cerebrovascular accidents, the relative anemia should be treated with oral supplemental iron.

6.1.3.4 Echocardiogram

The echo is very helpful in confirming the diagnosis and in evaluating several of the issues related to TOF. Enlargement of the right ventricle, large VSD, aortic over-ride and right ventricular outflow tract obstruction can be imaged. Shunting across the VSD and increased Doppler flow velocity across the right ventricular outflow tract can be demonstrated. Size of the main and proximal branch pulmonary arteries can be evaluated although the distal pulmonary arteries cannot easily be seen by echocardiogram.

6.1.4 Cardiac catheterization and angiography

Oxygen saturation data reveal systemic venous and arterial desaturation, usually proportional to the degree of right ventricular outflow obstruction. Usually no left-to-right shunts are demonstrated. Pulmonary venous and left atrial saturations are usually normal. The left ventricular and aortic saturations are diminished because of right-to-left shunt across the VSD. Aortic saturation is a better (than left ventricular) indicator of the degree of desaturation because of better mixing distally. The peak systolic pressures in both ventricles are equal because of a large VSD. The top of the right ventricular pressure curve is flat when compared to that of patients with PS with intact ventricular septum in which it is triangular. The pulmonary arterial pressures are low to normal with demonstrable peak systolic gradients across the pulmonary valve and infundibulum. However, multiple gradients may not be demonstrable in all patients either because of technical (multiple holes in the catheter or rapid withdrawal) or physiologic reasons. Angiographic data should be used to supplement pressure information for assessment of degree and level of right ventricular outflow obstruction. The left ventricular and aortic pressures are normal without any gradient across the aortic valve.

Angiographic evaluation of anatomy of TOF is generally recommended prior to total surgical correction, although at some centers detailed echocardiographic data may be considered adequate. Selective left ventricular angiography in a left axial oblique view to demonstrate the size and function of the left ventricle and the size and location of the VSD, particularly to exclude muscular VSD is important. Similarly selective right ventricular angiography to study its architecture, size and function and to evaluate right ventricular outflow obstruction is recommended. Pulmonary arteriogram in a sitting up view to visualize the size of the main and branch pulmonary arteries and to exclude branch pulmonary artery stenosis should be obtained. Aortic root angiography is also necessary to visualize coronary artery anatomy, especially to exclude coronary arteries crossing the right ventricular infundibulum. Origin of the left anterior descending coronary artery from the right coronary artery occurs in a significant number of cases of TOF and should be excluded, if necessary, by selective coronary angiography.

Management

The goal of management of TOF patients is to allow total surgical correction with minimal mortality and morbidity and to prevent or treat complications inherent to cyanotic heart defects in general and TOF in particular. Protection against subacute bacterial endocarditis, prevention and/or prompt treatment of dehydration, and periodic monitoring for relative anemia secondary to iron deficiency and prompt treatment when found should be undertaken. Palliative or corrective surgical procedures should be performed prior to development of significant polycythemia. Exercise, as tolerated should be permitted unless symptoms develop with activity.

Treatment of an infant with cyanotic spell may be summarized (Rao 1989a) as follows:

1. The infant should be placed in a knee-chest position. The reason for its effectiveness appears to be related to its effect in increasing the systemic vascular resistance and thus decreasing the right-to-left shunt and improving the pulmonary flow.
2. Humidified oxygen via a facemask should be administered. Since the major defect in the spell syndrome is pulmonary oligemia rather than alveolar hypoxia, oxygen administration has limited usefulness. If the infant is unduly disturbed by the facemask, oxygen therapy may be discontinued.
3. Morphine sulfate, 0.1 mg/kg subcutaneously, may be effective in aborting the spell. The mechanism of action is not clearly delineated, but its depressive effect on the central nervous system respiratory drive (thus reducing hyperpnea) and sedation of the infant may be important.
4. Once the physical examination is completed (and the limited but important laboratory studies are obtained) the infant should be left undisturbed and allowed to rest; this in itself may improve the infant's condition.
5. Correction of metabolic acidosis (with sodium bicarbonate), anemia (by blood transfusion), and dehydration (by appropriate fluids), if present, is very important at this stage.
6. If the spell continues, vasopressors to increase the systemic vascular resistance and thus increase the pulmonary blood flow may be tried. In our experience, methoxamine (Vasoxyl) an alpha agonist has been most helpful. It is a pure peripheral vascular stimulator without any direct action on the heart. Methoxamine 20-40 mg in 250 ml of 5% dextrose in water may be administered intravenously; the rate of infusion should be adjusted to increase the systolic blood pressure by 15 to 20% of the control value. Instead, phenylephrine may be given to increase systemic vascular resistance.
7. Alternatively, propranolol, 0.1 mg/kg body weight, diluted in 50 ml of 5% dextrose in water, may be slowly administered intravenously while monitoring the heart rate (by ECG if possible). Should there be marked bradycardia, propranolol should be stopped. Once it is found to be effective, the infant may be switched to oral propranolol 1-4 mg/kg/day in three and four divided doses. The mechanism of action of propranolol is not clearly understood, but may include negative inotropic effect on the right ventricular infundibular myocardium, prevention of decrease in systemic vascular resistance and/or prevention of ventilatory response (hyperpnea) to hypoxia, all through beta adrenergic blockade. Esmolol, a rapid acting beta blocker, may also be

used. The recommended loading dose of Esmolol is 500 mcg/kg followed by 50-100 mcg/kg/min.

8. Infrequently, general anesthesia may be necessary to break the spell.
9. If the infant does not improve with any of the aforementioned measures, an emergency systemic-to-pulmonary artery shunt (the author prefers modified Blalock-Taussig anastomosis) should be performed. Occasionally, total correction, if the anatomy is adequate, may he performed on an emergency basis. The important principle is that the infant requires more pulmonary blood flow.

If the infant improves with the management outlined above, total surgical correction of the cardiac defects, if anatomically feasible, or a systemic-to-pulmonary artery shunt to improve pulmonary blood flow on an elective basis within the next day or so may be performed. More recently, we have used balloon pulmonary valvuloplasty as an alternative to Blalock-Taussig shunt, especially if valvar obstruction is a significant component of right ventricular outflow obstruction (Rao et al 1992). Another alternative to surgery is oral propranolol (dosage as above) which may help postpone surgery by several months to years.

Total surgical correction to include closure of VSD in such a manner as to direct left ventricular output into the aorta and resection of the infundibulum and/or relief of pulmonary valvar obstruction can be performed almost at any age. Enlargement of the right ventricular outflow tract with a pericardial patch (or other prosthetic material) may be necessary in some cases. Sometimes total corrective procedures are not feasible with "respectable" mortality either because of pulmonary arterial (and/or annular) hypoplasia, "smallish" left ventricle, and/or anomalous course of a major coronary artery in the right ventricular infundibulum. Size and age of the patients also enter into such decision making. If it is deemed that a given patient is not suitable for total surgical correction, palliative surgery may be utilized to augment pulmonary blood flow and to allow the patients to grow into an age, size and anatomy that are more likely suitable for complete correction. Classic or modified Blalock-Taussig shunt is clearly a preferred surgical method for this purpose. We have used balloon pulmonary valvuloplasty in TOF patients to augment pulmonary blood flow and to allow for growth and development of the pulmonary arterial system and left ventricle so that a total surgical corrective procedure could be performed at a later time with a greater chance for success (Rao et al 1992).

Discussion of the management of TOF with pulmonary atresia, TOF with MAPCAs (multiple aorto-pulmonary collateral arteries) and TOF with syndrome of absent pulmonary valve is beyond the scope of this chapter and the reader is referred elsewhere (Alapati and Rao 2011) or to the standard textbooks.

6.2 Transposition of the great arteries

Transposition of the great arteries (TGA) is the most common cyanotic congenital heart defect presenting in the newborn period. It constitutes 5% of all CHD and 10% of all cyanotic CHD. There are multiple definitions used to describe TGA. Perhaps, the most accurate description is "a condition in which the aorta arises from the morphologic right ventricle and the pulmonary artery from the morphologic left ventricle". In the most common form, usually referred to as complete transposition, the atria are normal in position (situs solitus of the atria), there is atrioventricular concordance (right atrium connected to the right ventricle and the left atrium to the left ventricle), d loop of the ventricles (right ventricle on the right and left ventricle on the left), and ventriculo-arterial discordance (aorta arising from the right ventricle and the pulmonary artery from the ventricle). The systemic venous blood from the vena cavae enters the right atrium and right ventricle and from there into the aorta while the pulmonary venous blood enters the left atrium and left ventricle and from there into the pulmonary artery. Thus, the circulation is parallel instead of normal in-series circulation. Because of this reason, the systemic venous blood does not get oxygenated and the pulmonary venous blood does not get delivered to the body. The infant will not survive unless there are intercirculatory shunts such as atrial or ventricular septal defect or patent ductus arteriosus.

6.2.1 Symptoms

Clinical features depend upon the anatomic type, namely Group I, TGA with intact ventricular septum; Group II, TGA with VSD, and Group III, TGA with VSD and PS (Rao 2010).

In group I with intact septum, the infants usually present with cyanosis within the first week of life. They may otherwise be asymptomatic. However, they will soon become tachypnoeic and develop respiratory distress. If they are not appropriately treated, they become acidotic and go on to become lethargic without lack of spontaneous movement, and eventually die.

Group II TGA patients with VSD present with symptoms of congestive heart failure (tachypnea, tachycardia, sweating, and poor feeding) between 4 to 8 weeks of life, but the cyanosis is minimal.

Group III patients (TGA with VSD and PS) have variable presentation, depending upon the severity of PS. If there is poor mixing, they may present early in life and mimic TGA with intact septum. If the PS is severe, the presentation is essentially similar to that described in the TOF section. With moderate PS the presentation is late with longer survival. With mild PS, congestive heart failure signs may be present, similar to group II patients.

6.2.2 Physical examination

The group I patients with intact septum are usually severely cyanotic but are without distress until severe hypoxemia and acidosis develop. Clubbing is not present in the newborn period and may not develop until 3 to 6 months. The right ventricular impulse is increased and the second heart sound is single. Either no murmur or a grade I-II/VI nonspecific ejection systolic murmur may be auscultated. In group II patients, tachypnea, tachycardia, minimal cyanosis, hepatomegaly, increased right and left ventricular impulses, single second sound, a grade III-IV/VI holosystolic murmur at the left lower sternal border and a mid-diastolic flow rumble (murmur) at the apex may be present. In group III patients, the findings are similar to TGA with intact septum, TGA with VSD, or TOF depending upon the degree of mixing and severity of PS.

6.2.3 Noninvasive evaluation

6.2.3.1 Chest roentgenogram

Chest x-ray in the intact septum group is benign with normal to minimal cardiomegaly and normal to slightly increased pulmonary vascular marking. The thymic shadow may rapidly involute and a narrow pedicle (superior mediastinum) may be seen. A combination of the above signs may sometimes assume "egg-shaped" appearance on a postero-anterior chest roentgenogram. In group II patients with VSD, moderate to severe cardiomegaly and increased pulmonary vascular markings are usually seen. In group III patient, mild to at worst moderate cardiomegaly may be observed. The pulmonary vascular marking may be increased, normal or decreased, dependent upon the severity of PS.

6.2.3.2 Electrocardiogram

The ECG in a neonate with TGA and intact septum (Group I) may be normal with the usual right ventricular preponderance seen during this age. In older infants clear-cut right ventricular hypertrophy is seen and in addition right atrial enlargement may be observed. In group II patients, biventricular hypertrophy and left atrial enlargement are usual. In group III, right ventricular or biventricular enlargement is seen.

6.2.3.3 Echocardiogram

The echo is usually helpful in the diagnosis and assessment. Demonstration of transposition of the great arteries is somewhat difficult in view of the fact that atrial and ventricular anatomy is normal and the aortic and pulmonary valves look similar on echocardiographic study. If one can follow the great vessel arising from the left ventricle and demonstrate its bifurcation, identifying it as a pulmonary artery, the diagnosis is easy. One of the helpful indirect signs is somewhat a posterior course the great vessel off of the left ventricle in a precordial long axis view, indicating pulmonary artery in contradistinction to anteriorly coursing ascending aorta. On-end visualization of the aorta and pulmonary artery on a precordial short axis view of the heart is also helpful in suggesting TGA. The presence of an inter-atrial communication and patent ductus arteriosus and shunt across them by color and pulsed Doppler can also be evaluated. In addition to these, demonstration of VSD and PS will place the patients into the respective groups.

6.2.3.4 Other laboratory data

Blood gas values are useful in demonstrating the degree of hypoxemia and ventilatory status. Hemoglobin and hematocrit are particularly useful in the follow-up of older children.

6.2.4 Cardiac catheterization and angiography

With the increasing accuracy of echocardiographic diagnosis, invasive studies are not necessary for diagnosing TGA. Need for rapid relief hypoxemia and acidosis by balloon atrial septostomy and the need for a greater definition of coronary artery anatomy prior to arterial switch procedure may necessitate catheterization and angiography.

In group I patients, vena caval, right atrial, right ventricular and aortic saturations are moderately to severely diminished unless atrial, ventricular or ductal shunting is present. Similarly, the pulmonary venous, left atrial, left ventricular and pulmonary arterial saturations are high with minimal, if any right-to-left shunt. In TGA, the pulmonary artery saturations are higher than those in the aorta.

The left atrial pressure is usually high with a pressure gradient across the atrial septum. The right ventricular pressure is at systemic level without any gradient across the aortic valve. In TGA with intact septum the left ventricular and pulmonary artery pressure are normal without any gradient across the pulmonary valve. However, in the early neonatal period, prior to involution of the pulmonary vasculature, these pressures are elevated, compared to normal. In the presence of significant VSD and/or PS, the left ventricular pressure is elevated and this is usually proportional to the size of VSD and severity of PS. The pulmonary artery pressure is usually increased with associated VSD while with PS it may be low to normal.

Selective right ventricular angiography reveals a morphologically right ventricle with opacification of an anteriorly and superiorly displaced aorta. The aortic valve is located to the right of the pulmonary valve (d-TGA). The aorta ascends in a normal fashion and usually descends on the left side of the spine. The size and function of the right ventricle and presence of tricuspid insufficiency should be evaluated. If a VSD is present, it may be visualized. A laid-back view of the aortic root angiography along with a lateral view may be useful in demonstrating coronary artery anatomy. Aortography may, in addition, be useful in demonstrating PDA and CoA. Left ventricular cineangiogram reveals a morphologic left ventricle with prompt opacification of the pulmonary artery. The pulmonary valve is located posterior, inferior and to the left of the aortic valve. Left ventricular angiography should be scrutinized for subvalvar and valvar PS. A VSD may be visualized, if present.

6.2.5 Management

Untreated, TGA with intact septum carries a poor prognosis. The initial management of this and other cyanotic neonates is similar. Monitoring the infant's temperature and maintenance of neutral thermal environment is extremely important. In hypoxemic infants, ambient oxygen should be administered. In cyanotic CHD patients, no more than 0.4 FIO_2 is necessary. Metabolic acidosis (pH < 7.25), if any, should be corrected with sodium bicarbonate (usually 1-2 mEq/kg diluted half and half with 5% or 10% dextrose solution) immediately. Respiratory acidosis should be cared for by appropriate suctioning, intubation and assisted ventilation. Hypoglycemia may be a significant problem; therefore, the infant's serum glucose should be monitored and the neonates should routinely receive 10% dextrose in water intravenously. If hypoglycemia (<30 mg/100ml) occurs, 15% to 20% dextrose solution should be administered. Similarly hypocalcemia should be monitored for and treated, if found. If an infant is getting progressively hypoxemic, it is likely that the intercirculatory pathways (patent foramen ovale and patent ductus arteriosus) are closing. Prostaglandin E_I (PGE_I) (0.05 to 0.1 mcg/kg/min) intravenously may help open the ductus, thus improve oxygenation. Balloon atrial septostomy may be necessary to improve hypoxemia even after PGE_1. Total surgical correction by arterial switch procedure (Jatene) is the treatment of choice in these neonates and will be discussed here-under.

TGA patients with VSD usually present with heart failure and aggressive anticongestive measures are indeed needed. Balloon atrial septostomy may help relieve pulmonary venous congestion and improve oxygenation. These patients will require Jatene procedure with closure of VSD.

TGA patients with VSD and PS may have varying presentation. If the reason for hypoxemia is poor mixing, balloon atrial septostomy is the treatment of choice. If the hypoxemia is secondary to decreased pulmonary flow, a Blalock-Taussig type of shunt may be needed. Sometimes both balloon septostomy and balloon dilatation of pulmonary valve may be performed via catheters in some of these children. Eventually these patients require a Rastelli type of repair.

Mustard procedure, which was originally described in 1964 was the most commonly used operation for TGA in the past. In this operation, hemodynamic correction of the defect is achieved by re-directing the systemic and pulmonary venous returns by means of an intra-atrial baffle. Better understanding of the conduction system and its blood supply coupled with the use of a pericardial baffle (instead of Dacron baffle) has significantly reduced post-operative complications such as arrhythmia and baffle obstruction. Other types of atrial switch operations, originally described by Senning and by Shumacker have also been used in several centers. When venous switch procedure is opted for, Mustard and Senning procedures appear to be selected with equal frequency, depending upon the institution/surgeon. In 1975, Jatene described anatomical corrections for TGA by arterial switch with relocation of the coronary arteries. Initially this procedure was performed for TGA with non-restrictive VSD and subsequently was adapted to TGA with intact septum. The arterial switch procedure has several advantages over the venous switch procedure in that the arrhythmias are less frequent, and the left ventricle rather than the right ventricle serves as a pump to systemic circuit. Arterial switch procedure, however, must be performed in the early neonate prior to deconditioning the left (pulmonary) ventricle in TGA patients with intact septum. Although there are no extensive long term follow-up results available, the short term and medium-term follow-up results are very encouraging and, at this time, the arterial switch procedure with or without LeCompte maneuver is considered the preferable operation for patients with TGA.

6.3 Tricuspid atresia

Tricuspid atresia (TA) is a cyanotic, congenital cardiac anomaly and has been commonly defined as congenital absence or agenesis of the morphologic tricuspid valve. It is the third most common cyanotic CHD and is the most common cause of cyanosis with left ventricular hypertrophy. Tricuspid atresia accounts for 1.4% of subjects with CHD. The most common type of TA, muscular variety, is characterized by a dimple or a localized fibrous thickening in the floor of the right atrium at the expected site of the tricuspid valve. The right atrium is usually enlarged and its wall thickened and hypertrophied. An inter-atrial communication, which is necessary for survival, is usually a stretched patent foramen ovale. The left atrium is enlarged and may be more so if the pulmonary blood flow is increased. The mitral valve is morphologically a mitral valve, usually bicuspid but its orifice is large and rarely incompetent. The left ventricle is clearly a morphologic left ventricle with only occasional abnormality; however, it is enlarged and hypertrophied. The VSD may be large, small or non-existent (intact ventricular septum) or multiple VSDs may be present. While a variety of VSDs are seen in TA hearts, muscular defects are most common. Also, most of these VSDs are restrictive and produce subpulmonary stenosis in patients with normally related great arteries and subaortic stenosis in patients with transposed great arteries. The right ventricle is small and hypoplastic; its size, by and large, is determined by the anatomic type. The relative position of the great vessels is quite variable and has been the basis for classification of' this anomaly: Type I, normally related great arteries; Type II, d-transposition of the great arteries; Type III, malpositions of the great arteries other than d-transposition; and Type IV, Truncus arteriosus (Table III) (Rao 1980).
Pulmonary outflow tract obstruction may be either subvalvar or valvar in patients with transposition while in patients with normally related great arteries, it is often at the VSD level although, in a few cases, subvalvar pulmonary stenosis, narrow tract of the hypoplastic right ventricle and, rarely, valvar PS may also be responsible for pulmonary outflow tract obstruction. The pulmonary artery may be atretic and in such cases a PDA or aorto-pulmonary collateral vessels may be present. Association with aortic coarctation is rare with type I patients and is more common in patients with transposition of the great arteries.

An obligatory right-to-left shunt occurs it the atrial level in most types and subtypes of TA. Thus, the systemic and coronary venous blood mixes with pulmonary venous return in the left atrium and exits into the left ventricle. In type I (normally related great arteries) patients with a VSD, left-to-right ventricular shunt occurs, thus perfusing the lungs. In the absence of a VSD (i.e., intact ventricular septum), the pulmonary circulation is derived either via a PDA or through aorto-pulmonary collateral vessels. The presence of either a VSD or other means of blood supply to the lungs is essential for the patient's survival. The aortic blood flow is derived directly from the left ventricle. In type II (with d-transposition of the great arteries), the pulmonary blood flow is directly divided from the left ventricle. The systemic blood flow is via the VSD and right ventricle.

Type I	Normally related great arteries	Each Type and Subtype are divided
Type II	D-transposition of the great arteries	Subgroup a. Pulmonary atresia
Type III	Malpositions of the great arteries other than D-transposition	Subgroup b. Pulmonary stenosis or hypoplasia
		Subgroup c. Normal pulmonary arteries (no pulmonary stenosis)
Subtype 1.	L-transposition of the great arteries	
Subtype 2.	Double outlet right ventricle	
Subtype 3.	Double outlet left ventricle	
Subtype 4.	D-malposition of the great arteries (anatomically corrected malposition)	
Subtype 5.	L-malposition of the great arteries (anatomically corrected malposition)	
Type IV	Persistent truncus arteriosus	

Table 3. A Unified Classification of Tricuspid Atresia

6.3.1 Symptoms

Approximately one-half of the patients with TA present with symptoms on the first day of life and 80% would have had symptoms by the end of the first month of life. The magnitude of pulmonary blood flow determines the timing of and, type of clinical presentation. Two modes of presentation are recognized; those with decreased pulmonary blood flow and those with increased pulmonary blood flow.

Infants with pulmonary oligemia present with symptoms of cyanosis within the first few days of life; the more severe the pulmonary oligemia, the earlier is the clinical presentation. These hypoxemic infants may have hyperpnea and acidosis if the pulmonary blood flow is markedly diminished. The majority of the infants belong to type Ib (no transposition and pulmonary hypoplasia with a small VSD). Patients with pulmonary atresia (subgroup a, of all types) irrespective of great vessel relationship will also present with early cyanosis, especially when the ductus begins to close. Hypoxic spells are not common in the neonate although the spells can occur later in infancy.

Infants with pulmonary plethora usually present with signs of heart failure within the first few weeks of life although an occasional infant may present within the first few days of life. They are only minimally cyanotic, but present with symptoms of dyspnea, fatigue, difficulty to feed, and perspiration. Recurrent respiratory tract infections and failure to thrive are other modes of presentation. The majority of these patients belong to type II (transposition with a large VSD) although a small number of patients may be of type Ic (no transposition but a large VSD). The association of aortic coarctation with type II patients has already been mentioned and coarctation, when present, makes them vulnerable to early cardiac failure.

6.3.2 Physical findings

In infants (and children) with pulmonary oligemia, physical examination reveals central cyanosis, clubbing (in older infants and children), tachypnea or hyperpnea, normal pulses, prominent "a" wave in the jugular venous pulse (if there is inter-atrial obstruction), and no hepatic enlargement. Quiet precordium, and absence of thrills are usual. The second heart sound is usually single. A holosystolic murmur suggestive of VSD may be heard at the left lower or mid sternal border. No diastolic murmurs are heard. In patients with associated pulmonary atresia, no murmurs are usually heard, although in an occasional patient a continuous murmur of PDA may be heard. Signs of clinical congestive heart failure are notably absent.

In the group with pulmonary plethora, examination reveals tachypnea, tachycardia, decreased femoral pulses (if associated with CoA), minimal cyanosis and hepatomegaly. Prominent "a" waves in the jugular veins and/or presystolic hepatic pulsations may be observed with associated inter-atrial obstruction. The second heart sound may be single or split. A holosystolic murmur of VSD is usually heard at the left lower sternal border. An apical mid-diastolic flow murmur may be heard. Clear-cut signs of congestive heart failure are usually present.

6.3.3 Non-invasive evaluation

6.3.3.1 Chest x-ray

Chest film appearance is, by and large, dependent upon the total pulmonary blood flow. In patients with diminished pulmonary blood flow (the majority of infants fall into this group), the heart size is either normal or minimally enlarged. Several patterns of cardiac configuration have been described but in the author's experience and that of others, there is no consistent pattern that would be diagnostic of TA. There may be concavity in the region of pulmonary artery segment in patients with pulmonary oligemia and small pulmonary artery. The right atrial shadow may be prominent. In patients with increased pulmonary blood flow, cardiomegaly and prominent pulmonary vasculature are seen.

6.3.3.2 Electrocardiogram

The ECG can be virtually diagnostic of tricuspid atresia in an infant with cyanotic CHD. The characteristic features include right atrial enlargement, an abnormal, superiorly oriented major QRS vector (so called left axis deviation) in the frontal plane, left ventricular hypertrophy and diminished right ventricular forces. Abnormally superior vector (left axis deviation) is present in excess of 80% of patients with type I (normally related great vessels) anatomy while only less than 50% of patients with type II (transposition) anatomy show such a typical electrocardiographic pattern.

6.3.3.3 Echocardiogram

The echo is reasonably characteristic for TA. Two-dimensional echocardiography, apart from showing enlarged right atrium, left atrium, and left ventricle and a small right ventricle, will demonstrate the atretic tricuspid valve directly. In the most common muscular type, a dense band of echoes is seen at the site where the tricuspid valve should be and the anterior leaflet of the detectable atrioventricular valve is attached to the left side of the inter-atrial septum. Apical and subcostal four-chambered views are best to demonstrate the anatomy. Atrial and ventricular septal defects can also be demonstrated by 2-D echocardiography and shunting across these defects can be demonstrated by Doppler echocardiography. Semilunar valves can be identified as pulmonary or aortic by following the great vessel until the bifurcation of the pulmonary artery or arch of the aorta is seen, this will help decide whether there is associated transposition of the great arteries. Measurement of peak Doppler flow velocities across the VSD and right ventricular outflow tract will not only reveal if obstruction is present at these sites but will also allow estimation of pulmonary artery pressures. Suprasternal notch imaging will be of use in demonstrating CoA, which is often seen in type II (transposition) patients. Contrast echocardiography with two-dimensional imaging will clearly demonstrate sequential opacification of the right atrium, left atrium, left ventricle and then the right ventricle. However, such a study is not always necessary for diagnosis.

6.3.4 Cardiac catheterization and selective cineangiography

The diagnosis of TA based on clinical, electrocardiographic, and echocardiographic features is relatively simple, and cardiac catheterization and selective cineangiography, rarely, if ever, are essential for arriving at the diagnosis. However, these procedures are useful and should be undertaken to resolve issues not clarified by non-invasive studies and to evaluate multiple physiologic and anatomic features prior to planned Fontan-Kreutzer operation (Rao 1992).

Oxygen saturation data reveal diminished systemic venous saturation; the extent of decrease is related to the systemic arterial desaturation and the severity of congestive heart failure. The pulmonary venous saturation is usually in the normal range. A significant decrease in left atrial saturation is expected because of obligatory right-to-left shunting across the patent foramen ovale. Falsely high or falsely low saturations may be measured in the left atrium because of streaming. The left ventricular saturations are usually well mixed and are more reliable. The saturations in the left atrium, left ventricle and aorta as well as those in the right ventricle and pulmonary artery are nearly equal. Systemic arterial (aortic) desaturation is always present and the extent of desaturation is proportional to the Qp:Qs.

The right atrial pressure may be mildly increased. If the foramen ovale is restrictive the pressure in the right atrium is markedly elevated; a mean pressure gradient of 5 mmHg across the patent foramen ovale in favor of the right atrium and giant "a" waves in the right atrium are indicative of an obstructive foramen ovale. The left atrial mean and left ventricular end-diastolic pressures are usually normal, but may be elevated if there is increased pulmonary blood flow, poor left ventricular function or significant mitral insufficiency. The right ventricular pressure is proportional to the size of the VSD in type I (normally related great arteries) patients while it is at systemic level in type II (transposition) patients. Systolic pressure gradient across the VSD may be seen if it is restrictive. The pulmonary artery pressure may be normal or increased depending upon the size of the VSD

(and associated PS) in type I patients and upon the presence or absence of subvalvar or valvar PS in type II patients. Aortic pressures are usually normal. If CoA is present, systolic hypertension and pressure gradient across the coarctation will be present.
Of all the calculated values, Qp:Qs and pulmonary vascular resistance are most useful. The Qp:Qs is diminished in type I hypoxemic patients with small or no VSD while it is markedly increased in type I patients with moderate to large VSDs and in most patients with type II anatomy. Pulmonary vascular resistance is an important factor to be taken into consideration for deciding to go ahead with Fontan-Kreutzer operation; elevated resistance adversely affects the outcome of the operation.
Selective right atrial angiography will confirm the diagnosis. Following right atrial injection, successive opacification of the left atrium and left ventricle without direct opacification of the right ventricle occurs and this negative shadow of the unopacified right ventricle, the so called right ventricular window is considered characteristic for TA. Selective left ventricular angiography is also recommended and is useful in evaluating its size and function, size and type of VSD, anatomy and size of the right ventricle, relationship of the great arteries and the source of pulmonary blood flow. Selective right ventricular and pulmonary arterial angiograms are possible with the currently available catheter/guide wire technology and may be necessary in some cases for better definition prior to considering "corrective" surgical procedures.

6.3.5 Management

Physiologically "corrective" operation for TA, namely, Fontan-Kreutzer procedure and its modifications, have improved the prognosis of patients with tricuspid atresia. Such physiologic correction is usually performed in patients older than 2 years. As stated above, most patients with TA present with symptoms in the neonatal period and should be effectively palliated to enable them to reach the age at which surgical correction could be undertaken. The objective of any management plan, apart from providing symptomatic relief and increased survival rate, should be to preserve, protect, and restore anatomy (good sized and undistorted pulmonary arteries) and physiology (normal pulmonary artery pressures and preserved left ventricular function) to normal such that a "corrective" procedure could later be performed safely.
Medical management of the neonate, just as for TGA patients, includes maintenance of neutral thermal environment, normal acid-base status, normoglycemia and normocalcemia by appropriate monitoring and correction, if needed. No more than 0.4 FI02 is necessary unless there is associated pulmonary pathology.
In neonates with low arterial PO_2 and O_2 saturation with ductal dependent pulmonary blood flow, the ductus should be kept open by intravenous infusion of PGE_1, in doses similar to that described in TOF and TGA sections. Once the infant is stabilized and appropriate diagnostic studies are performed, a Blalock-Taussig type of shunt is performed in the group with pulmonary oligemia.
In neonates and infants with pulmonary plethora and congestive heart failure, aggressive anticongestive therapy must be instituted. In type I (normally related great arteries) patients, the natural history of the VSD is such that it closes spontaneously and the infants will go on to develop pulmonary origemia (Rao 1977b). Because of these reasons, it is recommended that banding of the pulmonary artery not be routinely performed in this group of patients. If optimal anticongestive therapy with some delay does not produce adequate relief of

symptoms, pulmonary artery banding should then be considered. Alternatively, an absorbable band may be used (Rao 2001). By contrast, in type II (transposition) patients, banding of the pulmonary artery should be performed once the infant is stabilized with anticongestive measures. If there is associated CoA, it should also be relieved.

In infants with evidence for interatrial obstruction, balloon and/or blade atrial septostomy may be necessary.

Following initial palliation, the children should be followed under close cardiologic supervision. Currently, preferred "corrective" procedure is staged total cavopulmonary anastomosis. A bi-directional Glenn procedure (superior vena cava to pulmonary artery anastomois) may be performed around the age of six months. Preoperative catheter evaluation to define the pulmonary artery pressure and anatomy and to exclude a persistent left superior vena cava (because it may divert blood away from the pulmonary arteries) prior to bidirectional Glenn surgery should be undertaken. At the time of bidirectional Glenn procedure, stenoses, if any, of the pulmonary artery should be repaired. Issues related to subaortic obstruction and mitral valve regurgitation should also be addressed.

When the patients reach the age and size (approximately 15 Kg) suitable for Fontan-Kreutzer operation, diversion of inferior vena caval blood into the pulmonary artery either by a lateral tunnel or extracardiac conduit is recommended. At the present time extracardiac conduit diversion of inferior vena caval blood into the pulmonary artery) is preferred by most surgeons.. Immediately prior to Fontan conversion, cardiac catheterization should be undertaken to ensure normal anatomy and pressure of the pulmonary artery as well as normal left ventricular end-diastolic pressure. At the same time, aortopulmonary collaterals should be evaluated by means of selective subclavian artery and descending thoracic aortic angiography. If collateral vessels are present, they should be occluded with coils or devices, as appropriate.

In patients with transposition of the great arteries, early pulmonary artery banding, treatment of aortic coarctation, and relieving or bypassing subaortic obstruction should also be incorporated into the treatment plan.

If the patient has risk factors for poor outcome (for e.g., elevated pulmonary pressure/resistance, pulmonary artery distortion, and left ventricular dysfunction) for the corrective procedure, a fenestrated Fontan procedure should be considered. Some surgeons prefer fenestration for all patients. Six to twelve months later, transcatheter closure of the fenestration may be undertaken if the fenestration did not spontaneously close.

Close follow-up after correction is indicated. While most of these patients will do well, some may develop arrhythmia (atrial flutter or fibrillation, paroxysmal supraventricular tachycardia), obstructed Fontan pathways, branch pulmonary artery stenosis, thrombo-embolism, persistent right to left shunts (Fontan fenestrations or atrial septal defects), systemic venous to pulmonary venous collateral vessels and protein-losing enteropathy. Detailed evaluation of these problems and appropriate treatment is mandatory

7. Conclusions

Congenital heart defect is an anatomic malformation of the heart and/or great vessel, which occurs during intrauterine development. The incidence of CHD is 0.6 to 0.8% of live-births. The exact etiology of CHD is not known and the majority of cardiac defects can be explained by multifactorial inheritance hypothesis. The CHD may be classified as acyanotic and cyanotic defects and the former is further divided into obstructive and left-to-right shunt lesions. Pathologic, physiologic, clinical and laboratory features of nine most common CHD, described in this chapter are distinctive. Methods of management for each of these defects are outlined. Based on this review, it appears that while the etiology of CHD is not clearly identified, their recognition by clinical evaluation and non-invasive laboratory tests is possible and their treatment with currently available transcatheter and surgical methods is feasible, effective and safe.

8. References

Alapati, S. & Rao, P. S. (2011). Tetralogy of Fallot in the neonate. *Neonatology Today,* Vol. 6, No. 5, pp. 1-8

Amin, Z.; Cao, Q. L. & Hijazi, Z. M. (2008). Closure of muscular ventricular septal defects: Transcatheter and hybrid techniques. Catheter *Cardiovasc Interv* Vol. 72, No. 1, pp. 102-111

Chopra, P. S. & Rao P. S. (2000). History of the development of atrial septal defect occlusion devices. *Current Intervent Cardiol Reports,* Vol. 2. No. 1. pp. 63-69

Fu, Y. C.; Bass, J.; Amin, Z.; et al. (2006). Transcatheter closure of perimembranous ventricular septal defects using the new Amplatzer membranous VSD occluder. Results of the U.S. Phase I trial. *J Am Coll Cardiol,* Vol. 47, No. 2 , pp. 319– 325

Fyler, D. C. (Ed) (1992). *Nadas' Pediatric Cardiology,* Hanly & Belfus, Inc., Philadelphia, PA

Galal, O.; Rao, P.S.; Al-Fadley, F. & Wilson, A. D. (1997). Follow-up results of balloon aortic valvuloplasty in children with special reference to causes of late aortic insufficiency. *Am Heart J,* Vol. 133. No. 4, pp. 418-427

Guntheroth, W. G.; Morgan, B. C. & Mullin, G. L. (1965). Physiologic studies of paroxysmal hyperpnea in cyanotic congenital heart disease. *Circulation,* Vol. 31. No. 1, pp. 70-76

Holzer, R.; de Giovanni, J.; Walsh, K.P. et al. (2006). Transcatheter closure of perimembranous ventricular septal defects using the Amplatzer membranous VSD occluder: Immediate and midterm results of an international registry. *Catheter Cardiovasc Interv,* Vol. 68. No. 4, pp. 620–628

Nora, J. J. (1968). Multifactorial inheritance hypothesis for etiology of congenital heart disease: the genetic- environmental interaction. *Circulation,* Vol. 38. No. 3, pp. 604-617

Nugent, E. W.; Freedom, R. M.; Nora, J. J. et al (1977). Clinical course in pulmonary stenosis. Circulation. Vol 56. No.1, (Suppl), pp. I38-147

Rao, P. S. (1977a). Prevention of heart disease in infants and children. *Current Prob Pediat,* Vol. 7. No. 7, pp. l-48, Year Book Medical Publishers, Inc., Chicago, IL

Rao, P. S. (1977b) Natural history of the ventricular septal defect in tricuspid atresia and its surgical implications. *Brit Heart J,* Vol. 39, No. 3, pp. 276-288

Rao, P. S. (1980). A unified classification of tricuspid atresia. *Am Heart J,* Vol. 99. No. 6, pp. 799-804

Rao, P. S. (1983). Pathophysiologic consequences of cyanotic heart disease. *Indian J Pediat,* Vol.50. No. 406, pp. 479-487

Rao, P. S. (1988). Indications for balloon pulmonary valvuloplasty. *Am Heart J,* Vol. 116. No. 6, pp. 1661-1662

Rao, P. S. (1989a): Congenital heart disease. In: *Conn's Current Therapy,* Rakel, R. E. (ed), pp. 2010-213, W.B. Saunders. ISBN 0-7216-2581-9, Philadelphia, PA

Rao, P. S. (1989b). Balloon angioplasty and valvuloplasty in infants, children and adolescents. *Current Prob Cardiol,* Vol. 14. No. 8, pp. 417-500, Year Book Medical Publishers, Inc., Chicago, IL.

Rao, P. S. (1990). Balloon aortic valvuloplasty: a review. *Clin Cardiol,* Vol. 13. No. 7, pp. 458-466

Rao, P. S. (1991a). Perinatal circulatory physiology. *Indian J Pediat,* Vol. 58, No. 4, pp. 441-451

Rao, P. S. (1991b). Evaluation of cardiac murmurs in children. *Indian J Pediat,* Vol. 58, No. 4, pp. 471-491

Rao, P. S. (Ed) (1992). *Tricuspid Atresia, 2nd ed.,* Futura Publishing Co., ISBN 0-87993-5189, New York, NY.

Rao, P. S. (Ed) (1993). *Transcatheter Therapy in Pediatric Cardiology.* Wiley-Liss, Inc, ISBN 0-471-58827-X, New York, NY

Rao, P. S. (1995). Coarctation of the aorta: In: *Secondary Forms of Hypertension.* Ram CVC (ed), *Seminars in Nephrology,* Kurtzman NA (ed), Vol. 15, No. 2, pp. 81-105, W.B. Saunders, Philadelphia, PA

Rao, P. S. (1998). Interventional pediatric cardiology: State of the art and future directions. *Pediat Cardiol,* Vol. 19, No. 1, pp. 107-124

Rao, P. S. (1999). Long-term follow-up results after balloon dilatation of pulmonic stenosis, aortic stenosis and coarctation of the aorta; a review. *Progr Cardiovasc Dis,* Vol. 42. No. 1, pp. 59-74

Rao, P. S. (2000a): Pulmonary valve disease. In: *Valvular Heart Disease. 3rd edition,* Alpert JS, Dalen JE, Rahimtoola S. (Eds), pp. 339-376, Lippincott, Williams and Wilkins, ISBN 0-7817-2310-8, Philadelphia, PA

Rao, P. S. (2000b). Late pulmonary insufficiency after balloon dilatation of the pulmonary valve (Letter). *Cathet Cardiovasc Intervent, Vol.* 49, No. , pp. 118-119

Rao, P. S. (2001). Absorbable pulmonary artery band in tricuspid atresia (Editorial). *Ann Thorac Surg,* Vol. 71, No. 1, pp. 361-362

Rao, P. S. (2007a). Percutaneous balloon pulmonary valvuloplasty: State of the art. *Cath Cardiovasc Intervent,* Vol. 69, No. 5, pp. 747-763

Rao, P. S. (2007b). Pulmonary valve stenosis. In: *Percutaneous Interventions in Congenital Heart Disease,* Sievert, H.; Qureshi, S. A.; Wilson, N. & Hijazi, Z. (Eds), pp 185-195, Informa Health Care, ISBN 10:1-884184-566-6, Oxford, UK

Rao, P. S. (2008). Perimembraneous ventricular septal defect closure with the Amplatzer device. (Editorial). *J Invasive Cardiol,* Vol. 20, No. 5, pp. 217-218,

Rao, P. S. (2010). Transposition of the great arteries in the neonate. *Neonatology Today,* Vol. 5, No. 8, pp. 1-8

Rao, P. S. & Carey, P. (1989). Doppler ultrasound in the prediction of pressure gradients across the aortic coarctation. *Am Heart J, Vol.* 118, No. 2, pp. 299-307

Rao, P. S.; Galal, O,; Patnana, M. et al. (1998). Three-to-ten-year follow-up results of balloon pulmonary valvuloplasty. *Heart,* Vol. 80, No. 6, pp. 591-595

Rao, P. S.; Galal, O.; Smith, P. A. & Wilson, A. D. (1996). Five-to-nine-year follow-up results of balloon angioplasty of native aortic coarctation in infants and children. *J Am Coll Cardiol,* Vol. 27, No. 2, pp. 462-470

Rao, P. S. & Sideris, E. B. (1996). Transcatheter occlusion of patent ductus arteriosus: state of the art. *J Invasive Cardiol,* Vol. 8, No. 7, pp. 278-288

Rao, P. S.; Sideris, E. B.; Hausdorf, G. et al. (1994). International experience with secundum atrial septal defect occlusion by buttoned device. *Am Heart J, Vol.* 128, No. 5, pp. 1022-1035

Rao, P. S.; Wilson, A. D.; Thapar, M. K. & Brais, M. (1992). Balloon pulmonary valvuloplasty in the management of cyanotic congenital heart defects. *Cathet Cardiovasc Diagn,* Vol. 25, No. 1, pp. 16-24

Singh, G. K. & Rao, P. S. (2010). Left heart outflow obstructions. In: *Cardiology, Third Edition,* Crawford, M. H, DiMarco, J. P. & Paulus, W. J. (Eds), pp. 1507-1518, Mosby Elsevier, ISBN 978-0-7234-3485-6, Edinburgh, UK

Thapar, M. K.; Rao, P. S.; Rogers, J. H. Jr. et al. (1978). Changing murmur of patent ductus arteriosus. *J Pediat, Vol.* 92. No. 6, pp. 939-941

Thanopoulos, B. D.; Tsaousis, G. S.; Konstantopoulou, G.I. et al. (1999). Transcatheter closure of muscular ventricular septal defects with the Amplatzer ventricular septal defect occluder: Initial clinical application in children. *J Am Coll Cardiol,* Vol. 33, No. 5, pp. 1395- 1399

Vogelpoel, L. & Schrire, V. (1960): Auscultatory and phonocardiographic assessment of pulmonary stenosis with intact ventricular septum. *Circulation,* Vol. 22, No. 1, pp. 55-72

Part 2

Prevalence and Etiology

2

Epidemiology and Etiology of Congenital Heart Diseases

Jarun Sayasathid[1], Kanchapan Sukonpan[2] and Naraporn Somboonna[3]
[1]*Cardiac Center, Faculty of Medicine, Naresuan University,*
[2]*Department of Obstetrics and Gynecology, Buddhachinaraj Hospital,*
[3]*Department of Microbiology, Faculty of Science, Chulalongkorn University*
Thailand

1. Introduction

Congenital heart disease (CHD), the most common type of birth defect, is an abnormal cardio-circulatory structure or function present at birth, although the disease is often discovered later in life. During prenatal life, the incidence of cardiac defect is higher due to affected fetuses that are aborted. CHD stems from an alteration in the embryonic development from a normal structure, or a failure of a structure to properly develop beyond an early stage of embryonic and fetal development. The non-typical patterns of cardio-circulatory flow owning to an anatomical defect may significantly influence the structural and functional development of the remainder of the circulatory system. Additionally, postnatal events have a marked impact on the clinical presentation of a specific isolated malformation.

As CHD accounts for the most frequent cause of lethal malformation among infants, CHD is also considered a major problem affecting public health worldwide (Bernier et al., 2010). Despite the continuing progress in non-surgical and surgical treatments that allow for the survival of the majority of patients, some complex heart diseases are still associated with substantial morbidity and mortality. According to a report, 45% of infant deaths owing to congenital anomalies were caused by CHD in Western Europe. In Latin America, North America, Eastern Europe and the South Pacific region (including Japan) this proportion has been reported to be 35%, 37%, 42% and 48%, respectively (Botto, 2003). 20% of spontaneous abortions and 10% of stillbirths are attributed to CHD (Botto, 2001). CHD causes high morbidity and mortality among infants, and affects the quality of life during childhood and adulthood, depending on the progression of the disease (Majnener et al., 2008). It also affects social interactions and the quality of life for parents of children with CHD.

While newborns with the cardiac disorder are symptomatic and identified soon after birth, many others are not diagnosed until the disease progresses into a severe stage. Data from the Northern Region Pediatric Cardiology database suggest around 1 in 4 cases of congenital heart disease in the UK are diagnosed later in childhood (Petersen et al., 2003). The signs and symptoms of heart disease depend on the type and severity of the disease. Children with critical cardiac lesion generally exhibit high morbidity and mortality because the risk of morbidity and mortality increases as treatment and diagnosis is delayed.

The screening process is very important to detect congenital heart malformations. One of the major contributors to increased mortality and morbidity is clinical deterioration and heart failure prior to diagnosis and treatment. Early detection of CHD in the fetus or in the asymptomatic period immediately after birth will reduce clinical deterioration by instigation of appropriate management of the disease. Technical improvements in sonographic systems during the past two decades have helped the obstetric sonographers detect congenital heart anomalies, especially in experienced hands. A fetal cardiac screening with fetal echocardiography allows for early detection of CHD allowing for the option of pregnancy termination in cases of complicated defects. In areas where termination of pregnancy is a realistic and supported option, a universal sonographic screening of all pregnancies with an average reported sensitivity of 35% and a termination rate of 43% following prenatal diagnosis, would result in a 15% overall reduction of the prevalence of most severe forms of CHD (Germanakis & Sifakis, 2006). The information from 20 registries of congenital malformation in 12 European countries demonstrated the overall prenatal detection rate of CHD was 25% (Garne et al, 2001). Echocardiography can be used for screening in live birth infants. Newborn echocardiographic screening enables pediatricians to detect abnormal cardiac characteristics early and accurately, especially heart diseases without murmur such as coarctation of the aorta (Coarc), atrial septal defect (ASD), atrioventricular septal defect (AVSD), hypertrophic cardiomyopathy and cardiac tumor. In addition, cardiopulmonary information obtained from the echocardiographic examination can be useful for neonatal care providers (Wang et al., 2007).

The echocardiographic screening in developing countries may be difficult due to lack of echocardiographic machines and sonographers. Fortunately, most of patients with CHDs can be detected by clinical presentations and physical examinations. Approximately 90% of patients with CHDs were referred for cardiovascular evaluation with cardiac murmur, arrhythmia, cyanosis, palpitation and chest pain. False positives occurred 22.3% of the time with innocent (functional) murmur, and non organic chest pain or other non cardiac diagnosis (Borzouee & Jannati, 2008). In a Toronto study, 0.28% of the school-age children were found to have innocent murmurs (Rose et al., 1964). Currently, infants are screened to detect CHD by clinical and physical examination after birth and another examination at 6-8 weeks. However, this screening program can detect only 50% of congenital defects (Knowles et al., 2005). Thailand has a lack of pediatric doctors and cardiologists, and, therefore, there has been training available for qualified nurses and health officers to screen patients for CHD using clinical and physical examinations. These screenings are not only for infants, but also for school-age children and adults too. Although we detected a lot of false positives from innocent murmurs and abnormal clinical presentations, we recognized many undiagnosed CHD patients and have found many CHD patients who choose to undergo proper treatment (Sayasathid et al., 2009, 2010). Another tool to recognize CHD is pulse oximetry. It can detect cyanotic CHD which are not detected by routine examination with high specificity (99.8%) and very low false positive rate (2%) although the sensitivity was only 63%. Either functional or fractional oxygen saturation was measured by pulse oximetry with oxygen saturation below 95% as the cut-off level in most studies (Thangaratinam et al., 2007). Children who are suspected of having CHD should be referred to a pediatric cardiologist for definitive diagnosis, suitable treatment and follow up.

Nonetheless, the cost-effectiveness remains a concern, especially in developing countries. Costs are very different between screening using echocardiography versus clinical examination. A cost-effectiveness analysis study for screening 100,000 newborns in the UK showed the total program cost £300,000 for clinical examination, £480,000 for pulse oximetry and £3.54 million for screening echocardiography. The addition cost per additional timely diagnosis of life-threatening CHD ranges from £4,900 for pulse oximetry to £4.5 million for screening echocardiography (Knowles et al., 2005). Hence, the public health officers need to consider appropriate methods of CHD detections for their countries.

Although, there have been many studies to find the etiology of CHD, the cause of most CHDs continues to be unknown. Some reports suggested the cause to be a combination between genetic and environmental factors. Heart disease symptoms in a child are generally simple when compared with an adult, and have widely different pathology and physiology. Heart disease in an adult is a disease that often happens later in life (acquired heart disease) in the blood vessels (coronary artery disease) and heart valves. In this chapter, we will describe the possible causes and risk factors of CHD.

The first corrective surgery with cardiopulmonary bypass for intra-cardiac malformations began at the Mayo Clinic and the University of Minnesota Hospital in the 1950s (Lillehei, 1956). Through the past half century, the diagnosis and treatment of CHDs have markedly improved. The rapid evolution of diagnosis, medical and surgical therapies has reduced the morbidity and mortality rate. The surgical mortality has decreased from an average of 15% in 1990 to an average of 5% in 2000 (Kenny, 2008, as cited in Gibbs et al., 2004). The majority of infants with CHD are now expected to survive into adolescence and adulthood. Currently, the number of adults diagnosed with CHD exceeds the number of children diagnosed with CHD.

Hence, the objectives of this chapter are to describe epidemiology and etiology of CHD, including preventative guidelines for pregnant mothers. The authors hope this will provide essential overview to not only physicians and public health officers but also pregnant women, interested readers and societal awareness for the possibility of CHD in newborns. We also hope to provide appropriate strategies for managing the problem. This would lead to an appropriate health care budget and plan for diseased children in the future.

Abbreviations

AR	=	aortic regurgitation
AS	=	aortic stenosis
ASD	=	atrial septal defect
AVSD	=	atrioventricular septal defect
BAV	=	bicuspid aortic valve
CHD	=	congenital heart disease
Coarc	=	coarctation of the aorta
DORV	=	double outlet right ventricle
HLH	=	hypoplastic left heart
HRH	=	hypoplastic right heart
IAA	=	interrupted aortic arch
MR	=	mitral regurgitation, (MVP = mitral valve prolapse)
PA	=	pulmonary atresia
PDA	=	patent ductus arteriosus
PS	=	pulmonary stenosis
SV	=	single ventricle
TA	=	tricuspid atresia
T/PAPVR	=	total/partial anomalous pulmonary venous return
TGA	=	transposition of great arteries
TOF	=	tetralogy of Fallot
VSD	=	ventricular septal defect

2. Epidemiology of congenital heart diseases

2.1 Incidence rate

The incidence of CHD refers to the number of newly identified cases, children or adult, depending on the degree of defective development of the individuals' heart, per unit of time or population. Incidence demonstrates the rate of disease. The incidence of congenital heart defect is difficult to precisely determine, partly because of difficulties in definition. However, not all cases of congenital heart disease are diagnosed in infancy. Incidence rates based on diagnoses in pregnant women and the first 12 months of the baby's life will, therefore, be an underestimate of true incidence. Accurate assessment of incidence of CHD is important in determining the etiology of CHD, and in comparisons between populations over time, which might reflect population genetics or environment factors to a region or country. The incidence of CHD ranges from 4 to 85.9 per 1,000 pregnancies. Many congenital heart defects have been detected in stillbirths, particularly by an early loss in gestation due to chromosome anomalies. According to Hoffman (1978), the incidence of CHD among stillbirths is 79 per 1,000, whereas Mitchell (1972) reported an incidence of CHD in stillbirths and neonatal death (death after birth and before 28 days of age) to be 27.5 per 1,000 and 73.2 per 1,000, respectively. Yet, this number is likely an underestimate to the actual incidence of CHD because of difficulties in definition and unrecognized live births. The increasing incidence of CHD is primarily because of better methods of detection and data collection, as well as more advanced instruments, i.e. echocardiography, and highly skilled health officers. The increasing incidence of CHD could be due to more teratogenic environments affecting pregnant women and their offspring. Although an increased use of fetal echocardiography in pregnant women can help detect more CHD cases, many pregnancies are aborted prior to the mothers' awareness of the pregnancy and the effective assessment of a structural heart defect is still impossible for the early gestation phase. Moreover, the detection of heart malformation via fetal autopsy and heart examination remains rarely performed among the stillborns especially in developing country due to the lack of pathologists and the additional process for health professionals to request an autopsy.

2.2 Birth prevalence

Unlike incidence, the prevalence for CHD is the number of existing cases in the population of interest at one point in time. Prevalence represents the probability that a person in a given population will have the disease at a given time. Prevalence is a function of the incidence of the disease in a population and the duration of that disease. The sooner the recognition of birth prevalence of CHD, the better the planning will be by hospitals, health officers, pediatricians, pediatric cardiologists and pediatric cardiac surgeons. Social and economic support can also be found early for the patients' families. The global prevalence of CHD among newborns ranges from approximately 3.7 to 17.5 per 1,000, which account for 30-45% of all congenital defects. In Northern England, birth prevalence of CHD was as high as 79.7 per 1,000 live births (Dadvand et al., 2008). The extreme variation of the birth prevalence might be owed to a single or a combination of the following factors: inclusion criteria, for example that reports include bicuspid aortic valve and tiny muscular VSD or not, specificity and sensitivity of the diagnostic methodologies, properly trained and technique specialty of examiners, and ethnic and regional backgrounds of the examinees. Additional factors might be associated with the unavoidable limits of the retrospective studies that the data depend on previous medical records, possibly incorrect registration, missing or insufficient coordination of cardiac pediatricians between outpatient and private clinics, and absence of autopsy to determine the cause of certain fetal death in stillbirths. Nonetheless, the estimation for birth prevalence of CHD remains simpler and more precise compared with the estimation for incidence of CHD from the baby population. Hence, most epidemiological studies report the birth prevalence rather than the baby incidence of CHD. Table 1 compares the birth prevalence of all CHD subtypes from 4 recent studies by Hoffman & Kaplan, 2002 (review literatures); Reller et al., 2008 (Metropolian Atlanta Congenital Defects Program, MACDP); Dolk & Loane, 2009 (European Surveillance of Congenital Anomalies, Eurocat) and Wu et al., 2010 (Asian population, Taiwan). Table 2 shows different percent distribution of CHD lesions in live births from various countries

Cardiac Lesion	Hoffman & Kaplan, 2002* Mean/Median	Reller, 2008* (MACDP)	Dolk & Loane, 2009** (Eurocat)	Wu, 2010* (Asian population)
VSD	3.57 / 2.83	4.18	3.06	4.01
PDA	0.80 / 0.57	0.29	---	2.01
ASD	0.94 / 0.56	1.31	2.05	3.23
AVSD	0.35 / 0.34	0.41	0.19	0.20
PA	0.13 / 0.08	0.04	0.09	---
PS	0.73 / 0.53	0.55	0.40	1.22
AS	0.40 / 0.26	0.11	0.14	0.16
Coarc	0.41 / 0.36	0.44	0.34	0.25
TOF	0.42 / 0.36	0.47	0.28	0.63
TGA	0.32 / 0.30	0.23	0.35	0.21
HRH	0.22 / 0.16	---	0.04	---
HLH	0.27 / 0.27	0.23	0.26	0.06
TA	0.08 / 0.09	0.05	0.08	0.05
Ebstein's	0.11 / 0.04	0.06	0.05	0.05
Truncus	0.11 / 0.09	0.06	0.09	0.08
DORV	0.16 / 0.13	---	---	0.15
SV	0.11 / 0.09	0.10	0.07	---
TAPVR	0.09 / 0.09	0.08	0.05	0.11
All CHD	9.60 / 7.67***	8.14	7.05	13.08
BAV	13.56/9.24	---	---	---

*Live births
**Non-chromosomal CHD prevalence (Includes: Live birth, Fetal death and Termination of pregnancy for fetal anomaly)
***Excluding bicuspid non-stenosis aortic valves, isolated partial anomalous pulmonary venous connection and silent ductus arteriosus

Table 1. Prevalence of CHD based on CHD subtypes and per 1,000 births compared among the four recent studies.

More importantly, the trend for birth prevalence of CHD was found to be increasing, highlighting three chief concerns. First, the increased number of CHD prevalence among the newborns could represent the greater number of adults with CHD and the likely increased number of CHD in their offspring in the future. This poses the concern about the overall increasing prevalence of CHD. A study in Hungary, estimates the prevalence of CHD to be 4.9% in offspring of individuals with CHD. More than half of these had the same malformation as the parent (Ceizel et al., 1981). Another study in 2001 showed the prevalence of CHD was 3.1% in offspring of individuals with CHDs and 1.3% in offspring of individuals without CHDs. The adjusted risk for offspring of parents with CHDs was 1.73 (95% CI, p=0.02) (Romano-Zelekha et al., 2001). On the other hand, if the high prevalence is due to the more common use of postnatal echocardiography for abnormal heart diagnosis, the greater birth prevalence of CHD signifies an underestimation of CHD among live births in the past and the importance for public health officers to have an accurate number of cases. For instance, fetal echocardiography screening could be performed to decide pregnancy termination of fetuses with severe cardiac malformation, and thereby reduce the birth prevalence of CHD. Finally, the rapid development of the world may increase many risk factors to develop CHD such as pollutants and teratogens. The number of births with CHD in Dallas county suggests an apparent increase in prevalence from approximately 5% in 1971 to 8% in 1984 (Fixler et al., 1990). Within the Baltimore-Washington Infant Study Group, the prevalence of CHD increased from 2.8 per 1,000 live births in 1981 to 4.3 per 1,000 live births in 1988 (Ferencz et al., 1989) and a recent report from North England demonstrated the total prevalence of CHD increased from 5.4 per 1,000 births and terminations of pregnancy in 1985 to 11.6 per 1,000 births and terminations of pregnancy in 2003 (Dadvand et al., 2008).

Cardiac Lesion	USA[1]	UK[2]	UK[3]	USA[4]	India[5]	Saudi[6*]	Jordan[7]	Bangla[8*]	Germany[9]
VSD	29.1	28.1	32.5	26.3	34.8	33.9	43.4	16.9	48.9
VSD+PS	2.4	8.6	---	---	---	---	---	---	---
PDA	7.6	6.5	11.9	2.6	18.6	11.6	8.3	12.7	4.3
ASD	7.4	8.3	5.9	7.5	2.3	18.1	13.6	26.0	17.0
AVSD	4.3	7.4	2.4	---	2.3	3.5	3.6	3.5	2.7
PA	---	---	0.8	---	---	---	---	2.8	0.9
PS	8.1	2.7	7.5	7.0	---	12.4	6.2	7.8	6.1
AS	3.5	4.1	5.1	3.3	2.3	2.5	4.3	1.4	2.2
Coarc	4.3	5.6	6.3	6.8	---	2.3	3.4	2.1	3.6
TOF	3.5	---	5.9	9.2	4.6	3.5	9.5	9.9	2.5
d-TGA	2.4	5.6	5.0	5.0	---	2.1	5.5	4.2	2.2
HLH	---	3.3	2.8	5.7	---	---	---	---	1.4
TA	1.1	1.5	1.7	1.5	2.3	---	3.7	3.5	---
Ebstein's	---	---	---	---	---	---	---	---	0.4
Truncus	---	1.2	1.1	---	---	---	---	0.7	0.5
DORV	1.1	---	---	---	---	---	---	---	1.0
SV	0.9	1.5	1.7		2.3	---	---	1.4	---
TAPVR	---	2.1	1.3	1.7	---	---	---	1.4	0.6
MR	0.6	---	---	---	---	---	---	---	---

[1]Mitchell et al., 1971, [2]Bound & Logan, 1977, [3]Dickinson et al., 1981, [4]Ferncz et al., 1985, [5]Khalil et al., 1994, [6]Alabdulgader, 2006, [7]Amro, 2009, [8] Fatema et al., 2008, [9]Lindinger et al., 2010
*Saudi = Saudi Arabia, and Bangla = Bangladesh

Table 2. Percent distribution of CHD lesions in live births in USA, UK, India, Saudi Arabia, Jordan, Bangladesh and Germany.

2.3 Adult prevalence

Similar to the knowledge of birth prevalence, the knowledge of adult prevalence can estimate the need for adult cardiology services. The accurate prevalence of CHD in the adult population is difficult to know. Although some patients with CHD have spontaneous recovery, for instance 35% of infants with VSD had their lesion close spontaneously (Mitchell et al., 1971), an overall number of adult diagnosed with CHD continues to rise and is now higher than that of the diagnosed pediatric cases. It was estimated that in 2000 there were fewer than 150,000 adults diagnosed with CHD in the UK. Of these, around 11,500 had the more complex forms of the disease, requiring life-long expert supervision and intervention (Report of the British Cardiac Society Working Party, 2002). It was also further estimated that by the year 2010 there would be over 185,000 adults in the UK living with CHD (over 17,000 with the complex form), a rise of around 25% in simple and 50% in complex conditions since 2000. Using a birth prevalence of CHD of 8.8 per 1,000 live births, it is estimated that more than 8,500 individuals with surgical repair of congenital heart defects reach adulthood each year in the USA (Morris, 2004). In year 2000, approximately 500,000 American adults were reported to have moderate to complex congenital heart defects. By 2020, nearly 760,000 adults will have CHD in the USA, with 200,000 having severe CHD, disregarding all those born before 1990 (Webb et al., 2002). Our review has only one study that reports exactly the adult prevalence of CHD. This study was done in a general population from 1985 to 2000 in Canada, it revealed the prevalence of CHD was 4.09 per 1,000 adults for all CHD and 0.38 per 1,000 for those with severe lesions (Table3). 57% of the adult CHD population was female (Marelli et al., 2007). The authors extrapolated a prevalence of 4.09 per 1,000 to a Canadian and US population corresponds to 96,000 patients in Canada and 856,000 patients in the United States. A recent study in the Netherlands studied 8,595 adults with CHD, and found the most common defects in the distribution of CHD were ASD (17%), VSD (16%), AS/BAV (14%), TOF (10%) and Coarc (10%) but the highest mortality was found in patients with TA (14.7%) and patients with UV and double inlet left ventricle (11.4%)(Zomer et al., 2010).

Two main reasons can explain this situation. First, there is the process of natural selection in which children with previously undetected CHD or children with inoperable CHD survive into adulthood with uncorrected lesions. Up to 75%of children with CHD did not exhibit clinical signs of diseases until the diseases became severe. Moreover, around 10% of CHD are not diagnosed until adulthood (Mettler & Peeler, 2009), in particular secundum atrial septum defect, ventricular septal defect, pulmonary stenosis, anormalous coronary arteries, Ebstein's anomaly and congenitally corrected transposition of great arteries. One of the more recent CHD studies in Thailand reported 0.41 to 1.05 prevalent cases of unrecognized CHD for every 1,000 elementary-age students. This variation was due to the topography and the limitation of medical staff and facilities in the study areas. In this population, the most frequently identified heart defects were VSD 41.4%, PS 16.1%, PDA 12.6% and ASD 9.2% (Sayasathid, et al., 2010). The second reason is the improvement of surgical therapy and postoperative care of neonates and infants in the past few decades, this has led to increased survival of children with CHD. Currently, more than 90% of children born with CHD can survive into adulthood (Moons et al., 2009). From 1979 through 1997, mortality associated with CHD (all ages) declined 39% from 2.5 to 1.5 per 100,000 (Boneva et al., 2001). Although many children with CHD cannot be cured, the initial therapy, including corrective and palliative, allows the adult prevalence of CHD to continue to increase. At Mayo clinic, the number of adult patients with CHD who undergo operation has grown to approximately

300-400 patients per year (Brown et al., 2009). These patients have elevated risk of premature morbidity and mortality. CHD is often more severe and has more complicated treatment in adults than children. Moreover, a recent analysis of the United States administrative database found that mortality was greater for adults with CHD when the operations were performed by adult cardiac surgeons, compared with pediatric (congenital-trained) heart surgeons (4.8% versus 1.9%, $P<0.001$) (Brown et al., 2009, as cited in Karamalou et al., 2008). For CHD adults, arrhythmias are more common, cardiac chambers often enlarge, and ventricles tend to develop systolic dysfunction. The main causes of death were progressive heart failure 26% and sudden cardiac arrest 22% (Zomer et al., 2010). Multidisciplinary care may also be required.

Lesion		prevalence per 1,000 adults
Severe lesion		
	TOF or truncus	0.17
	AVSD	0.14
	TGA	0.04
	SV	0.03
	All severe lesions	0.38
Other lesion		
	ASD	0.88
	VSD	0.78
	PDA	0.02
	AS or AR	0.11
	Coarc	0.07
	Ebstein's	0.01
	All other lesions	3.71
All CHD		4.09

Table 3. The prevalence of adult CHD based on subtypes in year 2000, Canada (Marelli et al., 2007).

Another problem that should be of concern is the transfer system from pediatric to adult health care. Many children with CHD did not follow-up when they were discharged from pediatric care and referred to adult care. In a Canadian study, only 47% of teenagers with CHD had transferred successfully to adult care (Reid et al., 2004). The results were similar in a German study, 76% of patients with CHD did not have follow-up care as an adult in a 5-year period (Wacker et al., 2005). The prevalence of adults with CHD is underestimated if it does not include this group of patients. These patients received medical care again when their diseases had progressed and their symptoms had become severe. This lack of care as an adult made it difficult to manage the disease and resulted in high morbidity & mortality in these patients. Patients with CHD must recognize the necessesity of ongoing surveillance and the transfer system must be developed to prevent the loss of follow-up patients.

3. Etiology of congenital heart diseases

The heart development, which initiates at embryonic day 15 in vertebrates, comprises an organized series of molecular and morphologic events that involve five primary steps: (1)

migration of pre-cardiac cells from the primitive streak and assembly of the paired cardiac crescents at the myocardial plate, (2) coalescence of the cardiac crescents to form the primitive heart tube, establishment of the definitive heart, (3) cardiac looping, assurance of proper alignment of the future cardiac chambers, (4) septation and heart chamber formation, and (5) development of the cardiac conduction system and coronary vasculature (McFadden & Olson, 2002; Moorman & Christoffels, 2003; Gittenberger-de Groot et al., 2005). From a series of complex processes, each component occurs at the right time under the orchestration of a cascade of genes and gene products, resulting in the coordination of cell migration and the formation of the extracellular matrix. Thus, CHD is usually caused by altered development of embryonic structure, or a failure of the structure to develop beyond an early embryonic or fetal stage. The anatomical defect generally influences further structural and functional development. Although descriptions of abnormal heart development in fetuses and babies have remained unclearly defined, substantial knowledge about the etiology of CHD have been made during the last decade. Some malformations may be directly inherited through vertical gene transfer, underlying the individuals' genetic disorder, or be associated with the consequences of an environmental toxin or diet. Alternatively, random errors in cell migration leading to improper cardiac development are possible. Together, the findings emphasize the complex and multifactorial causes of the CHD where additional research remain needed.

Better understanding for the etiology and risk factors of CHD is important, and will help pave the way for proper preventative measures and treatment guidelines by physicians as well as public health officers. The followings represent all reported potential causes of CHD to date.

3.1 Genetic disorders

The human genome, which contains approximately 20,000 to 25,000 genes, is comprised of coding and non-coding regions that are essential for proper protein structure and expression. The coding DNA sequence determines the amino acid sequence and subsequently the protein structure, and structure determines function (Lander, 2011; Reid-Lombardo & Bartelings, 2010). The non-coding sequences may contain promoters and regulation of transcription. In general, the DNA sequences remain relatively unchanged during vertical genetic transfer to the offspring. Nonetheless, occasional changes in the nucleotide sequences, referred to as mutations, and horizontal gene transfer do occur. Mutations range from a single nucleotide substitution, also called single nucleotide polymorphism (SNP), to a deletion or insertion of a DNA fragment. Some mutations only appear visible at the level of the chromosome (chromosome abnormalities), while some mutations cause phenotypic changes and a heritable trait to the offspring.

Any change in the DNA sequence, including SNPs, insertion, deletion and shuffling of DNA fragment, that results in frameshift mutation of the gene-encoding sequence likely affects protein folding and protein function. Abnormal protein folding structure and function can cause an improper development of many organs, including the heart. Hence, genetics is responsible for one major role in cardiovascular malformation, and indeed the genetic disorders represent the most common cause of CHD. Certain chromosome abnormities were linked to specific types of congenital heart lesions, and several types have been reported to be associated with specific gene defects. For instances, AVSD are often diagnosed in patients with trisomy 21.

Moreover, CHD that occur in multiple members of a family increases the incidence of CHD in familial lines, and support evidences of inherited genetic disorders towards the heart abnormities. Molecular genetics in conjunction with cytogenetics provide an opportunity to decipher the genetic basis and pathogenesis of CHD. With the rapid era of DNA sequencing and genetic discoveries, it is expected that genetic diagnosis and screening will become incorporated into standard practice in the near future. Consequently, it is imperative that cardiologists understand the basis for genetic disorders, and the medical and ethical implications relevant to the genetic information. Today, genetics are predisposed to malformation of the hearts and blood vessels, and account for the highest number of human birth defects. Thus, hereditary and congenital diseases are classified into three broad categories

3.1.1 Chromosome defect

Defects in chromosomes associated with CHD are diverse; some examples are aneuploidy or polyploidy, improper rearrangement during mitosis and meiosis, translocation, inversion or deletions. Importantly, certain chromosomes were reported to have a greater degree of significance and of percentages to heart development, and thus the same defects in different chromosomes may not result in similar defects (Table 4). About 0.30-2.0% of all live births have chromosomal defects, usually the chromosomal defects were aneuploidy and trisomy 21, 18, 13 (Dolk et al., 2010). Among all CHDs detected during infant period, the chromosomal defects account for approximately 6 - 10% (Ferencz et al., 1989; Tennstedt et al., 1999; Zhang et al., 2010). In Table 4, defects in chromosomes X, 3, 4, 5, 7, 8, 9, 10, 11, 13, 17, 18, 21 and 22 showed association with CHD.

Nonetheless, the table summarizes the data reported by different studies, some conducted in different times and places. The incidence of CHD generally depends on multiple factors besides the type of genetic disorders and the chromosome where the disorders take place. The other factors include how many fetuses are conceived by the mothers, and how many of these fetuses reach term alive. Further, the affected number of fetuses also depends on the rate of the survival of the affected fetuses and the increased use of therapeutic abortion.

3.1.2 Single gene disorder

Heart development is controlled by multiple genes regulating a complicated network of transcription regulation, translation regulation, and signal transduction pathways, ranging from a control of muscle growth, patterning to contractility, to name a few. However, mutations in only one or a few components of the cardiac gene network can result in the improper development of the heart. One type of heart defect could also be caused by different types of single gene disorders. Since the 1990s, researchers have identified more than 10 different single gene mutations that can lead to heart defects. To date, many genes responsible for several congenital heart defects have been identified (table 5).

Transcription Factor Genes transcribe and translate proteins that serve to interact cooperatively with each other to control gene expression.

- **NKX2-5, the NK family, on chromosome 5q35;** Homeobox-containing genes play critical roles in regulating tissue-specific gene expression essential for specification of heart muscle progenitors (Komuro & Izumo, 1993; Toko et al., 2002). Mutations in NKX2-5 result in loss of heart formation in the embryo and have been found in sporadic

CCVM. Although the contributions of these variants to the disease phenotype remains uncertain, the linkage between this gene disorder and the atrioventricular conduction defect, ASD, VSD or TOF, have been found (Elliott et al., 2003; McElhinney et al., 2003; Stallmeyer et al., 2010).

- **TBX1, T-box 1 transcription factor, the T-box family;** The human TBX1 gene encodes another T-box transcription factor, expressed in neural crest and the developing cardiac outflow tract (conotruncus) (Calmont et al., 2009). Microdeletion TBX1 gene, located on chromosomal 22q11, causes DiGeorge syndrome, also known as Velocardiofacial syndrome. There are variable ranges of clinical phenotypes for DiGeorge syndrome, including IAA, truncus arteriosus, TOF, DORV and TGA (Jerome & Papaioannou, 2001; Xu et al., 2004; Yagi et al., 2003).
- **TBX5, T-box 5 transcription factor, the T-box family;** is a member of a phylogenetically conserved family of genes that share a common DNA-binding domain, the T-box. TBX5 was found expressed in embryonic human heart and limb. Mutations in this gene have been associated with Holt-Oram syndrome (Fan et al., 2003), which is characterized by skeletal malformations of the upper extremities and CHD, most commonly secundum ASD but also VSD and TOF (Basson et al., 1999; Faria et al., 2008; Li et al., 1997; Xin et al., 2009).
- **GATA4, GATA binding protein 4;** is related to zinc finger transcription factors. This protein is thought to regulate genes involved in embryogenesis and in myocardial differentiation and function. Furthermore, GATA4 interacts with Tbx5 and with Nkx2-5 to regulate cardiac gene expression. This provides evidence that a transcriptional complex including all three proteins may be necessary for proper septation of the human heart. Mutations in this gene have been associated with non-syndromic CHD cardiac septal defects (Gang et al., 2003; Tomita-Mitchell et al., 2007).
- **TFAP2B, transcription factor AP-2 beta;** This gene encodes a member of the AP-2 family of transcription factors. This protein functions in the differentiation of neural crest cell derivatives, and contributes to the embryogenesis of the ductus arteriosus (Hilger-Eversheim et al., 2000). Mutations in this gene result in autosomal dominant Char syndrome, a dominant disorder comprised of facial dysmorphism, hand anomalies, and patent ductus arteriosus (Mani et al., 2005; Satoda et al., 2000; Zhao et al., 2001).
- **ZFPM2/FOG2, zinc finger protein, multitype 2;** The zinc finger protein encoded by this gene is a widely expressed member of the FOG family of transcription factors. The FOG family members modulate the activity of co-factors with the GATA family of proteins, which are important regulators of hematopoiesis and cardiogenesis in mammals. In experimental gene targeting of ZFPM2/FOG2 in mice, the mutation resulted in cardiac malformation including TOF, endothelial specific disruption (DORV, a common AV valve), VSD and ASD as well as left ventricular wall hypoplasia, and the failure to form coronary arteries (Tevosian et al., 2000). Recent reports found mutations of the ZFPM2/FOG2 gene associated with TOF (De Luca et al., 2010; Pizzuti et al., 2003).
- **ZIC3, Zic family member 3 heterotaxy 1;** This gene encodes a member of the ZIC family of C2H2- type zinc finger proteins. Mutations in ZIC3 gene, located at chromosome Xq24-q27.1 (Casey et al., 1993), cause X-linked visceral heterotaxy and

complex CHD including ASD, AVSD, TGA, PS, and TAPVR (Zhu et al., 2007; Grinberg & Millen, 2005).

Cell signaling genes produce proteins involved in cell signal transduction, which allow cells to respond to their environment and are therefore involved in regulation of many important biological functions.

- **JAG1, Jagged 1;** The jagged 1 protein encoded by JAG1 is the human homolog of the Drosophila jagged protein. Human jagged 1 is the ligand for the receptor NOTCH, which is essential in many organ developmental programs. Analysis of JAG1 expression during mammalian embryogenesis showed its high level of gene expression during the heart and vessel developing periods, and the finding was consistent with the crucial role of its patterning of the right heart and pulmonary vasculature (Loomes et al., 1999). Mutations in the jagged 1 protein cause Alagille syndrome, a complex disease characterized by liver problem, PS, and with or without TOF (Heritage et al., 2002; McElhinney et al., 2002; Colliton et al., 2001).
- **NOTCH1, NOTCH2, The NOTCH family receptors;** The NOTCH gene encodes a single-pass transmembrane protein receptor that interacts with the ligands named Delta and Serrate/Jagged, and perform many cellular regulatory function. Mutations in NOTCH1 have been shown to cause autosomal-dominant aortic valve defects, and bicuspid (two-leaflet) aortic valve (Grag et al., 2005; McKellar et al., 2007; Mohamed et al., 2006). Because BAV is a risk factor for valve calcification, it has previously been hypothesized that calcification was due to increased blood flow turbulence across the valve leaflets (Robicsek et al., 2004), leading to progressive aortic stenosis and regurgitation in later life. Furthermore, mutation in NOTCH2 receptor was recently found to be able to cause Alagille syndrome even in the patients with no Jagged1 mutations (El-Rassy et al., 2008; McDaniell et al., 2006).
- **PTPN11;** The protein encoded by this gene is a member of the protein tyrosine phosphatase (PTP) family. PTPs are known to be signaling molecules that regulate a variety of cellular processes including cell growth, differentiation, mitotic cycle, and oncogenic transformation. Mutations in this gene are a cause of Noonan syndrome, located on chromosome 12q24 (Jamieson et al., 1994), it is an autosomal dominant disorder characterized by dysmorphic facial features, skeletal malformations, short stature, and cardiac abnormalities, most characteristic are PS, ASD, AVSD and hypertrophic cardiomyopathy (Jongmans et al., 2005; Sarkozy et al., 2003).
- **CFC1, cryptic family 1;** This gene encodes a member of the EGF-Cripto, Frl-1, and Cryptic (CFC) family. These proteins play key roles in intercellular signaling pathways during vertebrate embryogenesis. This protein is involved in left-right asymmetric morphogenesis during organ development. Mutations in this gene can cause autosomal visceral heterotaxy with complex CHD including TGA, septal defects and systemic vein anomalies (Goldmuntz et al., 2002; Ozcelik et al., 2006; Yan et al., 1999).
- **SOS1, son of sevenless homolog 1;** This gene encodes a protein that is a guanine nucleotide exchange factor for RAS proteins, membrane proteins that bind guanine nucleotides and participate in signal transduction pathways. Mutations in this gene are associated with gingival fibromatosis 1 and Noonan syndrome (Serrano-Martin et al., 2008).

- **PROSIT240, also known as THRAP2**; An evolutionarily conserved THRAP genes encode a family of proteins that regulate embryonic development. Missense mutation PROSIT240 gene has been identified as a cause of transposition of the great arteries (Muncke et al., 2003).
- **CRELD1, cysteine-rich with EGF-like domains 1;** CRELD1 is the member of a family of matrix cellular proteins. Matrix cellular proteins contain epidermal growth factor-like repeats, and are grouped in a class of cysteine-rich domains that mediate interactions between proteins of diverse functions. Mutation in CRELD1 genes, locating on chromosome 3p25 locus, represents a vital gene position for AVSD (Guo et al., 2010; Zatyka et al., 2005; Robinson et al., 2003).
- **EVC, EVC2;** This gene encodes a protein containing a leucine zipper and a transmembrane domain. The functions of EVC and EVC2, which share a promoter, are aligned in control limb, skeleton and teeth development. Mutation of this gene has been implicated in both Ellis-van Creveld syndrome and Weyers acrodental dysostosis, the disease locus mapped to chromosome 4p16 (Polymeropoulos et al., 1996). Ellis-van Creveld syndrome is an autosomal recessive disorder characterized by chondrodysplasia and CHD, typically a common atrium of the atrioventricular septal defect type or secundum type atrial septal defects (Ali et al., 2010; Hills et al., 2011; Tompson et al., 2007). Some heterozygous carriers of these mutations manifested Weyers acrodental dysostosis suggesting it is allelic with Ellis-van Creveld syndrome (Riiz-Perez et al., 2000).
- **TGFBR1 and TGFBR2, transforming growth factor receptor 1 and 2;** This gene encodes a member of the Ser/Thr protein kinase family and the TGFB receptor subfamily. Mutations in this gene have been associated with Marfan syndrome, Loeys-Deitz Aortic Aneurysm syndrome (Loeys et al., 2006; Singh et al., 2006).

Extracellular Matrix Protein Genes encode extracellular matrix proteins which cause congenital syndromes involving arteriopathies of different forms.

- **ELN, elastin;** This gene encodes a protein is one of the two components of elastic fibers. It resides in the Williams critical region on 7q11.23. Deletions and mutations in this gene are associated with Williams or Williams-Beuren syndrome in which the phenotype is comprised of characteristic endocrine, cognitive, and facial features in association with areas of arterial narrowing, most typically non-syndromic supravalvular AS (Micale et al., 2010; Rodriguez-Revenga et al., 2005; Arrington et al., 2006).
- **FBN1, fibrillin 1;** This gene encodes a member of the fibrillin family. This fibrillin has long been assumed to be critical in the aortic wall and other connective tissues as a structural protein. Mutations in this gene are associated with Marfan syndrome (Brautbar et al., 2010; De Backer, 2009; Li et al., 2008). Marfan syndrome is an autosomal dominant disease of connective tissue principally involving the skeletal, ocular systems and cardiovascular malformation whose manifestations include mitral valve prolapse and regurgitation, presenting in infancy in the most severe cases, and progressive aneurismal dilation of the aortic root with the potential for catastrophic aortic dissection and rupture. Marfan syndrome was first mapped to chromosome 15 using traditional genetic linkage analysis (Dietz et al., 1991). Other studies have revealed that fibrillin has a regulatory role in TGF- signaling, and dysregulation of the pathway may instead underlie Marfan pathogenesis (Neptune et al., 2003).

Type of abnormality	Predominant of CHD	Percentage of CHD	Reference
Numeric aberrations; Autosomes:			
• **Monosomy**			
X (Turner syndrome)	Left-sided obstruction, PAPVR, MVP, aortic route dilatation	35	1 - 5
• **Trisomy**			
13 (Patau syndrome)	VSD, PDA, ASD, dextroposition	80-90	6 - 8
18 (Eward syndrome)	VSD, PDA, ASD, TOF, DORV, CPVD	80-100	9 - 11
21 (Down syndrome)	VSD, AVSD, ASD	40-50	12, 13
• **Tetrasomy**			
22pter-q11 (Cat-Eye syndrome)	TAPVR, HLH	40	14 - 16
Structural aberrations;			
• **Duplication**			
3q26-27 (Cornelia de Lange)	PS, VSD, ASD, DORV	40	17 - 19
8q	VSD, TA	45	20, 21
9p	ASD	40	22
11q	ASD	35	22
• **Deletion**			
3p (3p-syndrome)	AVSD	25	23, 24
4p (Wolf-Hirschhorn)	ASD, VSD, PDA, PS	30-50	25
4q	ASD, VSD, PS	50	26 - 28
5p (Cri du chat syndrome)	VSD, PDA, TOF	30	29
8p (8p-syndrome)	AVSD	65-80	30, 31
10p	VSD, ASD, PS	50	32, 33
11q (Jacobsen syndrome)	VSD, left heart obstructive malformations, HLH	60	34, 35
18p	VSD, PDA, PS, heterotaxy phenotype	10	36, 37
18q	ASD, VSD, PS	30	38, 39
• **Microdeletion**			
7q11 (Williams syndrome)	SVAS, PS	60	40, 41
17p11.2 (Smith-Magenis syndrome)	VSD, ASD, PS, AV malformation	30	42, 43
22q11.2 (DiGeorge syndrome)	TOF, TAPVR Aortic arch anomalies, IAA type B, TOF, TA, ASCA	75-85	44, 45

ASCA: aberrant subclavian artery, CPVD: congenital polyvalvular disease, CVM: cardiovascular malformations, DCM: dilated cardiomyopathy, RAA: right aortic arch, SVAS: supravalvular aortic stenosis (Ref: [1]Douchin et al., 2000; [2]Lichiardopol & Morta, 2004; [3]Mazzanti & Cacciari, 1998; [4]Poprawski et al., 2009; [5]Tan & Yeo, 2009; [6]Lin et al., 2007; [7]Lizarraga et al., 1991; [8]Musewe et al., 1990; [9]Van Praagh et al., 1989; [10]Matsuka et al., 1981; [11]Musewe et al., 1990; [12]Paladini et al., 2000; [13]Weijerman et al., 2010; [14]Berends et al., 2001; [15]Rosias et al., 2001; [16]Wilson et al., 1984; [17]Akdeniz et al., 2009; [18]Barisic et al., 2008; [19]Selicorni et al., 2009; [20]Digilio et al., 2003; [21]Giltay et al., 1998; [22]Roskers et al., 1990; [23]Green et al., 2000; [24]Shuib et al., 2009; [25]Battaglia et al., 1999; [26]Tsai et al., 1999; [27]Strehle & Bantock, 2003; [28]Huang et al., 2002; [29]Hills et al., 2006; [30]Devriendt et al., 1999; [31]Wat et al., 2009; [32]Lindstrand et al., 2010; [33]Van Esch et al., 1999; [34]Grossfeld et al., 2004; [35]Mattina et al., 2009; [36]Digilio et al., 2000; [37]Movahhedian et al., 1991; [38]Cody et al., 1999; [39]Linnandivi et al., 2006; [40]Eronen et al., 2002;[41]Ferrero et al., 2007; [42]Edelman et al., 2007;[43]Potocki et al., 2003; [44]Ballesta et al., 2008; [45]Shprintzen, 2008)

Table 4. Chromosome abnormality associated with congenital heart anomalies and their percentages.

Gene	Syndrome	Chromosome location	Inheritance	Congenital heart malformation
Transcription Factor Gene				
NKX2-5	Non-syndromic	5q34	AD	ASD, AVB, VSD, TOF, HCM, TV abnormality
TBX1	DiGeorge Syndrome	22q11.21	Sporadic	VSD, PTA, IAA, TOF
TBX5	Holt-Oram Syndrome	12q24.1	AD	HOS, ASD, AVSD, AVB, TOF, TAPVR, TA, PS
GATA4	Non-syndromic	8p23.1p22	AD	ASD
TFAP2B	Char syndrome	6p12	AD	PDA
ZFPM2/FOG2	Non-syndromic	8q23	Sporadic	TOF
ZIC3	HeterotaxySyndrome	Xq26	X-linked	Heterotaxy, ASD, AVSD, TGA, PS, DORV, TAPVR
Cell signaling Genes				
Jagged 1	Alagille Syndrome	20p12	AD	PS, TOF
NOTCH1	Non-syndromic	9q34-35	Sporadic	BAV
NOTCH2	Alagille Syndrome	1p12	AD	PS, TOF
PTPN11	Noonan syndrome	12q24	AD	PS, PV dysplasia, ASD, AVSD, HCM
CFC1	Heterotaxy syndrome	2q21	Unknown	Heterotaxy, TGA, DORV
SOS1	Noonan syndrome	2p21	AD	PS, septal defect, HCM
PROSIT240	Non-syndromic	12q24	Unknown	TGA
CRELD1	Non-syndromic	3p21	Sporadic	AVSD
EVC/EVC2	Ellis- van Creveld syndrome	4p16	AR	Common atrium, ASD
TGFBR2	Marfan syndrome	3p22	AD	Aortic aneurysm
Extracellular Matrix Protein Genes				
FBN1	Marfan Syndrome	15q21.1	AD	MVP, aortic root dilatation
ELN	Williams Syndrome	7q11.23	AD	SVAS

AD: autosomal dominant, AR: autosomal recessive, AVB: atrioventricular block; HCM: hypertrophic cardiomyopathy, HOS: Holt-Oram syndrome, SVAS: supravalvular aortic stenosis

Table 5. Gene abnormality and contiguous gene syndromes associated with congenital heart anomalies.

3.1.3 Polygenic / Multifactorial inheritance

Multifactor inheritance, also known as polygeny, relies on the concept of threshold limit, when the threshold limit of the combined genetic and environmental factors is reached, malformation results. Below the threshold level, the malformation is absent. One common key risk is that the babies are genetically oriented towards some level of atypical cardiovascular formation and/or development, together with the exposure to other causative factors. Different stages of cardiac development possess various degrees of vulnerability to environmental factors. Some clues to multifactorial inheritances are a reason for CHD, including a lack of consistent CHD people in the pedigree of the family, and an occasional abnormality with no recognizable pattern in the pedigree of the family.

3.2 Maternal factors

Various teratogenic agents have been implicated as the etiologic agents of CHD. For example, women who have insulin-dependent diabetes mellitus, and those who take certain medications, such as acne and epilepsy medication, have a higher risk for having babies with CHD. Women with drug or alcohol abuse also have predisposing risks. The basic biological principle mechanism of teratogens action that cause CHD include susceptible stage of organogenesis development, genetic differences in susceptibility, dose response relationships, and specific actions of the teratogenic agent. The highest degree of embryonic and fetal sensitivity or susceptibility to adverse effects of exposure to teratogens occurs during the first trimester, especially during the 2nd to 8th week of embryonic life. Dose response relationship implies that for each teratogen there is a dose threshold, theoretic dose below which no adverse effects can be observed.

3.2.1 Maternal health and medical disease

Certain chronic illnesses in the mother (table 6), such as diabetes, and other viral infections, such as the flu, may contribute to heart defects.

- **Maternal diabetes mellitus;** The study by Correa et al. found odds ratios for pre-gestational diabetes mellitus (PGDM) and all cardiac defects was 4.64 (2.87-7.51), while gestational diabetes mellitus (GDM) was associated with cardiac defects found 1.59 (1.27-1.99) (Correa et al., 2008). This excess risk is related to the level of maternal hyperglycemia during the embryonic period. The overall risk of one or more major anomalies is 6 to 7 percent, which is double the risk in the general obstetric population (Wyatt et al., 2005). Congenital heart defects increased in diabetic pregnancy include heterotaxy, TOF, TGA, septal defects, anomalous pulmonary venous return, and various defects causing left or right outflow obstruction (Lisowski et al., 2010; Corrigan et al., 2003; Wren et al., 2003). The possible mechanism is that embryonic hyperglycemia may cause disturbances in metabolism of arachidonic acid, inositol and promote excessive formation of oxygen free radicals which causes mitochondrial damage, and activation of apoptotic pathways.
- **Maternal phenylketonuria;** One of the most common teratogen of pregnancy complications, when these pregnancies are untreated, 90% of the offspring suffer microcephaly, mental retardation and increased risk of heart defects through increased blood levels of phenylalanine and phenyl pyruvic acid (Rouse & Azen, 2004). Frequencies of congenital abnormalities increased with increasing maternal phenylalanine levels. The MPKUCS has demonstrated an increased rate of CHD (7.5%), the most frequent cardiac defects are TOF, Coarc, PDA, HLH and VSD (Levy et al., 2001). Diet control before conception and during pregnancy reduces the risk of CHD (Matalon et al., 2003; Michals-Matalon et al., 2002).

- **Maternal connective tissue diseases;** Connective tissue disease is a group of multi-system disorder, such as systemic lupus erythematosus (SLE), which have been associated with congenital complete atrioventricular heart block in offspring. With regard to maternal anti-Ro and anti-La autoantibodies can transmit from a mother to the fetus, which causes a fetal inflammatory response that damages the AV nodal and myocardial tissue in susceptible fetus' which may result in myocarditis, endocardial fibroelastosis and cardiac arrhythmias (Buyon et al., 2009; Clancy & Buyon, 2004).
- **Maternal rubella;** Women who contract rubella during pregnancy have a high risk of having a baby with congenital rubella syndrome (CRS) which will cause effects such as miscarriage, stillbirth, and a series of birth defects. The risk of fetal infection varies according to the time of onset of maternal infection. Infection rates are highest during the first trimester. The most common manifestations of CRS are congenital cataracts, sensorineural deafness, and congenital heart defects (especially PDA). When the heart is targeted, there is direct viral damage to the myocardium, affecting primarily the left atrium and the heart septa, leading to thrombosis, necrosis, and hemorrhage that cause of PDA, PS, and ASD (De Santis et al., 2006; Webster, 1998).
- **Maternal febrile illness**; Influenza during the first trimester of pregnancy is associated with febrile illness, which appears to cause more right-sided obstructive heart defects, especially TA and PA, some left obstructive defects and VSD (Oster et al., 2011; Tikkanen & Heinonen, 1991; Yu et al., 2008; Botto et al., 2001). In both hyperthermia and infection there have been documented biological effects on developmental apoptosis pathways. It has been suggested that altered apoptosis may cause birth defects, and apoptosis is known to be involved in cardiac morphogenesis, such as in the development of the cardiac outflow tract.
- **Maternal Stress;** Intense maternal stress during the periconceptional period was associated with increased risk of delivering infants with certain congenital anomalies particularly with conotruncal heart defects and neural tube defects (Carmichael & Shaw, 2000; Adams et al., 1989).
- **Maternal obesity;** Many studies have examined the association between maternal prepregnancy and during pregnant obesity (elevated BMI >25.0 Kg/m^2) with CHD such as ASD, VSD, conotruncal defects and right ventricular outflow tract defects (Cedergren & Kallen, 2003; Mills et al., 2010; Oddy et al., 2009; Gilboa et al., 2010). Several aspects of such potential associations between obesity and heart defects remain unclear due to studies of obesity and heart defects which are difficult to assess and compare because of the possibility of bias in obesity that may associated with unrecognized diabetes. While some literature found no association between maternal weight and isolated CHDs (Khalil et al., 2008; Watkins & Botto, 2001).

3.2.2 Maternal drug and medical use

Consumption of many drugs, such as thalidomide and isotretinoin, during early gestationcan interfere with the normal cardiogenesis of the fetus. This list of definite and potential human cardiac teratogens was showed in table 6.

3.2.3 Maternal drugs abuse

Some studies suggest that drinking alcohol or using cocaine, especially during the pregnancy, can increase the risk of congenital heart defects (table 6).

- **Caffeine;** Caffeine can cross the placenta, and the concern that caffeine may causes birth defects prompted the FDA to caution pregnant women to limit their caffeine intake. Today, there is no evidence associating caffeine ingestion during pregnancy and teratogenicity of congenital heart disease (Pejtsik et al., 1992; Linn et al., 1982).
- **Alcohol;** Maternal alcohol use during pregnancy is associated with fetal alcohol syndrome which comprise a spectrum of abnormal face, growth restriction, central nervous system abnormality and cardiac defects with VSDs occurring most commonly (Pejtsik et al., 1992; Carmichael et al, 2003; Burd et al., 2007; Loser et al., 1992). In Spain, a case-control study by Martinez-Frias et al. reported that a higher risk of developing CHDs was found in the group with the highest-level daily doses of alcohol consumption (the absolute alcohol ingestion was more than 92 gram per day. However, mechanism in teratogenic effect of alcohol on the developing heart malformation is as of now unclear.
- **Cocaine;** Maternal cocaine ingestion was reported to induce coronary thrombosis in the developing fetal heart leading to formation of a single ventricle, other defects were also reported, such as Ebstein's anomaly, VSD, heterotaxy (Linn et al., 1982; Kueh & Loffredo, 2002; Lipshultz et al., 1991; Martin & Khoury, 1992).
- **Cigarette Smoking;** Smoking during pregnancy enhances the risk of adverse pregnancy outcomes such as low birth weight. The relationship between gestational smoking and congenital heart defects has been studied, however the information is inconclusive. Some studies have reported associations between maternal smoking and ASD, AVSD, TOF (Alverson et al., 2011; Malik et al., 2008; Kallen, 1999). A recent study in Greece found that periconceptional tobacco smoking was associated with increased risk of CHD in the offspring (OR=2.7) and has been associated with a quantity of cigarette smoking (Karatza et al., 2011). However, no associations were found (Kallen, 1999) so research on large population-based studies is required to evaluate.

3.3 Environment or lifestyle factors

Evidence of teratogenic contamination in certain environments and workplaces is sporadic, albeit environmental factors are a more common cause for multifactorial inheritance CHD. Definitive evidence for the causal relationship between certain exposure and CHD is still unavailable. Available evidence suggests the finding of the higher incidence of CHD babies from women who reside in area with drinking water contaminated by trichloroethylene, dichloroethylene and chromium. While maternal exposure to paint, lacquer, agricultural chemicals, organic solvents, dyes and lead have also been occasionally found statistically associated with CHD. Ingestion of heavy metals and lifetime accumulation of a considerable amount of heavy metals through diet also affects CHD development in babies (table 6).

- **Organic Solvents;** A few studies reported increased risk of HLH, Coarc, PS, TGA with intact ventricular septum, TOF, TAPVR, non-chromosomal AVSD and Ebstein's anomaly. Other reports of occupational exposure to organic solvents have been associated with an increased risk of VSD (Tikkanen & Heinonen, 1991, 1992; Shaw et al., 2003). However the precise links are difficult to clarify, because solvent composition varies between different commercial preparations.
- **Pesticides & Other Toxic Substances;** A study by Adam et al suggests an association of maternal employment in the agricultural industry with an increased risk of conotruncal defects that suggests a possible association with chemicals used in agriculture (Adams

Risk factor	Common lesion of CHD	Estimated risk of CHD (OR)	Reference
Maternal health:			
• Diabetis mellitus in pregnancy	Heterotaxy, TOF, TGA, septal defects, left or right outflow obstruction	4.6-10.0	1 - 3
• Phenylketonuria	TOF, COA, PDA, VSD. HLH	>6	4
• Connective tissue disease	Complete atrioventricular heart block	Increased	5, 6
• Rubella infection	PDA, PS, ASD	Increased	7 - 9
• Febrile illness	Tricuspid or pulmonary atresia ,VSD	1.8-2.8	10
• Stress	Conotruncal heart defects	Increased	11, 12
• Obesity	Conotruncal heart defects , TAPVR, HLH, septal defects	1-3	13 - 16
Maternal medical use:			
• Lithium	Ebstein's anomaly, MR,TR	7.7	17, 18
• Vitamin A >10,000 IU/d	Outflow tract defect	increased	19, 20
• Isotretinoin (RoAccutane)	Overriding aorta, interrupted, hypoplastic aortic arch, ASD ,VSD	increased	21, 22
• Trimethadione	TOF, HLH, TGA,	increased	23
• Phenytoin	Coarc, PDA,AS, PS	increased	24
• Valproic acid	Outflow tract, VSD TOF	increased	25, 26
• Coumadin	PDA	increased	27
• Thalidomide	PS, TGA, TAPVR,VSD, ASD, TA, TOF	increased	28
• Ibuprofen	TGA, AVSD, VSD	1.8	29
• Naproxen	Any defects	1.7	29
• Trimethoprim -Sulfonamide	Any defects	2.1-4.8	30
• Sulfasalazine	Any defects	3.4	31
• Nitrofurantoin	HLH, ASD, VSD	1.6	32
• Angiotensin-converting Enzyme inhibitors	ASD, VSD, PS, PDA	3.7	33
• Tricyclic /tetracyclic Antidepressant	VSD	2.2	34
• Paroxitine	VSD, ASD	1.3-1.7	35, 36
Maternal illegal drug:			
• Alcohol	VSD	1.3-1.7	37 - 40
• Cigarette Smoking	ASD, AVSD, TOF	1.0-3.0	41 - 43
• Cocaine and Marijuana	Single ventricle , Ebstein's anomaly, VSD, heterotaxy	Increased	44 - 47
Environmental:			
• Organic Solvents	TGA, HLH, Coarc, TOF, PS	2.3-3.9	48 - 50
• Pesticides	TGA, TAPVR, VSD	Increased	12
• Air pollution:			
-CO	VSD, TOF, PS	1.2-2.6	51, 52
-NO	TOF	1.1	51, 52

(Ref: [1]Lisowski et al., 2010; [2]Corrigan et al., 2009; [3]Wren et al., 2003; [4]Rouse & Azen, 2004; [5]Buyon et al., 2009; [6]Clancy & Buyon, 2004; [7]Row, 1973; [8]De Santis et al., 2006; [9]Webster, 1998; [10]Botto et al., 2001; [11]Carmichael & Shaw, 2000; [12]Adam et al., 1989; [13]Cedergren & Kallen, 2003; [14]Mills et al., 2010; [15]Oddy et al., 2009; [16]Gilboa et al., 2010; [17]Cohen et al., 1994; [18]Jacobson et al., 1992; [19]Rothman et al., 1995; [20]Botto et al., 2001; [21]Lammer et al., 1985; [22]Willhite et al., 1986; [23]Rischbieth, 1979; [24]O'Brien & Gilmour-White, 1993; [25]Sonoda et al., 1993; [26]Winter et al., 1987; [27]Hou, 2004; [28]Smithells & Newman, 1992; [29]Ericson & Kallen, 2001; [30]Czeizel et al., 2001; [31]Newman & Correy, 1983; [32]Crider et al., 2009; [33]Cooper et al., 2006; [34]Kallen & Otterblad Olausson, 2006; [35]Bar-Oz et al., 2007; [36]Berard et al., 2007; [37]Pejtsil et al., 1992; [38]Carmichael et al., 2003; [39]Burd et al., 2007; [40]Loser et al., 1992; [41]Alverson et al., 2011; [42]Malik et al., 1999; [43]Kallen, 1999; [44]Linn et al., 1982; [45]Kuehl & Loffredo, 2002; [46]Lipshultz et al., 1991; [47]Martin & Khoury, 1992; [48]Tikkanen & Heinonen, 1991; [49]Shaw et al., 2003; [50]Tikkanen et al., 1992; [51]Gilboa et al., 2005; [52]Dadvand et al., 2011)

Table 6. Risk factors that are known or believed to be associated with the congenital heart defects.

et al., 1989). In the Baltimore-Washington Infant Study (BWIS), potential exposure to herbicides and rodenticides was associated with an increased risk of TGA, while potential exposure to pesticides was associated with TAPVR and VSD. A case-control study of various end-product uses reported an increased risk of conotruncal defects with maternal reports of exposure to insecticides (Shaw et al., 1999).

- **Air Pollution;** Ambient air pollution such carbon monoxide (CO), nitric oxide (NO), ozone (O_3), and sulfur dioxide (SO_2) may cause CHD dependent on pollutant levels (Ritz et al., 2002; Rankin et al., 2009). A study by Gilboa et al, observed positive associations between carbon monoxide and isolated ASD, TOF, particulate matter < 10 µm in diameter and isolated ASD as well as between ozone and VSD (Gilboa et al., 2005). From a study by Dadvand et al, exposure to CO and NO has been associated with ventricular septal defect and cardiac septa malformations. CO was also associated with congenital pulmonary valve stenosis and NO was associated TOF (Dadvand et al., 2011). Further studies are also required to clarify if air pollution exposure influences the risk for CHD.
- **Maternal Home Tap Water Consumption;** It has a positive association between a mother's consumption of home tap water during the first trimester of pregnancy and cardiac anomalies. This was unrelated to water contamination, mother's race, or her educational level (Shaw et al., 1990).
- **Waste Sites;** Many of the recent studies about possible increased risk of CHD in communities situated near hazardous waste sites are inconsistent (Croen et al., 1997) and may not ultimately prove to be causal.
- **Ionizing Radiation**; there are few reports on possible associations of CHD with maternal exposure to ionizing radiation in occupational settings or as part of medical or dental evaluations. Studies found no clear evidence of any association. Further studies are also required to clarify the precise relationship between these factors and CHD.

4. Prevention

Excluding genetic counseling, the genetic disorder cannot be protected against; simple guidelines to pregnant mothers for prevention of CHD in their newborns are good diet, physical activity, lifestyle, environments and occupation that the parents should discuss with their primary care provider or obstetrician. Women of childbearing age also should obtain prenatal care, including testing for diabetes and past rubella immunization, they should also discuss any medication use with their obstetrician; and should avoid contact with ill people, especially those with rubella or influenza. Women of childbearing age should take 400 micrograms of folic acid on a daily basis starting before pregnancy, which can reduce congenital heart and neural tube defects, and should avoid certain types of behaviors such as exposure to organic solvents, smoking and heavy alcohol use. If a woman has no immunity to rubella, she should get vaccinated prior to pregnancy. Preconception care and appropriate dietary management for women with phenylketonuria should be an important strategy. Detection and appropriate management of diabetes before and during pregnancy should be an important step for reducing risk of CHD in offspring. Avoidance of medications that are suspected to cause congenital defects, including congenital heart disease, should be taken, and the medications should have warnings about that risk to allow mothers and physicians to make informed decisions about the risks and benefits of the use of the medication during pregnancy. Recommendations also are possible for screening for possible cardiac defects using fetal echocardiography during pregnancy when warranted by reports of prenatal maternal illnesses or exposures. The need for screening any individual should be made on an individual basis from the type, likelihood, and level of potential exposure, as well as the time of gestation during which it occurred. This decision typically will be made as a result of the obstetrical history. Because congenital heart defects represent some of the more prevalent birth defects, that result in significant lifelong morbidity, and are an important cause of mortality attributed to birth defects, the development of effective prevention interventions is paramount from a public health perspective.

5. Conclusion

The number of patients, both children and adults, with CHD has continued to rise. The most common reasons for CHD are associated with multiple factors. Epidemiology studies reveal underestimated cases of CHD, and together with the etiology the studies help to define potential risk factors for CHD. The epidemiology and etiology of CHD also help prioritize the areas needed for intervention and additional regulations the public health officers may impose. Patients and parents of babies with CHD must understand the significance of routine medical checkups, which can be accomplished though an effective transition program and collaboration among healthcare providers.

6. Acknowledgement

The authors thank Sarah Hof and Randall Jones for their supports in proofreading.

7. References

Adams, MM.; Mulinare, J. & Dooley, K. (1989). Risk factors for conotruncal cardiac defects in Atlanta. *Journal of the American College of Cardiology*, Vol.14, No.2, (August 1989), pp. 432-442, ISSN 0735-1097

Akazawa, H. & Komuro, I. (2005). Cardiac transcription factor Csx/Nkx2-5: Its role in cardiac development and diseases. *Pharmacology & therapeutics*, Vol.107, No.2, (Ausgust 2005), pp. 252-268, ISSN 1879-016X

Akdeniz, C.; Odemis, E.; Erdem, A. & Celebi, A. (2009). Double outlet right ventricle and aortopulmonary window in a patient with Cornelia de Lange syndrome: a novel association. *Genetic counseling*, Vol.20, No.2, pp. 161-166, ISSN 1015-8146

Alabdulgader, AAA. (2006). Congenital heart disease in Saudi Arabia: current epidemiology and future projects. *Eastern Mediterranean Health Journal*, Vol.12, No.2, pp. 157-167, ISSN 1020-3397

Alverson, CJ.; Strickland, MJ.; Gilboa, SM. & Correa, A. (2011). Maternal smoking and congenital heart defects in the Baltimore-Washington Infant Study. *Pediatrics*, Vol.127, No.3, (March 2011), pp. e647-e653, ISSN 1098-4275

Ali, BR.; Akawi, NA.; Chedid, F.; Bakir, M.; Ur Rehman, M.; Rahmani, A. & Al-Gazali, L. (2010). Molecular and clinical analysis of Ellis-van Creveld syndrome in the United Arab Emirates. *BMC Medical Genetics*, Vol.11, (Febuary 2010), pp. 33, ISSN 1471-2350

Amro, K. (2009). Pattern of Congenital Heart Disease in Jordan. *European Journal of General Medicine,* Vol.6, No.3, pp. 161-165, ISSN 1304-3897

Arrington, CB.; Nightengale, D.; Lowichik, A.; Rosenthal, ET.; Christian-Ritter, K. & Viskochil, DH. (2006). Pathologic and molecular analysis in a family with rare mixed supravalvar aortic and pulmonic stenosis. *Pediatric and Devopmental Pathology*, Vol.9, No.4, (July-August 2006), pp. 297-306, ISSN 1615-5742

Ballesta Martinez, MJ.; Guillen Navarro, E.; Lopez Exposito, I.; Bafalliu Vidal, JA.; Domingo Jimenez, R.; Guia Torrent, JM.; Robles Sanchez, F. & Sanchez Solis de Querol, M. (2008). [Review of 22 patients with 22q11.2 deletion syndrome: phenotype spectrum]. *Anales de pediatria (Barcelona, Spain: 2003)*, Vol.69, No.4, (October 2008), pp. 304-310, ISSN 1695-9531

Bar-Oz, B.; Einarson, T.; Einarson, A.; Boskovic, R.; O'Brien, L.; Malm, H.; Berard, A. & Koren, G. (2007). Paroxetine and congenital malformations: meta-Analysis and consideration of potential confounding factors. *Clinical Therapeutics*, Vol.29, No.5, (May 2007), pp. 918-926, ISSN 0149-2918

Barisic, I.; Tokic, V.; Loane, M.; Bianchi, F.; Calolari, E.; Game, E.; Wellesley, D. & Dolk, H. (2008). Descriptive epidemiology of Cornelia de Lange syndrome in Europe. *American Journal of Medical Genetics Part A*, Vol.146A, No.1, (January 2008), pp. 51-59, ISSN 1552-4833

Basson, CT.; Huang, T.; Lin, RC.; Bachinsky, DR.; Weremowicz, S.; Vaglio, A.; Bruzone, R.; Quadrelli, R.; Lerone, M.; Romeo, G.; Silengo, M.; Pereira, A.; Krieger, J.; Mesquita, SF.; Kamisago, M.; Morton, CC.; Pierpont, ME.; Muller, CW.; Seidman, JG. & Seidman, CE. (1999). Different TBX5 interactions in heart and limb defined by Holt-Oram syndrome mutations. *Proceedings of the National Academy of Sciencs of the United States of America*, Vol.96, No.6, (March 1999), pp. 2919-2924, ISSN 1091-6490

Battaglia, A.; Carey, JC.; Cederholm, P.; Viskochil, DH.; Brothman, AR. & Galasso, C. (1999). Natural history of Wolf-Hirschhorn syndrome: experience with 15 cases. *Pediatrics*, Vol.103, No.4 Pt 1, (April 1999), pp. 830-836, ISSN 1098-4275

Berard, A.; Ramos, E.; Rey, E.; Blais, L.; St-Andre, M. & Oraichi, D. (2007). First trimester exposure to paroxetine and risk of cardiac malformations in infants: the importance of dosage. *Birth Defects Research. Part B, Developmental and Reproductive Toxicology*, Vol.80, No.1, (Febuary 2007), pp. 18-27, ISSN 1542-9733

Berends, MJ.; Tan-Sindhunata, G.; Leegte, B. & van Essen, AJ. (2001). Phenotypic variability of Cat-Eye syndrome. *Genetic counseling*, Vol.12, No.1, pp. 23-34, ISSN 1015-8146

Bernier, PL.; Stefanescu, A.; Samoukovic, G. & Tchervenkov, CI. (2010). The Challenge of Congenital Heart diease Worldwide: Epidemiologic and Demographic Facts. *Pediatric Cardiac Surgery Annual*, pp. 26-34, ISSN 1092-9126

Boneva, RS.; Botto, LD.; Moore, CA.; Yang, Q, Correa, A. & Erickson, JD. (2001). Mortality Associated With Congenital Heart Defects in the United States: Trends and Racial Disprities, 1979-1997. *Circulation*, Vol.103, (May 2001), pp. 2376-2381, ISSN 1524-4539

Borzouee, M. & Jannati, M. (2008). Distribution and Characteristecs of the Heart Disease in Pediatric Age Group in Southern Iran. *Iranian Cardiovascular Research Journal*, Vol.2, No.1, pp. 48-51, ISSN 1735-8868

Botto, LD.; Correa, A. & Erickson, JD. (2001). Racial and Temporal Variations in The Prevalence of Heart Defects. *Pediatrics*, Vol.107, No.3, (March 2001), pp. 1-8, ISSN 1098-4275

Botto, LD. & Correa, A. (2003). Decreasing the burden of congenital heart anomalies: an epidemiologic evaluation of risk factors and survival. *Progress in Pediatric Cardiology*, Vol.18, pp. 111–121, ISSN 1058-9813

Botto, LD.; Lynberg, MC. & Erickson, JD. (2001). Congenital heart defects, maternal febrile illness, and multivitamin use: a population-based study. *Epidemiology*, Vol.12, No.5, (September 2001), pp. 485-490, ISSN 1531-5487

Botto, LD.; Loffredo, C.; Scanlon, KS.; Ferencz, C.; Khoury, MJ.; David Wilson, P. & Correa, A. (2001). Vitamin A and cardiac outflow tract defects. *Epidemiology*, Vol.12, No.5, (September 2001), pp. 491-496, ISSN 1531-5487

Bound, JP. & Logan, WF. (1977). Incidence of congenital heart disease in Blackpool 1957-1971. *British Heart Journal*, Vol.39, pp. 445-450, ISSN 0007-0769

Brautbar, A.; LeMaire, SA.; Franco, LM.; Coselli, JS.; Milewicz, DM. & Belmont, JW. FBN1 mutations in patients with descending thoracic aortic dissections. *American Journal of Medical Genetics Part A*, Vol.152A, No.2, (Febuary 2010), pp. 413-416, ISSN 1552-4833

Brown, ML.; Dearani, JA. & Burkhart, HM. (2009). The adult with congenital disease: medical and surgical considerations for management. *Current Opinion in Pediatrics*, Vol.21, pp. 561-564, ISSN 1040-8703

Burd, L.; Deal, E.; Rios, R.; Adickes, E.; Wynne, J. & Klug, MG. (2007). Congenital heart defects and fetal alcohol spectrum disorders. *Congenital Heart Disease*, Vol.2, No.4, (August 2007), pp. 250-255, ISSN 1747-0803

Buyon, JP.; Clancy, RM. & Friedman, DM. (2009). Autoimmune associated congenital heart block: integration of clinical and research clues in the management of the maternal / foetal dyad at risk. *Journal of Internal Medicine*, Vol.265, No.6, (June 2009), pp. 653-662, ISSN 1365-1796

Ceizel, A.; Pornoi, A.; Peterffy, E. & Tarcal, E. (1982). Study of children of parents operated on for congenital cardiovascular malformations. *British Heart Journal*, Vol.47, No.3, (March, 2001), pp. 290-293, ISSN 0007-0769

Calmont, A.; Ivins, S.; Van Bueren, KL.; Papangeli, I.; Kyriakopoulou, V.; Andrews, WD.; Matin, JF.; Moon, AM.; Illingworth, EA.; Basson, A. & Scambler, PJ. (2009). Tbx1 controls cardiac neural crest cell migration during arch artery development by regulating Gbx2 expression in the pharyngeal ectoderm. *Development*, Vol.136, No.18, (September 2009), pp. 3173-3183, ISSN 1461-7072

Carmichael, SL. & Shaw, GM. (2000). Maternal life event stress and congenital anomalies. *Epidemiology*, Vol.11. No.1, (January 2000), pp. 30-35, ISSN 1531-5487

Carmichael, SL.; Shaw, GM.; Yang, W. & Lammer, EJ. (2003). Maternal periconceptional alcohol consumption and risk for conotruncal heart defects. *Birth Defects Reserch Part A. Clinical and Molecular Teratology*, Vol.67, No.10, (October 2003), pp. 875-878, ISSN 1542-0760

Casey, B.; Devoto, M.; Jones, KL. & Ballabio, A. (1993). Mapping a gene for familial situs abnormalities to human chromosome Xq24-q27.1. *Nature Genetics*, Vol.5, No.4, (December 1993), pp. 403-407, ISSN 1546-1718

Cedergren, MI. & Kallen, BA. (2003). Maternal obesity and infant heart defects. *Obesity Research*, Vol.11, No.3, (September 2003), pp. 1065-1071, ISSN 1550-8528

Clancy, RM. & Buyon, JP. (2004). Autoimmune-associated congenital heart block: dissecting the cascade from immunologic insult to relentless fibrosis. *The anatomicla record.*

Part A, Discoveries in molecular, cellular, and evolutionary biology, Vol.280, No.2, (October 2004), pp. 1027-1035, ISSN 1552-4884

Cody, JD.; Ghidoni, PD.; DuPont, BR.; Hale, DE.; Hilsenbeck, SG.; Stratton, RF.; Hoffman, DS.; Muller, S.; Schaub, RL.; Leach, RJ. & Kaye, CI. (1999).. Congenital anomalies and anthropometry of 42 individuals with deletions of chromosome 18q. *American Journal of Medical Genetics*, Vol.85. No.5, (August 1999), pp. 455-462, ISSN 0148-7299

Cohen, LS.; Friedman, JM.; Jefferson, JW.; Johnson, EM. & Weiner, ML. (1994). A reevaluation of risk of in utero exposure to lithium. *Journal of the American Medical Association*, Vol.271, No.2, (January 1994), pp. 146-150, ISSN 1538-3598

Colliton, RP.; Bason, L.; Lu, FM.; Piccoli, DA.; Krantz, ID. & Spinner, NB. (2001). Mutation analysis of Jagged1 (JAG1) in Alagille syndrome patients. *Human Mutation*, Vol.17, No.2, (Febuary 2001), pp. 151-152, ISSN 1098-1004

Cooper, WO.; Hernandez-Diaz, S.; Arbogast, PG.; Dudley, JA.; Dyer, S.; Gideon, PS.; Hall, K. & Ray, WA. (2006). Major congenital malformations after first-trimester exposure to ACE inhibitors. *The New England Journal of Medicine*, Vol.354, No.23, (June 2006), pp. 2443-2451, ISSN 1533-4406

Correa, A.; Gilboa, SM.; Besser, LM.; Botto, LD.; Moore, CA.; Hobbs, CA.; Cleves, MA.; Reihle-Colarusso, TJ.; Waller, DK. & Reece, EA. (2008). Diabetes mellitus and birth defects. *American Journal of Obestetrics and Gynecology*, Vol.199, No.3, (September 2008), pp. e1-e9, ISSN 1097-6886

Corrigan, N.; Brazil, DP. & McAuliffe, F. (2009). Fetal cardiac effects of maternal hyperglycemia during pregnancy. *Birth Defects Research Part A. Clinical and Molecular Teratology*, Vol.85, No.6, (June 2009), pp. 523-530, ISSN 1542-0760

Crider, KS.; Cleves, MA.; Reefhuis, J.; Berry, RJ.; Hobbs, CA. & Hu, DJ. (2009). Antibacterial medication use during pregnancy and risk of birth defects: National Birth Defects Prevention Study. *Archives of Pediatrics and Adolescent Medicine*, Vol.163, No.11, (November 2009), pp. 978-985, ISSN 1538-3628

Croen, LA.; Shaw, GM.; Sanbonmatsu, L.; Selvin, S. & Buffler, PA. (1997). Maternal residential proximity to hazardous waste sites and risk for selected congenital malformations. *Epidemiology*, Vol.8, No.4, (July 1997), pp. 347-354, ISSN 1531-5487

Czeizel, AE.; Rockenbauer, M.; Sorensen, HT. & Olsen, J. (2001). The teratogenic risk of trimethoprim-sulfonamides: a population based case-control study. *Reproductive Toxicology*, Vol.15, No.6, (November-December 2001), pp. 637-646, ISSN 1873-1708

Dadvand, P.; Rankin, J.; Shitley, MDF.; Rushton, S. & Pless-Mulloli, T. (2008). Descriptive epidemiology of congenital heart disease in Northern England. *Paediatric and Perinatal Epidemiology*, Vol.23, pp. 58-65, ISSN 1365-3016

Dadvand, P.; Rankin, J.; Rushton, S. & Pless-Mulloli, T. (2011). Association between maternal exposure to ambient air pollution and congenital heart disease: A register-based spatiotemporal analysis. *American Journal of Epidemiology*, Vol.173, No.2, (January 2011), pp. 171-182, ISSN 0002-9262

De Backer, J. (2009). Cardiovascular characteristics in Marfan syndrome and their relation to the genotype. *Verhandelingen-Koninklijke Academie voor Geneeskunde van Belgie*, Vol.71, No.6, pp. 335-371, ISSN 0302-6469

De Luca, A.; Sarkozy, A.; Ferese, R.; Consoli, F.; Lepri, F.; Dentici, ML.; Vergara, P.; De Zorzi, A.; Versacci, P.; Digilio, MC.; Marino, B. & Dallapiccola, B. (2010). New mutations

in ZFPM2/FOG2 gene in tetralogy of Fallot and double outlet right ventricle. *Clinical Genetics*, Vol.3, pp. 1-7, ISSN 1399-0004
De Santis, M.; Cavaliere, AF.; Straface, G. & Caruso, A. (2006). Rubella infection in pregnancy. *Reproductive Toxicology*, Vol.21, No.4, (May 2006), pp. 390-398, ISSN 1873-1708
Devriendt, K.; Matthijs, G.; Van Dael, R.; Gewillig, M.; Eyskens, B.; Hjalgrim, H.; Dolmer, B.; McGaughran, J.; Brondum-Nielsen, K.; Marynen, P.; Fryns, JP. & Vermeesch, JR. (1999). Delineation of the critical deletion region for congenital heart defects, on chromosome 8p23.1. *American Journal of Heman Genetics*, Vol.64. No.4, (April 1999), pp. 1119-1126, ISSN 0002-9297
Dickinson, DF.; Arnold, R. & Wilkinson, JL. (1981). Congenital heart disease among 160480 liveborn children in Liverpool 1960 to 1969 Implications for surgical treatment. *British Heart* Journal, Vol.46, pp. 55-62, ISSN 0007-0769
Dietz, HC.; Pyeritz, RE.; Hall, BD.; Cadle, RG.; Hamosh, A.; Schwartz, J.; Meyers, DA. & Francomano, CA. (1991). The Marfan syndrome locus: confirmation of assignment to chromosome 15 and identification of tightly linked markers at 15q15-q21.3. *Genomics*, Vol.9, No.2, (Febuary 1991), pp. 355-361, ISSN 0888-6717
Digilio, MC.; Marino, B.; Giannotti, A.; Di Donato, R. & Dallapiccola, B. (2000). Heterotaxy with left atrial isomerism in a patient with deletion 18p. *American Journal of Medical Genetics*, Vol.94, No.3, (September 2000), pp. 198-200, ISSN 0148-7299
Digilio, MC.; Angioni, A.; Giannotti, A.; Dallapiccola, B. & Marino, B. (2003). Truncus arteriosus and duplication 8q. *American Journal of Medical Genetics Part A*, Vol.121A, No.1, (August 2003), pp. 79-81, ISSN 1552-4833
Dolk, H. & Loane, M. (March, 2009). *EUROCAT Steering Committee: Congenital heart defects in Europe: 2000-2005*, April 2011, Available from:
http://eurocat.bio-medical.co.uk/content/Special-Report-CHD.pdf
Dolk, H.; Loane, M. & Game, E. (2010). The prevalence of congenital anomalies in Europe. *Advances in Experimental Medicine and Biology*, Vol.686, pp. 349-364, ISSN 0065-2598
Douchin, S.; Rossignol, AM.; Klein, SK.; Siche, JP.; Baguet, JP. & Bost, M. (2000). [Heart malformations and vascular complications associated with Turner's syndrome. Prospective study of 26 patients]. *Archives des maladies du Coeur et des vaisseaux*, Vol.93, No.5, (May 2000), pp. 565-570, ISSN 0003-9683
Edelman, EA.; Girirajan, S.; Finucane, B.; Patel, PI.; Lupski, JR.; Smith, AC. & Elsea, SH. (2007). Gender, genotype, and phenotype differences in Smith-Magenis syndrome: a meta-analysis of 105 cases. *Clinical Genetics*, Vol.71, No.6, (June 2007), pp. 540-550, ISSN 0009-9163
Elliott, DA.; Kirk, EP.; Yeoh, T.; Chandar, S.; McKenzie, F.; Taylor, P.; Grossfeld, P.; Fatkin, D.; Jones, O.; Hayes, P.; Feneley, M. & Harvey, RP. (2003). Cardiac homeobox gene NKX2-5 mutations and congenital heart disease: associations with atrial septal defect and hypoplastic left heart syndrome. *Journal of the American College of Cardiology*, Vol.41, No.11, (June 2003), pp. 2072-2076, ISSN 0735-1097
El-Rassy, I.; Bou-Abdallah, J.; Al-Ghadban, S.; Bitar, F. & Nemer, G. (2008). Absence of NOTCH2 and Hey2 mutations in a familial Alagille syndrome case with a novel frameshift mutation in JAG1. *American Journal of Medical Genetics Part A*, Vol.146, No.7, (April 2008), pp. 937-939, ISSN 1552-4833

Ericson, A. & Kallen, BA. (2001). Nonsteroidal anti-inflammatory drugs in early pregnancy. *Reproductive Toxicology*, Vol.15, No.4, (July-August 2001), pp. 371-375, ISSN 1873-1708

Eronen, M.; Peippo, M.; Hiippala, A.; Raatikka, M.; Arvio, M.; Johansson, R. & Kahkonen, M. (2002). Cardiovascular manifestations in 75 patients with Williams syndrome. *Journal of Medical Genetics*, Vol.39, No.8, (August 2002), pp. 554-558, ISSN 1468-6244

Fan, C.; Liu, M. & Wang, Q. (2003). Functional analysis of TBX5 missense mutations associated with Holt-Oram syndrome. *Journal of Boiological Chemistry, Vol.278, No.10, (March 2003), pp. 8780-8785, ISSN 0021-9258*

Faria, MH.; Rabenhorst, SH.; Pereira, AC. & Krieger, JE. (2008). A novel TBX5 missense mutation (V263M) in a family with atrial septal defects and postaxial hexodactyly. *Intenal Journal of Cardiology*, Vol.130, No.1, (October 2008), pp. 30-35, ISSN 0167-1718

Fatema, NN.; Chowdhury, RB. & Chowdhury, L. (2008). Incidence of Congenital Heart Disease among Hospital Live Birth in a Tertiar Hospital of Bangladesh. *Cardiovascular Journal*, Vol.1, No.1, pp. 14-20, ISSN 2071-0917

Ferencz, C.; Rubin, JD.; McCarter, RJ.; Brenner, JI.; Neil, CA.; Perry, LW.; Hepner, SI. & Downing, JW. (1985). Congenital heart disease: prevalence at birth. The Baltimore-Washington Infant Study. *American Journal of* Epidemiology, Vol.121, No.1, pp. 31-16, ISSN0002-9262

Ferencz, C.; Boughman, JA.; Neill, CA.; Brenner, JI. & Perry, LW. (1989). Congenital cardiovascular malformations: questions on inheritance. Baltimore-Washington Infant Study Group. *Journal of the American College of Cardiology*, Vol.14, No.3, pp. 756-763, ISSN 0735-1097

Ferrero, GB.; Biamino, E.; Sorasio, L.; Banaudi, E.; Peruzzi, L.; Forzano, S.; Di Cantogno, LV. & Silengo, MC. (2007). Presenting phenotype and clinical evaluation in a cohort of 22 Williams-Beuren syndrome patients. *European Journal of Medical Genetics*, Vol.50, No.5, (September-October 2007), pp. 327-337, ISSN 1769-7212

Fixler, DE.; Pastor, P.; Chamberlin, M.; Sigman, E. & Eifler, CW. (1990). Trend in Congenital Heart Disease in Dallas County Births. 1971-1984. *Circulation*, Vol.81, No.1, (January 1990), pp. 137-142, ISSN 1524-4539

Garg, V.; Kathiriya, IS.; Barnes, R.; Schluterman, MK.; King, IN.; Butler, CA.; Rothrock, CR.; Eapen, RS.; Hirayama-Yamada, K.; Joo, K.; Matsuka, R.; Cohen, JC. & Ssrivastava, D. (2003). GATA4 mutations cause human congenital heart defects and reveal an interaction with TBX5. *Nature*, Vol.424, No.6947, (July 2003), pp. 443-447, ISSN 1476-4687

Garg, V.; Muth, AN.; Ransom, JF.; Schluterman, MK.; Barnes, R.; King, IN.; Grossfeld, PD. & Srivastva, D. (2005). Mutations in NOTCH1 cause aortic valve disease. *Nature*, Vol.437, No.7056, (September 2005), pp. 270-274, ISSN 1476-4687

Garne, E.; Stoll, C. & Clementi, M. (2001). Evaluation of prenatal diagnosis of congenital heart disease by ultrasound: experience from 20 European registries. *Ultrasound in Obstetrics & Gynecology*, Vol.17, (May 2001), pp. 386-391, ISSN 1469-0705

Giltay, JC.; Bokma, JA.; de France, H. & Beemer, FA. (1998). VSD, hypospadias and normal psychomotor development in a patient with inv dup 8(13-q21.2). *Clinical Genetics*, Vol.53, No.1, (January 1998), pp. 74-78, ISSN 0009-9163

Gittenberger-de Groot, AC; Bartelings, MM; Deruiter, MC & Poelmann, RR. (2005). Basics of cardiac development for the understanding of congenital heart malformations. *Pediatric Research*, Vol.57, No.2, (February 2005), pp. 169-176, ISSN 0031-3998

Germanakis, I. & Sifakis, S. (2006). The Impact of Fetal Echocardiography on the Prevalence of Liveborn Congenital Heart Disease. *Pediatric Cardiology*, Vol. 27, No.4, pp. 465-472, ISSN 1432-1971

Gilboa, SM.;, Correa, A.; Botto, LD.; Rasmussen, SA.; Waller, DK.; Hobbs, CA.; Cleves, MA. & Riehle-Colarusso, TJ. (2010). Association between prepregnancy body mass index and congenital heart defects. *American Journal of Obstetrics & Gynecology*, Vol.202, No.1, (January 2010), pp. e1-e10, ISSN 1097-6868

Gilboa, SM.; Mendola, P.; Olshan, AF.; Langlois, PH.; Savitz, DA.; Loomis, D.; Herring, AH. & Fixler, DE. (2005). Relation between ambient air quality and selected birth defects, seven county study, Texas, 1997-2000. *American Journal of Epidemiology*, Vol.162, No.3, (August 2005), pp. 238-252, ISSN 0002-9262

Goldmuntz, E.; Bamford, R.; Karkera, JD.; dela Cruz, J.; Roessler, E. & Muenke, M. (2002). CFC1 mutations in patients with transposition of the great arteries and double-outlet right ventricle. *American Journal of Human Genetics*, Vol.70, No.3, (March 2002), pp. 776-780, ISSN 0002-9297

Green, EK.; Priestley, MD.; Waters, J.; Maliszewska, C.; Latif, F. & Maher, ER. (2000). Detailed mapping of a congenital heart disease gene in chromosome 3p25. *Journal of Medical Genetics*, Vol.37, No.8, (August 2000), pp. 581-587, ISSN 1468-6244

Grinberg, I. & Millen, KJ. (2005). The ZIC gene family in development and disease. *Clinical Genetics*, Vol.67, No.4, (April 2005), pp. 290-296, ISSN 0009-9163

Grossfeld, PD.; Mattina, T.; Lai, Z.; Favier, R.; Jones, KL.; Cotter, F. &Jones, C. (2004). The 11q terminal deletion disorder: a prospective study of 110 cases. *American Journal of Medical Genetics Part A*, Vol.129A, No.1, (August 2004), pp. 51-61, ISSN 1552-4833

Guo, Y.; Shen, J.; Yuan, L.; Li, F.; Wang, J. & Sun, K. (2010). Novel CRELD1 gene mutations in patients with atrioventricular septal defect. *World Journal of Pediatrics*, Vol.6, No.4, (November 2010), pp. 348-52, ISSN 1708-8569

Heritage, ML.; MacMillan, JC. & Anderson, GJ. (2002). DHPLC mutation analysis of Jagged1 (JAG1) reveals six novel mutations in Australian alagille syndrome patients. *Human Molecular Genetics*, Vol.20, No.6, (December 2002), pp. 481, ISSN 0964-6906

Hilger-Eversheim, K.; Moser, M.; Schorle, H. & Buettner, R. (2000). Regulatory roles of AP-2 transcription factors in vertebrate development, apoptosis and cell-cycle control. *Gene*, Vol.260, No.1-2, (December 2000), pp. 1-12, ISSN 1769-7212

Hills, C.; Moller, JH.; Finkelstein, M.; Lohr, J. & Schimmenti, L. (2006). Cri du chat syndrome and congenital heart disease: a review of previously reported cases and presentation of an additional 21 cases from the Pediatric Cardiac Care Consortium. *Pediatrics*, Vol.117, No.5, (May 2006), pp. e924-e927, ISSN 1098-9163

Hoffman, JIE. & Christianson, R. (1978). Congenital heart disease in a cohort of 19502 births with long-term follow-up. *The American journal of cardiology*, Vol.42, No.4, (October 1978), pp. 641-647, ISSN 0002-9149

Hoffman, JIE. & Kaplan, S. (2002). The Incidence of Congenital Heart Disease. *Journal of the American College of Cardiology*, Vol.39, No.12, (June 2002), pp. 1890-1900, ISSN 0735-1097

Hou, JW. (2004). Fetal warfarin syndrome. *Chang Gung Medical Journal*, Vol.27, No.9, (September 2004), pp. 691-695, ISSN 2072-0939

Huang, T.; Lin, AE.; Cox, GF.; Golden, WL.; Feldman, GL.; Ute, M.; Schrander-Stumpel, C.; Kamisago, M. & Vermeulen, SJ. (2002). Cardiac phenotypes in chromosome 4q-syndrome with and without a deletion of the dHAND gene. *Genetics in Medicine*, Vol.4. No.6, (November-December 2002), pp. 464-467, ISSN 1530-0366

Jacobson, SJ.; Jones, K.; Johnson, K.; Ceolin, L.; Kaur, P.; Sahn, D.; Donnenfeld, AE.; Rieder, M, Santelli, R. & Smythe, J. (1992). Prospective multicentre study of pregnancy outcome after lithium exposure during first trimester. *Lancet*, Vol.339, No.8792, (Febuary 1992), pp. 530-533, ISSN 1474-547X

Jamieson, CR.; van der Burgt, I.; Brady, AF.; van Reen, M.; Elsawi, MM.; Hol, F.; Jeffery, S.; Patton, MA. & Mariman, E. (1994). Mapping a gene for Noonan syndrome to the long arm of chromosome 12. *Nature Genetics*, Vol.8, No.4, (December 1994), pp. 357-360, ISSN 1546-1718

Jerome, LA. & Papaioannou, VE. (2001). DiGeorge syndrome phenotype in mice mutant for the T-box gene, Tbx1. *Nature Genetics*, Vol.27, No.3, (March 2001), pp. 286-291, ISSN 1546-1718

Jongmans, M.; Sistermans, EA.; Rikken, A.; Nillesen, WM.; Tamminga, R.; Patton, M.; Maier, EM.; Tartaqlia, M.; Noordam, K. & van der Burgt, I. (2005). Genotypic and phenotypic characterization of Noonan syndrome: new data and review of the literature. *American Journal of Medical Genetics Part A*, Vol.134A, No.2, (April 2005), pp. 165-170, ISSN 1552-4833

Kallen, B. & Otterblad Olausson, P. (2006). Antidepressant drugs during pregnancy and infant congenital heart defect. *Reproductive Toxicology*, Vol.21, No.3, (April 2006), pp. 221-222, ISSN 1873-1708

Kallen, K. (1999). Maternal smoking and congenital heart defects. *European Journal of Epidemiology*, Vol.15, No.8, (September 1999), pp. 731-737, ISSN 0393-2990

Khalil, HS.; Saleh, AM. & Subhani, SN. (2008). Maternal obesity and neonatal congenital cardiovascular defects. *International Journal of Gynaecolgy and Obstetrics*, Vol.102, No.3, (September 2008), pp. 232-236, ISSN 1879-3479

Karatza, AA.; Giannakopoulos, I.; Dassios, TG.; Belavgenis, G.; Mantagos, SP.; Varvarigou AA. (2011). Periconceptional tobacco smoking and Xisolated congenital heart defects in the neonatal period. *Internal Journal of Cardiology*, Vol.105, No.2, (May 2011), pp. 295-299, ISSN0167-5273

Kenny, D. (2008). Long-term outcome of the child with congenital heart disease. *Paediatrics and child health*, Vol.19, No.1, pp. 37-42, ISSN 1205-7088

Khalil, A.; Aggarwal, R.; Thirupuram, S. & Arora, R. (1994). INCIDENCE OF CONGENITAL HEART DISEASE AMONG HOSPITAL LIVE BIRTHS IN INDIA. *INDIAN PEDIATRICS*, Vol.31, (May 1994), pp. 519-527 ISSN 0019-6061

Knowles, R.; Griebsch, I.; Dezateux, C. & Brown, J. (2005). Newborn screening for congenital heart defects: a systemic review and cost-effectiveness analysis. *Health Technology Assessment*, Vol.9, No.44, pp. 1-6, ISSN 1366-5278

Komuro, I. & Izumo, S. (1993). Csx: a murine homeobox-containing gene specifically expressed in the developing heart. *Proceedings of the NationalAcedemy of Sciencs of the United States of America*, Vol.90, No.17, (Septeber 1993), pp. 8145-8149, ISSN 1091-6490

Kuehl, KS. & Loffredo, C. (2002). Risk factors for heart disease associated with abnormal sidedness. *Teratology*, Vol.66, No.5, (November 2002), pp. 242-248, ISSN 0040-3709

Lammer, EJ.; Chen, DT.; Hoar, RM.; Agnish, ND.; Benke, PJ.; Braun, JT.; Curry, CJ.; Fernhoff, PM.; Grix, AW Jr. & Lott, IT. (1985). Retinoic acid embryopathy. *The New England Journal of Medicine*, Vol.13, No.14, (October 1985), pp. 837-841, ISSN 1533-4406

Levy, HL.; Guldberg, P.; Guttler, F.; Hanley, WB.; Matalon, R.; Rouse, BM.; Trefz, F.; Azen, C.; Allred, EN.; de la Cruz, F. & Koch, R. (2001). Congenital heart disease in maternal phenylketonuria: report from the Maternal PKU Collaborative Study. *Pediatric Research*, Vol.49, No.5, (May 2001), pp. 636-642, ISSN 0031-3998

Lichiardopol, C. & Mota, M. (2004). Cardiovascular risk factors in Turner's syndrome. *Romanian Journal of Internal Medicine*, Vol.42, No.2, pp. 371-379, ISSN 1220-4749

Li, D.; Yu, J.; Gu, F.; Pang, X.; Ma, X.; Li, R.; Liu, N. & Ma, X. (2008). The roles of two novel FBN1 gene mutations in the genotype-phenotype correlations of Marfan syndrome and ectopia lentis patients with marfanoid habitus. *Genetic Testing*, Vol.12, No.2, (June 2008), pp. 325-330, ISSN 1557-7473

Li, QY.; Newbury-Ecob, RA.; Terrett, JA.; Wilson, DI.; Curtis, AR.; Yi, CH.; Gebuhr, T.; Bullen, PJ.; Robson, SC.; Strachan, T.; Bonnet, D.; Lyonnet, S.; Young, ID.; Raeburn, JA.; Buckler, AJ.; Law, DJ. & Brook, JD. (1997). Holt-Oram syndrome is caused by mutations in TBX5, a member of the Brachyury (T) gene family. *Nature Genetics*, Vol.15, No.1, (January 1997), pp. 21-29, ISSN 1546-1718

Lillehei, CW.; Dewall, RA.; Read, RC.; Warden, HE. & Varco, RL. (1956). Direct Vision Intracardiac Surgery in Man Using a Simple, Disposable Artificial Oxygenator. *DISEASES of the CHEST*, Vol.29, No.1, January 1956, pp. 1-8, ISSN 0096-0217

Lin, HY.; Lin, SP.; Chen, YJ.; Hsu, CH.; Kao, HA.; Chen, MR.; Hung, HY.; Ho, CS.; Chang, JH.; Huang, FY.; Tsai, TC.; Lin, DS. & Chan, WY. (2007). Clinical characteristics and survival of trisomy 13 in a medical center in Taiwan, 1985-2004. *Pediatrics International*, Vol.49, No.3, (June 2007), pp. 380-386, ISSN 1442-200X

Lindinger, A.; Schwedler, G. & Hense, HW. (2010). Prevalence of Congenital Heart Defect in Newborns in Germany: Results of the First Registration Year of the PAN Study (July 2006 to June 2007). *Klinische Padiatr*ie, Vol.222, pp. 321-326, ISSN 0300-8630

Linn, S.; Schoenbaum, SC.; Monson, RR.; Rosner, B.; Stubblefield, PG. & Ryan, KJ. (1982). No association between coffee consumption and adverse outcomes of pregnancy. *The New England Journal of Medicine*, Vol.306, No.3, (January 1982), pp. 141-145, ISSN 1533-4406

Linnankivi, T.; Tienari, P.; Somer, M.; Kahkonen, M.; Lonnqvist, T.; Valanne, L. & Pigko, H. (2006).. 18q deletions: clinical, molecular, and brain MRI findings of 14 individuals. *American Journal of Medical Genetics Part A*, Vol.140, No.4, (Febuary 2006), pp. 331-339, ISSN 1552-4833

Lipshultz, SE.; Frassica, JJ. & Orav, EJ. (1991). Cardiovascular abnormalities in infants prenatally exposed to cocaine. *The Journal of Pediatrics*, Vol.118, No.1, (January 1991), pp. 44-51, ISSN 1097-6833

Lisowski, LA.; Verheijen, PM.; Copel, JA.; Kleinman, CS.; Wassink, S.; Visser, GH. & Meijboom, EJ. (2010). Congenital heart disease in pregnancies complicated by maternal diabetes mellitus. An international clinical collaboration, literature review, and meta-analysis. *Herz*, Vol.35, No.1, (January 2010), pp. 19-26, ISSN 0946-1299

Lizarraga, MA.; Mintegui, S.; Sanchez Echaniz, J.; Galdeano, JM.; Pastor, E. & Cabrera, A. (1991). [Heart malformations in trisomy 13 and trisomy 18]. *Revista Espanola de Cardiologia*, Vol.44, No.9, (November 1991), pp. 605-610, ISSN 0300-8932

Loeys, BL.; Schwarze, U.; Holm, T.; Callewaert, BL.; Thomas, GH.; Pannu, H.; De Backer, JF.; Oswald, GL.; Symoens, S.; Manouvier, S.; Roberts, AE.; Faravelli, F.; Greco, MA.; Pyeritz, RE.; Milewic, DM.; Coucke, PJ.; Cameron, DE.; Braverman, AC.; Byers, PH.; De Paepe, AM. & Dietz, HC. (2006). Aneurysm syndromes caused by mutations in the TGF-beta receptor. *The New England Journal of Medicine*, Vol.355, No.8, (August 2006), pp. 788-798, ISSN 1533-4406

Loomes, KM.; Underkoffler, LA.; Morabito, J.; Gottlieb, S.; Piccoli, DA.; Spinner, NB.; Baldwin, HS. & Oakey, RJ. (1999). The expression of Jagged1 in the developing mammalian heart correlates with cardiovascular disease in Alagille syndrome. *Human Molecular Genetics*, Vol.8, No.13, (December 1999), pp. 2442-2449, ISSN 0964-6906

Loser, H.; Pfefferkorn, JR. & Themann, H. (1992). [Alcohol in pregnancy and fetal heart damage]. *Klinische Padiatrie*, Vol.204, No.5, (September-October 1992), pp. 335-339, ISSN 0300-8630

Majnener, A.; Limperopoulos, C.; Shevell, M.; Rohlicek, C.; Rosenblatt, B. & Tchervenkov, C. (2008). Developmental and Functional Outcomes at School Entry in Children with Congenital Heart Defects. *The Journal of Pediatrics*, Vol.153, No.1, (July 2008), pp. 55-60 ISSN 0022-3476

Malik, S.; Cleves, MA.; Honein, MA.; Romitti, PA.; Botto, LD.; Yang, S. & Hobbs, CA. (2008). Maternal smoking and congenital heart defects. *Pediatrics*, Vol.121, No.4, (April 2008), pp. e810-e816, ISSN 1098-4275

Mani, A.; Radhakrishnan, J.; Farhi, A.; Carew, KS.; Warnes, CA.; Nelson-Williams, C.; Day, RW.; Pober, B.; State, MW. & Lifton, RP. (2005). Syndromic patent ductus arteriosus: evidence for haploinsufficient TFAP2B mutations and identification of a linked sleep disorder. *Proceedings of the National Academy of Sciencs of the United States of America*, Vol.102, No.8, (Febuary 2005), pp. 2975-2979, ISSN 1091-6490

Marelli, AJ.; Mackie, AS.; Ionescu-Ittu, R.; Rahme, E. & Pilote, L. (2007). Congenital Heart Disease in the General Population: Changing Prevalence and Age Distribution. *Circulation*, Vol.115, No.2, (January 2007), pp. 163-172, ISSN 1524-4539

Martin, ML. & Khoury, MJ. (1992). Cocaine and single ventricle: a population study. *Teratology*, Vol.46, No.3, (September 1992), pp. 267-270, ISSN 0040-3709

Matalon, KM.; Acosta, PB. & Azen, C. (2003). Role of nutrition in pregnancy with phenylketonuria and birth defects. *Pediatrics*, Vol.112, No.6 Pt 2, (December 2003), pp. 1534-1536, ISSN 1098-9163

Matsuoka, R.; Matsuyama, S.; Yamamoto, Y.; Kuroki, Y. & Matsui, I. (1981). Trisomy 18q. A case report and review of karyotyope-phenotype correlations. *Human Genetics*, Vol.57, No.1, pp. 78-82, ISSN 0340-6717

Mattina, T.; Perrotta, CS. & Grossfeld, P. (2009). Jacobsen syndrome. *Orphanet Journal of Rare Disease*, Vol.4, pp. 9, ISSN 1750-1172

Mazzanti, L. & Cacciari, E. (1998). Congenital heart disease in patients with Turner's syndrome. Italian Study Group for Turner Syndrome (ISGTS). *The Journal of pediatrics*, Vol.133, No.5, (November 1998), pp. 688-698, ISSN 1097-6833

McDaniell, R.; Warthen, DM.; Sanchez-Lara, PA.; Pai, A.; Krantz, ID.; Piccoli, DA. & Spinner, NB. (2006). NOTCH2 mutations cause Alagille syndrome, a heterogeneous disorder of the NOTCH signaling pathway. *American Journal of Human Genetics*, Vol.79, No.1, (July 2006), pp. 169-173, ISSN 0002-9297

McElhinney, DB.; Geiger, E.; Blinder, J.; Benson, DW. & Goldmuntz, E. (2003). NKX2.5 mutations in patients with congenital heart disease. *Journal of American College of Cardiology*, Vol.42, No.9, (November 2003), pp. 1650-1655, ISSN 0735-1097

McElhinney, DB.; Krantz, ID.; Bason, L.; Piccoli, DA.; Emerick, KM.; Spinner, NB. & Goldmuntz, E. (2002). Analysis of cardiovascular phenotype and genotype-phenotype correlation in individuals with a JAG1 mutation and/or Alagille syndrome. *Circulation*, Vol.106, No.20, (November 2002), pp. 2567-2574, ISSN 0007-7322

McFadden, DG. & Olson, EN. (2002). Heart development: learning from mistakes. *Current Option in Genetics & Development.* Vol.12, No.3, (June 2002), pp. 328-335, ISSN 0959-437X

McKellar, SH.; Tester, DJ.; Yagubyan, M.; Majumdar, R.; Ackerman, MJ. & Sundt, TM. (2007). 3rd. Novel NOTCH1 mutations in patients with bicuspid aortic valve disease and thoracic aortic aneurysms *Journal of Thoracic and Cardiovascular Surgery*, Vol.134, No.2, (August 2007), pp. 290-296, ISSN 0022-5223.

Mettler, BA. & Peeler, BB. (2009). Congenital Heart Disease: Surgery in Adult. *Surgical Clinics of North America*, Vo.l89, pp. 1021-1032, ISSN 0039-6109

Micale, L.; Turturo, MG.; Fusco, C.; Augello, B.; Jurado, LA.; Izzi, C.; Digilio, MC.; Milani, D.; Lapi, E.; Zelante, L. & Merla, G. (2010). Identification and characterization of seven novel mutations of elastin gene in a cohort of patients affected by supravalvular aortic stenosis. *European Journal of Human Genetics, Vol.18, No.3, (March 2010), pp. 317-323, ISSN 1476-5438*

Michals-Matalon, K.; Platt, LD.; Acosta, PP.; Azen, C. & Walla, CA. (2002). Nutrient intake and congenital heart defects in maternal phenylketonuria. *American Journal of Obestetrics and Gynecology*, Vol.187, No.2, (August 2002), pp. 441-444, ISSN 1097-6868

Mills, JL.; Troendle, J.; Conley, MR.; Carter, T. & Druschel, CM. (2010). Maternal obesity and congenital heart defects: a population-based study. *The American Journal of Clinical Nutrition*, Vol.91, No.6, (June 2010), pp. 1543-1549, ISSN 1938-3207

Mitchell, SC.; Korones, SB. & Berendes, HW. (1971). Congenital Heart Disease in 56,109 Birhts: Incidence and Natural History. *Circulation*, Vol.43, (March 1971), pp. 323-332, ISSN 1524-4539

Mohamed, SA.; Aherrahrou, Z.; Liptau, H.; Erasmi, AW.; Hagemann, C.; Wrobel, S.; Borzym, K.; Schunkert, H.; Sievers, HH. & Erdmann, J. (2006). Novel missense mutations (p.T596M and p.P1797H) in NOTCH1 in patients with bicuspid aortic valve. *Biochemical and Biophysical Research Communications*, Vol.345, No.4, (July 2006), pp. 1460-1465, ISSN 0006-291X

Moons, P.; Pinxten, S.; Dedroog, D.; Deyk, KV.; Gewillig, M.; Hilderson, D. & Budts, W. (2009). Expectations and Experiences of Adolescents with Congenital Heart Disease on Being Transferred from Pediatric Cardiology to an Adult Congenital Heart Disease Program. *Journal of Adolescent Health*, Vol.44, No.4, (April, 2009), pp. 307-412, ISSN 1054-139X

Morris, CD. (2004). Lessons from epidemiology for the care of women with congenital heart disease. *Progress in Pediatric Cardiology,* Vol.19, pp. 5-13, ISSN 1058-9813

Movahhedian, HR.; Kane, HA.; Borgaonkar, D.; McDermott, M. & Septimus, S. (1991). Heart disease associated with deletion of the short arm of chromosome 18. *Delaware Medical Journal,* Vol.63, No.5, (May 1991), pp. 285-289, ISSN 0011-7781

Muncke, N.; Jung, C.; Rudiger, H.; Ulmer, H.; Roeth, R.; Hubert, A.; Goldmuntz, E.; Driscoll, D.; Goodship, J.; Schon, K. & Rappold, G. (2003). Missense mutations and gene interruption in PROSIT240, a novel TRAP240-like gene, in patients with congenital heart defect (transposition of the great arteries). *Circulation,* Vol.108,No.23, (December 2003), pp. 2843-2850, ISSN 0009-7322

Musewe, NN.; Alexander, DJ.; Teshima, I.; Smallhorn, JF. & Freedom, RM. (1990). Echocardiographic evaluation of the spectrum of cardiac anomalies associated with trisomy 13 and trisomy 18. *Journal of the American College of Cardiology,* Vol.15, No.3, (March 1990), pp. 673-677, ISSN 0735-1097

Neptune, ER.; Frischmeyer, PA.; Arking, DE.; Myers, L.; Bunton, TE.; Gayraud, B.; Ramirez, F.; Sakai, LY. & Dietz, HC. (2003). Dysregulation of TGF-beta activation contributes to pathogenesis in Marfan syndrome. *Nature Genetics,* Vol.33, No.3, (March 2003), pp. 407-411, ISSN 1546-1718

Newman, NM. & Correy, JF. (1983). Possible teratogenicity of sulphasalazine. *The Medical Journal of Australia,* Vol.1, No.11, (May 1983), pp. 528-529, ISSN 1326-5377

O'Brien, MD. & Gilmour-White, S. (1993). Epilepsy and pregnancy. *BMJ,* Vol.307, No.6902, (August 1993), pp. 492-495, ISSN 1468-5833

Oddy, WH.; De Klerk, NH.; Miller, M.; Payne, J. & Bower, C. (2009). Association of maternal pre-pregnancy weight with birth defects: evidence from a case-control study in Western Australia. *The Australian & Nezeland Journal of Obstetrics & Gynaecology,* Vol.49, No.1, (Febuary 2009), pp. 11-15, ISSN 1497-828X

Oster, ME.; Riehle-Colarusso, T.; Alverson, CJ. & Correa, A. (2011). Associations between maternal Fever and influenza and congenital heart defects. *The Journal of Pediatrics,* Vol.158, No.6, (June 2011), pp. 990-995, ISSN 1097-6833

Ozcelik, C.; Bit-Avragim, N.; Panek, A.; Gaio, U.; Geier, C.; Lange, PE.; Dietz, R.; Posch, MG.; Perrot, A. & Stiller, B. (2006). Mutations in the EGF-CFC gene cryptic are an infrequent cause of congenital heart disease. *Pediatric Cardiology, Vol.27, No.6, (November-December 2006), pp. 695-698, ISSN 1432-1971*

Paladini, D.; Tartaglione,, A.; Agangi, A.; Teodoro, A.; Forleo, F.; Borghese, A. & Martinelli, P. (2000). The association between congenital heart disease and Down syndrome in prenatal life. *Ultrasound in Obstetrics & Gynecology,* Vol.15, No.2, (February 2000), pp. 104-108, ISSN 1469-0705

Pejtsik, B.; Pinter, J.; Horvath, M. & Hadnagy, J. (1992). [Relationship between congenital heart disease and various factors affecting pregnancy]. *Orvosi Hetilap,* Vol.133, No.3, (January 1992), pp. 155-158, ISSN 1788-6120

Petersen, S.; Peto, V. & Rayner, M. (2003). *Congenital heart disease statistics 2003, 19 April 2011,* Available from: http: www.heratstats.org

Pizzuti, A.; Sarkozy, A.; Newton, AL.; Conti, E.; Flex, E.; Digilio, MC.; Amati, F.; Gianni, D.; Tandoi, C.; Marino, B.; Crossley, M. & Dallapiccola, B. (2003). Mutations of ZFPM2/FOG2 gene in sporadic cases of tetralogy of Fallot. *Human Genetics,* Vol.22, No.5, (November 2003), pp. 372-377, ISSN 1098-1004

Polymeropoulos, MH.; Ide, SE.; Wright, M.; Goodship, J.; Weissenbach, J.; Pyeritz, RE.; Da Silva, EO.; Ortiz De Luna, RI. & Francomano, CA. (1996). The gene for the Ellis-van Creveld syndrome is located on chromosome 4p16. *Genomics*, Vol.35, No.1, (July 1996), pp. 1-5, ISSN 0888-7543

Potocki, L.; Shaw, CJ.; Stankiewicz, P. & Lupski, JR. (2003). Variability in clinical phenotype despite common chromosomal deletion in Smith-Magenis syndrome [del(17)(p11.2p11.2)]. *Genetics in Medicine*, Vol.5, No.6, (November-December 2003), pp. 430-434, ISSN 1530-0366

Poprawski, K.; Michalski, M.; Lawniczak, M. & Lacka, K. (2009). Cardiovascular abnormalities in patients with Turner syndrome according to Karyotype: own experience and literature review. *Polskie archiwum medycyny wewnetrznej*, Vol.119, No.7-8, (July-August 2009), pp. 453-460, ISSN 0032-3772

Reid, GJ.; Irvine, MJ.; McCrindle, BW.; Sananes, R.; Ritvo, PG.; Siu, SC. & Webb, GD. (2004). Prevalence and Correlates of Successful Transfer From Pediatric to Adult Health Care Among a Cohort of Young Adults With Complex Congenital Heart Defects. *Pediatrics*, Vol.113, No.3, (March 2004), pp. e197-e205, ISSN 1098-4275

Rankin, J.; Chadwick, T.; Natarajan, M.; Howel, D.; Pearce, MS. & Pless-Mulloli, T. (2009). Maternal exposure to ambient air pollutants and risk of congenital anomalies. *Environmental Research*, Vol.109, No.2, pp. 181-187, ISSN 0013-9351

Reid-Lombardo, KM. & Petersen, GM. (2010). Understanding genetic epidermiologic association studies Part 1: fundamentals. *Surgery*, Vol.147, No.4, (April 2010), pp. 469-474, ISSN

Reller, MD.; Stricklland, MJ.; Richle-Colarusso, T.; Mahle, WT. & Correa, A. (2008). Prevalence of Congenital Heart Defect in Metropolitan Atlanta, 1998-2005. *The Journal of Pediatrics*, Vol.153, No.6, (December 2008), pp. 803-813, ISSN 00022-3476

Report of the British Cardiac Society Working Party. (2002). Grown-up congenital heart (GUCH) disease: current needs and provision of service for adolescents and adults with congenital heart disease in the UK. *Heart*, Vol.88, No.1, pp. i1-i4, ISSN 1355-6037

Rischbieth, RH. (1979). Troxidone (trimethadione) embryopathy: case report with reveiw of the literature. *Clinical and Experimental Neurology*, Vol.16, pp. 251-256, ISSN 0196-6383

Ritz, B.; Yu, F.; Fruin, S.; Chapa, G.; Shaw, GM. & Harris, JA. (2002). Ambient air pollution and risk of birth defects in Southern California. *American Journal of Epidemiology*, Vol.155, No.1, (January 2002), pp. 17-25, ISSN 0002-9262

Robicsek, F.; Thubrikar, MJ.; Cook, JW. & Fowler, B. (2004). The congenitally bicuspid aortic valve: how does it function? Why does it fail? *The Annals of Thoracic Surgery*, Vol.77, No.1, (January 2004), pp. 177-185, ISSN 0003-4975

Robinson, SW.; Morris, CD.; Goldmuntz, E.; Reller, MD.; Jones, MA.; Steiner, RD. & Maslen, CL. (2003). Missense mutations in CRELD1 are associated with cardiac atrioventricular septal defects. *American Journal of Human Genetics*, Vol.72, No.4, (April 2003), pp. 1047-1052, ISSN 0002-9297

Rodriguez-Revenga, L.; Badenas, C.; Carrio, A. & Mila, M. (2005). Elastin mutation screening in a group of patients affected by vascular abnormalities. *Pediatric Cardiology*, Vol.26, No.6, (November-December 2005), pp. 827-831, ISSN 1432-1971

Romana-Zelekha, O.; Hirsh, R.; Blieden, L.; Green, MS. & Shohat, T. (2001). The risk for congenital heart defects in offspring of individuals with congenital heart defects. *Clinical Genetics,* Vol.59, (May 2001), pp. 325-329 ISSN 1399-0004

Roisas, PR.; Sijstermans, JM.; Theunissen, PM.; Pulles-Heintberger, CF.; De Die-Smulders, CE.; Engelen, JJ. & Van Der Meer, SB. (2001). Phenotypic variability of the cat eye syndrome. Case report and review of the literature. *Genetic counseling,* Vol.12, No.3, pp. 273-282, ISSN 1015-8146

Rose, V.; Boyd, ARJ. & Ashton, TE. (1964). Incidence of Heart Disease in Children in the City of Toronto. *The Canadian Medical Association* Journal, Vol.91, No.3, (July 1964), pp. 95-100, ISSN 1488-2329

Roskes, EJ.; Boughman, JA.; Schwartz, S. & Cohen, MM. (1990). Congenital cardiovascular malformations (CCVM) and structural chromosome abnormalities: a report of 9 cases and literature review. *Cinical Genetics,* Vol.38, No.3, (September 1990), pp. 198-210, ISSN 0009-9163

Rothman, KJ.; Moore, LL.; Singer, MR.; Nguyen, US.; Mannino, S. & Milunsky, A. (1995). Teratogenicity of high vitamin A intake. *The New England Journal of Medicine,* Vol.333, No.21, (November 1995), pp. 1369-1373, ISSN 1533-4406

Rouse, B. & Azen, C. (2004). Effect of high maternal blood phenylalanine on offspring congenital anomalies and developmental outcome at ages 4 and 6 years: the importance of strict dietary control preconception and throughout pregnancy. *The Journal of Pediatrics,* Vol.44, No.2, (Febuary 2004), pp. 235-239, ISSN 1097-6833

Ruiz-Perez, VL.; Ide, SE.; Strom, TM.; Lorenz, B.; Wilson, D.; Woods, K.; King, L.; Francomano, C.; Freisinger, P.; Spranger, S.; Marino, B.; Dallapiccola, B.; Wright, M.; Meitinger, T.; Polymeropoulos, MH. & Goodship, J. (2000). Mutations in a new gene in Ellis-van Creveld syndrome and Weyers acrodental dysostosis. *Natur Genetics,* Vol.24, No.3, (March 2000), pp. 283-286, ISSN 1546-1718

Satoda, M.; Zhao, F.; Diaz, GA.; Burn, J.; Goodship, J.; Davidson, HR.; Pierpont, ME. & Gelb, BD. (2000). Mutations in TFAP2B cause Char syndrome, a familial form of patent ductus arteriosus. *Nature Genetics,* Vol.25, No.1, (May 2000), pp. 42-46, ISSN 1546-1718

Sarkozy, A.; Conti, E.; Seripa, D.; Digilio, MC.; Grifone, N.; Tandoi, C.; Fazio, VM.; Di Ciommo, V.; Marino, B.; Pizzuh, A. & Dallapiccola, B. (2003). Correlation between PTPN11 gene mutations and congenital heart defects in Noonan and LEOPARD syndromes. *Journal of Medical Genetics,* Vol.40, No.9, (September 2003), pp. 704-708, ISSN 1468-6244

Sayasathid, J.; Tantiwongkosri, K. & Somboonna, N. (2009). Unrecognied Congenital Heart Disease among Thai Children. *Journal of The Medical Association of Thailand,* Vol.92, No.3, (March 2009), pp. 356-359, ISSN 0125-2208

Sayasathid, J.; Supachokchaipattanna, P.; Pipatvech, K.; Sukonpan, K.; Somboonna, N. & Pannarunothai, S. (2010). The prevalence of unrecognized congenital heart disease among healthy elementary school students in northern Thailand. *Asian Biomedicine,* Vol.4, No.1, (February 2010), pp. 171-175, ISSN 1905-7415

Selicomi, A.; Colli, AM.; Passarini, A.; Milani, D.; Cereda, A.; Cerutti, M.; Maitz, S.; Alloni, V.; Salvini, L.; Galli, MA.; Ghiglia, S.; Salice, P. & Danzi, GB. (2009). Analysis of congenital heart defects in 87 consecutive patients with Brachmann-de Lange syndrome. *American Journal of Medical Genetics Part A*, Vol.149A, No.6, (June 2009), pp. 1268-1272, ISSN 1552-4833

Serrano-Martin, MM.; Martinez-Aedo, MJ.; Tartaglia, M. & Lopez-Siguero, JP. (2008). [SOS1 mutation: a new cause of Noonan syndrome]. *Anales de Pediatria (Barcelona, Spain: 2003)*, Vol.68, No.4, (April 2008), pp. 365-368, ISSN 1695-9531

Shaw, GM.; Nelson, V.; Iovannisci, DM.; Finnell, RH. & Lammer, EJ. (2003). Maternal occupational chemical exposures and biotransformation genotypes as risk factors for selected congenital anomalies. *American Journal of Epidemiology*, Vol.157, No.6, (March 2003), pp. 475-484, ISSN 0002-9262

Shaw, GM.; Swan, SH.; Harris, JA. & Malcoe, LH. (1990). Maternal water consumption during pregnancy and congenital cardiac anomalies. *Epidemiology*, Vol.1, No.3, (May 1990), pp. 206-211, ISSN 1531-5487

Shaw, GM.; Wasserman, CR.; O'Malley, CD.; Nelson, V. & Jackson, RJ. (1999). Maternal pesticide exposure from multiple sources and selected congenital anomalies. *Epidemiology*, Vol.10, No.1, (January 1999), pp. 60-66, ISSN 1531-5487

Shprintzen, RJ. (2008). Velo-cardio-facial syndrome: 30 Years of study. *Development Disabilities Research Reviews*, Vol.14, No.1, pp. 3-10, ISSN 1080-4013

Shuib, S.; McMullan, D.; Rattenberry, E.; Barber, RM.; Rahman, F.; Zatyka, M.; Chapman, C.; Macdonald, F.; Latif, F.; Davison, V. & Maher, ER. (2009). Microarray based analysis of 3p25-p26 deletions (3p- syndrome). *American Journal of Medical Genetics Part A*, Vol.149A, No.10, (October 2009), pp. 2099-2105, ISSN 1552-4833

Smithells, RW. & Newman, CG. (1992). Recognition of thalidomide defects. *Journal of Medical Genetics*, Vol.29, No.10, (October 1992), pp. 716-723, ISSN 1468-6244

Singh, KK.; Rommel, K.; Mishra, A.; Karck, M.; Haverich, A.; Schmidtke, J. & Arslan-Kirchner, M. (2006). TGFBR1 and TGFBR2 mutations in patients with features of Marfan syndrome and Loeys-Dietz syndrome. *Human Mutation*, Vol.27, No.8, (August 2006), pp. 770-777, ISSN 1098-1004

Sonoda, T.; Ohdo, S.; Ohba, K.; Okishima, T. & Hayakawa, K. (1993). Sodium valproate-induced cardiovascular abnormalities in the Jcl:ICR mouse fetus: peak sensitivity of gestational day and dose-dependent effect. *Teratology*, Vol.48, No.2, (August 1993), pp. 127-132, ISSN 0040-3709

Stallmeyer, B.; Fenge, H.; Nowak-Gottl, U. & Schulze-Bahr, E. (2010). Mutational spectrum in the cardiac transcription factor gene NKX2.5 (CSX) associated with congenital heart disease. *Cinical Genetics*, Vol.78, No.6, (December 2010), pp. 533-540, ISSN 0009-9163

Strehle, EM. & Bantock, HM. (2003). The phenotype of patients with 4q-syndrome. *Genetic Counseling*, Vol.14, No.2, pp. 195-205, ISSN 1015-8146

Tan, KB. & Yeo, GS. (2009). Pattern of Turner syndrome in Singapore (1999-2004). *Singapore Medical Journal*, Vol.50, No.6, (June 2009), pp. 587-590, ISSN 0037-5675

Tennstedt, C., Chaoui, R.; Korner, H. & Dietel, M. (1999). Spectrum of congenital heart defects and extracardiac malformations associated with chromosomal abnormalities: results of a seven year necropsy study. *Heart*, Vol.82, No.1, (July 1999), pp. 34-39, ISSN 1468-201X

Tevosian, SG.; Deconinck, AE.; Tanaka, M.; Schinke, M.; Litovsky, SH.; Izumo, S.; Fujiwara, Y. & Orkin, SH. (2000). FOG-2, a cofactor for GATA transcription factors, is essential for heart morphogenesis and development of coronary vessels from epicardium. *Cell*, Vol.101, No.7, (June 2000), pp. 729-739, ISSN 0092-8674

Thangaratinam, S.; Daniels, J.; Ewer, AK.; Zamora, J. & Khan, K. (2007). Accuracy of pulse oximetry in screening for congenital disease in asymptomatic newborns: a systematic review. *Archives of Disease in Childhood – Fetal and Neonatal Edition*, Vol.92, (May, 2007), pp. F176-F180, ISSN 1468-2052

Tikkanen, J. & Heinonen, OP. (1991). Maternal hyperthermia during pregnancy and cardiovascular malformations in the offspring. *European Journal of Epidemiology*, Vol.7, No.6, (November 1991), pp. 628-635, ISSN 0393-2990

Tikkanen, J. & Heinonen, OP. (1991). Risk factors for ventricular septal defect in Finland. *Public Health*, Vol.105, No.2, (March 1991), pp. 99-112, ISSN 0033-3506

Tikkanen, J. & Heinonen, OP. (1992). Risk factors for conal malformations of the heart. *European Journal of Epidemiology*, Vol.8, No.1, (January 1992), pp. 48-57, ISSN 0393-2990

Toko, H.; Zhu, W.; Takimoto, E.; Shiojima, I.; Hiroi, Y.; Zou, Y.; Oka, T.; Akazawa, H.; Mizukami, M.; Sakamoto, M.; Terasaki, F.; Kitaura, Y.; Takano, H.; Nagai, T.; Nagai, R. & Komuro, I. (2002). Csx/Nkx2-5 is required for homeostasis and survival of cardiac myocytes in the adult heart. *Journal of Biological Chemistry*, Vol.227, No.27, (July 2002), pp. 24735-24743, ISSN 0021-9258

Tomita-Mitchell, A.; Maslen, CL.; Morris, CD.; Garg, V. & Goldmuntz, E. (2007). GATA4 sequence variants in patients with congenital heart disease. *Journal of Medical Genetics*, Vol.44, No.12, (December 2007), pp. 779-783, ISSN 1468-7212

Tompson, SW.; Ruiz-Perez, VL.; Blair, HJ.; Barton, S.; Navarro, V.; Robson, JL.; Wright, MJ. & Goodship, JA. (2007). Sequencing EVC and EVC2 identifies mutations in two-thirds of Ellis-van Creveld syndrome patients. *Human Genetics*, Vol.120, No.5, (January 2007), pp. 663-670, ISSN 0340-6717

Tsai, CH.; Van Dyke, DL. &, Feldman, GL. (1999). Child with velocardiofacial syndrome and del (4)(q34.2): another critical region associated with a velocardiofacial syndrome-like phenotype. *American Journal of Medical Genetics Part A*, Vol.82, No.4, (Febuary 1999), pp. 336-339, ISSN 0148-7299

Van Esch, H.; Groenen, P.; Fryns, JP.; Van de Ven, W. & Devriendt, K. (1999). The phenotypic spectrum of the 10p deletion syndrome versus the classical DiGeorge syndrome. *Genetic Counseling*, Vol.10, No.1, pp. 59-65, ISSN 1015-8146

Van Praagh, S.; Truman, T.; Firpo, A.; Bano-Rodrigo, A.; Freied, R.; McManus, B.; Engle, MA. & Van Praagh, R. (1989). Cardiac malformation in trisomy-18: a study of 41 postmortem cases. *Journal of the American College of Cardiology*, Vol.13, No.7, (June 1989), pp. 1586-1597, ISSN 1558-3597

Wacker, A.; Kaemmerer, H.; Hollweek, R.; Hauser, M.; Deutsch, MA.; Brodherr, H.; Eicken, A. & Hess, J. (2005). Outcome of operated and unoperated adults with congenital cardiac disease lost to follow-up for more than five years. *American Journal of Cardiology*, Vol.95, No.6, (March 2005), pp. 776-779, ISSN 0002-9149

Wang, NK.; Shen, CT. & Lin, MS. (2007). Results of Echocardiographic Screening in 10,000 Newborns. *Acta Paediatric Taiwan*, Vol.48, No.1, pp. 7-9, ISSN 1608-8115

Wat, MJ.; Shchelochkov, OA.; Holder, AM.; Breman, AM.; Dagli, A.; Bacino, C.; Scaglia, F.; Zori, RT.; Cheung, SW.; Scott, DA. & Kang, SHL. (2009). Chromosome 8p23.1 deletions as a cause of complex congenital heart defects and diaphragmatic hernia.

American Journal of Medical Genetics Part A, Vol. 149A, No.8, (August 2009), pp. 1661-1677, ISSN 1552-4833

Watkins, ML. & Botto, LD. (2001). Maternal prepregnancy weight and congenital heart defects in offspring. *Epidemiology*, Vol.12, No.4, (July 2001), pp. 439-446, ISSN 1531-5487

Webster, WS. (1998). Teratogen update: congenital rubella. *Teratology*, Vol.58, No.1, (July 1998), pp. 13-23, ISSN 0040-3709

Webb, CL.; Jenkin, KJ.; Parpawich, PP.; Bolger, AF.; Conner, RM.; Allen, HD. & Barst, RJ. (2002). Collaborative Care for Adults With Congenital Heart Disease. *Circulation*, Vol.105, No.23, (May 2002), pp. 2318-2323, ISSN 1524-4539

Weijerman, ME.; van Furth, AM.; van der Mooren, MD.; van Weissenbruch, MM.; Rammeloo, L. & Broers, CJ. (2010). Prevalence of congenital heart defects and persistent pulmonary hypertension of the neonate with Down syndrome. *European Journal of Pediatrics*, Vol.169, No.10, (October 2010), pp. 1195-1199, ISSN 1432-1076

Willhite, CC.; Hill, RM. & Irving, DW. (1986). Isotretinoin-induced craniofacial malformations in humans and hamsters. *Journal of Craniofacial Genetics and Development Biology – Supplement*, Vol.2, pp. 193-209, ISSN 0890-6661

Wilson, GN.; Baker, DL.; Schau, J. & Paker, J. (1984). Cat eye syndrome owing to tetrasomy 22pter leads to q11. *Journal of Medical Genetics*, Vol.21, No.1, (February 1984), pp. 60-63, ISSN 1468-6244

Winter, RM.; Donnai, D.; Burn, J. & Tucker, SM. (1987). Fetal valproate syndrome: is there a recognisable phenotype? *Journal of Medical Genetics*, Vol.24, No.11, (November 1987), pp. 692-695, ISSN 1468-6244

Wren, C.; Birrell, G. & Hawthorne, G. (2003). Cardiovascular malformations in infants of diabetic mothers. *Heart*, Vol89, No.10, (October 2003), pp. 1217-1220, ISSN 1355-6037

Wu, MH.; Chen, HC.; Lu, CW.; Wang, JK.; Huang, SC. & Huang, SK. (2010). Prevalence of Congenital Heart Disease at Live Birth in Taiwan. *The Journal of Pediatrics*, Vol.156, No.5, (May 2010). pp. 782-785, ISSN 0022-3476

Wyatt, JW.; Frias, JL.; Hoyme, HE.; Jovanovic, L.; Kaaja, R.; Brown, F.; Garg, S.; Lee-Parritz, A.; Seely, EW.; Kerr, L.; Mattoo, V. & Tan, M. (2005). Congenital anomaly rate in offspring of mothers with diabetes treated with insulin lispro during pregnancy. *Diabetic Medicine*, Vol.22, No.6, (June 2005), pp. 803-807, ISSN 1464-5491

Xin, N.; Qiu, GR.; Gong, LG.; Xu, XY. & Sun, KL.(2009). [The mechanism of TBX5 abnormal expression in simple congenital heart disease]. Yi Chuan. 2009 Apr;31(4):374-80. *YiChuan*, Vol.31, No.4, (April 2009), pp. 374-380, ISSN 0253-9772

Xu, H.; Morishima, M.; Wylie, JN.; Schwartz, RJ.; Bruneau, BG.; Lindsay, EA. & Baldini, A. (2004). Tbx1 has a dual role in the morphogenesis of the cardiac outflow tract. *Development*, Vol.131, No.13, (July 2004), pp. 97-101, ISSN 1461-7072

Yagi, H.; Furutani, Y.; Hamada, H.; Sasaki, T.; Asakawa, S.; Minoshima, S.; Ichida, F.; Joo, K.; Kimura, M.; Imamura, S.; Kamatani, N.; Momma, K.; Takao, A.; Nakazawa, M.; Shimizu, N. & Matsuoka, R. (2003). Role of TBX1 in human del22q11.2 syndrome. *Lancet*, Vol.362, No.9393, (October 2003), pp. 1366-1373, ISSN 0140-6736

Yan, YT.; Gritsman, K.; Ding, J.; Burdine, RD.; Corrales, JD.; Price, SM.; Talbot, WS.; Schier, AF. & Shen, MM. (1999). Conserved requirement for EGF-CFC genes in vertebrate left-right axis formation. *Gene & Development*, Vol.13, No.19, (October 1999), pp. 2527-2537, ISSN 1549-5477

Yu, ZB.; Han, SP. & Guo, XR. (2008). [A Meta-analysis on the risk factors of perinatal congenital heart disease in Chinese people]. *Zhonghua Liuxingbingxue Zazhi*, Vol.29, No.11, (November 2008), pp. 1137-1140, ISSN 0254-6450

Zatyka, M.; Priestley, M.; Ladusans, EJ.; Fryer, AE.; Mason, J.; Latif, F. & Maher, ER. (2005). Analysis of CRELD1 as a candidate 3p25 atrioventicular septal defect locus (AVSD2). *Clinical Genetics*, Vol.67, No.6, (June 2005), pp. 526-528, ISSN 0009-9163

Zhang, L.; Zhang, XH.; Ren, MH. & Song, GN. (2010). [Chromosomosome abnormalities and congenital heart diseases: a retrospective on 49 cases]. *Journal of Sichuan University. Medical science edition*, Vol.41, No.2, (March 2010), pp. 312-315, ISSN 1672-173X

Zhao, F.; Weismann, CG.; Satoda, M.; Pierpont, ME.; Sweeney, E.; Thompson, EM. & Gelb, BD. (2001). Novel TFAP2B mutations that cause Char syndrome provide a genotype-phenotype correlation. *American Journal of Human Genetics*, Vol.69, No.4, (October 2001), pp. 695-703, ISSN 0002-9297

Zhu, L.; Harutyunyan, KG.; Peng, JL.; Wang, J.; Schwartz, RJ. & Belmont, JW. (2007). Identification of a novel role of ZIC3 in regulating cardiac development. *Human Molecular Genetics*, Vol.16, No.14, (July 2007), pp. 1649-1660, ISSN 0964-6906

Zomer, AC.; Vaartjes, I.; Uiterwaal, CS.; Van der Velde, ET.; Van der Merkhof, LF.; Baur, LH.; Ansink, TJ.; Cozijnsen, L.; Pieper, PG.; Meijboom, FJ.; Grobbee, DE. & Mulder, BJ. (2010). Circumstances of death in adult congenital heart disease. *International Journal of Cardiology*, (October 2010), doi:10.1016/j.ijcard.2010.09.015

3

Recent Advances Concerning the Molecular Mechanism of Patent Ductus Arteriosus

Susumu Minamisawa[1] and Utako Yokoyama[2]
[1]*Waseda University*
[2]*Yokohama City University*
Japan

1. Introduction

The ductus arteriosus (DA), a fetal arterial shunt between the main pulmonary artery and the descending aorta, is a normal and essential fetal structure. Normally, the DA begins to close immediately after birth, but in some cases it remains patent after birth. Postnatal patent DA (PDA) is a major cause of morbidity and mortality in premature infants, leading to severe complications including pulmonary hypertension, right ventricular dysfunction, postnatal infections, and respiratory failure (Hermes-DeSantis & Clyman, 2006). The incidence of PDA among full-term newborns has been estimated at one in 500, and in preterm newborns it accounts for the majority of all congenital heart disease cases (Mitchell, 1971). The incidence of PDA exceeds 30% in preterm babies with birth weights <1,500 g (Van Overmeire, 2004). Curiously, patent DA can be essential for patients with complex congenital heart diseases in which the systemic or pulmonary circulation is dependent on the passage of blood through the DA. Therefore, a thorough understanding of the precise molecular mechanism underlying DA closure is very important in pediatric cardiovascular medicine.

Closure of the human DA occurs in two phases: functional closure of the lumen within the first hours after birth by smooth muscle constriction, and anatomic occlusion of the lumen over the next several days due to extensive neointimal thickening and vascular remodelling. Although this overall process is similar among all mammals, the time course of the two phases varies among species.

DA constriction after birth is induced by an increase in arterial oxygen tension, a dramatic decline in circulating prostaglandinE_2 (PGE_2), and a decrease in blood pressure within the DA lumen (Smith 1998; Clyman 2006). Anatomical closure of the DA is associated with a unique system of differentiation of the vessel wall. The most prominent phenotypic change is intimal thickening, a process characterized by (a) an area of subendothelial deposition of extracellular matrix, (b) the disassembly of the internal elastic lamina and loss of elastic fiber in the medial layer, and (c) the migration of undifferentiated medial smooth muscle cells (SMCs) into the subendothelial space. The DA later undergoes permanent closure through structural remodelling and fibrosis. The resulting fibrous band with no lumen persists in the adult as the ligamentum arteriosum (Fay & Cooke 1972). The cascade of events is thought to orchestrate the activation of subsequent signalling pathways, leading finally to the complete obliteration of the DA. In this chapter, we focus on reviewing the current state of knowledge regarding the mechanisms by which vascular remodelling of the DA is regulated.

2. Anatomical closure of the DA

After birth, extensive remodelling of the DA wall occurs, leading to permanent closure of the DA. Although these rapid changes are readily apparent after birth, the structural remodelling of the DA has already begun in late gestation, under the control of the abovementioned unique differentiation system. Therefore, the DA has a distinct structural character from its neighboring arteries. For example, smooth muscle myosin isoform SM2, which is predominantly expressed in adult arteries, is highly expressed in the fetal DA (Kim, 1993).

2.1 Physiological intimal thickening of the DA

Intimal thickening, though often observed in pathological arteries, such as injured or atherosclerotic arteries, is also a characteristic developmental structural change in the DA. The intimal thickening that occurs in the DA is physiological in nature and is required for postnatal DA closure (Rabinovitch, 1996; Yokoyama. 2006a). In rats, intimal thickening can be observed in the mature DA on the 21st day of gestation, though it is not observed in the immature DA on the 19th day of gestation. Intimal thickening starts with a lifting of the endothelial cells. Accumulations of hyaluronan and other extracellular matrices in the subendothelial region and fragmention of the inner elastic lamina provide optimal conditions for the migration of SMCs into the subendothelial region (De Reeder, 1988). These changes in DA structure have been well investigated both in rodents and in humans. Given that intimal thickening is poorly developed in patients with PDA and in animal models of PDA (Gittenberger-de Groot, 1980; Gittenberger-de Groot,1985; Tada,1985), this process must play a critical role in permanent closure of the DA after birth. Therefore, a common molecular mechanism must underlie the development of intimal thickening of the DA in humans and animals alike.

2.2 Molecular mechanisms underlying intimal thickening

Intimal thickening is associated with many characteristic phenomena such as the proliferation and migration of SMCs, the accumulation of extracellular matrix in the subendothelial region, and the fragmention of the inner elastic lamina. Analysis of the causal genes of this complex process in patients with PDA and animal models of PDA is resulting in significant progress toward understanding the molecular mechanism underlying it.

2.2.1 Cyclooxygenase (COX): The generator of PGE_2

The cyclooxygenases COX1 and COX2 catalyze the synthesis of prostaglandin H, a precursor of biologically active prostaglandins including PGE_2, from arachidonic acid. Therefore COX inhibitors such as indomethacin are often used for treatment of PDA to induce vasoconstriction of the DA by attenuating the synthesis of PGE_2. Exposure *in utero* to indomethacin induces premature closure of the DA. Interestingly, it has been reported that infants of mothers who received indomethacin tocolysis are susceptible to symptomatic PDA. These contradictory observations suggest that a relatively complex mechanism underlies the role of COX1 and COX2 in the DA. Furthermore, genetic disruption of COX1 and COX2 results in postnatal PDA (Loftin, 2001). As seen in COX-deleted mice, COX2 plays a primary role in DA closure after birth, and its effect is attenuated in cases of preterm gestation. In addition to COX2, COX1 also contributes to DA closure in a gene dosage-dependent manner (Loftin, 2001; Loftin, 2002). Although it is not apparent from the literature why COX deletion causes PDA in mice, we assume that the same mechanism should work as described below in mice harboring deletion of the EP4 gene, a predominant PGE_2 receptor in the DA. Trivedi et al. have demonstrated that COX2 expression is attenuated in EP4-deleted mice (Trivedi,. 2006), suggesting the existence of a positive feedback loop in COX-PGE_2 cascades.

2.2.2 Prostacyclin (PGI_2)

Dogs have been studied as an animal model of inherited PDA because their histological features of normal DA and PDA closely resemble those of humans. Through such studies, De Reeder et al. have demonstrated that the expression of PGI_2 synthase is high in the endothelium and low in vascular SMCs in PDA and other patent neighboring arteries. In normally closing DA, in contrast, high amounts of PGI_2 are found in the vascular SMCs of the intimal cushions, suggesting that PGI_2 plays a role in the onset of intimal thickening (de Reeder, 1989).

2.2.3 PGE_2 – EP4: A critical player in regulating intimal thickening

PGE_2, the most potent vasodilator affecting the DA, is produced in the placenta (Smith 1998) and in the DA itself (Clyman, 1978; Coceani, 1978). During gestation, PGE_2 contributes to DA patency *in utero*. Stimulation of PGE_2 receptors activates adenylyl cyclases (ACs). The resulting increased intracellular concentrations of cyclic AMP (cAMP) inhibit myosin light chain kinase, inducing DA relaxation (Smith 1998). The dilator effect of PGE_2 on the mammalian DA is mediated mainly by the PGE_2 receptor, EP4. After birth, the concentration of circulating PGE_2 declines dramatically as the placenta is removed and PGE_2 is rapidly catabolised through lung circulation. Furthermore, the expression levels of PGE_2 receptors are decreased in the DA wall (Smith 1998).

Although PGE_2 plays a primary role in maintaining the patency of the DA, previous studies have demonstrated that genetic disruption of EP4 paradoxically results in fatal PDA in mice (Nguyen, 1997; Segi, 1998). We have found that intimal thickening was completely absent in DA from EP4-disrupted neonatal mice (Yokoyama, 2006a). Moreover, a marked reduction in hyaluronan production was found in EP4-disrupted DA, whereas a thick layer of hyaluronan deposit was present in wild-type DA. PGE_2-EP4-cAMP-protein kinase A (PKA) signalling up-regulates hyaluronan synthase type 2 mRNA, which increases hyaluronan production in the DA. Accumulation of hyaluronan then promotes SMCs migration into the subendothelial layer to induce intimal thickening (Yokoyama, 2006a). Therefore, signalling through PGE_2-EP4 plays two essential roles in DA development, namely, vascular dilation and intimal thickening.

2.2.4 Specific adenylyl cyclases regulate intimal thickening of the DA

Chronic PGE_2-EP4-AC-cAMP-PKA signalling during gestation induces vascular remodelling of the DA and thereby promotes hyaluronan-mediated intimal thickening and structural closure of the vascular lumen. Both PGE_1 and PGE_2 also induce vasodilation in the DA. Since intracellular cAMP is synthesized by ACs, which are transmembrane enzymes activated by G protein-coupled receptors, including PGE receptors, ACs must play an important role in regulating vasodilation and remodelling in the DA. To date, nine different isoforms of membrane-bound forms of ACs (AC1 through AC9) have been identified in vertebrate tissues. Most tissues express several AC isoforms, which exhibit remarkable diversity in their biochemical properties (Sunahara & Taussig 2002). Since SMCs in the DA exhibit biological properties distinct from those of SMCs in other vessels such as the aorta, it is possible to identify specific AC isoforms that play a distinct role in the DA. Recent advances concerning AC isoform-selective activation or inhibition have allowed us to investigate the role of AC isoforms and the availability of AC isoform-selective activators in regulating DA vascular tone and remodelling. AC2 and AC6, for example, are more highly expressed in rat DA than in the aorta during the perinatal period (Yokoyama, 2010). AC6-targeted siRNA counteracts PGE-induced hyaluronan production in rat DA SMCs. Overexpression of AC6 enhances PGE-induced hyaluronan production and induces intimal thickening in DA explants. Furthermore, intimal thickening of the DA is less marked in mice lacking AC6 than in wild-type mice. Interestingly, stimulation of AC2 attenuates AC6-induced hyaluronan production via inhibition of the p38 mitogen-activated protein kinase pathway and AC6-induced intimal thickening of the DA. The AC2/6 activator 6-[N-(2-isothiocyanatoethyl) aminocarbonyl] forskolin (FD1) does not induce hyaluronan-mediated intimal thickening in DA explants, though the AC5/6 activator 6-[3-(dimethylamino)propionyl]-14 15-dihydroforskolin (FD6) does. Therefore AC6 must be responsible for hyaluronan-mediated intimal thickening of the DA, while AC2 inhibits AC6-induced hyaluronan production. It should be noted that the DA is dilated by stimulation with both FD1 and FD6, the effect of which is longer than that of stimulation with PGE_1 (Yokoyama, 2010). These data suggest that the activation of both AC2 and AC6 induces vasodilation, although the effectiveness of AC2 and AC6 activation has not yet been directly investigated. Administration of FD1 induces vasodilation without intimal thickening of the DA, suggesting that combinative stimulation with AC2 and AC6 or AC2-specific stimulation may be a novel alternative therapy to current PGE therapy for patients with DA-dependent congenital heart disease.

2.2.5 Epac (Exchange Protein Activated by cAMP): A novel target of cAMP

A new target of cAMP, i.e., a new exchange protein activated by cAMP, has recently been discovered and is called Epac. Epac has been known to utilize a distinct cAMP signalling pathway that is independent of PKA (Bos 2006). Epac is a guanine nucleotide exchange protein that regulates the activity of small G proteins. There are two variants: Epac1 is expressed in most tissues, including the heart and blood vessels, whereas Epac2 is expressed in the adrenal gland and the brain. Although both Epac1 and Epac2 are up-regulated during the perinatal period, Epac1, but not Epac2, acutely promotes SMC migration and thus intimal thickening in the DA (Yokoyama, 2008). Since Epac stimulation does not increase hyaluronan production, the effect of Epac1 on SMC migration is independent of that of hyaluronan accumulation, which operates through a mechanism different from that underlying PKA stimulation. Epac stimulation improves the organization of actin stress fibers and enhances focal adhesion of DA SMCs. Therefore, the EP4-cAMP signal pathway can induce intimal thickening in the DA via a PKA-dependent mechanism or an Epac-dependent mechanism.

2.2.6 Oxygen and reactive oxygen species

The DA is an oxygen-sensitive tissue, and oxygen is its most potent vasoconstrictor. The DA senses the change in oxygen tension through the change in redox status. Redox and reactive oxygen species are known to play an important role in vascular remodelling of pathological arteries. Therefore, the change in oxygen tension that occurs after birth should affect postnatal vascular remodelling of the DA. In this regard, Clyman's group has demonstrated that muscular constriction produces a region of ischemic hypoxia in the middle of the ductus muscle media and that intense hypoxia within the constricted vessel wall of the DA induces vascular endothelial cell growth factor (VEGF), which in turn stimulates neointimal proliferation and vasa vasorum ingrowth (Waleh, 2010; Clyman, 2002). They have also emphasized that hypoxia in the vessel wall plays a role in permanent DA closure. Yet before the blood flow through the DA is completely obstructed, the DA is exposed to blood containing higher oxygen content after birth compared to the blood passing through it during the fetal period. Recently we have found that oxygenation promotes migration of DA SMCs followed by intimal thickening of the rat DA (unpublished data). Accordingly, oxygenation, in addition to inducing contraction, plays an important role in completing DA closure through promoting intimal thickening after PGE_2 removal. Further investigation is warranted to elucidate the molecular mechanism by which oxygenation promotes intimal thickening of the DA.

2.2.7 Calcium channel

A growing body of evidence has demonstrated that voltage-dependent calcium channels (VDCCs), in addition to their role in determining the contractile state, play an important role in regulating differentiation, proliferation, migration, and gene expression in vascular SMCs. VDCCs are classified according to their distinct electrophysiological and pharmacological properties into low-voltage-activated (T-type) and high-voltage-activated (L-, N-, P-, Q-, and R-type) VDCCs. VDCCs consist of different combinations of α1 subunits and auxiliary subunits. Among the α1 subunits, α1C and α1G are the most predominant isoforms in the rat DA (Yokoyama, 2006b). In addition to a conventional α1C subunit, a novel alternatively spliced variant of the α1C isoform is highly expressed in the neointimal cushion of the rat DA, although the role of the spliced variant of the α1C isoform in neointimal cushion formation has not yet been investigated (Yokoyama, 2006b). Interestingly, α1G, a T-type VDCC, is significantly up-regulated in oxygenated rat DA tissue and in the region of intimal thickening in the DA (Akaike, 2009). α1G plays a role in migration of DA SMCs and neointimal cushion formation. *R(-)*-efonidipine, a T-type VDCC-specific antagonist, delays the closure of the rat DA through inhibiting the contraction and neointimal formation of the DA (Akaike, 2009). Therefore, isoform-specific inhibition of VCDD may be an alternative therapeutic strategy to regulate the patency of the DA.

2.2.8 Cytokines

Inflammatory responses to vascular injury or atherosclerosis are known to be associated with the pathogenesis of neointimal thickening. Given that several proinflammatory cytokines are known to play an essential role during vascular remodelling, it is reasonable to assume that cytokines might contribute to physiological vascular remodelling processes as well, in particular, the permanent closure of the DA. Accordingly, it is likely that VEGF stimulates neointimal proliferation and vasa vasorum ingrowth during permanent DA closure, as described above (Waleh, 2010; Clyman, 2002). In addition, transforming growth factor-beta (TGF-β) 1 in endothelial cells and SMCs probably regulates vascular remodelling of the DA, though the function and expression of TGF-β 1 in the DA are controversial (Tannenbaum, 1996; Zhou, 1998).

Clyman's group has demonstrated that the expression levels of vascular cell adhesion molecule (VCAM)-1 (an important ligand for the mononuclear cell adhesion receptor VLA4), E-selectin, IL-8, macrophage colony stimulating factor-1, CD154, interferon-gamma, IL-6, and tumor necrosis factor-alpha are increased in the ductus wall. They have also found that VLA4+ monocytes/macrophages (CD68+ and CD14+) and, to a lesser extent, T-lymphocytes adhere to the postnatal DA (Waleh, 2005).

The expression of IL-15 mRNA is significantly higher in rat DA than in the aorta. IL-15 immunoreactivity is detected predominantly in the internal elastic laminae, and to a lesser extent in SMCs, in the rat DA. IL-15 attenuates PDGF-BB-mediated SMC proliferation and PGE_1-induced hyaluronan production in a dose-dependent manner. Accordingly, IL-15 might have an inhibitory effect on the physiological vascular remodelling processes involved in closing the DA (Iwasaki, 2007).
Moreover, growth hormones promote the migration of DA SMCs, thus enhancing intimal cushion formation in the DA. Growth hormones also regulate the expression of cytoskeletal, genes in DA SMCs, which may retain a synthetic phenotype in the smooth muscle-specific cytoskeletal genes (Jin, 2011).

2.3 Vascular smooth muscle differentiation

SMCs retain the ability to reversibly alter their phenotype in response to various environmental and physiological changes (McDonald and Owens 2007). This property has been termed phenotypic switching or SMC plasticity. Contractile SMCs express high levels of contractile proteins involved in establishing and maintaining myofilament structure and function, including SM22α, SMA and SMMHC. In contrast, synthetic SMCs express lower levels of contractile muscle proteins and have higher rates of proliferation, migration and production of extracellular matrix components. The DA is a very specialized blood vessel, with a vascular wall composed of highly differentiated and contractile smooth muscle (Slomp, 1997). A unique transcriptional program is probably responsible for generating this particular artery during fetal development (Ivey, 2008). A growing body of evidence has demonstrated that maturation and differentiation of DA SMCs is essential for postnatal DA closure. Deletion of several factors that are required for DA SMCs to adopt a contractile phenotype results in PDA. It should be noted, however, that neointimal thickening is induced by migrating and proliferating vascular SMCs, which are characterized as a dedifferentiated (synthetic) phenotype. Therefore, the DA must consist of SMCs exhibiting phenotypic heterogeneity.

2.3.1 Myocardin

Myocardin is a remarkably potent transcriptional coactivator that regulates SMC contractile proteins. Myocardin-null mouse embryos exhibit a block in vascular SMC differentiation as well as defects in the yolk sac vasculature (Li, 2003). Importantly, mice generated after selective myocardin ablation of cardiac neural crest-derived vascular SMCs exhibit PDA and die at postnatal day 3 (Huang, 2008). In these mutant mice, the *myocardin*-deficient vascular SMCs populating the DA exhibit ultrastructural features generally associated with the synthetic, rather than the contractile, SMC phenotype. In addition, the architecture of the neointima and tunica media of the DA is markedly disturbed in association with a dramatic increase in extracellular matrix and a relative decrease in vascular SMC volume. These data demonstrate that myocardin regulates the expression of genes required to induce the contractile phenotype in neural crest–derived SMCs and provide new insights into the molecular and genetic systems that underlie the vascular remodeling of the DA.

2.3.2 TFAP2B

Identifying gene mutations in TFAP2B, a neural crest cell-specific transcription factor involved in Char syndrome, is one of the most important discoveries regarding the molecular mechanism of PDA. Char syndrome is a genetic syndrome consisting of PDA in association with facial anomalies and minor skeletal anomalies (Chen, 2011; Satoda, 2000; Khetyar, 2008). In addition, Ivey et al. has demonstrated that TFAP2B disruption affects the development of vascular SMCs in the DA (Ivey, 2008), although they did not observe morphological differences between TFAP2B-/- and wild-type mice at embryonic days 13.5, 15.5 and 18.5. It will be intriguing to examine in future studies whether TFAP2B plays a role in neointimal formation of the DA.

2.3.3 Jag1

The evolutionarily conserved Notch signaling pathway plays a major role in vascular development in mammals and other vertebrates (Kurpinski, 2010; High, 2008). Mice with SMC-specific deletion of Jag1, which encodes a Notch ligand, die postnatally from PDA (Feng, 2010). These mice exhibit defects in contractile SMC differentiation in the medial vascular wall of the DA, which therefore fails to express contractile SMC proteins. However, the differentiation of contractile vascular SMCs is confined to the region adjacent to the endothelial cell layer in the DA. Therefore, propagation of the Jag1-Notch signal throughout the width of the vascular wall is required for contractile SMC differentiation of the DA.

2.4 Extracellular matrix involved in vascular remodelling of the DA

Vascular cells are defined by the ways in which they regulate their extracellular matrix, and changes in the extracellular matrix, in turn, determine vascular cell phenotype, i.e. the ability to differentiate, proliferate, and migrate (Rabinovitch, 1996). As described in section 2.2.3, PGE-induced hyarulonan plays a critical role in the onset of intimal thickening of the DA (De Reeder, 1988; Yokoyama, 2006a). In addition, it has been reported that DA SMCs produce twice as much fibronectin as aortic SMCs do (Rabinovitch, 1996). Mason et al. have demonstrated that preventing fibronectin-dependent intimal thickening would be a feasible manipulation to cause PDA as a mode of treatment of congenital heart diseases (Mason, 1999). TGF β and nitric oxide induce extracellular matrix, including hyaluronan and fibronectin, in DA SMCs (Rabinovitch, 1996). Future studies will be needed to determine the other constituents of extracellular matrix that play a role in vascular remodelling of the DA.

2.5 Disassembly of the internal elastic lamina and loss of elastic fiber in the medial layer of the DA

The disassembly and fragmentation of the internal elastic lamina and sparse elastic fibers in the middle layer of the DA is a hallmark of vascular remodelling in the DA. In the normally closing DA, impaired elastogenesis coincides with increased SMC migration and proliferation, contributing to physiological occlusion. The reduced elasticity of the DA wall may help its structure collapse easily as a prelude to postnatal permanent closure of the DA. In PDA, in contrast, an abundance of elastin lamellae in the intima, a subendothelial elastic lamina, and a failure of intimal SMC migration are found in humans and animal models (de Reeder, 1990; Hinek, 1991; Slomp, 1992). In humans and in animal models such as canine puppies and the inbred Brown-Norway (BN) rat (Bokenkamp, 2006), the subendothelial elastic lamina is thought to limit the passage of SMCs from the media to the intima. In PDA in BN rats, the media of elastin lamellae are absent, and the intima contains many elastic fibers. The abnormal distribution of elastin in the PDA of BN rats suggests that impaired elastin metabolism is related to the persistence of the DA and implicates a genetic factor that may link the PDA with aortic fragility. In this regard, recent studies have identified a new aortic aneurysm syndrome that is due to mutations in the TGF β receptors 1 and 2 and is associated with PDA and ductal aneurysm (Loeys, 2005). Further investigation is required to identify the molecular mechanism underlying the impaired elastogenesis in cases of DA.

3. Conclusion

Ductal closure occurs in two phases. In full-term newborns, the first few hours after birth see acute and functional closure as a result of smooth muscle contraction of the DA, which is triggered by an increase in oxygen tension and a decline in levels of circulating PGE_2. Importantly, prior to this, anatomical vascular remodelling occurs under the control of highly conserved yet complex molecular mechanisms. This remodelling requires a specific sequence of processes, which includes the differentiation of vascular SMCs and endothelial cells, the accumulation of extracellular matrix, vascular SMC migration into the subendothelial region, impaired elastogenesis, and eventually fibrotic changes due to apoptosis and necrosis. Recent advances in high-throughput genetic screening for human diseases and genetically manipulated animal models of PDA have facilitated the identification of pathways and genes involved in development and closure of the DA. As seen in the PGE_2-EP4-cAMP signal pathway as well as in the oxygen and calcium channels, multiple vasoreactive stimulations can serve as an important modulator of vascular remodelling of the DA. In this regard, endothelin-1, nitric oxide, and other vasoreactive factors in the DA that we have not discussed here in detail may play a role in vascular remodelling of the DA. Thus, it is reasonable to infer that endothelial cells in the DA may also play an important role in the differentiation of vascular SMCs, which are considered to be a pivotal cellular structure in the pathogenesis of PDA. In addition to its role in controlling vascular tone in the functional closure of the DA, the vascular remodelling of the DA is now attracting considerable attention as a target for novel therapeutic strategies for patients with PDA and DA-dependent cardiac anomalies.

4. Acknowledgments

This work was supported by grants from the Grant-in-Aid for Scientific Research (KAKENHI) (U.Y.), the Ministry of Health, Labor and Welfare of Japan (S.M. U.Y.), the Ministry of Education, Culture, Sports, Science and Technology of Japan (S.M.), the Yokohama Foundation for Advanced Medical Science (S.M., U.Y.), the Kanae Foundation for the Promotion for Medical Science (U.Y.), the Miyata Cardiology Research Promotion Funds (S.M., U.Y.), the Takeda Science Foundation (S.M., U.Y.), the Sumitomo Foundation (U.Y.), the Japan Heart Foundation Research Grant (U.Y.), the Kowa Life Science Foundation (U.Y.), the Uehara Memorial Foundation (U.Y.), "High-Tech Research Center" Project for Private Universities: MEXT (S.M.), a Waseda University Grant for Special Research Projects (S.M.), and the Vehicle Racing Commemorative Foundation (S.M.).

5. References

Akaike, T., Jin, M. H., Yokoyama, U., Izumi-Nakaseko, H., Jiao, Q., Iwasaki, S., Iwamoto, M., Nishimaki, S., Sato, M., Yokota, S., Kamiya, Y., Adachi-Akahane, S., Ishikawa, Y. & Minamisawa, S. (2009). T-type Ca2+ channels promote oxygenation-induced closure of the rat ductus arteriosus not only by vasoconstriction but also by neointima formation.*J Biol Chem* Vol.284, No.36, Sep 4 2009.pp.24025-34, ISSN 0021-9258

Bokenkamp, R., Gittenberger-De Groot, A. C., Van Munsteren, C. J., Grauss, R. W., Ottenkamp, J. & Deruiter, M. C. (2006). Persistent ductus arteriosus in the Brown-Norway inbred rat strain.*Pediatr Res* Vol.60, No.4, Oct 2006.pp.407-12, ISSN 0031-3998

Bos, J. L. (2006). Epac proteins: multi-purpose cAMP targets.*Trends Biochem Sci* Vol.31, No.12, Dec 2006.pp.680-6, ISSN 0968-0004

Chen, Y. W., Zhao, W., Zhang, Z. F., Fu, Q., Shen, J., Zhang, Z., Ji, W., Wang, J. & Li, F. (2011) Familial Nonsyndromic Patent Ductus Arteriosus Caused by Mutations in TFAP2B.*Pediatr Cardiol* Jun 4. 2011. ISSN 1432-1971

Clyman, R. I. (2006). Mechanisms regulating the ductus arteriosus.*Biol Neonate* Vol.89, No.4, 2006.pp.330-5, ISSN 0006-3126

Clyman, R. I., Mauray, F., Roman, C. & Rudolph, A. M. (1978). PGE2 is a more potent vasodilator of the lamb ductus arteriosus than is either PGI2 or 6 keto PGF1alpha.*Prostaglandins* Vol.16, No.2, Aug 1978.pp.259-64, ISSN 0090-6980

Clyman, R. I., Seidner, S. R., Kajino, H., Roman, C., Koch, C. J., Ferrara, N., Waleh, N., Mauray, F., Chen, Y. Q., Perkett, E. A. & Quinn, T. (2002). VEGF regulates remodeling during permanent anatomic closure of the ductus arteriosus.*Am J Physiol Regul Integr Comp Physiol* Vol.282, No.1, Jan 2002.pp.R199-206, ISSN 0363-6119

Coceani, F., Bodach, E., White, E., Bishai, I. & Olley, P. M. (1978). Prostaglandin I2 is less relaxant than prostaglandin E2 on the lamb ductus arteriosus.*Prostaglandins* Vol.15, No.4, Apr 1978.pp.551-6, ISSN 0090-6980

De Reeder, E. G., Girard, N., Poelmann, R. E., Van Munsteren, J. C., Patterson, D. F. & Gittenberger-De Groot, A. C. (1988). Hyaluronic acid accumulation and endothelial cell detachment in intimal thickening of the vessel wall. The normal and genetically defective ductus arteriosus.*Am J Pathol* Vol.132, No.3, Sep 1988.pp.574-85, ISSN 0002-9440

de Reeder, E. G., Gittenberger-de Groot, A. C., van Munsteren, J. C., Poelmann, R. E., Patterson, D. F. & Keirse, M. J. (1989). Distribution of prostacyclin synthase, 6-keto-prostaglandin F1 alpha, and 15-hydroxy-prostaglandin dehydrogenase in the normal and persistent ductus arteriosus of the dog.*Am J Pathol* Vol.135, No.5, Nov 1989.pp.881-7, ISSN 0002-9440

de Reeder, E. G., van Munsteren, C. J., Poelmann, R. E., Patterson, D. F. & Gittenberger-de Groot, A. C. (1990). Changes in distribution of elastin and elastin receptor during intimal cushion formation in the ductus arteriosus.*Anat Embryol (Berl)* Vol.182, No.5, 1990.pp.473-80, ISSN 0340-2061

Fay, F. S. & Cooke, P. H. (1972). Guinea pig ductus arteriosus. II. Irreversible closure after birth.*Am J Physiol* Vol.222, No.4, Apr 1972.pp.841-9, ISSN 0002-9513

Feng, X., Krebs, L. T. & Gridley, T. Patent ductus arteriosus in mice with smooth muscle-specific Jag1 deletion. (2010). *Development* Vol.137, No.24, Dec.pp.4191-9, ISSN 1477-9129

Gittenberger-de Groot, A. C., Strengers, J. L., Mentink, M., Poelmann, R. E. & Patterson, D. F. (1985). Histologic studies on normal and persistent ductus arteriosus in the dog.*J Am Coll Cardiol* Vol.6, No.2, Aug 1985.pp.394-404, ISSN 0735-1097

Gittenberger-de Groot, A. C., van Ertbruggen, I., Moulaert, A. J. & Harinck, E. (1980). The ductus arteriosus in the preterm infant: histologic and clinical observations.*J Pediatr* Vol.96, No.1, Jan 1980.pp.88-93, ISSN 0022-3476

Hermes-DeSantis, E. R. & Clyman, R. I. (2006). Patent ductus arteriosus: pathophysiology and management.*J Perinatol* Vol.26 Suppl 1, May 2006.pp.S14-8; discussion S22-3, ISSN 0743-8346

High, F. A., Lu, M. M., Pear, W. S., Loomes, K. M., Kaestner, K. H. & Epstein, J. A. (2008). Endothelial expression of the Notch ligand Jagged1 is required for vascular smooth muscle development.*Proc Natl Acad Sci U S A* Vol.105, No.6, Feb 12 2008.pp.1955-9, ISSN 1091-6490

Hinek, A., Mecham, R. P., Keeley, F. & Rabinovitch, M. (1991). Impaired elastin fiber assembly related to reduced 67-kD elastin-binding protein in fetal lamb ductus arteriosus and in cultured aortic smooth muscle cells treated with chondroitin sulfate.*J Clin Invest* Vol.88, No.6, Dec 1991.pp.2083-94, ISSN 0021-9738

Huang, J., Cheng, L., Li, J., Chen, M., Zhou, D., Lu, M. M., Proweller, A., Epstein, J. A. & Parmacek, M. S. (2008). Myocardin regulates expression of contractile genes in smooth muscle cells and is required for closure of the ductus arteriosus in mice.*J Clin Invest* Vol.118, No.2, Feb 2008.pp.515-25, ISSN 0021-9738

Ivey, K. N., Sutcliffe, D., Richardson, J., Clyman, R. I., Garcia, J. A. & Srivastava, D. (2008). Transcriptional regulation during development of the ductus arteriosus.*Circ Res* Vol.103, No.4, Aug 15 2008.pp.388-95, ISSN 1524-4571

Iwasaki, S., Minamisawa, S., Yokoyama, U., Akaike, T., Quan, H., Nagashima, Y., Nishimaki, S., Ishikawa, Y. & Yokota, S. (2007). Interleukin-15 inhibits smooth muscle cell proliferation and hyaluronan production in rat ductus arteriosus.*Pediatr Res* Vol.62, No.4, Oct 2007.pp.392-8, ISSN 0031-3998

Jin, M. H., Yokoyama, U., Sato, Y., Shioda, A., Jiao, Q., Ishikawa, Y. & Minamisawa, S. (2011). DNA microarray profiling identified a new role of growth hormone in vascular remodeling of rat ductus arteriosus.*J Physiol Sci* Vol.61, No.3, May.pp.167-79, ISSN 1880-6562

Khetyar, M., Syrris, P., Tinworth, L., Abushaban, L. & Carter, N. (2008). Novel TFAP2B mutation in nonsyndromic patent ductus arteriosus.*Genet Test* Vol.12, No.3, Sep 2008.pp.457-9, ISSN 1090-6576

Kim, H. S., Aikawa, M., Kimura, K., Kuro-o, M., Nakahara, K., Suzuki, T., Katoh, H., Okamoto, E., Yazaki, Y. & Nagai, R. (1993). Ductus arteriosus. Advanced differentiation of smooth muscle cells demonstrated by myosin heavy chain isoform expression in rabbits.*Circulation* Vol.88, No.4 Pt 1, Oct 1993.pp.1804-10, ISSN 0009-7322

Kurpinski, K., Lam, H., Chu, J., Wang, A., Kim, A., Tsay, E., Agrawal, S., Schaffer, D. V. & Li, S. (2010). Transforming growth factor-beta and notch signaling mediate stem cell differentiation into smooth muscle cells.*Stem Cells* Vol.28, No.4, Apr.pp.734-42, ISSN 1549-4918

Li, S., Wang, D. Z., Wang, Z., Richardson, J. A. & Olson, E. N. (2003). The serum response factor coactivator myocardin is required for vascular smooth muscle development.*Proc Natl Acad Sci U S A* Vol.100, No.16, Aug 5 2003.pp.9366-70, ISSN 0027-8424

Loeys, B. L., Chen, J., Neptune, E. R., Judge, D. P., Podowski, M., Holm, T., Meyers, J., Leitch, C. C., Katsanis, N., Sharifi, N., Xu, F. L., Myers, L. A., Spevak, P. J., Cameron, D. E., De Backer, J., Hellemans, J., Chen, Y., Davis, E. C., Webb, C. L., Kress, W., Coucke, P., Rifkin, D. B., De Paepe, A. M. & Dietz, H. C. (2005). A syndrome of altered cardiovascular, craniofacial, neurocognitive and skeletal development caused by mutations in TGFBR1 or TGFBR2.*Nat Genet* Vol.37, No.3, Mar 2005.pp.275-81, ISSN 1061-4036

Loftin, C. D., Trivedi, D. B. & Langenbach, R. (2002). Cyclooxygenase-1-selective inhibition prolongs gestation in mice without adverse effects on the ductus arteriosus.*J Clin Invest* Vol.110, No.4, Aug 2002.pp.549-57, ISSN 0021-9738

Loftin, C. D., Trivedi, D. B., Tiano, H. F., Clark, J. A., Lee, C. A., Epstein, J. A., Morham, S. G., Breyer, M. D., Nguyen, M., Hawkins, B. M., Goulet, J. L., Smithies, O., Koller, B. H. & Langenbach, R. (2001). Failure of ductus arteriosus closure and remodeling in neonatal mice deficient in cyclooxygenase-1 and cyclooxygenase-2.*Proc Natl Acad Sci U S A* Vol.98, No.3, Jan 30 2001.pp.1059-64, ISSN 0027-8424

Mason, C. A., Bigras, J. L., O'Blenes, S. B., Zhou, B., McIntyre, B., Nakamura, N., Kaneda, Y. & Rabinovitch, M. (1999). Gene transfer in utero biologically engineers a patent ductus arteriosus in lambs by arresting fibronectin-dependent neointimal formation.*Nat Med* Vol.5, No.2, Feb 1999.pp.176-82, ISSN 1078-8956

McDonald, O. G. & Owens, G. K. (2007). Programming smooth muscle plasticity with chromatin dynamics.*Circ Res* Vol.100, No.10, May 25 2007.pp.1428-41, ISSN 1524-4571

Mitchell, S. C., Korones, S. B. & Berendes, H. W. (1971). Congenital heart disease in 56,109 births. Incidence and natural history.*Circulation* Vol.43, No.3, Mar 1971.pp.323-32, ISSN 0009-7322

Nguyen, M., Camenisch, T., Snouwaert, J. N., Hicks, E., Coffman, T. M., Anderson, P. A., Malouf, N. N. & Koller, B. H. (1997). The prostaglandin receptor EP4 triggers remodelling of the cardiovascular system at birth.*Nature* Vol.390, No.6655, Nov 6 1997.pp.78-81, ISSN 0028-0836

Rabinovitch, M. (1996). Cell-extracellular matrix interactions in the ductus arteriosus and perinatal pulmonary circulation.*Semin Perinatol* Vol.20, No.6, Dec 1996.pp.531-41, ISSN 0146-0005

Satoda, M., Zhao, F., Diaz, G. A., Burn, J., Goodship, J., Davidson, H. R., Pierpont, M. E. & Gelb, B. D. (2000). Mutations in TFAP2B cause Char syndrome, a familial form of patent ductus arteriosus.*Nat Genet* Vol.25, No.1, May 2000.pp.42-6, ISSN 1061-4036

Segi, E., Sugimoto, Y., Yamasaki, A., Aze, Y., Oida, H., Nishimura, T., Murata, T., Matsuoka, T., Ushikubi, F., Hirose, M., Tanaka, T., Yoshida, N., Narumiya, S. & Ichikawa, A. (1998). Patent ductus arteriosus and neonatal death in prostaglandin receptor EP4-deficient mice.*Biochem Biophys Res Commun* Vol.246, No.1, May 8 1998.pp.7-12, ISSN 0006-291X

Slomp, J., Gittenberger-de Groot, A. C., Glukhova, M. A., Conny van Munsteren, J., Kockx, M. M., Schwartz, S. M. & Koteliansky, V. E. (1997). Differentiation, dedifferentiation, and apoptosis of smooth muscle cells during the development of the human ductus arteriosus.*Arterioscler Thromb Vasc Biol* Vol.17, No.5, May 1997.pp.1003-9, ISSN 1079-5642

Slomp, J., van Munsteren, J. C., Poelmann, R. E., de Reeder, E. G., Bogers, A. J. & Gittenberger-de Groot, A. C. (1992). Formation of intimal cushions in the ductus arteriosus as a model for vascular intimal thickening. An immunohistochemical study of changes in extracellular matrix components.*Atherosclerosis* Vol.93, No.1-2, Mar 1992.pp.25-39, ISSN 0021-9150

Smith, G. C. (1998). The pharmacology of the ductus arteriosus.*Pharmacol Rev* Vol.50, No.1, Mar 1998.pp.35-58, ISSN 0031-6997

Sunahara, R. K. & Taussig, R. (2002). Isoforms of mammalian adenylyl cyclase: multiplicities of signaling.*Mol Interv* Vol.2, No.3, Jun 2002.pp.168-84, ISSN 1534-0384

Tada, T., Wakabayashi, T., Nakao, Y., Ueki, R., Ogawa, Y., Inagawa, A., Shibata, T. & Kishimoto, H. (1985). Human ductus arteriosus. A histological study on the relation between ductal maturation and gestational age.*Acta Pathol Jpn* Vol.35, No.1, Jan 1985.pp.23-34, ISSN 0001-6632

Tannenbaum, J. E., Waleh, N. S., Mauray, F., Gold, L., Perkett, E. A. & Clyman, R. I. (1996). Transforming growth factor-beta protein and messenger RNA expression is increased in the closing ductus arteriosus.*Pediatr Res* Vol.39, No.3, Mar 1996.pp.427-34, ISSN 0031-3998

Trivedi, D. B., Sugimoto, Y. & Loftin, C. D. (2006). Attenuated cyclooxygenase-2 expression contributes to patent ductus arteriosus in preterm mice.*Pediatr Res* Vol.60, No.6, Dec 2006.pp.669-74, ISSN 0031-3998

Van Overmeire, B., Allegaert, K., Casaer, A., Debauche, C., Decaluwe, W., Jespers, A., Weyler, J., Harrewijn, I. & Langhendries, J. P. (2004). Prophylactic ibuprofen in premature infants: a multicentre, randomised, double-blind, placebo-controlled trial.*Lancet* Vol.364, No.9449, Nov 27-Dec 3 2004.pp.1945-9, ISSN 1474-547X

Waleh, N., Seidner, S., McCurnin, D., Giavedoni, L., Hodara, V., Goelz, S., Liu, B. M., Roman, C. & Clyman, R. I. (2010). Anatomic Closure of the Premature Patent Ductus Arteriosus: The Role of CD14+/CD163+ Mononuclear Cells and Vascular Endothelial Growth Factor (VEGF) in Neointimal Mound Formation.*Pediatr Res* Jun 17. ISSN 1530-0447

Waleh, N., Seidner, S., McCurnin, D., Yoder, B., Liu, B. M., Roman, C., Mauray, F. & Clyman, R. I. (2005). The role of monocyte-derived cells and inflammation in baboon ductus arteriosus remodeling.*Pediatr Res* Vol.57, No.2, Feb 2005.pp.254-62, ISSN 0031-3998

Yokoyama, U., Minamisawa, S., Quan, H., Ghatak, S., Akaike, T., Segi-Nishida, E., Iwasaki, S., Iwamoto, M., Misra, S., Tamura, K., Hori, H., Yokota, S., Toole, B. P., Sugimoto, Y. & Ishikawa, Y. (2006a). Chronic activation of the prostaglandin receptor EP4 promotes hyaluronan-mediated neointimal formation in the ductus arteriosus.*J Clin Invest* Vol.116, No.11, Nov 2006.pp.3026-34, ISSN 0021-9738

Yokoyama, U., Minamisawa, S., Adachi-Akahane, S., Akaike, T., Naguro, I., Funakoshi, K., Iwamoto, M., Nakagome, M., Uemura, N., Hori, H., Yokota, S. & Ishikawa, Y. (2006b). Multiple transcripts of Ca^{2+} channel alpha1-subunits and a novel spliced variant of the alpha1C-subunit in rat ductus arteriosus.*Am J Physiol Heart Circ Physiol* Vol.290, No.4, Apr 2006.pp.H1660-70, ISSN 0363-6135

Yokoyama, U., Minamisawa, S., Quan, H., Akaike, T., Suzuki, S., Jin, M., Jiao, Q., Watanabe, M., Otsu, K., Iwasaki, S., Nishimaki, S., Sato, M. & Ishikawa, Y. (2008). Prostaglandin E2-activated Epac promotes neointimal formation of the rat ductus arteriosus by a process distinct from that of cAMP-dependent protein kinase A.*J Biol Chem* Vol.283, No.42, Oct 17 2008.pp.28702-9, ISSN 0021-9258

Yokoyama, U., Minamisawa, S., Katayama, A., Tang, T., Suzuki, S., Iwatsubo, K., Iwasaki, S., Kurotani, R., Okumura, S., Sato, M., Yokota, S., Hammond, H. K. & Ishikawa, Y. (2010). Differential regulation of vascular tone and remodeling via stimulation of type 2 and type 6 adenylyl cyclases in the ductus arteriosus.*Circ Res* Vol.106, No.12, Jun 25.pp.1882-92, ISSN 1524-4571

Zhou, B., Coulber, C. & Rabinovitch, M. (1998). Tissue-specific and developmental regulation of transforming growth factor-beta1 expression in fetal lamb ductus arteriosus endothelial cells.*Pediatr Res* Vol.44, No.6, Dec 1998.pp.865-72, ISSN 0031-3998

4

Bone Morphogenetic Protein Signaling Pathways in Heart Development and Disease

Cristina Harmelink and Kai Jiao
The University of Alabama at Birmingham
USA

1. Introduction

The heart is the first organ to develop and its proper formation is requisite for survival of the embryo. Heart development relies on exquisitely controlled signaling cascades that together weave the temporal and spatial cardiac gene expression patterns required for normal heart morphogenesis and function. Aberrations in cardiogenic signaling pathways or in cardiac gene expression patterns can result in congenital heart defects (CHDs), the most common type of birth defect worldwide and the leading noninfectious cause of infant death in the Western world (Hoffman 1995; Hoffman and Kaplan 2002). This review provides evidence from multiple experimental models that demonstrates the conserved, critical roles of Bone Morphogenetic Protein (BMP) signaling pathways throughout heart development, from induction of the cardiac mesoderm to the formation of the four-chambered heart. BMP signaling pathways have roles in developmental processes that can contribute to CHDs, including formation of the septa, valves, and outflow tract.

2. Overview

2.1 Heart development

During gastrulation, cardiac progenitors within the lateral plate mesoderm migrate in bilateral sheets of cells to the anterior of the embryo. Within the cardiac mesoderm, there are two populations of cells that contribute to the developing heart called the first and second heart fields (FHF and SHF, respectively). At embryonic (E) day 7.5 in mice, cells of the FHF form the cardiac crescent. At this stage, the second population of cardiac cells, the SHF, is medial and anterior to the FHF. As the embryo folds, at mouse E8.0, the cardiac crescent fuses along the midline and forms the heart tube while the SHF moves dorsally. The heart tube consists of an outer myocardial layer and an inner endocardial layer, separated by an extracellular matrix (ECM) called the cardiac jelly. SHF cells migrate through the pharyngeal mesoderm to populate the anterior and posterior regions of the heart tube. Starting from E8.5 in the mouse, the heart undergoes rightward looping. Regional proliferation along the myocardium of the outer curvature of the heart tube demarcates the future atrial and ventricular chambers. The myocardium of the inflow tract (IFT), outflow tract (OFT), atrioventricular canal (AVC) and inner curvature of the heart tube is characteristically non-proliferative. The FHF contributes primarily to the left ventricle as well as to part of the atrium, and the SHF contributes to the atria, right ventricle, and OFT. At about E9.5 in the

AVC, the endocardial cells respond to signals from the myocardium and undergo epithelial to mesenchymal transition (EMT) to form the cushions, the primordial valve structures. Cushions are also formed in the proximal region of the OFT at a slightly later stage. Around E10.0, another population of cells called the cardiac neural crest cells (CNCC) migrates from the dorsal neural tube and contributes to the developing OFT. By E11.5, the proepicardial cells have migrated around and enveloped the heart, forming the epicardium. Finally, septation and valve development result in a four-chambered heart with right, pulmonary, and left, systemic, halves by mouse E14.5. For a review, see (Evans et al. 2010).

2.2 BMP signaling pathways

BMP ligands are conserved growth factors that belong in the Transforming Growth Factor-β (TGFβ) superfamily. More than twenty BMPs have been identified and they have a myriad of functions during development. BMP precursor proteins are activated via endoproteolytic cleavage, glycosylated, and then secreted as homo- or hetero-dimers (Derynck et al. 1985; Derynck et al. 1986; Wozney et al. 1990). Once processed and secreted, BMP ligands relay their signal to the nucleus through signaling cascades that utilize unique combinations of serine threonine kinase receptors which respond to specific ligand combinations. There are three type I receptors (out of seven) and three type II receptors (out of five) that transduce the BMP signals. The type I receptors are ALK2 (ACVRI, ACTRI), ALK3 (BMPRIA/BRK-1), and ALK6 (BMPRIB, BRK-2) (Macías-Silva et al. 1998; Koenig et al. 1994; ten Dijke et al. 1994). The type II receptors are BMPR2 (BMPRII, BRK-3), ACVR2A (ACTRIIA), and ACVR2B (ACTRIIB) (Yamashita et al. 1995; Nohno et al. 1995; Rosenzweig et al. 1995; Kawabata, Chytil, and Moses 1995). The BMP dimer binds a type II receptor, which recruits and phosphorylates a type I receptor in its intracellular kinase domain (Yamashita et al. 1995). The type I receptor then phosphorylates an intracellular receptor-regulated SMAD protein (R-SMAD). SMAD1, SMAD5, and SMAD8 are activated specifically by BMP signals (Cárcamo, Zentella, and Massagué 1995; Wieser, Wrana, and Massagué 1995; Hoodless et al. 1996; Nishimura et al. 1998; Chen, Bhushan, and Vale 1997). After phosphorylation, activated R-SMADs form a complex with the common SMAD, SMAD4 (Zhang, Musci, and Derynck 1997). The R-SMAD-SMAD4 complex translocates to the nucleus, where it cooperates with other cofactors to regulate gene transcription; an example is illustrated elsewhere (Jiao, Zhou, and Hogan 2002). BMP signaling can occur independently of SMAD proteins in non-canonical pathways. For example, BMPs can activate MAP kinase pathways, resulting in the activation of p38 MAPK, PI3K, ERK, and JNK with downstream effects on cell proliferation and differentiation (Yamaguchi et al. 1995; Shibuya et al. 1998; Kimura et al. 2000; Lou et al. 2000; Lai and Cheng 2002; Yanagisawa et al. 2001; Xu et al. 1996).

It has recently been demonstrated that BMP signaling can regulate microRNA (miRNA) biosynthesis. miRNAs are short non-coding RNA that target messenger RNA (mRNA) in a sequence-specific manner for post-transcriptional degradation and translational inhibition. miRNAs are transcribed as primary miRNAs (pri-miRNAs), which are processed by the Drosha complex within the nucleus. pri-miRNA processing results in a shorter pre-miRNA, which is exported from the nucleus to the cytoplasm where it is cleaved into its mature miRNA structure by Dicer. For a review on miRNA during cardiovascular development and disease, the reader is referred to Liu and Olson (2010). Activated R-SMADs can directly interact with the microprocessor complex, Drosha, independent of the common SMAD, SMAD4, to promote the biosynthesis of miRNAs such as *miR-21* (Davis et al. 2008; Ji et al.

2007; Warner et al. 2004; Fukuda et al. 2007; Davis et al. 2010). *miR-21* is upregulated in damaged cardiovascular tissue (Ji et al. 2007).

The timing, duration, and gradient of BMP ligands affect the outcomes and add to the complexity of BMP signaling pathways. After BMP processing and secretion, access to the receptors and retention in the ECM are inhibited by extracellular factors such as noggin, chordin, follistatin, cerberus, and gremlin (McMahon et al. 1998; Streit et al. 1998; Sasai et al. 1995; Hemmati-Brivanlou, Kelly, and Melton 1994; Fainsod et al. 1997; Bouwmeester et al. 1996; Hsu et al. 1998). These inhibitors bind BMP ligands, interfering with ligand-receptor interaction (Zimmerman, De Jesús-Escobar, and Harland 1996; Hsu et al. 1998; Yamashita et al. 1995; Piccolo et al. 1996; Iemura et al. 1998). BMP signaling is also regulated at the membrane, for instance by the pseudoreceptor BAMBI (BMP and Activin membrane bound inhibitor). BAMBI lacks the intracellular domain needed to transduce the signal and, upon binding BMP receptors, it inhibits the formation of an active BMP receptor complex (Onichtchouk et al. 1999; Grotewold et al. 2001). Alternatively, BMP signaling can be enhanced at the membrane level by modulators such as DRAGON, which acts as a co-receptor and presents BMPs to the receptors (Samad et al. 2005; Babitt et al. 2005; Babitt et al. 2006). Another example is endoglin, a transmembrane protein that binds to BMP ligands and enhances BMP signaling (Barbara, Wrana, and Letarte 1999; Scherner et al. 2007). Intracellularly, BMP signaling can be downregulated by SMURF, an E3 ubiquitin ligase that promotes R-SMAD degradation, receptor turnover, and facilitates inhibition by the inhibitory SMADs, SMAD6 and SMAD7 (Murakami et al. 2003; Kavsak et al. 2000; Ebisawa et al. 2001). SMAD6 and SMAD7 inhibit BMP signaling cascades through binding active type I BMP receptors and preventing R-SMAD activation, and by competing with SMAD4 for R-SMADs (Imamura et al. 1997; Hata et al. 1998; Hanyu et al. 2001). Lastly, crosstalk with other signaling pathways affects R-SMAD phosphorylation, activity, turnover and nuclear accumulation (Pera et al. 2003; Sapkota et al. 2007; Fuentealba et al. 2007; Suzawa et al. 2002).

3. BMP signaling in heart development

3.1 Cardiac specification and heart tube formation

In this section, we will review the functions of different components of BMP signaling during the initial stages of heart development.

3.1.1 BMP ligands

Initial insight into the roles of BMP signaling pathways in cardiac specification came from studying the *BMP2/4* ortholog, *Dpp*, in *Drosophila melanogaster*. *Dpp*-deficient larva did not form the precursor cells for the heart organ, the dorsal vessel, while ectopic DPP caused ectopic formation of the dorsal vessel precursor cells (Xu et al. 1998; Frasch 1995; Yin and Frasch 1998). In the anterior region of chick embryos, the endoderm expresses BMP2 and 5, and the ectoderm expresses BMP4 and BMP7 (Schultheiss, Burch, and Lassar 1997; Somi et al. 2004). *In vivo* and *in vitro* experiments using chicken embryos revealed that both the FHF and the SHF pre-cardiac mesodermal cells differentiate in response to BMP signals (Waldo et al. 2001; Tirosh-Finkel et al. 2006). In mice, BMP2, BMP4, BMP5, and BMP7 are expressed in the anterior mesoderm (Zhang and Bradley 1996; Dudley and Robertson 1997; Solloway and Robertson 1999). Regardless of the differences in BMP expression patterns between species, it has been well-established that BMP signaling pathways induce precardiac mesoderm to undergo cardiac differentiation (Alsan and Schultheiss 2002; Barron, Gao, and Lough 2000; Tirosh-Finkel et al. 2010). *Bmp2* deletion in mice causes embryonic lethality between E7.5-E9.0 (Zhang and Bradley 1996). Some mutant embryos lack hearts altogether and others develop ectopic heart tubes in the exocoelomic cavity, suggesting a critical role of BMP signaling for heart formation (Zhang and Bradley 1996).

BMP signaling pathways induce cardiac differentiation through upregulation of cardiogenic genes. Expression of the cardiac transcription factors *Nkx2.5* and *Gata4* is initiated by BMP signaling (Frasch 1995; Schultheiss, Burch, and Lassar 1997; Andrée et al. 1998; Schlange et al. 2000; Jamali et al. 2001; Liberatore et al. 2002; Shi et al. 2000; Lien et al. 2002; Reiter, Verkade, and Stainier 2001; Schultheiss, Xydas, and Lassar 1995). The *Nkx2.5* promoter region contains evolutionary conserved BMP-response elements that are necessary for its cardiac expression (Lien et al. 2002; Liberatore et al. 2002; Brown et al. 2004). BMP signaling also activates the expression of myocardin, a cardiac and smooth muscle-specific transcriptional cofactor for serum response factor, a regulator of cardiac differentiation (Arsenian et al. 1998; Wang et al. 2001; Callis, Cao, and Wang 2005). SMAD1 is also a transcriptional cofactor for myocardin to activate downstream gene expression (Callis, Cao, and Wang 2005).

3.1.2 BMP receptors

The BMP type I receptor ALK3 is widely expressed in mouse embryos and *Alk3* deletion causes embryonic lethality at E8.0 with no mesoderm formation (Mishina et al. 1995; Dewulf et al. 1995). ALK2, another type I receptor, is expressed in Hensen's node and in the primitive streak (Gu et al. 1999; Mishina et al. 1999). Deleting *Alk2* in mouse embryos results in gastrulation defects and embryonic lethality before E9.5 (Gu et al. 1999; Mishina et al. 1999). The third type I receptor, ALK6, is not expressed during early heart development and disrupting its function does not affect mouse cardiogenesis or viability (Dewulf et al. 1995; Yi et al. 2000). Knockout of the type II receptor, BMPR2, which is expressed widely throughout chicken embryos and during mouse cardiomyogenesis, causes embryonic lethality at gastrulation (Ehrman and Yutzey 1999; Stern et al. 1995; Feijen, Goumans, and van den Eijnden-van Raaij 1994; Beppu et al. 2000). In mice, ACVR2A is expressed after cardiomyocyte formation at E9.5 and ACVR2B is ubiquitously expressed during cardiomyogenesis (Feijen, Goumans, and van den Eijnden-van Raaij 1994; Beppu et al. 2000). Disruption of *Acvr2a* alone does not cause heart defects and disruption of *Acvr2b* causes heart defects later in development (Matzuk, Kumar, et al. 1995; Oh and Li 1997). However, deletion of both *Acvr2a* and *Acvr2b* results in embryonic death at gastrulation, suggesting functional redundancy of these type II receptors (Song et al. 1999).

3.1.3 SMAD proteins

In chicken embryos, the receptor-regulated SMAD proteins, SMAD1, SMAD5, and SMAD8, are enriched in the heart forming region (Faure et al. 2002). In mice, *Smad1* and *Smad5* mRNA are expressed in the mesoderm during cardiomyocyte formation (Tremblay, Dunn, and Robertson 2001). *Smad1* disruption in mice results in embryonic lethality at E10.5 from failure of umbilical-placental connections to form (Tremblay, Dunn, and Robertson 2001). Germline deletion of *Smad5* results in defective left-right symmetry with a heart looping abnormality and defective angiogenesis (Chang et al. 2000; Yang et al. 1999). Deletion of *Smad4*, the gene encoding the common SMAD, causes death before E7.5, with reduced size and failure to gastrulate (Sirard et al. 1998). Conditional deletion of *Smad4* from the epiblast causes embryonic lethality by E8.5, but the heart tube forms and *Nkx2.5* is expressed (Chu et al. 2004). Heart tube formation and cardiac gene expression may occur in these mice because canonical BMP signaling occurs before *Smad4* deletion or because other R-SMAD transcriptional cofactors compensate for the loss of SMAD4.

3.1.4 BMP inhibitors

Inhibition of BMP during gastrulation restricts the heart forming fields to discrete territories in the anterior of the embryo. Noggin, chordin, and follistatin are secreted from the notochord and bind BMP ligands, preventing receptor activation (McMahon et al. 1998; Streit et al. 1998; Sasai et al. 1995; Hemmati-Brivanlou, Kelly, and Melton 1994; Fainsod et al. 1997). The responsiveness of pre-cardiac mesoderm to inhibitory signals from the notochord is developmentally regulated. Ectopic application of noggin to stage 4 chick mesendoderm prevents the initiation of the cardiac gene expression and development of the contracting cardiomyocytes (Schultheiss, Burch, and Lassar 1997; Schlange et al. 2000). If noggin is applied to explants a stage later, the cardiac gene expression is initiated without spontaneous contraction of myocytes. If noggin is applied at stage 6, differentiation occurs normally (Nakajima et al. 2002). In mice, deletion of noggin or follistatin individually does not cause heart defects, but deletion of both reverses heart looping (Bachiller et al. 2000; McMahon et al. 1998; Matzuk, Lu, et al. 1995). Deleting chordin causes defects phenocopying those in DiGeorge syndrome (Bachiller et al. 2003).

3.2 Cardiogenesis after heart tube formation

In this section, we will discuss BMP signaling during different cardiogenic processes after heart tube formation.

3.2.1 Myocardial wall morphogenesis

During early heart development, myocardial walls expand through cardiomyocyte proliferation and differentiation. The ventricle chamber myocardium develops a latticework of muscular projections on the subendocardial surface called trabeculae. Trabecular myocardium generates contractile force, coordinates intraventricular conduction, and helps diffuse nutrients to the cardiomyocytes within the expanding heart wall prior to vascularization. Later in heart development, the trabecular myocardium undergoes remodeling and is incorporated into the compact myocardium, the interventricular septum, and the papillary muscles of the atrioventricular valves. For a review, see Dunwoodie (2007). Proper formation of myocardial walls is essential for embryo viability and postnatal cardiac function. Abnormal myocardial wall morphogenesis can result in left ventricular noncompaction, which may lead to cardiomyopathy (Pignatelli et al. 2003; Xing et al. 2006).
BMP10 is initially expressed in the looping mouse heart within regions destined to be the atrial and ventricular chambers, and its expression is maintained in the chamber myocardium during heart development. (Neuhaus, Rosen, and Thies 1999; Somi et al. 2004; Chen et al. 2004) Also, *Bmp10* is upregulated in mouse models of hypertrabeculation (Chen et al. 2004). Myocardial expression of BMP10 during chamber formation relies on endocardial expression of notch (Grego-Bessa et al. 2007). Deleting *Bmp10* in mice causes embryonic lethality at E9.0 with decreased cardiomyocyte proliferation, downregulation of cardiac genes *Nkx2.5* and *Mef2c*, and loss of trabecular myocardium (Chen et al. 2004).

Removing both *Bmp6* and *Bmp7* in mice causes embryonic lethality at midgestation with hypoplastic ventricles and reduced trabeculations (Kim, Robertson, and Solloway 2001). Mice with conditional deletion of the BMP receptor *Alk3* from the myocardium die during embryogenesis and display underdeveloped myocardial walls and ventricle septal defects (VSD) (Gaussin et al. 2002). Specific inactivation of the common Smad, *Smad4,* from the myocardium likewise causes embryonic lethality at midgestation and disrupts myocardial wall formation and ventricle septation (Azhar et al. 2010; Song, Yan, et al. 2007; Qi et al. 2007; Wang, Xu, et al. 2005). Myocardial deletion of *Smad4* causes downregulation of genes encoding cell cycle regulators, cardiac structural proteins, and transcription factors. Together, these studies provide multiple lines of evidence that show BMP signaling is required for ventricular myocardial wall morphogenesis through regulation of cardiomyocyte proliferation, differentiation, and gene expression.

3.2.2 Conduction system development

In vertebrates, regional differentiation of the myocardium allows for development of slow-conducting, nonchamber myocardium (IFT, AVC, and OFT) and fast-conducting chamber myocardium (atria and ventricles). Proper formation of the AVC is important for establishment of the primary conduction system. The primary conduction system includes the atrioventricular node (AVN) and its associated structures. In mice, AVN precursor cells are observed in the AVC at E9.5. The AVN subsequently extends into the left ventricle and connects with the trabecular myocardium and the interventricular septum. (See reviews, (Christoffels et al. 2010; Moorman and Christoffels 2003)). The electrical impulse is carried from the atria, across the AVC to the ventricles (Valderrábano et al. 2006; Rentschler et al. 2002; de Jong et al. 1992). The AVC has a slower conduction rate than the atria and delays the atrial-ventricular electrical impulse (de Jong et al 1992).

BMP2 is necessary for AVC specification and expression of *Tbx2* (Yamada et al. 2000; Ma et al. 2005). TBX2 is a transcriptional repressor of chamber-specific genes and is specifically expressed in nonchamber myocardium of the IFT and the AVC (Aanhaanen et al. 2009; Habets et al. 2002; Yamada et al. 2000; Christoffels et al. 2004; Harrelson et al. 2004). In the AVC, BMP2 activates *Tbx2* transcription to suppress proliferation and inhibit the expression of chamber-specific genes *Nppa, Cx40, Cx43,* and *Chisel* (Ma et al. 2005; Shirai et al. 2009; Christoffels et al. 2004). BMP2 can directly regulate *Tbx2* through a SMAD-dependent enhancer upstream of its transcription start site (Singh et al. 2009). BMP signaling also promotes *Tbx2* transcription through SMAD1 inhibition of TBX20, a *Tbx2* repressor (Singh et al. 2009). The BMP2-TBX2 pathway is restricted to the AVC region by notch/HEY signaling in the developing heart chambers (Rutenberg et al. 2006; Kokubo et al. 2005).

Deletion of *Bmp2* from mouse myocardium decreases *Tbx2* expression and results in the expansion of chamber myocardium into the AVC region (Ma et al. 2005). Inactivation of the BMP receptor *Alk3* specifically in the AVC myocardium disrupts AV valve development and AVN morphogenesis, resulting in ventricular pre-excitation (Gaussin et al. 2005; Stroud et al. 2007). Lastly, removal of myocardial *Tbx2* results in abnormal AVC patterning and ventricular pre-excitation (Aanhaanen et al. 2011). Taken together, these data suggest that BMP2 regulation of *Tbx2* expression and AVC myocardial patterning is important for development of the AVN and proper atrial-ventricular conduction. Indeed, the phenotype resulting from AVC-depletion of *Alk3* resembles Wolff-Parkinson-White syndrome (WPWS, OMIM 224700), a pre-excitation syndrome that can present as tachycardia due to an abnormal connection between the atria and ventricles (Gaussin et al. 2005). Recently, a heterozygous microdeletion was identified in a chromosomal region encompassing *BMP2* that is associated with predisposition to WPWS (Lalani et al. 2009).

3.2.3 Valvulo-septal development of the atrioventricular canal and outflow tract

The AVC and OFT are septated by endocardial cushion maturation into valvulo-septal structures. Cushions develop in the AVC and OFT through the expansion of the ECM. Induction of cushion formation occurs within the looped heart, when the myocardium signals through the cardiac jelly to the endocardium. Endocardial cells then delaminate and invade the cardiac jelly to form the mesenchymal cells of the endocardial cushions. For reviews, see Person, Klewer, and Runyan (2005) and Butcher and Markwald (2007). The AVC cushions form earlier than the OFT cushions and develop into the mitral (left) and tricuspid (right) valves at the junction of the atria and ventricles. The OFT cushions, but not the AVC cushions, have a CNCC contribution (Kirby, Gale, and Stewart 1983; Waldo et al. 1998; Jiang et al. 2000). The cushions in the OFT develop into the semilunar valves in the aorta (left) and pulmonary artery (right). Congenital defects in valve formation and septation comprise the most common CHDs, while defects involving the OFT are found in 4 per 10,000 live births and are often lethal (Hoffman 1995; Edmonds and James 1993). Pathological mutations in the BMP receptor *ALK2* have been found in patients with congenital defects in atrioventricular septum development, providing evidence for the importance of BMP signaling pathways in human heart development (Smith et al. 2009; Joziasse et al. 2011).

At E9.5 in mice, BMP2 has weak expression in OFT myocardium which disappears by E10.5 (Lyons, Pelton, and Hogan 1990). BMP2 is strongly and persistently expressed in AVC and atrial myocardium at E10.5 (Lyons, Pelton, and Hogan 1990; Abdelwahid et al. 2001). It is also expressed in the cushion mesenchyme during valve remodeling and in adult mouse valves (Sugi et al. 2004). In mice, BMP2 enhances cardiac jelly formation, endocardial EMT, and AVC myocardial patterning (Ma et al. 2005; Rivera-Feliciano and Tabin 2006; Sugi et al. 2004; Camenisch et al. 2002). BMP2 upregulates *Twist1*, an inducer of EMT, and *Has2*, a component of the cardiac jelly necessary for EMT (Camenisch et al. 2000; Ma et al. 2005; Yang et al. 2004). Myocardial deletion of *Bmp2* decreases ECM in the AVC cushions, however the OFT cushions develop normally (Ma et al. 2005; Rivera-Feliciano and Tabin 2006). This suggests a compensatory mechanism in the OFT such as BMP4 signaling. Data suggests that BMP2 signaling interacts with notch1 and TGFβ signaling pathways to coordinate EMT (Luna-Zurita et al. 2010; Boyer et al. 1999; Yamagishi et al. 1999).

BMP4 is expressed in AVC myocardium in mice at E9.5, but at E10.5 its expression is largely restricted to the myocardium of the OFT (Jones, Lyons, and Hogan 1991; Abdelwahid et al. 2001). It is also expressed in the chicken OFT (Somi et al. 2004). BMP4 is 92% identical in the C-terminus to BMP2, and they have overlapping functions (Goldman, Donley, and Christian 2009; Uchimura et al. 2009). Conditional deletion of *Bmp4* from mouse myocardium causes atrioventricular septation defects, double outlet right ventricle (DORV, both arteries are connected to the right ventricle), and aortic arch artery malformations (Jiao et al. 2003; Liu et al. 2004). Mouse models with myocardial-specific deletion of *Bmp4* or with hypomorphic *Bmp4* alleles have impaired AVC cushion mesenchymal cell proliferation (Jiao et al. 2003; Kulessa and Hogan 2002). Mice compound heterozygous for *Bmp2*-null and *Bmp4*-null or *Bmp4*-hypomorphic alleles have VSD (Goldman, Donley, and Christian 2009). Decreased expression of myocardial BMP4 does not affect OFT development, but it increases BMP7 expression (Liu et al. 2004). On a *Bmp7*-null background, BMP4 reduction causes a shortened OFT with hypoplastic OFT cushions, revealing dose-dependence and functional redundancy of BMP signaling in the OFT morphogenesis (Liu et al. 2004).

Despite being expressed during early heart development, single gene deletions of *Bmp5*, *Bmp6*, or *Bmp7* do not cause heart defects, likely due to redundancy of the BMP signaling family members (Kingsley et al. 1992; Jena et al. 1997; Dudley and Robertson 1997; Luo et al. 1995; Solloway et al. 1998; Kim, Robertson, and Solloway 2001). BMP5 is expressed throughout the heart tube myocardium and later becomes restricted to the myocardium of the AVC and OFT in mouse and chicken embryos (Yamagishi et al. 2001; Solloway and Robertson 1999; Somi et al. 2004). In mice, BMP6 is expressed in OFT endocardium and myocardium, and within the OFT and AVC mesenchyme (Kim, Robertson, and Solloway 2001; Jones, Lyons, and Hogan 1991; Solloway and Robertson 1999; Yamagishi et al. 2001). BMP6 is not expressed in the developing chicken heart (Somi et al. 2004). BMP7 is robustly expressed throughout the myocardium of the developing hearts of mice and chickens (Solloway and Robertson 1999; Lyons, Hogan, and Robertson 1995; Somi et al. 2004). Combinations of gene deletions in mouse models reveal their essential roles in chamber formation and septal-valvulogenesis. *Bmp5* and *Bmp7* double deletion causes embryonic lethality at E10.5, with delayed heart development, no endocardial cushion formation or chamber septation, and abnormal pericardium (Solloway and Robertson 1999). Removal of *Bmp6* and *Bmp7* results in defects in OFT cushion development, chamber septation, and myocardial wall formation (Kim, Robertson, and Solloway 2001). Deletion of *Bmp5* and *Bmp6* does not cause heart defects (Solloway et al. 1998).

Deletion of *Alk3* from the myocardium or the endocardium disrupts endocardial cushion formation (Gaussin et al. 2002; Song, Fässler, et al. 2007; Ma et al. 2005). Myocardial deletion of *Alk3* causes VSD and hypoplastic AVC cushions, with decreased TGFβ signaling in the AVC myocardium (Gaussin et al. 2002). Deleting *Alk3* specifically from the AVC myocardium disrupts AV valve maturation (Gaussin et al. 2005). Endocardial deletion of *Alk3* causes hypoplastic cushions with reduced cushion mesenchyme to about 20% of normal (Ma et al. 2005; Song, Fässler, et al. 2007; Park et al. 2006; Rivera-Feliciano and Tabin 2006). Endocardial deletion of *Alk2* causes failure of EMT in AVC cushions along with decreased expression of EMT proteins MSX1 and SMAD2, an intracellular modulator of TGFβ signaling (Wang, Sridurongrit, et al. 2005). The role of ALK2 in cushion formation appears to be specific to the endocardium, as conditional deletion of *Alk2* from the myocardium has no effect on cushion development (Wang, Sridurongrit, et al. 2005). Ectopic expression of active ALK2 in the chicken ventricle endocardium induces EMT (Desgrosellier et al. 2005). CNCC-depletion of *Alk3* or *Alk2* disrupts CNCC invasion, resulting in a shortened OFT with defective proximal septation (Stottmann et al. 2004; Kaartinen et al. 2004). Hypomorphic *Bmpr2* alleles cause defects in proximal OFT septation and loss of semilunar valve formation, while AVC cushions form normally (Délot et al. 2003). However, completely abrogating *Bmpr2* in mouse hearts causes an array of CHDs, such as DORV, VSD, and AVC cushion defects (Beppu et al. 2009). Disruption of *Acvr2b* causes postnatal death with abnormal cardiac septation (Oh and Li 1997). Deletion of *Smad4* from the myocardium affects OFT positioning, with a DORV phenotype in one mouse model (Azhar et al. 2010). Conditional deletion of *Smad4* in CNCC reduced the contribution of CNCC to OFT, causing defects in OFT cushion formation, septation, elongation, and positioning (Jia et al. 2007; Ko et al. 2007; Nie et al. 2008). Deletion of *Smad8* does not affect viability or heart development, but mice display defects in pulmonary vascular remodeling (Huang et al. 2009).

BMP signaling regulates SHF myocardialization and OFT morphogenesis in part by promoting *miR-17-92* cluster transcription (Wang et al. 2010). The *miR-17-92* cluster has roles in lung and heart development (Lu et al. 2007; Ventura et al. 2008). It is expressed as a primary transcript that encodes six miRNAs *(miR-17, -18a, -19a, -20a, -19b-1,* and *-92a-1*). BMP regulates the transcription of *miR-17-92* through SMAD binding sites in the 5′ region (Wang et al. 2010). In turn, *miR-17-92* negatively regulates *Isl1* and *Tbx1* mRNA stability and translation (Wang et al. 2010). Deleting BMP reduces *miR-17-92,* causes misexpression of *Isl1* and *Tbx1,* and leads to defects in proximal OFT septation (Wang et al. 2010).

Inhibition of BMP signaling is also critical for normal valvulo-septal formation. For example, *Nkx2.5* is required for OFT development, in part by repressing BMP signaling (Prall et al. 2007). Deleting *Nkx2.5* results in expansion of SHF specification due to increased BMP expression, decreased proliferation, and failed OFT truncation. Disrupting the misregulated BMP signaling in the *Nkx2.5* mutants by deleting *Smad1* effectively rescues the proliferation and the OFT defects. Mutations in the BMP-inhibitor *Smad6* cause hyperplasia of cardiac valves and OFT septation defects, due to unregulated BMP signaling (Galvin et al. 2000). Noggin blocks EMT in mouse explants and overexpression of noggin in chicken embryos causes OFT septation defects (Sugi et al. 2004; Allen et al. 2001). Mutations in chordin cause abnormal OFT septation, resembling syndromes associated with loss of CNCC (Bachiller et al. 2003).

4. BMP induction of stem cells and progenitor cells to a cardiac fate

Controlled differentiation of stem cells has relevance in translational research for pre-clinical cell grafting and for establishing cardiomyocyte cultures for drug discovery and toxicology. As primary inducers of cardiac differentiation, BMP cytokines have important roles in growth factor-based stem cell therapies for cardiac tissue repair. Use of growth factor peptides to induce cardiac muscle formation from embryonic stem (ES) cells has been researched for over a decade. BMP ligands have been proven to be important inductors of cardiac fate in multiple ES cell types. In mouse ES cells (mESC), BMP2 or BMP4 can activate cardiac differentiation, in combination with other factors such as Activin A or fibroblast growth factor 2 (FGF2) (Johansson and Wiles 1995; Kawai et al. 2004; Behfar et al. 2002). In the pluripotent mouse embryonal carcinoma cell line, P19CL6, treatment with BMP4 promotes cardiomyocyte formation and expression of α-MHC (Monzen et al. 1999; Monzen et al. 2001). Addition of noggin, a BMP inhibitor, prevents differentiation and this can be abolished by overexpressing BMP2, or SMAD1 and SMAD4 (Monzen et al. 1999; Monzen et al. 2001). In human ES cells (hESC), BMP4 promotes a cardiac fate (Takei et al. 2009; Kattman et al. 2011). BMP stimulation induces *Sox17* expression, which is important for directing mesoderm toward a cardiac fate (Stefanovic et al. 2009). Addition of BMP2 or BMP4 in hESC, along with Activin A and other factors, can reliably induce multipotent cardiovascular progenitors that can generate multiple cell lineages such as cardiomyocytes, smooth muscle cells, and endothelial cells *in vitro* and *in vivo* (Laflamme et al. 2007; Tomescot et al. 2007; Yang et al. 2008; Liu et al. 2007). Human induced pluripotent stem cells (iPSC) can also be induced to undergo cardiomyogenesis using similar multistep additions of factors, including BMP4 (Takahashi et al. 2007; Carvajal-Vergara et al. 2010; Kattman et al.

2011). BMP2 stimulation with FGF inhibition also induces multipotent cardiovascular progenitor cells in hESC, human iPSC, and primate ESC (Blin et al. 2010). BMP4 enhances simian ESC differentiation into cardiomyocytes as well (Hosseinkhani et al. 2007). Future studies of stem cells and progenitor cells may help develop peptide therapies to stimulate the proliferation and differentiation of self-renewing stem cells within the postnatal heart.

5. Conclusion

CHDs occur in nearly 1% of newborns and in over 5% of fetuses that do not survive to term in the Western world (Hoffman 1995; Hoffman and Kaplan 2002). Due to advances in medicine, there is a growing number of children and adults living with CHDs who require lifelong healthcare (Hoffman and Kaplan 2002). Therefore, understanding the molecular mechanisms of heart development and the underlying causes of CHDs has immediate translational significance. BMP signaling pathways are critical regulators of heart development in species as varied as fruit flies, chickens, mice, and humans. Mutations in the BMP pathway have been identified in humans with CHDs. This review discussed the critical roles of BMP signaling pathways in cardiac specification from the mesoderm, myocardial wall formation, valve development, chamber septation, and outflow tract morphogenesis. Because cardiac morphogenesis and BMP signaling pathways are evolutionarily conserved, information gleaned from a variety of model systems provides valuable insight into human heart development and CHDs. In the future this insight may help develop diagnostic tests and therapeutic options for people with CHDs.

6. References

Aanhaanen, W. T., B. J. Boukens, A. Sizarov, V. Wakker, C. de Gier-de Vries, A. C. van Ginneken, A. F. Moorman, R. Coronel, and V. M. Christoffels. 2011. Defective Tbx2-dependent patterning of the atrioventricular canal myocardium causes accessory pathway formation in mice. *J Clin Invest* 121 (2):534-44.

Aanhaanen, W. T., J. F. Brons, J. N. Domínguez, M. S. Rana, J. Norden, R. Airik, V. Wakker, C. de Gier-de Vries, N. A. Brown, A. Kispert, A. F. Moorman, and V. M. Christoffels. 2009. The Tbx2+ primary myocardium of the atrioventricular canal forms the atrioventricular node and the base of the left ventricle. *Circ Res* 104 (11):1267-74.

Abdelwahid, E., D. Rice, L. J. Pelliniemi, and E. Jokinen. 2001. Overlapping and differential localization of Bmp-2, Bmp-4, Msx-2 and apoptosis in the endocardial cushion and adjacent tissues of the developing mouse heart. *Cell Tissue Res* 305 (1):67-78.

Allen, S. P., J. P. Bogardi, A. J. Barlow, S. A. Mir, S. R. Qayyum, F. J. Verbeek, R. H. Anderson, P. H. Francis-West, N. A. Brown, and M. K. Richardson. 2001. Misexpression of noggin leads to septal defects in the outflow tract of the chick heart. *Dev Biol* 235 (1):98-109.

Alsan, B. H., and T. M. Schultheiss. 2002. Regulation of avian cardiogenesis by Fgf8 signaling. *Development* 129 (8):1935-43.

Andrée, B., D. Duprez, B. Vorbusch, H. H. Arnold, and T. Brand. 1998. BMP-2 induces ectopic expression of cardiac lineage markers and interferes with somite formation in chicken embryos. *Mech Dev* 70 (1-2):119-31.

Arsenian, S., B. Weinhold, M. Oelgeschläger, U. Rüther, and A. Nordheim. 1998. Serum response factor is essential for mesoderm formation during mouse embryogenesis. *EMBO J* 17 (21):6289-99.

Azhar, M., P. Y. Wang, T. Frugier, K. Koishi, C. Deng, P. G. Noakes, and I. S. McLennan. 2010. Myocardial deletion of Smad4 using a novel α skeletal muscle actin Cre recombinase transgenic mouse causes misalignment of the cardiac outflow tract. *Int J Biol Sci* 6 (6):546-55.

Babitt, J. L., F. W. Huang, D. M. Wrighting, Y. Xia, Y. Sidis, T. A. Samad, J. A. Campagna, R. T. Chung, A. L. Schneyer, C. J. Woolf, N. C. Andrews, and H. Y. Lin. 2006. Bone morphogenetic protein signaling by hemojuvelin regulates hepcidin expression. *Nat Genet* 38 (5):531-9.

Babitt, J. L., Y. Zhang, T. A. Samad, Y. Xia, J. Tang, J. A. Campagna, A. L. Schneyer, C. J. Woolf, and H. Y. Lin. 2005. Repulsive guidance molecule (RGMa), a DRAGON homologue, is a bone morphogenetic protein co-receptor. *J Biol Chem* 280 (33):29820-7.

Bachiller, D., J. Klingensmith, C. Kemp, J. A. Belo, R. M. Anderson, S. R. May, J. A. McMahon, A. P. McMahon, R. M. Harland, J. Rossant, and E. M. De Robertis. 2000. The organizer factors Chordin and Noggin are required for mouse forebrain development. *Nature* 403 (6770):658-61.

Bachiller, D., J. Klingensmith, N. Shneyder, U. Tran, R. Anderson, J. Rossant, and E. M. De Robertis. 2003. The role of chordin/Bmp signals in mammalian pharyngeal development and DiGeorge syndrome. *Development* 130 (15):3567-78.

Barbara, N. P., J. L. Wrana, and M. Letarte. 1999. Endoglin is an accessory protein that interacts with the signaling receptor complex of multiple members of the transforming growth factor-beta superfamily. *J Biol Chem* 274 (2):584-94.

Barron, M., M. Gao, and J. Lough. 2000. Requirement for BMP and FGF signaling during cardiogenic induction in non-precardiac mesoderm is specific, transient, and cooperative. *Dev Dyn* 218 (2):383-93.

Behfar, A., L. V. Zingman, D. M. Hodgson, J. M. Rauzier, G. C. Kane, A. Terzic, and M. Pucéat. 2002. Stem cell differentiation requires a paracrine pathway in the heart. *FASEB J* 16 (12):1558-66.

Beppu, H., M. Kawabata, T. Hamamoto, A. Chytil, O. Minowa, T. Noda, and K. Miyazono. 2000. BMP type II receptor is required for gastrulation and early development of mouse embryos. *Dev Biol* 221 (1):249-58.

Beppu, H., R. Malhotra, Y. Beppu, J. J. Lepore, M. S. Parmacek, and K. D. Bloch. 2009. BMP type II receptor regulates positioning of outflow tract and remodeling of atrioventricular cushion during cardiogenesis. *Dev Biol* 331 (2):167-75.

Blin, G., D. Nury, S. Stefanovic, T. Neri, O. Guillevic, B. Brinon, V. Bellamy, C. Rücker-Martin, P. Barbry, A. Bel, P. Bruneval, C. Cowan, J. Pouly, S. Mitalipov, E. Gouadon, P. Binder, A. Hagège, M. Desnos, J. F. Renaud, P. Menasché, and M. Pucéat. 2010. A purified population of multipotent cardiovascular progenitors derived from primate pluripotent stem cells engrafts in postmyocardial infarcted nonhuman primates. *J Clin Invest* 120 (4):1125-39.

Bouwmeester, T., S. Kim, Y. Sasai, B. Lu, and E. M. De Robertis. 1996. Cerberus is a head-inducing secreted factor expressed in the anterior endoderm of Spemann's organizer. *Nature* 382 (6592):595-601.

Boyer, A. S., I. I. Ayerinskas, E. B. Vincent, L. A. McKinney, D. L. Weeks, and R. B. Runyan. 1999. TGFbeta2 and TGFbeta3 have separate and sequential activities during epithelial-mesenchymal cell transformation in the embryonic heart. *Dev Biol* 208 (2):530-45.

Brown, C. O., X. Chi, E. Garcia-Gras, M. Shirai, X. H. Feng, and R. J. Schwartz. 2004. The cardiac determination factor, Nkx2-5, is activated by mutual cofactors GATA-4 and Smad1/4 via a novel upstream enhancer. *J Biol Chem* 279 (11):10659-69.

Butcher, J. T., and R. R. Markwald. 2007. Valvulogenesis: the moving target. *Philos Trans R Soc Lond B Biol Sci* 362 (1484):1489-503.

Callis, T. E., D. Cao, and D. Z. Wang. 2005. Bone morphogenetic protein signaling modulates myocardin transactivation of cardiac genes. *Circ Res* 97 (10):992-1000.

Camenisch, T. D., D. G. Molin, A. Person, R. B. Runyan, A. C. Gittenberger-de Groot, J. A. McDonald, and S. E. Klewer. 2002. Temporal and distinct TGFbeta ligand requirements during mouse and avian endocardial cushion morphogenesis. *Dev Biol* 248 (1):170-81.

Camenisch, T. D., A. P. Spicer, T. Brehm-Gibson, J. Biesterfeldt, M. L. Augustine, A. Calabro, S. Kubalak, S. E. Klewer, and J. A. McDonald. 2000. Disruption of hyaluronan synthase-2 abrogates normal cardiac morphogenesis and hyaluronan-mediated transformation of epithelium to mesenchyme. *J Clin Invest* 106 (3):349-60.

Carvajal-Vergara, X., A. Sevilla, S. L. D'Souza, Y. S. Ang, C. Schaniel, D. F. Lee, L. Yang, A. D. Kaplan, E. D. Adler, R. Rozov, Y. Ge, N. Cohen, L. J. Edelmann, B. Chang, A. Waghray, J. Su, S. Pardo, K. D. Lichtenbelt, M. Tartaglia, B. D. Gelb, and I. R. Lemischka. 2010. Patient-specific induced pluripotent stem-cell-derived models of LEOPARD syndrome. *Nature* 465 (7299):808-12.

Chang, H., A. Zwijsen, H. Vogel, D. Huylebroeck, and M. M. Matzuk. 2000. Smad5 is essential for left-right asymmetry in mice. *Dev Biol* 219 (1):71-8.

Chen, H., S. Shi, L. Acosta, W. Li, J. Lu, S. Bao, Z. Chen, Z. Yang, M. D. Schneider, K. R. Chien, S. J. Conway, M. C. Yoder, L. S. Haneline, D. Franco, and W. Shou. 2004. BMP10 is essential for maintaining cardiac growth during murine cardiogenesis. *Development* 131 (9):2219-31.

Chen, Y., A. Bhushan, and W. Vale. 1997. Smad8 mediates the signaling of the ALK-2 [corrected] receptor serine kinase. *Proc Natl Acad Sci U S A* 94 (24):12938-43.

Christoffels, V. M., W. M. Hoogaars, A. Tessari, D. E. Clout, A. F. Moorman, and M. Campione. 2004. T-box transcription factor Tbx2 represses differentiation and formation of the cardiac chambers. *Dev Dyn* 229 (4):763-70.

Christoffels, V. M., G. J. Smits, A. Kispert, and A. F. Moorman. 2010. Development of the pacemaker tissues of the heart. *Circ Res* 106 (2):240-54.

Chu, G. C., N. R. Dunn, D. C. Anderson, L. Oxburgh, and E. J. Robertson. 2004. Differential requirements for Smad4 in TGFbeta-dependent patterning of the early mouse embryo. *Development* 131 (15):3501-12.

Cárcamo, J., A. Zentella, and J. Massagué. 1995. Disruption of transforming growth factor beta signaling by a mutation that prevents transphosphorylation within the receptor complex. *Mol Cell Biol* 15 (3):1573-81.

Davis, B. N., A. C. Hilyard, G. Lagna, and A. Hata. 2008. SMAD proteins control DROSHA-mediated microRNA maturation. *Nature* 454 (7200):56-61.

Davis, B. N., A. C. Hilyard, P. H. Nguyen, G. Lagna, and A. Hata. 2010. Smad proteins bind a conserved RNA sequence to promote microRNA maturation by Drosha. *Mol Cell* 39 (3):373-84.

de Jong, F., T. Opthof, A. A. Wilde, M. J. Janse, R. Charles, W. H. Lamers, and A. F. Moorman. 1992. Persisting zones of slow impulse conduction in developing chicken hearts. *Circ Res* 71 (2):240-50.

Derynck, R., J. A. Jarrett, E. Y. Chen, D. H. Eaton, J. R. Bell, R. K. Assoian, A. B. Roberts, M. B. Sporn, and D. V. Goeddel. 1985. Human transforming growth factor-beta complementary DNA sequence and expression in normal and transformed cells. *Nature* 316 (6030):701-5.

Derynck, R., J. A. Jarrett, E. Y. Chen, and D. V. Goeddel. 1986. The murine transforming growth factor-beta precursor. *J Biol Chem* 261 (10):4377-9.

Desgrosellier, J. S., N. A. Mundell, M. A. McDonnell, H. L. Moses, and J. V. Barnett. 2005. Activin receptor-like kinase 2 and Smad6 regulate epithelial-mesenchymal transformation during cardiac valve formation. *Dev Biol* 280 (1):201-10.

Dewulf, N., K. Verschueren, O. Lonnoy, A. Morén, S. Grimsby, K. Vande Spiegle, K. Miyazono, D. Huylebroeck, and P. Ten Dijke. 1995. Distinct spatial and temporal expression patterns of two type I receptors for bone morphogenetic proteins during mouse embryogenesis. *Endocrinology* 136 (6):2652-63.

Dudley, A. T., and E. J. Robertson. 1997. Overlapping expression domains of bone morphogenetic protein family members potentially account for limited tissue defects in BMP7 deficient embryos. *Dev Dyn* 208 (3):349-62.

Dunwoodie, S. L. 2007. Combinatorial signaling in the heart orchestrates cardiac induction, lineage specification and chamber formation. *Semin Cell Dev Biol* 18 (1):54-66.

Délot, E. C., M. E. Bahamonde, M. Zhao, and K. M. Lyons. 2003. BMP signaling is required for septation of the outflow tract of the mammalian heart. *Development* 130 (1):209-20.

Ebisawa, T., M. Fukuchi, G. Murakami, T. Chiba, K. Tanaka, T. Imamura, and K. Miyazono. 2001. Smurf1 interacts with transforming growth factor-beta type I receptor through Smad7 and induces receptor degradation. *J Biol Chem* 276 (16):12477-80.

Edmonds, L. D., and L. M. James. 1993. Temporal trends in the birth prevalence of selected congenital malformations in the Birth Defects Monitoring Program/Commission on Professional and Hospital Activities, 1979-1989. *Teratology* 48 (6):647-9.

Ehrman, L. A., and K. E. Yutzey. 1999. Lack of regulation in the heart forming region of avian embryos. *Dev Biol* 207 (1):163-75.

Evans, S. M., D. Yelon, F. L. Conlon, and M. L. Kirby. 2010. Myocardial lineage development. *Circ Res* 107 (12):1428-44.

Fainsod, A., K. Deissler, R. Yelin, K. Marom, M. Epstein, G. Pillemer, H. Steinbeisser, and M. Blum. 1997. The dorsalizing and neural inducing gene follistatin is an antagonist of BMP-4. *Mech Dev* 63 (1):39-50.

Faure, S., P. de Santa Barbara, D. J. Roberts, and M. Whitman. 2002. Endogenous patterns of BMP signaling during early chick development. *Dev Biol* 244 (1):44-65.

Feijen, A., M. J. Goumans, and A. J. van den Eijnden-van Raaij. 1994. Expression of activin subunits, activin receptors and follistatin in postimplantation mouse embryos suggests specific developmental functions for different activins. *Development* 120 (12):3621-37.

Frasch, M. 1995. Induction of visceral and cardiac mesoderm by ectodermal Dpp in the early Drosophila embryo. *Nature* 374 (6521):464-7.

Fuentealba, L. C., E. Eivers, A. Ikeda, C. Hurtado, H. Kuroda, E. M. Pera, and E. M. De Robertis. 2007. Integrating patterning signals: Wnt/GSK3 regulates the duration of the BMP/Smad1 signal. *Cell* 131 (5):980-93.

Fukuda, T., K. Yamagata, S. Fujiyama, T. Matsumoto, I. Koshida, K. Yoshimura, M. Mihara, M. Naitou, H. Endoh, T. Nakamura, C. Akimoto, Y. Yamamoto, T. Katagiri, C. Foulds, S. Takezawa, H. Kitagawa, K. Takeyama, B. W. O'Malley, and S. Kato. 2007. DEAD-box RNA helicase subunits of the Drosha complex are required for processing of rRNA and a subset of microRNAs. *Nat Cell Biol* 9 (5):604-11.

Galvin, K. M., M. J. Donovan, C. A. Lynch, R. I. Meyer, R. J. Paul, J. N. Lorenz, V. Fairchild-Huntress, K. L. Dixon, J. H. Dunmore, M. A. Gimbrone, D. Falb, and D. Huszar. 2000. A role for smad6 in development and homeostasis of the cardiovascular system. *Nat Genet* 24 (2):171-4.

Gaussin, V., G. E. Morley, L. Cox, A. Zwijsen, K. M. Vance, L. Emile, Y. Tian, J. Liu, C. Hong, D. Myers, S. J. Conway, C. Depre, Y. Mishina, R. R. Behringer, M. C. Hanks, M. D. Schneider, D. Huylebroeck, G. I. Fishman, J. B. Burch, and S. F. Vatner. 2005. Alk3/Bmpr1a receptor is required for development of the atrioventricular canal into valves and annulus fibrosus. *Circ Res* 97 (3):219-26.

Gaussin, V., T. Van de Putte, Y. Mishina, M. C. Hanks, A. Zwijsen, D. Huylebroeck, R. R. Behringer, and M. D. Schneider. 2002. Endocardial cushion and myocardial defects after cardiac myocyte-specific conditional deletion of the bone morphogenetic protein receptor ALK3. *Proc Natl Acad Sci U S A* 99 (5):2878-83.

Goldman, D. C., N. Donley, and J. L. Christian. 2009. Genetic interaction between Bmp2 and Bmp4 reveals shared functions during multiple aspects of mouse organogenesis. *Mech Dev* 126 (3-4):117-27.

Grego-Bessa, J., L. Luna-Zurita, G. del Monte, V. Bolós, P. Melgar, A. Arandilla, A. N. Garratt, H. Zang, Y. S. Mukouyama, H. Chen, W. Shou, E. Ballestar, M. Esteller, A. Rojas, J. M. Pérez-Pomares, and J. L. de la Pompa. 2007. Notch signaling is essential for ventricular chamber development. *Dev Cell* 12 (3):415-29.

Grotewold, L., M. Plum, R. Dildrop, T. Peters, and U. Rüther. 2001. Bambi is coexpressed with Bmp-4 during mouse embryogenesis. *Mech Dev* 100 (2):327-30.

Gu, Z., E. M. Reynolds, J. Song, H. Lei, A. Feijen, L. Yu, W. He, D. T. MacLaughlin, J. van den Eijnden-van Raaij, P. K. Donahoe, and E. Li. 1999. The type I serine/threonine kinase receptor ActRIA (ALK2) is required for gastrulation of the mouse embryo. *Development* 126 (11):2551-61.

Habets, P. E., A. F. Moorman, D. E. Clout, M. A. van Roon, M. Lingbeek, M. van Lohuizen, M. Campione, and V. M. Christoffels. 2002. Cooperative action of Tbx2 and Nkx2.5 inhibits ANF expression in the atrioventricular canal: implications for cardiac chamber formation. *Genes Dev* 16 (10):1234-46.

Hanyu, A., Y. Ishidou, T. Ebisawa, T. Shimanuki, T. Imamura, and K. Miyazono. 2001. The N domain of Smad7 is essential for specific inhibition of transforming growth factor-beta signaling. *J Cell Biol* 155 (6):1017-27.

Harrelson, Z., R. G. Kelly, S. N. Goldin, J. J. Gibson-Brown, R. J. Bollag, L. M. Silver, and V. E. Papaioannou. 2004. Tbx2 is essential for patterning the atrioventricular canal and for morphogenesis of the outflow tract during heart development. *Development* 131 (20):5041-52.

Hata, A., G. Lagna, J. Massagué, and A. Hemmati-Brivanlou. 1998. Smad6 inhibits BMP/Smad1 signaling by specifically competing with the Smad4 tumor suppressor. *Genes Dev* 12 (2):186-97.

Hemmati-Brivanlou, A., O. G. Kelly, and D. A. Melton. 1994. Follistatin, an antagonist of activin, is expressed in the Spemann organizer and displays direct neuralizing activity. *Cell* 77 (2):283-95.

Hoffman, J. I. 1995. Incidence of congenital heart disease: II. Prenatal incidence. *Pediatr Cardiol* 16 (4):155-65.

Hoffman, J. I., and S. Kaplan. 2002. The incidence of congenital heart disease. *J Am Coll Cardiol* 39 (12):1890-900.

Hoodless, P. A., T. Haerry, S. Abdollah, M. Stapleton, M. B. O'Connor, L. Attisano, and J. L. Wrana. 1996. MADR1, a MAD-related protein that functions in BMP2 signaling pathways. *Cell* 85 (4):489-500.

Hosseinkhani, M., H. Hosseinkhani, A. Khademhosseini, F. Bolland, H. Kobayashi, and S. P. Gonzalez. 2007. Bone morphogenetic protein-4 enhances cardiomyocyte differentiation of cynomolgus monkey ESCs in knockout serum replacement medium. *Stem Cells* 25 (3):571-80.

Hsu, D. R., A. N. Economides, X. Wang, P. M. Eimon, and R. M. Harland. 1998. The Xenopus dorsalizing factor Gremlin identifies a novel family of secreted proteins that antagonize BMP activities. *Mol Cell* 1 (5):673-83.

Huang, Z., D. Wang, K. Ihida-Stansbury, P. L. Jones, and J. F. Martin. 2009. Defective pulmonary vascular remodeling in Smad8 mutant mice. *Hum Mol Genet* 18 (15):2791-801.

Iemura, S., T. S. Yamamoto, C. Takagi, H. Uchiyama, T. Natsume, S. Shimasaki, H. Sugino, and N. Ueno. 1998. Direct binding of follistatin to a complex of bone-morphogenetic protein and its receptor inhibits ventral and epidermal cell fates in early Xenopus embryo. *Proc Natl Acad Sci U S A* 95 (16):9337-42.

Imamura, T., M. Takase, A. Nishihara, E. Oeda, J. Hanai, M. Kawabata, and K. Miyazono. 1997. Smad6 inhibits signalling by the TGF-beta superfamily. *Nature* 389 (6651):622-6.

Jamali, M., C. Karamboulas, P. J. Rogerson, and I. S. Skerjanc. 2001. BMP signaling regulates Nkx2-5 activity during cardiomyogenesis. *FEBS Lett* 509 (1):126-30.

Jena, N., C. Martín-Seisdedos, P. McCue, and C. M. Croce. 1997. BMP7 null mutation in mice: developmental defects in skeleton, kidney, and eye. *Exp Cell Res* 230 (1):28-37.

Ji, R., Y. Cheng, J. Yue, J. Yang, X. Liu, H. Chen, D. B. Dean, and C. Zhang. 2007. MicroRNA expression signature and antisense-mediated depletion reveal an essential role of MicroRNA in vascular neointimal lesion formation. *Circ Res* 100 (11):1579-88.

Jia, Q., B. W. McDill, S. Z. Li, C. Deng, C. P. Chang, and F. Chen. 2007. Smad signaling in the neural crest regulates cardiac outflow tract remodeling through cell autonomous and non-cell autonomous effects. *Dev Biol* 311 (1):172-84.

Jiang, X., D. H. Rowitch, P. Soriano, A. P. McMahon, and H. M. Sucov. 2000. Fate of the mammalian cardiac neural crest. *Development* 127 (8):1607-16.

Jiao, K., H. Kulessa, K. Tompkins, Y. Zhou, L. Batts, H. S. Baldwin, and B. L. Hogan. 2003. An essential role of Bmp4 in the atrioventricular septation of the mouse heart. *Genes Dev* 17 (19):2362-7.

Jiao, K., Y. Zhou, and B. L. Hogan. 2002. Identification of mZnf8, a mouse Krüppel-like transcriptional repressor, as a novel nuclear interaction partner of Smad1. *Mol Cell Biol* 22 (21):7633-44.

Johansson, B. M., and M. V. Wiles. 1995. Evidence for involvement of activin A and bone morphogenetic protein 4 in mammalian mesoderm and hematopoietic development. *Mol Cell Biol* 15 (1):141-51.

Jones, C. M., K. M. Lyons, and B. L. Hogan. 1991. Involvement of Bone Morphogenetic Protein-4 (BMP-4) and Vgr-1 in morphogenesis and neurogenesis in the mouse. *Development* 111 (2):531-42.

Joziasse, I. C., K. A. Smith, S. Chocron, M. van Dinther, V. Guryev, J. J. van de Smagt, E. Cuppen, P. Ten Dijke, B. J. Mulder, C. L. Maslen, B. Reshey, P. A. Doevendans, and J. Bakkers. 2011. ALK2 mutation in a patient with Down's syndrome and a congenital heart defect. *Eur J Hum Genet* 19 (4):389-93.

Kaartinen, V., M. Dudas, A. Nagy, S. Sridurongrit, M. M. Lu, and J. A. Epstein. 2004. Cardiac outflow tract defects in mice lacking ALK2 in neural crest cells. *Development* 131 (14):3481-90.

Kattman, S. J., A. D. Witty, M. Gagliardi, N. C. Dubois, M. Niapour, A. Hotta, J. Ellis, and G. Keller. 2011. Stage-specific optimization of activin/nodal and BMP signaling promotes cardiac differentiation of mouse and human pluripotent stem cell lines. *Cell Stem Cell* 8 (2):228-40.

Kavsak, P., R. K. Rasmussen, C. G. Causing, S. Bonni, H. Zhu, G. H. Thomsen, and J. L. Wrana. 2000. Smad7 binds to Smurf2 to form an E3 ubiquitin ligase that targets the TGF beta receptor for degradation. *Mol Cell* 6 (6):1365-75.

Kawabata, M., A. Chytil, and H. L. Moses. 1995. Cloning of a novel type II serine/threonine kinase receptor through interaction with the type I transforming growth factor-beta receptor. *J Biol Chem* 270 (10):5625-30.

Kawai, T., T. Takahashi, M. Esaki, H. Ushikoshi, S. Nagano, H. Fujiwara, and K. Kosai. 2004. Efficient cardiomyogenic differentiation of embryonic stem cell by fibroblast growth factor 2 and bone morphogenetic protein 2. *Circ J* 68 (7):691-702.

Kim, R. Y., E. J. Robertson, and M. J. Solloway. 2001. Bmp6 and Bmp7 are required for cushion formation and septation in the developing mouse heart. *Dev Biol* 235 (2):449-66.

Kimura, N., R. Matsuo, H. Shibuya, K. Nakashima, and T. Taga. 2000. BMP2-induced apoptosis is mediated by activation of the TAK1-p38 kinase pathway that is negatively regulated by Smad6. *J Biol Chem* 275 (23):17647-52.

Kingsley, D. M., A. E. Bland, J. M. Grubber, P. C. Marker, L. B. Russell, N. G. Copeland, and N. A. Jenkins. 1992. The mouse short ear skeletal morphogenesis locus is associated with defects in a bone morphogenetic member of the TGF beta superfamily. *Cell* 71 (3):399-410.

Kirby, M. L., T. F. Gale, and D. E. Stewart. 1983. Neural crest cells contribute to normal aorticopulmonary septation. *Science* 220 (4601):1059-61.

Ko, S. O., I. H. Chung, X. Xu, S. Oka, H. Zhao, E. S. Cho, C. Deng, and Y. Chai. 2007. Smad4 is required to regulate the fate of cranial neural crest cells. *Dev Biol* 312 (1):435-47.

Koenig, B. B., J. S. Cook, D. H. Wolsing, J. Ting, J. P. Tiesman, P. E. Correa, C. A. Olson, A. L. Pecquet, F. Ventura, and R. A. Grant. 1994. Characterization and cloning of a receptor for BMP-2 and BMP-4 from NIH 3T3 cells. *Mol Cell Biol* 14 (9):5961-74.

Kokubo, H., S. Miyagawa-Tomita, M. Nakazawa, Y. Saga, and R. L. Johnson. 2005. Mouse hesr1 and hesr2 genes are redundantly required to mediate Notch signaling in the developing cardiovascular system. *Dev Biol* 278 (2):301-9.

Kulessa, H., and B. L. Hogan. 2002. Generation of a loxP flanked bmp4loxP-lacZ allele marked by conditional lacZ expression. *Genesis* 32 (2):66-8.

Laflamme, M. A., K. Y. Chen, A. V. Naumova, V. Muskheli, J. A. Fugate, S. K. Dupras, H. Reinecke, C. Xu, M. Hassanipour, S. Police, C. O'Sullivan, L. Collins, Y. Chen, E. Minami, E. A. Gill, S. Ueno, C. Yuan, J. Gold, and C. E. Murry. 2007. Cardiomyocytes derived from human embryonic stem cells in pro-survival factors enhance function of infarcted rat hearts. *Nat Biotechnol* 25 (9):1015-24.

Lai, C. F., and S. L. Cheng. 2002. Signal transductions induced by bone morphogenetic protein-2 and transforming growth factor-beta in normal human osteoblastic cells. *J Biol Chem* 277 (18):15514-22.

Lalani, S. R., J. V. Thakuria, G. F. Cox, X. Wang, W. Bi, M. S. Bray, C. Shaw, S. W. Cheung, A. C. Chinault, B. A. Boggs, Z. Ou, E. K. Brundage, J. R. Lupski, J. Gentile, S. Waisbren, A. Pursley, L. Ma, M. Khajavi, G. Zapata, R. Friedman, J. J. Kim, J. A. Towbin, P. Stankiewicz, S. Schnittger, I. Hansmann, T. Ai, S. Sood, X. H. Wehrens, J. F. Martin, J. W. Belmont, and L. Potocki. 2009. 20p12.3 microdeletion predisposes to Wolff-Parkinson-White syndrome with variable neurocognitive deficits. *J Med Genet* 46 (3):168-75.

Liberatore, C. M., R. D. Searcy-Schrick, E. B. Vincent, and K. E. Yutzey. 2002. Nkx-2.5 gene induction in mice is mediated by a Smad consensus regulatory region. *Dev Biol* 244 (2):243-56.

Lien, C. L., J. McAnally, J. A. Richardson, and E. N. Olson. 2002. Cardiac-specific activity of an Nkx2-5 enhancer requires an evolutionarily conserved Smad binding site. *Dev Biol* 244 (2):257-66.

Liu, N., and E. N. Olson. 2010. MicroRNA regulatory networks in cardiovascular development. *Dev Cell* 18 (4):510-25.

Liu, W., J. Selever, D. Wang, M. F. Lu, K. A. Moses, R. J. Schwartz, and J. F. Martin. 2004. Bmp4 signaling is required for outflow-tract septation and branchial-arch artery remodeling. *Proc Natl Acad Sci U S A* 101 (13):4489-94.

Liu, Y., M. Asakura, H. Inoue, T. Nakamura, M. Sano, Z. Niu, M. Chen, R. J. Schwartz, and M. D. Schneider. 2007. Sox17 is essential for the specification of cardiac mesoderm in embryonic stem cells. *Proc Natl Acad Sci U S A* 104 (10):3859-64.

Lou, J., Y. Tu, S. Li, and P. R. Manske. 2000. Involvement of ERK in BMP-2 induced osteoblastic differentiation of mesenchymal progenitor cell line C3H10T1/2. *Biochem Biophys Res Commun* 268 (3):757-62.

Lu, Y., J. M. Thomson, H. Y. Wong, S. M. Hammond, and B. L. Hogan. 2007. Transgenic over-expression of the microRNA miR-17-92 cluster promotes proliferation and inhibits differentiation of lung epithelial progenitor cells. *Dev Biol* 310 (2):442-53.

Luna-Zurita, L., B. Prados, J. Grego-Bessa, G. Luxán, G. del Monte, A. Benguría, R. H. Adams, J. M. Pérez-Pomares, and J. L. de la Pompa. 2010. Integration of a Notch-dependent mesenchymal gene program and Bmp2-driven cell invasiveness regulates murine cardiac valve formation. *J Clin Invest* 120 (10):3493-507.

Luo, G., C. Hofmann, A. L. Bronckers, M. Sohocki, A. Bradley, and G. Karsenty. 1995. BMP-7 is an inducer of nephrogenesis, and is also required for eye development and skeletal patterning. *Genes Dev* 9 (22):2808-20.

Lyons, K. M., B. L. Hogan, and E. J. Robertson. 1995. Colocalization of BMP 7 and BMP 2 RNAs suggests that these factors cooperatively mediate tissue interactions during murine development. *Mech Dev* 50 (1):71-83.

Lyons, K. M., R. W. Pelton, and B. L. Hogan. 1990. Organogenesis and pattern formation in the mouse: RNA distribution patterns suggest a role for bone morphogenetic protein-2A (BMP-2A). *Development* 109 (4):833-44.

Ma, L., M. F. Lu, R. J. Schwartz, and J. F. Martin. 2005. Bmp2 is essential for cardiac cushion epithelial-mesenchymal transition and myocardial patterning. *Development* 132 (24):5601-11.

Macías-Silva, M., P. A. Hoodless, S. J. Tang, M. Buchwald, and J. L. Wrana. 1998. Specific activation of Smad1 signaling pathways by the BMP7 type I receptor, ALK2. *J Biol Chem* 273 (40):25628-36.

Matzuk, M. M., T. R. Kumar, A. Vassalli, J. R. Bickenbach, D. R. Roop, R. Jaenisch, and A. Bradley. 1995. Functional analysis of activins during mammalian development. *Nature* 374 (6520):354-6.

Matzuk, M. M., N. Lu, H. Vogel, K. Sellheyer, D. R. Roop, and A. Bradley. 1995. Multiple defects and perinatal death in mice deficient in follistatin. *Nature* 374 (6520):360-3.

McMahon, J. A., S. Takada, L. B. Zimmerman, C. M. Fan, R. M. Harland, and A. P. McMahon. 1998. Noggin-mediated antagonism of BMP signaling is required for growth and patterning of the neural tube and somite. *Genes Dev* 12 (10):1438-52.

Mishina, Y., R. Crombie, A. Bradley, and R. R. Behringer. 1999. Multiple roles for activin-like kinase-2 signaling during mouse embryogenesis. *Dev Biol* 213 (2):314-26.

Mishina, Y., A. Suzuki, N. Ueno, and R. R. Behringer. 1995. Bmpr encodes a type I bone morphogenetic protein receptor that is essential for gastrulation during mouse embryogenesis. *Genes Dev* 9 (24):3027-37.

Monzen, K., Y. Hiroi, S. Kudoh, H. Akazawa, T. Oka, E. Takimoto, D. Hayashi, T. Hosoda, M. Kawabata, K. Miyazono, S. Ishii, Y. Yazaki, R. Nagai, and I. Komuro. 2001. Smads, TAK1, and their common target ATF-2 play a critical role in cardiomyocyte differentiation. *J Cell Biol* 153 (4):687-98.

Monzen, K., I. Shiojima, Y. Hiroi, S. Kudoh, T. Oka, E. Takimoto, D. Hayashi, T. Hosoda, A. Habara-Ohkubo, T. Nakaoka, T. Fujita, Y. Yazaki, and I. Komuro. 1999. Bone morphogenetic proteins induce cardiomyocyte differentiation through the mitogen-activated protein kinase kinase kinase TAK1 and cardiac transcription factors Csx/Nkx-2.5 and GATA-4. *Mol Cell Biol* 19 (10):7096-105.

Moorman, A. F., and V. M. Christoffels. 2003. Cardiac chamber formation: development, genes, and evolution. *Physiol Rev* 83 (4):1223-67.

Murakami, G., T. Watabe, K. Takaoka, K. Miyazono, and T. Imamura. 2003. Cooperative inhibition of bone morphogenetic protein signaling by Smurf1 and inhibitory Smads. *Mol Biol Cell* 14 (7):2809-17.

Nakajima, Y., T. Yamagishi, K. Ando, and H. Nakamura. 2002. Significance of bone morphogenetic protein-4 function in the initial myofibrillogenesis of chick cardiogenesis. *Dev Biol* 245 (2):291-303.

Neuhaus, H., V. Rosen, and R. S. Thies. 1999. Heart specific expression of mouse BMP-10 a novel member of the TGF-beta superfamily. *Mech Dev* 80 (2):181-4.

Nie, X., C. X. Deng, Q. Wang, and K. Jiao. 2008. Disruption of Smad4 in neural crest cells leads to mid-gestation death with pharyngeal arch, craniofacial and cardiac defects. *Dev Biol* 316 (2):417-30.

Nishimura, R., Y. Kato, D. Chen, S. E. Harris, G. R. Mundy, and T. Yoneda. 1998. Smad5 and DPC4 are key molecules in mediating BMP-2-induced osteoblastic differentiation of the pluripotent mesenchymal precursor cell line C2C12. *J Biol Chem* 273 (4):1872-9.

Nohno, T., T. Ishikawa, T. Saito, K. Hosokawa, S. Noji, D. H. Wolsing, and J. S. Rosenbaum. 1995. Identification of a human type II receptor for bone morphogenetic protein-4 that forms differential heteromeric complexes with bone morphogenetic protein type I receptors. *J Biol Chem* 270 (38):22522-6.

Oh, S. P., and E. Li. 1997. The signaling pathway mediated by the type IIB activin receptor controls axial patterning and lateral asymmetry in the mouse. *Genes Dev* 11 (14):1812-26.

Onichtchouk, D., Y. G. Chen, R. Dosch, V. Gawantka, H. Delius, J. Massagué, and C. Niehrs. 1999. Silencing of TGF-beta signalling by the pseudoreceptor BAMBI. *Nature* 401 (6752):480-5.

Park, C., K. Lavine, Y. Mishina, C. X. Deng, D. M. Ornitz, and K. Choi. 2006. Bone morphogenetic protein receptor 1A signaling is dispensable for hematopoietic development but essential for vessel and atrioventricular endocardial cushion formation. *Development* 133 (17):3473-84.

Pera, E. M., A. Ikeda, E. Eivers, and E. M. De Robertis. 2003. Integration of IGF, FGF, and anti-BMP signals via Smad1 phosphorylation in neural induction. *Genes Dev* 17 (24):3023-8.

Person, A. D., S. E. Klewer, and R. B. Runyan. 2005. Cell biology of cardiac cushion development. *Int Rev Cytol* 243:287-335.

Piccolo, S., Y. Sasai, B. Lu, and E. M. De Robertis. 1996. Dorsoventral patterning in Xenopus: inhibition of ventral signals by direct binding of chordin to BMP-4. *Cell* 86 (4):589-98.

Pignatelli, R. H., C. J. McMahon, W. J. Dreyer, S. W. Denfield, J. Price, J. W. Belmont, W. J. Craigen, J. Wu, H. El Said, L. I. Bezold, S. Clunie, S. Fernbach, N. E. Bowles, and J. A. Towbin. 2003. Clinical characterization of left ventricular noncompaction in children: a relatively common form of cardiomyopathy. *Circulation* 108 (21):2672-8.

Prall, O. W., M. K. Menon, M. J. Solloway, Y. Watanabe, S. Zaffran, F. Bajolle, C. Biben, J. J. McBride, B. R. Robertson, H. Chaulet, F. A. Stennard, N. Wise, D. Schaft, O. Wolstein, M. B. Furtado, H. Shiratori, K. R. Chien, H. Hamada, B. L. Black, Y. Saga, E. J. Robertson, M. E. Buckingham, and R. P. Harvey. 2007. An Nkx2-5/Bmp2/Smad1 negative feedback loop controls heart progenitor specification and proliferation. *Cell* 128 (5):947-59.

Qi, X., G. Yang, L. Yang, Y. Lan, T. Weng, J. Wang, Z. Wu, J. Xu, X. Gao, and X. Yang. 2007. Essential role of Smad4 in maintaining cardiomyocyte proliferation during murine embryonic heart development. *Dev Biol* 311 (1):136-46.

Reiter, J. F., H. Verkade, and D. Y. Stainier. 2001. Bmp2b and Oep promote early myocardial differentiation through their regulation of gata5. *Dev Biol* 234 (2):330-8.

Rentschler, S., J. Zander, K. Meyers, D. France, R. Levine, G. Porter, S. A. Rivkees, G. E. Morley, and G. I. Fishman. 2002. Neuregulin-1 promotes formation of the murine cardiac conduction system. *Proc Natl Acad Sci U S A* 99 (16):10464-9.

Rivera-Feliciano, J., and C. J. Tabin. 2006. Bmp2 instructs cardiac progenitors to form the heart-valve-inducing field. *Dev Biol* 295 (2):580-8.

Rosenzweig, B. L., T. Imamura, T. Okadome, G. N. Cox, H. Yamashita, P. ten Dijke, C. H. Heldin, and K. Miyazono. 1995. Cloning and characterization of a human type II receptor for bone morphogenetic proteins. *Proc Natl Acad Sci U S A* 92 (17):7632-6.

Rutenberg, J. B., A. Fischer, H. Jia, M. Gessler, T. P. Zhong, and M. Mercola. 2006. Developmental patterning of the cardiac atrioventricular canal by Notch and Hairy-related transcription factors. *Development* 133 (21):4381-90.

Samad, T. A., A. Rebbapragada, E. Bell, Y. Zhang, Y. Sidis, S. J. Jeong, J. A. Campagna, S. Perusini, D. A. Fabrizio, A. L. Schneyer, H. Y. Lin, A. H. Brivanlou, L. Attisano, and C. J. Woolf. 2005. DRAGON, a bone morphogenetic protein co-receptor. *J Biol Chem* 280 (14):14122-9.

Sapkota, G., C. Alarcón, F. M. Spagnoli, A. H. Brivanlou, and J. Massagué. 2007. Balancing BMP signaling through integrated inputs into the Smad1 linker. *Mol Cell* 25 (3):441-54.

Sasai, Y., B. Lu, H. Steinbeisser, and E. M. De Robertis. 1995. Regulation of neural induction by the Chd and Bmp-4 antagonistic patterning signals in Xenopus. *Nature* 376 (6538):333-6.

Scherner, O., S. K. Meurer, L. Tihaa, A. M. Gressner, and R. Weiskirchen. 2007. Endoglin differentially modulates antagonistic transforming growth factor-beta1 and BMP-7 signaling. *J Biol Chem* 282 (19):13934-43.

Schlange, T., B. Andrée, H. H. Arnold, and T. Brand. 2000. BMP2 is required for early heart development during a distinct time period. *Mech Dev* 91 (1-2):259-70.

Schultheiss, T. M., J. B. Burch, and A. B. Lassar. 1997. A role for bone morphogenetic proteins in the induction of cardiac myogenesis. *Genes Dev* 11 (4):451-62.

Schultheiss, T. M., S. Xydas, and A. B. Lassar. 1995. Induction of avian cardiac myogenesis by anterior endoderm. *Development* 121 (12):4203-14.

Shi, Y., S. Katsev, C. Cai, and S. Evans. 2000. BMP signaling is required for heart formation in vertebrates. *Dev Biol* 224 (2):226-37.

Shibuya, H., H. Iwata, N. Masuyama, Y. Gotoh, K. Yamaguchi, K. Irie, K. Matsumoto, E. Nishida, and N. Ueno. 1998. Role of TAK1 and TAB1 in BMP signaling in early Xenopus development. *EMBO J* 17 (4):1019-28.

Shirai, M., K. Imanaka-Yoshida, M. D. Schneider, R. J. Schwartz, and T. Morisaki. 2009. T-box 2, a mediator of Bmp-Smad signaling, induced hyaluronan synthase 2 and Tgfbeta2 expression and endocardial cushion formation. *Proc Natl Acad Sci U S A* 106 (44):18604-9.

Singh, R., T. Horsthuis, H. F. Farin, T. Grieskamp, J. Norden, M. Petry, V. Wakker, A. F. Moorman, V. M. Christoffels, and A. Kispert. 2009. Tbx20 interacts with smads to confine tbx2 expression to the atrioventricular canal. *Circ Res* 105 (5):442-52.

Sirard, C., J. L. de la Pompa, A. Elia, A. Itie, C. Mirtsos, A. Cheung, S. Hahn, A. Wakeham, L. Schwartz, S. E. Kern, J. Rossant, and T. W. Mak. 1998. The tumor suppressor gene

Smad4/Dpc4 is required for gastrulation and later for anterior development of the mouse embryo. *Genes Dev* 12 (1):107-19.
Smith, K. A., I. C. Joziasse, S. Chocron, M. van Dinther, V. Guryev, M. C. Verhoeven, H. Rehmann, J. J. van der Smagt, P. A. Doevendans, E. Cuppen, B. J. Mulder, P. Ten Dijke, and J. Bakkers. 2009. Dominant-negative ALK2 allele associates with congenital heart defects. *Circulation* 119 (24):3062-9.
Solloway, M. J., A. T. Dudley, E. K. Bikoff, K. M. Lyons, B. L. Hogan, and E. J. Robertson. 1998. Mice lacking Bmp6 function. *Dev Genet* 22 (4):321-39.
Solloway, M. J., and E. J. Robertson. 1999. Early embryonic lethality in Bmp5;Bmp7 double mutant mice suggests functional redundancy within the 60A subgroup. *Development* 126 (8):1753-68.
Somi, S., A. A. Buffing, A. F. Moorman, and M. J. Van Den Hoff. 2004. Dynamic patterns of expression of BMP isoforms 2, 4, 5, 6, and 7 during chicken heart development. *Anat Rec A Discov Mol Cell Evol Biol* 279 (1):636-51.
Repeated Author. 2004. Expression of bone morphogenetic protein-10 mRNA during chicken heart development. *Anat Rec A Discov Mol Cell Evol Biol* 279 (1):579-82.
Song, J., S. P. Oh, H. Schrewe, M. Nomura, H. Lei, M. Okano, T. Gridley, and E. Li. 1999. The type II activin receptors are essential for egg cylinder growth, gastrulation, and rostral head development in mice. *Dev Biol* 213 (1):157-69.
Song, L., R. Fässler, Y. Mishina, K. Jiao, and H. S. Baldwin. 2007. Essential functions of Alk3 during AV cushion morphogenesis in mouse embryonic hearts. *Dev Biol* 301 (1):276-86.
Song, L., W. Yan, X. Chen, C. X. Deng, Q. Wang, and K. Jiao. 2007. Myocardial smad4 is essential for cardiogenesis in mouse embryos. *Circ Res* 101 (3):277-85.
Stefanovic, S., N. Abboud, S. Désilets, D. Nury, C. Cowan, and M. Pucéat. 2009. Interplay of Oct4 with Sox2 and Sox17: a molecular switch from stem cell pluripotency to specifying a cardiac fate. *J Cell Biol* 186 (5):665-73.
Stern, C. D., R. T. Yu, A. Kakizuka, C. R. Kintner, L. S. Mathews, W. W. Vale, R. M. Evans, and K. Umesono. 1995. Activin and its receptors during gastrulation and the later phases of mesoderm development in the chick embryo. *Dev Biol* 172 (1):192-205.
Stottmann, R. W., M. Choi, Y. Mishina, E. N. Meyers, and J. Klingensmith. 2004. BMP receptor IA is required in mammalian neural crest cells for development of the cardiac outflow tract and ventricular myocardium. *Development* 131 (9):2205-18.
Streit, A., K. J. Lee, I. Woo, C. Roberts, T. M. Jessell, and C. D. Stern. 1998. Chordin regulates primitive streak development and the stability of induced neural cells, but is not sufficient for neural induction in the chick embryo. *Development* 125 (3):507-19.
Stroud, D. M., V. Gaussin, J. B. Burch, C. Yu, Y. Mishina, M. D. Schneider, G. I. Fishman, and G. E. Morley. 2007. Abnormal conduction and morphology in the atrioventricular node of mice with atrioventricular canal targeted deletion of Alk3/Bmpr1a receptor. *Circulation* 116 (22):2535-43.
Sugi, Y., H. Yamamura, H. Okagawa, and R. R. Markwald. 2004. Bone morphogenetic protein-2 can mediate myocardial regulation of atrioventricular cushion mesenchymal cell formation in mice. *Dev Biol* 269 (2):505-18.
Suzawa, M., Y. Tamura, S. Fukumoto, K. Miyazono, T. Fujita, S. Kato, and Y. Takeuchi. 2002. Stimulation of Smad1 transcriptional activity by Ras-extracellular signal-regulated

kinase pathway: a possible mechanism for collagen-dependent osteoblastic differentiation. *J Bone Miner Res* 17 (2):240-8.

Takahashi, K., K. Tanabe, M. Ohnuki, M. Narita, T. Ichisaka, K. Tomoda, and S. Yamanaka. 2007. Induction of pluripotent stem cells from adult human fibroblasts by defined factors. *Cell* 131 (5):861-72.

Takei, S., H. Ichikawa, K. Johkura, A. Mogi, H. No, S. Yoshie, D. Tomotsune, and K. Sasaki. 2009. Bone morphogenetic protein-4 promotes induction of cardiomyocytes from human embryonic stem cells in serum-based embryoid body development. *Am J Physiol Heart Circ Physiol* 296 (6):H1793-803.

ten Dijke, P., H. Yamashita, T. K. Sampath, A. H. Reddi, M. Estevez, D. L. Riddle, H. Ichijo, C. H. Heldin, and K. Miyazono. 1994. Identification of type I receptors for osteogenic protein-1 and bone morphogenetic protein-4. *J Biol Chem* 269 (25):16985-8.

Tirosh-Finkel, L., H. Elhanany, A. Rinon, and E. Tzahor. 2006. Mesoderm progenitor cells of common origin contribute to the head musculature and the cardiac outflow tract. *Development* 133 (10):1943-53.

Tirosh-Finkel, L., A. Zeisel, M. Brodt-Ivenshitz, A. Shamai, Z. Yao, R. Seger, E. Domany, and E. Tzahor. 2010. BMP-mediated inhibition of FGF signaling promotes cardiomyocyte differentiation of anterior heart field progenitors. *Development* 137 (18):2989-3000.

Tomescot, A., J. Leschik, V. Bellamy, G. Dubois, E. Messas, P. Bruneval, M. Desnos, A. A. Hagège, M. Amit, J. Itskovitz, P. Menasché, and M. Pucéat. 2007. Differentiation in vivo of cardiac committed human embryonic stem cells in postmyocardial infarcted rats. *Stem Cells* 25 (9):2200-5.

Tremblay, K. D., N. R. Dunn, and E. J. Robertson. 2001. Mouse embryos lacking Smad1 signals display defects in extra-embryonic tissues and germ cell formation. *Development* 128 (18):3609-21.

Uchimura, T., Y. Komatsu, M. Tanaka, K. L. McCann, and Y. Mishina. 2009. Bmp2 and Bmp4 genetically interact to support multiple aspects of mouse development including functional heart development. *Genesis* 47 (6):374-84.

Valderrábano, M., F. Chen, A. S. Dave, S. T. Lamp, T. S. Klitzner, and J. N. Weiss. 2006. Atrioventricular ring reentry in embryonic mouse hearts. *Circulation* 114 (6):543-9.

Ventura, A., A. G. Young, M. M. Winslow, L. Lintault, A. Meissner, S. J. Erkeland, J. Newman, R. T. Bronson, D. Crowley, J. R. Stone, R. Jaenisch, P. A. Sharp, and T. Jacks. 2008. Targeted deletion reveals essential and overlapping functions of the miR-17 through 92 family of miRNA clusters. *Cell* 132 (5):875-86.

Waldo, K. L., D. H. Kumiski, K. T. Wallis, H. A. Stadt, M. R. Hutson, D. H. Platt, and M. L. Kirby. 2001. Conotruncal myocardium arises from a secondary heart field. *Development* 128 (16):3179-88.

Waldo, K., S. Miyagawa-Tomita, D. Kumiski, and M. L. Kirby. 1998. Cardiac neural crest cells provide new insight into septation of the cardiac outflow tract: aortic sac to ventricular septal closure. *Dev Biol* 196 (2):129-44.

Wang, D., P. S. Chang, Z. Wang, L. Sutherland, J. A. Richardson, E. Small, P. A. Krieg, and E. N. Olson. 2001. Activation of cardiac gene expression by myocardin, a transcriptional cofactor for serum response factor. *Cell* 105 (7):851-62.

Wang, J., S. B. Greene, M. Bonilla-Claudio, Y. Tao, J. Zhang, Y. Bai, Z. Huang, B. L. Black, F. Wang, and J. F. Martin. 2010. Bmp signaling regulates myocardial differentiation from cardiac progenitors through a MicroRNA-mediated mechanism. *Dev Cell* 19 (6):903-12.

Wang, J., S. Sridurongrit, M. Dudas, P. Thomas, A. Nagy, M. D. Schneider, J. A. Epstein, and V. Kaartinen. 2005. Atrioventricular cushion transformation is mediated by ALK2 in the developing mouse heart. *Dev Biol* 286 (1):299-310.

Wang, J., N. Xu, X. Feng, N. Hou, J. Zhang, X. Cheng, Y. Chen, Y. Zhang, and X. Yang. 2005. Targeted disruption of Smad4 in cardiomyocytes results in cardiac hypertrophy and heart failure. *Circ Res* 97 (8):821-8.

Warner, D. R., V. Bhattacherjee, X. Yin, S. Singh, P. Mukhopadhyay, M. M. Pisano, and R. M. Greene. 2004. Functional interaction between Smad, CREB binding protein, and p68 RNA helicase. *Biochem Biophys Res Commun* 324 (1):70-6.

Wieser, R., J. L. Wrana, and J. Massagué. 1995. GS domain mutations that constitutively activate T beta R-I, the downstream signaling component in the TGF-beta receptor complex. *EMBO J* 14 (10):2199-208.

Wozney, J. M., V. Rosen, M. Byrne, A. J. Celeste, I. Moutsatsos, and E. A. Wang. 1990. Growth factors influencing bone development. *J Cell Sci Suppl* 13:149-56.

Xing, Y., F. Ichida, T. Matsuoka, T. Isobe, Y. Ikemoto, T. Higaki, T. Tsuji, N. Haneda, A. Kuwabara, R. Chen, T. Futatani, S. Tsubata, S. Watanabe, K. Watanabe, K. Hirono, K. Uese, T. Miyawaki, K. R. Bowles, N. E. Bowles, and J. A. Towbin. 2006. Genetic analysis in patients with left ventricular noncompaction and evidence for genetic heterogeneity. *Mol Genet Metab* 88 (1):71-7.

Xu, R. H., Z. Dong, M. Maeno, J. Kim, A. Suzuki, N. Ueno, D. Sredni, N. H. Colburn, and H. F. Kung. 1996. Involvement of Ras/Raf/AP-1 in BMP-4 signaling during Xenopus embryonic development. *Proc Natl Acad Sci U S A* 93 (2):834-8.

Xu, X., Z. Yin, J. B. Hudson, E. L. Ferguson, and M. Frasch. 1998. Smad proteins act in combination with synergistic and antagonistic regulators to target Dpp responses to the Drosophila mesoderm. *Genes Dev* 12 (15):2354-70.

Yamada, M., J. P. Revelli, G. Eichele, M. Barron, and R. J. Schwartz. 2000. Expression of chick Tbx-2, Tbx-3, and Tbx-5 genes during early heart development: evidence for BMP2 induction of Tbx2. *Dev Biol* 228 (1):95-105.

Yamagishi, T., Y. Nakajima, K. Miyazono, and H. Nakamura. 1999. Bone morphogenetic protein-2 acts synergistically with transforming growth factor-beta3 during endothelial-mesenchymal transformation in the developing chick heart. *J Cell Physiol* 180 (1):35-45.

Yamagishi, T., Y. Nakajima, S. Nishimatsu, T. Nohno, K. Ando, and H. Nakamura. 2001. Expression of bone morphogenetic protein-5 gene during chick heart development: possible roles in valvuloseptal endocardial cushion formation. *Anat Rec* 264 (4):313-6.

Yamaguchi, K., K. Shirakabe, H. Shibuya, K. Irie, I. Oishi, N. Ueno, T. Taniguchi, E. Nishida, and K. Matsumoto. 1995. Identification of a member of the MAPKKK family as a potential mediator of TGF-beta signal transduction. *Science* 270 (5244):2008-11.

Yamashita, H., P. ten Dijke, D. Huylebroeck, T. K. Sampath, M. Andries, J. C. Smith, C. H. Heldin, and K. Miyazono. 1995. Osteogenic protein-1 binds to activin type II receptors and induces certain activin-like effects. *J Cell Biol* 130 (1):217-26.

Yanagisawa, M., K. Nakashima, K. Takeda, W. Ochiai, T. Takizawa, M. Ueno, M. Takizawa, H. Shibuya, and T. Taga. 2001. Inhibition of BMP2-induced, TAK1 kinase-mediated neurite outgrowth by Smad6 and Smad7. *Genes Cells* 6 (12):1091-9.

Yang, J., S. A. Mani, J. L. Donaher, S. Ramaswamy, R. A. Itzykson, C. Come, P. Savagner, I. Gitelman, A. Richardson, and R. A. Weinberg. 2004. Twist, a master regulator of morphogenesis, plays an essential role in tumor metastasis. *Cell* 117 (7):927-39.

Yang, L., M. H. Soonpaa, E. D. Adler, T. K. Roepke, S. J. Kattman, M. Kennedy, E. Henckaerts, K. Bonham, G. W. Abbott, R. M. Linden, L. J. Field, and G. M. Keller. 2008. Human cardiovascular progenitor cells develop from a KDR+ embryonic-stem-cell-derived population. *Nature* 453 (7194):524-8.

Yang, X., L. H. Castilla, X. Xu, C. Li, J. Gotay, M. Weinstein, P. P. Liu, and C. X. Deng. 1999. Angiogenesis defects and mesenchymal apoptosis in mice lacking SMAD5. *Development* 126 (8):1571-80.

Yi, S. E., A. Daluiski, R. Pederson, V. Rosen, and K. M. Lyons. 2000. The type I BMP receptor BMPRIB is required for chondrogenesis in the mouse limb. *Development* 127 (3):621-30.

Yin, Z., and M. Frasch. 1998. Regulation and function of tinman during dorsal mesoderm induction and heart specification in Drosophila. *Dev Genet* 22 (3):187-200.

Zhang, H., and A. Bradley. 1996. Mice deficient for BMP2 are nonviable and have defects in amnion/chorion and cardiac development. *Development* 122 (10):2977-86.

Zhang, Y., T. Musci, and R. Derynck. 1997. The tumor suppressor Smad4/DPC 4 as a central mediator of Smad function. *Curr Biol* 7 (4):270-6.

Zimmerman, L. B., J. M. De Jesús-Escobar, and R. M. Harland. 1996. The Spemann organizer signal noggin binds and inactivates bone morphogenetic protein 4. *Cell* 86 (4):599-606.

5

Molecular Mechanisms of Congenital Heart Disease

Jing-bin Huang and Jian Liang
Department of Cardiothoracic Surgery, The Affiliated Ruikang Hospital of Guangxi Traditional Chinese Medical College, Nanning China

1. Introduction

Congenital heart disease (CHD) is the most common type of birth defect, affecting 1% of all live births, and is the leading non-infectious cause of death in the first year of life [1,2]. CHD is a multifactorial complex disease, with environmental and genetic factors playing important roles. It has been recognized that environmental factors/insults during fetal development increase the risk of CHD, including viral infections with rubella [3], exposure to chemical teratogens such as retinoic acid , lithium, dilantin [4]and halogenated hydrocarbon [5]and maternal diseases including diabetes and systemic lupus erythematosus [1, 6]. Epidemiologic studies of CHD have demonstrated an increased recurrence risk for cardiac malformations in sequent pregnancies, supporting the existence of gene predispositions.

Great progress in molecular genetics and developmental biology has been made. Current genetic techniques for evaluation of congenital heart defects include cytogenetic techniques, fluorescence in situ hybridization (FISH) and DNA mutation analysis. Most methods employ polymerase chain reaction–based assays. Indirect screening methods, such as denaturing high-performance liquid chromatography or single-strand conformation polymorphism have been used extensively. More expensive exon-by-exon sequencing of genomic DNA has recently emerged [7, 8]. It has been accepted that the intricate process of cardiac morphogenesis is controlled by a network of highly conserved genetic and molecular pathways. The origins of CHD are diverse, such as abnormal chromosome structure (eg. duplication or deletion), gene mutations, single nucleotide polymorphisms, abnormal RNA, epigenetics and so on, and they are summarized in Figure 1.

In humans, heart development begins at 15 to 16 days of gestation with the migration of precardiac stem cells, in five steps:(1)migration of precardiac cells from the primitive streak and assembly of the paired cardiac crescents at the myocardial plate, (2) coalescence of the cardiac crescents to form the primitive heart tube, establishing the definitive heart, (3) cardiac looping, assurance of proper alignment of the future cardiac chambers, (4) septation and heart chambers formation, and (5) development of the cardiac conduction system and coronary vasculature [9-11]. The establishment of left-right asymmetry is very important to the normal development of heart [12, 13]. Secreted FGF, BMP, Nodal, and Wnt act as input signal of symmetric cardiac morphogenesis, BMP2, FGF8, Shh/Ihh, and Nodal function as positive regulators, whereas Wnt and Ser are negative regulators [14-16]. The cardiogenic plate-specific expressed genes NKX2.5, SRF, GATA4, TBX5, and HAND2, compose the core regulatory network of cardiac morphogenesis, controlling heart looping, left-right symmetry and chambers formation. SRF regulates the differentiation of coronary vascular smooth muscle cells [17, 18]. Genes that involved in epicardial development include FOG-2, vascular cell adhesion molecule 1, integrins, erythropoietin, and erythropoietin receptor. Specific genes such as the NOTCH receptor, Jagged (JAG), WNT, transforming growth factor beta 2 (TGF ß2) and bone morphogenic proteins have been implicated in cardiac neural crest development in the mouse[12, 19-21]. Retinoic acid signal pathway is involved in the regulation of cardiac looping. Complex signal pathways are implicated in the crosstalk between endocardium and myocardium to form endocardial cushion and heart valves, including VEGF, NFATc1, Notch, Wnt/ß-catenin, BMP/TGF-ß, EGF, erbB, NF1 signal pathways [10, 22-24].

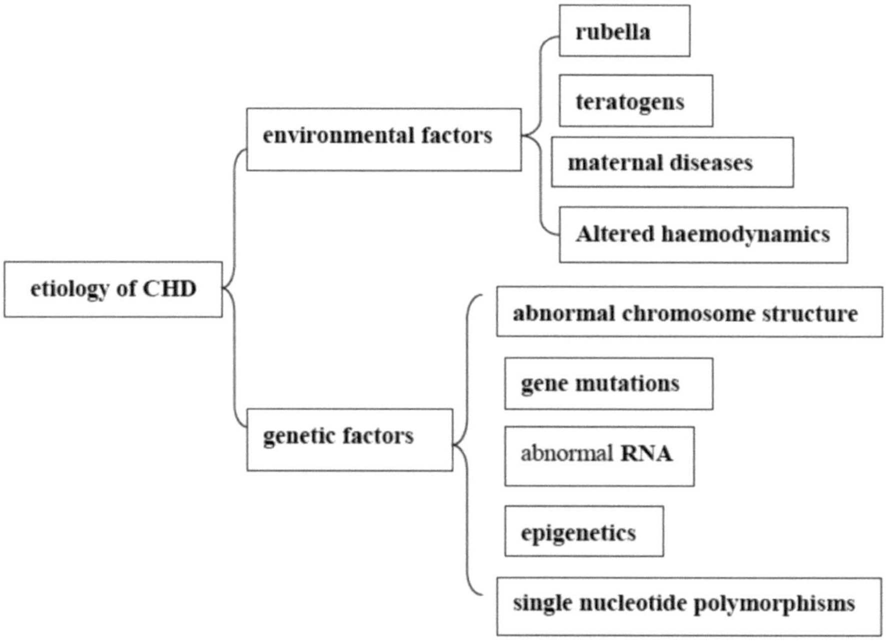

Fig. 1. Eteology of CHD

2. Molecular mechanisms of congenital heart disease

2.1.1 Causative genes of CHD

The etiological factors of many genetic syndromes and familial CHD have been identified, but the genetic basis of majority of "sporadic" CHD remains unknown. With the progress in molecular genetics and developmental biology, many genes associated heart development have been identified. When searching computer databases such as NCBI Gene Bank for "cardiac or heart", we can indentify 1154 loci in human. Search for"(heart or cardiac)and development", limited to human, 630 genes were found. A number of selected congenital heart defects and genetic syndromes have been found to be associated with mutations in a variety of single genes. The mutations were found only in affected individuals, were not present in control samples, and were demonstrated to change protein structure or function.

Disease genes of CHD identified to date are summarized in Table 1, and the functions of these causative genes are summarized as following [25].

disorder	Causative genes	Chromosome Location
Congenital heart defects		
Familial congenital heart diseas(ASD, atrioventricular block)	*NKX2.5*	5q34-q35
D-TGA, DORV	*CFC1*	2q21
D-TGA	*PROSIT240*	12q24
Tetralogy of Fallot	*ZFPM2*	8q23
	NKX2.5	5q34-q35
	JAG1	20p12
Atrioventricular septal defect	*CRELD1*	3p21
ASD/VSD	*GATA4*	8p23
Heterotaxy	*ZIC3*	Xq26
	CFC1	2q21
	ACVR2B	3p21.3-p221q42.1
	LEFTYA	
Supravalvar aortic stenosis Syndromes	*ELN*	7q11
Holt-Oram Syndromes	*TBX5*	12q24
Alagille Syndromes	*JAG1*	20p12
Char Syndromes (PDA)	*TFAP2B*	6p12
Noonan Syndromes	*PTPN11*	12q24
	KRAS	2p1.21
	SOS1	2p21
CHARGE Syndromes	*CHD7*	8q12
Ellis-van Creveld	*EVC, EVC2*	4p16
Martan Syndromes	*FBN1*	15q21.1
Marfan-like Syndromes	*TGFBR2*	3p22
Cardiofaciocutaneous Syndromes	*KRAS*	12p12.1
	BRAF	7q34
	MEK1	15q21
	MEK2	7q32
Costello Syndromes	*HRAS*	11p15.5

Table 1. Causative genes of CHD

For example, NKX2-5, Homeobox-containing genes play critical roles in regulating tissue-specific gene expression essential for tissue differentiation, as well as determining the temporal and spatial patterns of development. It has been demonstrated that a Drosophila

homeobox-containing gene called 'tinman' is expressed in the developing dorsal vessel and in the equivalent of the vertebrate heart. Mutations in tinman result in loss of heart formation in the embryo, suggesting that tinman is essential for Drosophila heart formation. Furthermore, abundant expression of Csx, the presumptive mouse homolog of tinman, is observed only in the heart from the time of cardiac differentiation. CSX, the human homolog of murine Csx, has a homeodomain sequence identical to that of Csx and is expressed only in the heart, again suggesting that CSX plays an important role in human heart formation. Studies have recently shown that nonsyndromic CHD can result from single-gene defects. Schott et al identified mutations in *NKX2.5* in 4 kindreds with atrial septal defects and atrioventricular conduction delay without other apparent syndromic features. The mutations were found only in affected individuals, were not present in control samples, and were demonstrated to change protein structure or function [26-28].
Noonan Syndrome is a genetic multiple malformation disorder that includes short stature, typical facial dysmorphism, webbed neck, chest deformity, and cardiovascular abnormalities. The cardiac involvement is observed in 80% to 90% of affected individuals, with valvar pulmonic stenosis and hypertrophic cardiomyopathy being the most common. Other congenital heart defects observed in Noonan Syndrome are secundum atrial septal defect, atrioventricular septal defect, mitral valve abnormalities, aortic coarctation, and tetralogy of Fallot. Noonan Syndrome is genetically heterogeneous, which means that there are at least 3 Noonan Syndrome disease genes, *PTPN11*, *SOS1*, and *KRAS* [29]. It is *PTPN11*, which encodes a protein tyrosine phosphatase called SHP-2. SHP-2 plays an important role in signal transduction for a wide variety of biological processes, including the formation of the semilunar valves. Mutations in the *PTPN11* gene are observed in 40% to 50% of Noonan Syndrome patients [25, 30].

2.1.2 Functions of the causative genes of CHD

Table2 shows the functions of the causative genes of CHD.

Genes affected		
Transcription factors	Signaling proteins	Vascular extracellular matrix
GATA4	PTPN11	FBN-1
TBX1	Jagged 1	Elastin
TBX5	DMPK	
NKX2.5	CFC1	
dHAND	SOS1	
TFAP2	TGFBR2	
ZFPM2	KRAS	
	BRAF	
	MEK1	
	MEK2	
	HRAS	
	ACVR2B	
	CRELD1	
	LEFTYA	

NKX2-5, NK2 transcription factor related, locus 5

Table 2. Inborn Errors Causing CHD

Homeobox-containing genes play critical roles in regulating tissue-specific gene expression essential for tissue differentiation, as well as determining the temporal and spatial patterns of development. Mutations in NKX2-5 result in loss of heart formation in the embryo, suggesting that NKX2-5 is essential for heart formation [31, 32].

CFC1, cripto, FRL-1, cryptic family 1

This gene encodes a member of the epidermal growth factor (EGF)- Cripto, Frl-1, and Cryptic (CFC) family. These proteins play key roles in intercellular signaling pathways during vertebrate embryogenesis. Mutations in this gene can cause autosomal visceral heterotaxy. This protein is involved in left-right asymmetric morphogenesis during organ development [33, 34].

PROSIT240, MED13L, mediator complex subunit 13-like

Also known as THRAP2, The evolutionarily conserved THRAP genes encode a family of proteins that regulate embryonic development. THRAP2 is involved in early development of the heart and brain [35].

ZFPM2, zinc finger protein, multitype 2

The zinc finger protein encoded by this gene is a widely expressed member of the FOG family of transcription factors. The family members modulate the activity of GATA family proteins, which are important regulators of hematopoiesis and cardiogenesis in mammals [36].

Jagged 1, jagged 1 (Alagille syndrome)

The jagged 1 protein encoded by JAG1 is the human homolog of the Drosophilia jagged protein. Human jagged 1 is the ligand for the receptor notch 1. Mutations that alter the jagged 1 protein cause Alagille syndrome [37].

CRELD1, cysteine-rich with EGF-like domains 1

Epidermal growth factor-like repeats are a class of cysteine-rich domains that mediate interactions between proteins of diverse function. CRELD1 is the founding member of a family of matricellular proteins [38].

GATA4, GATA binding protein 4

This gene encodes a member of the GATA family of zinc-finger transcription factors. This protein is thought to regulate genes involved in embryogenesis and in myocardial differentiation and function. Mutations in this gene have been associated with cardiac septal defects [39].

ZIC3, Zic family member 3 heterotaxy 1

This gene encodes a member of the ZIC family of C2H2-type zinc finger proteins. Mutations in this gene cause X-linked visceral heterotaxy [40].

ACVR2B, activin A receptor, type 2, beta

Activins are dimeric growth and differentiation factors which belong to the transforming growth factor-beta superfamily of structurally related signaling proteins. These receptors are all transmembrane proteins [41].

LEFTYA, left-right determination factor 2

This gene encodes a member of the TGF-beta family of proteins. The encoded protein is secreted and plays a role in left-right asymmetry determination of organ systems during development.Mutations in this gene have been associated with left-right axis malformations, particularly in the heart and lungs [42].

ELN, Elastin

This gene encodes a protein that is one of the two components of elastic fibers. Deletions and mutations in this gene are associated with supravalvular aortic stenosis (SVAS) and autosomal dominant cutis laxa [43].

TBX5, T-box 5

This gene is a member of a phylogenetically conserved family of genes that share a common DNA-binding domain, the T-box. The encoded protein may play a role in heart development and specification of limb identity. Mutations in this gene have been associated with Holt-Oram syndrome [44].

TFAP2B, transcription factor AP-2 beta

This gene encodes a member of the AP-2 family of transcription factors. This protein functions as both a transcriptional activator and repressor. Mutations in this gene result in autosomal dominant Char syndrome, suggesting that this gene functions in the differentiation of neural crest cell derivatives [45].

PTPN11, protein tyrosine phosphatase, non-receptor type 11

The protein encoded by this gene is a member of the protein tyrosine phosphatase (PTP) family. PTPs are known to be signaling molecules that regulate a variety of cellular processes including cell growth, differentiation, mitotic cycle, and oncogenic transformation. Mutations in this gene are a cause of Noonan syndrome as well as acute myeloid leukemia [46].

SOS1, son of sevenless homolog 1

This gene encodes a protein that is a guanine nucleotide exchange factor for RAS proteins, membrane proteins that bind guanine nucleotides and participate in signal transduction pathways. Mutations in this gene are associated with gingival fibromatosis 1 and Noonan syndrome type 4 [47].

CHD7, chromodomain helicase DNA binding protein 7

This gene encodes a protein that contains several helicase family domains. Mutations in this gene have been found in some patients with the CHARGE syndrome [48, 49].

EVC, Ellis van Creveld syndrome

This gene encodes a protein containing a leucine zipper and a transmembrane domain. This gene has been implicated in both Ellis-van Creveld syndrome (EvC) and Weyers acrodental dysostosis [50].

FBN1, fibrillin 1

This gene encodes a member of the fibrillin family. Mutations in this gene are associated with Marfan syndrome, isolated ectopia lentis, autosomal dominant Weill-Marchesani syndrome, MASS syndrome, and Shprintzen-Goldberg craniosynostosis syndrome [51].

TGFBR2, transforming growth factor receptor 2

This gene encodes a member of the Ser/Thr protein kinase family and the TGFB receptor subfamily. Mutations in this gene have been associated with Marfan Syndrome, Loeys-Deitz Aortic Aneurysm Syndrome, and the development of various types of tumors [52].

KRAS, v-Ki-ras2 Kirsten rat sarcoma viral oncogene homolog

This gene, encodes a protein that is a member of the small GTPase superfamily. The transforming protein that results is implicated in various malignancies, including lung adenocarcinoma, mucinous adenoma, ductal carcinoma of the pancreas and colorectal carcinoma [53].

BRAF, v-raf murine sarcoma viral oncogene homolog B1

This gene encodes a protein belonging to the raf/mil family of serine/threonine protein kinases. This protein plays a role in regulating the MAP kinase/ERKs signaling pathway, which affects cell division, differentiation, and secretion. Mutations in this gene are associated with cardiofaciocutaneous syndrome [53].

MEK1, MAP2K1, mitogen-activated protein kinase 1

The protein encoded by this gene is a member of the dual specificity protein kinase family, which acts as a mitogen-activated protein (MAP) kinase kinase. This kinase is involved in many cellular processes such as proliferation, differentiation, transcription regulation and development [54].

MEK2, MAP2K2, mitogen-activated protein kinase 2

The protein encoded by this gene is a dual specificity protein kinase that belongs to the MAP kinase kinase family. This kinase is known to play a critical role in mitogen growth factor signal transduction. Mutations in this gene cause cardiofaciocutaneous syndrome (CFC syndrome) [55].

HRAS, v-Ha-ras Harvey rat sarcoma viral oncogene homolog

This gene belongs to the Ras oncogene family. The products encoded by these genes function in signal transduction pathways. Mutations in this gene cause Costello syndrome. Defects in this gene are implicated in a variety of cancers [56].

2.2 Pathogenic mechanisms of congenital heart disease

Phenotypes of CHD vary from small ASD and VSD, which may go undetected throughout life, to large ASD and VSD, which are significantly symptomatic. Clinically significant anomalies range from persistence of fetal circulation (eg, patent ductus arteriosus) to complex defects such as transposition of the great vessels, single ventricle anomaly, hypoplastic left heart syndrome, and complex variants of heterotaxy. The etiological factors of many genetic syndromes and familial CHD have been identified, but the genetic basis of majority of "sporadic" CHD remains unknown. It is hypothesized that susceptibility resulted from single nucleotide polymorphisms or key gene(s), with the interaction of environmental factors, which disturb normal cardiac development, result in cardiac defects. There are six causative mechanisms according to pathogenetic classification of congenital cardiovascular malformations: ectomesenchymal tissue migration abnormalities (causing conotruncal malformations and aortic arch anomalies); intracardiac blood flow defects (causing septal defects and left or right heart obstructive malformations); cell death abnormalities (causing septal defects and valve abnormalities); extra cellular matrix abnormalities (causing atrioventricular canal defects); abnormal targeted growth (causing partial or total anomalous pulmonary venous return and cor triatriatum); and abnormal situs and looping (causing left–right positioning problems) [57, 58].

2.2.1 Mutations in components of the cardiac gene network cause CHD

Heart development is controlled by a highly conserved network of transcription factors that connect signaling pathways with genes of muscle growth, patterning, and contractility. The core transcription factor network consists of *NKX2, MEF2, GATA, TBX,* and *Hand.* Dozens of other transcription factors contribute to cardiogenesis, in many cases by serving as accessory factors for these core regulators. Autoregulatory and cross regulatory of the cardiac gene network maintain the cardiac phenotype once the network has been activated by upstream inductive signals. Mutations in components of the cardiac gene Network cause CHD [59, 60].

Mutations in *NKX2.5* cause a spectrum of congenital heart defects, including atrial-septal defects (ASDs), ventricular-septal defects (VSDs), and cardiac conduction abnormalities. Mutations in TBX5 cause the congenital disease Holt–Oram syndrome, which is characterized by truncations of the upper limbs and heart malformations [61, 62]. Mutations in *GATA4,* some of which disrupt its interaction with *TBX5,* cause ASDs and VSDs. In mouse models, haploinsufficiency for Nkx2-5 or Tbx5 resulted in an increased incidence of structural heart disease, confirming that normal heart development is sensitive to small changes in expression levels of Nkx2-5 and Tbx5. GATA4 also is an essential, dosage-dependent regulator of cardiac morphogenesis. The missense mutation in Gata4 specifically disrupted the Gata4-Tbx5 interaction while maintaining its ability to interact with Nkx2.5. In previous studies, Tbx5 had been shown to interact with Nkx2.5, demonstrating that all three transcription factors could physically interact *in vitro.* In summary, a mutation in any of these three genes can result in human CSD and suggests that these three genes may work to direct common molecular pathways critical for cardiac septum formation. [63, 64]. Consistent with this, mutations in *MYH6,* a downstream transcriptional target of GATA4 and TBX5, was implicated as a cause of human atrial septal defects .TBX5, GATA4 and NKX2-5 function together only to activate genes. The overlapping expression patterns and complex interactions of these transcription factors allow fine regulation of cardiac gene expression and morphogenesis [20, 65-67] (Figure 2).

2.2.2 Regulatory pathway of cardiac genes

Several types of congenital heart disease involve valve defects of varying severity. Notch signaling is an ancient intercellular signaling mechanism that plays an important role during valve development. Mutations affecting signaling proteins and downstream pathways can lead to valve disease. In mammals, four Notch family receptors have been described: NOTCH1 through to NOTCH4 [20, 68]. The Notch ligands are encoded by the Jagged (*JAG1* and *JAG2*) and Delta-like (*DLL1, DLL3* and *DLL4*) gene families. The Notch signaling pathway is an evolutionarily conserved mechanism used by metazoans to control cell fate decisions through local cell interactions. The notch gene encodes a single-pass transmembrane protein receptor that interacts with its ligands, Delta and Serrate/Jagged. Upon binding of the ligand, the intracellular domain of Notch (NIC) undergoes proteolytic cleavage, and is translocated to the nucleus. In the nucleus, NIC binds to its major downstream effector, Suppressor-of-

Hairless (Su(H)). Su(H) binds to the regulatory sequences of the Enhancer-of-Split locus, upregulating the expression of basic helix-loop-helix proteins, which in turn regulate the expression of downstream target genes. Upon ligand binding, a signal is transmitted intracellularly by a process involving the proteolytic cleavage of the receptor and the subsequent nuclear translocation of the Notch intracellular domain (NICD) (Figure 3) . Alagille syndrome is an autosomal dominant disorder characterized by developmental abnormalities of the liver, heart, eye, skeleton and, at lower penetrance, several other organs. Most cases of Alagille syndrome are caused by *JAG1* mutations, although a small number of Alagille syndrome patients with *NOTCH2* mutations have been identified. The cardiac defects associated with Alagille syndrome include pulmonary artery stenosis and hypoplasia, pulmonic valve stenosis, and tetralogy of Fallot. These defects are likely to be due to a requirement for Notch signaling-mediated differentiation of cardiac neural crest cells into smooth muscle cells, which has been demonstrated in a mouse model. Bicuspid aortic valve affects 1-2% of the population, making it the most common congenital cardiac malformation. Bicuspid aortic valve predisposes one to aortic valve calcification. Aortic valve calcification was linked to Notch regulation of the transcription factor RUNX2.Heterozygous mutations in the *NOTCH1* gene were found in two families with autosomal-dominant aortic valve disease. *NOTCH1* mutations are also found in 4% of sporadic bicuspid aortic valve patients. The formation of bicuspid aortic valve might reflect the role of Notch signaling in regulating the epithelial-mesenchymal transition required for the generation of the heart valves [20, 69, 70]. Recently, mutations in Notch1 in humans have been shown to cause aortic valve defects and activation of Notch1 in mouse leads to abnormal cardiogenesis characterized by deformities of the ventricles and atrioventricular canal. Additionally, mutations in various Notch signaling pathway genes, including Jagged1, mind bomb 1, Hesr1/Hey1, and Hesr2/Hey2, result in cardiac defects, such as pericardial edema, atrial and ventricular septal defects, cardiac cushion, and valve defects [71-74].

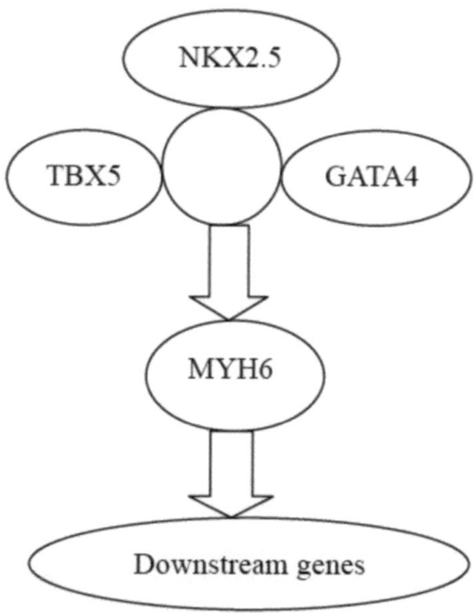

Fig. 2. Interaction of NKX2.5,TBX5 and GATA4

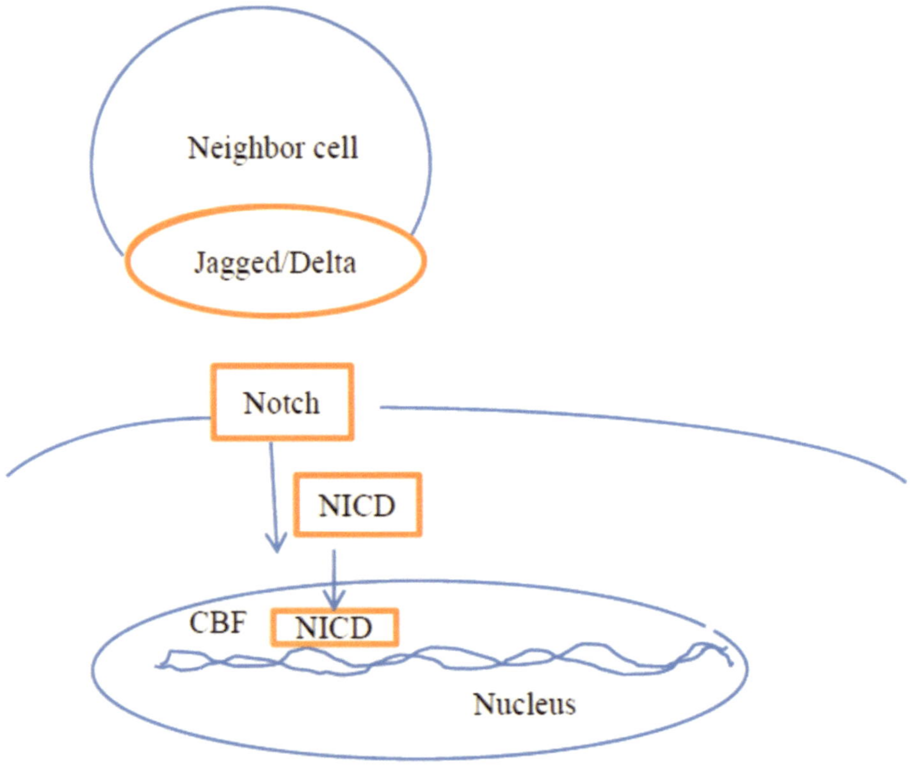

Fig. 3. Notch pathway

2.2.3 Altered haemodynamics

Haemodynamic forces have been demonstrated to play an important role in cardiac development. When these forces are impaired or when genes involved in growth and differentiation are not functioning correctly, malformations may arise. Shear stress is one of those haemodynamic forces, and the expression of many genes, including those of the endothelin pathway, changes in response to alterations in shear stress. For example, ligating the right lateral vitelline vein of chicken embryos results in cardiovascular malformations similar to those observed in knockout mice studies of components of the endothelin-1/endothelin-converting enzyme-1/ endothelin-A receptor pathway. In zebrafish, altering haemodynamics mechanically or genetically has profound consequences on heart morphology. In mice, a recent study pinpointed altered haemodynamics as a key intermediate between altered outflow tract morphogenesis and signaling events in branchial-arch artery remodeling. In human, complex congenital heart diseases with an outflow tract defect, such as tetralogy of Fallot, can be accompanied by 'accessory' congenital heart diseases, such as persistent right-sided aortic arch. Because the heart functions during its morphogenesis, haemodynamic forces might participate in cardiac morphogenesis [20, 71, 74] (Figure 4).

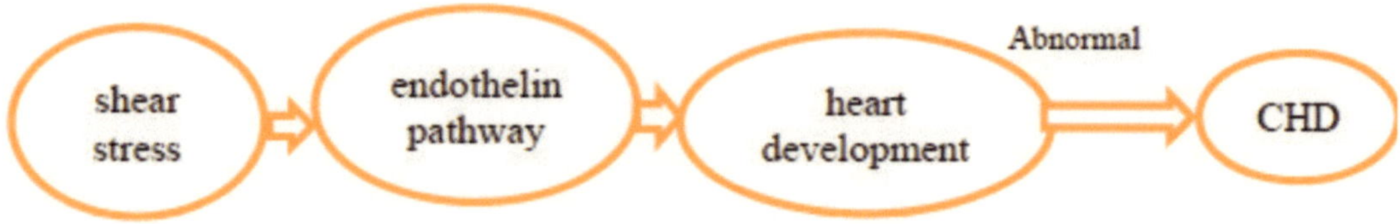

Fig. 4. Altered haemodynamics leads to CHD

2.2.4 MicroRNA dysfunction

MicroRNAs are natural, single-stranded, non-protein-coding small RNA molecules (~22 nucleotides) that regulate gene expression by binding to target mRNAs and suppress its translation or initiate its degradation. Mature miRNAs are processed from -70 nucleotides long precursor miRNA (pre-miRNAs) that form hairpin secondary structures and that are often evolutionarily conserved. Pre-miRNAs are transcribed from miRNA genes. Although the specific biological roles of most miRNAs are still unknown, functional characterizations of a few of them suggest that these small RNA molecules are involved in many processes of animal development and physiology[75-77] .For example, miR-1 and miR-133 control cardiac and skeletal muscle development [78, 79]. Both genes are under the control of serum response factor, indicating that they are part of a developmental programme regulated by cardiac transcription factors. It has been shown that miR-1 targets the cardiac transcription factor HAND2. Deletion of *miR-1-2* results in heart defects that include VSDs; surviving mice have conduction system defects and increased cardiomyocyte proliferation. Dysregulation of miRNAs might result in congenital heart disease in human [80, 81](Figure 5).

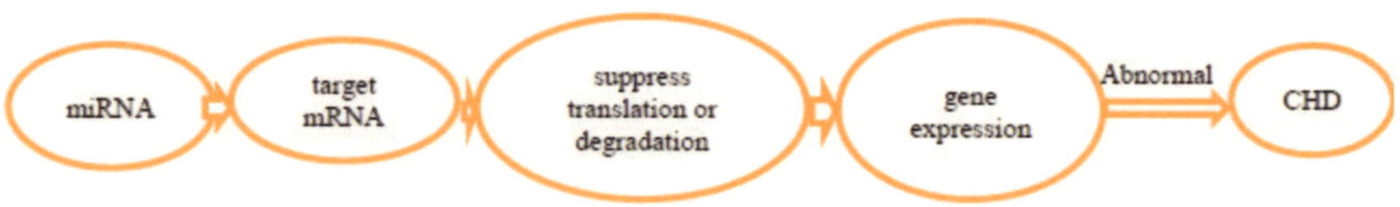

Fig. 5. MicroRNA dysfunction results in CHD

2.2.5 Epignetics

Epigenetics refers to DNA and chromatin modifications that play a critical role in regulation of various genomic functions, and it was then redefined as the study of heritable traits that are not dependent on the primary sequence of DNA. Although the genotype of most cells of a given organism is the same (with the exception of gametes and the cells of the immune system), cellular phenotypes and functions differ radically, and this can be (at least to some extent) controlled by differential epigenetic regulation that is set up during cell differentiation and embryonic morphogenesis [82,83]. Once the cellular phenotype is established, genomes of somatic cells are 'locked' in tissue-specific patterns of gene expression, generation after generation. This heritability of epigenetic information in somatic cells has been called an 'epigenetic inheritance system' [84]. Even after the epigenomic profiles are established, a substantial degree of epigenetic variation can be generated during the mitotic divisions of a cell in the absence of any specific environmental factors. Such variation is most likely to be the outcome of stochastic events in the somatic inheritance of epigenetic profiles. From the epigenetic point of view, phenotypic differences in monozygous twins could result, in part, from their epigenetic differences. It has recently become clear that epigenetic regulators play crucial roles in the global shaping and maintenance of developmental patterning. This involves dynamic tissue and cell type-specific changes during patterning, as well as the maintenance of the cellular memory that is required for developmental stability.BAF60C (also known as SMARCD3), a subunit of the Swi/Snf-like chromatin-remodelling complex BAF, physically links cardiac transcription factors to the BAF complex. Loss of BAF60C results in severe defects in cardiac morphogenesis and impaired activation of a subset of cardiac genes. The muscle-restricted histone methyltransferase SMYD1 (also known as BOP) is a crucial regulator of cardiac chamber growth and differentiation. Histone deacetylases have mostly been characterized as having an important role in heart hypertrophy and development [20] (Figure 6).

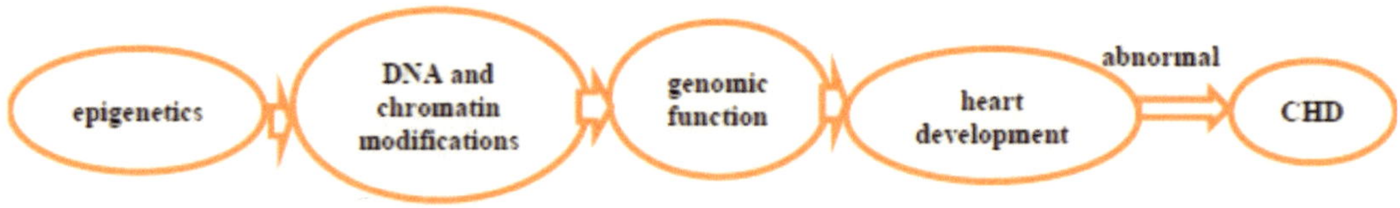

Fig. 6. Dysfunctions of epignetics leads to CHD

2.2.6 Adult congenital heart diseases

Individuals with congenital heart disease can suffer from secondary heart disease later in life, possibly as a result of corrective surgery during infancy. The sequelae are sometimes severe; for example, after closure of a septal defect, some patients can progress to heart failure. With improved surgical outcomes for those with congenital heart disease, the number of adults with such diseases now exceeds the number of children. The population of patients with adult congenital heart disease is approximately 800,000 in the U.S.A majority faces a lifetime of problems including arrhythmias, ventricular dysfunction, and one or more re-operations. Thus, it has become imperative to understand the postnatal consequences of congenital heart diseases [85]. Recent results suggest that these might be caused, at least in part, by the direct effects of mutations associated with congenital heart disease on postnatal heart morphology and function. For example, in a family with *GATA4* mutations, apart from having heart structural defects, some individuals developed dilated cardiomyopathy later in life. Indeed, data from mouse models support a connection between *GATA4* mutations and adult cardiomyopathy [86]. Similarly, mutations in *TBX20* were identified in patients with cardiomyopathy as well as in those with structural congenital heart diseases. Mouse studies have also revealed roles for other congenital-heart-disease-associated genes in cardiac function. Studies of mice in which *Nkx2-5* had been deleted only in the ventricles suggest a role for this gene in the function of the postnatal conduction system and in myocardial structure, and examination of patients with *NKX2-5* mutations revealed that some had aspects of cardiomyopathy, as predicted from the mouse data. Thus, embryonic patterning genes control structural components of the heart and can also have a separate role in heart function, for example by regulating *Serca2*.These genes can thus modulate important aspects of heart function that cause pathology in the postnatal heart when dysregulated. This concept has important implications for the clinical management of adults with congenital heart disease [20,87].

3. Strategies and future perspectives

The molecular mechanisms of congenital heart defects are so complex that we have to use diverse strategies to explore them. **Animal Models** Biomedical models have been defined as "surrogates for a human being, or a human biologic system, that can be used to understand normal and abnormal function from gene to phenotype and to provide a basis for preventive or therapeutic intervention in human diseases" . Because of the striking homology between mammalian genomes and the many similarities in anatomy, cell biology, and physiology, rat is an excellent animal model for studying of cardiac development and identifying novel genes that could contribute to human disease. The Human Genome Initiative is providing genetic information not only from humans, but also from animals traditionally used as models. In addition, related enabling technologies in transgenesis and animal cloning provide new approaches for designing and performing experiments to dissect complex biological systems. Because of these new technologies (e.g., transgenesis), scientists are no longer limited to the traditional methods of choosing naturally occurring models. Researchers can utilize genomic knowledge and available tools to create appropriate animal models. This approach is referred to as reverse genetics. In contrast to forward genetics in which the gene or genes responsible for a particular phenotype are identified by positional cloning (phenotype to genotype), the reverse genetics approach determines the function of a gene and predicts the phenotype of a cell, tissue, or organism (genotype to phenotype). **Genome-Wide Studies** Considerable progress has been made in understanding the pathophysiology of perioperative stress responses and their impact on the cardiovascular system; however, researchers are just beginning to unravel genetic and molecular determinants that predispose to increased risk for CHD. Recent improvements in genotyping technology and in our knowledge of human genetic variation have made it possible to carry out genome-wide genetic association studies to identify susceptibility genes for common disease. Multistage designs involving large numbers of coding sequence variants (300,000) and relatively large samples sizes (several hundred cases and control subjects) will be essential to reliably detect alleles with appreciable effect sizes (2-fold increase in relative risk). Direct sequencing of candidate genes in cases and control subjects provides an alternative approach that can reveal low-frequency alleles that influence disease susceptibility [88,89]. **Gene Expression (Microarrays)** Microarray analysis is a useful tool to obtain a gene expression profile of CHD. However, current estimates suggest that greater than 60% of human genes have more than one isoform. Alternatively, spliced isoforms from the same gene can produce proteins with different properties and distinct functions. The specific roles of gene expression and their splicing variants necessary for development need to be further delineated. **MicroRNA** Current research has revealed that the influence of RNA molecules on gene expression reaches beyond the realm of protein synthesis back into the nucleus, where it not only dictates the transcriptional activity of genes, but also shapes the chromatin architecture of extensive regions of DNA. Non-coding RNA, in the context of this review, refers to transcripts expressed and processed in the nucleus much like any protein coding gene, but lacking an open reading frame and often transcribed antisense to bona fide protein coding genes. Dysregulation of miRNAs might result in congenital heart disease in humans. Further studies of miRNAs in CHD are required. **Epigenetics** There is increasing evidence that epigenetic modifications, arising primarily through DNA methylation and histone modifications may have as important a role as genetics in certain diseases, such as cancer, birth defects, developmental disorders, and psychiatric disorders. **Bioinformatics** Unprecedented growth in the interdisciplinary domain of biomedical informatics reflects the recent advancements in genomic sequence availability, high-content biotechnology screening systems, as well as the expectations of computational biology to command a leading role in drug discovery and disease characterization. These forces have moved much of life sciences research almost completely into the computational domain. Human genome project has succeeded, and postgenome era is following. Human genome comprises 30, 000-40, 000 genes, but their functions, relation, interaction, and regulation remain unknown. Bioinformatics is a powerful and indispensable tool in exploring the molecular mechanisms of CHD [90, 91].

4. Conclusions

Congenital heart disease (CHD) is the most common type of birth defect. Despite of the many advances in our understanding of cardiac development and many genes related to cardiac development identified, the fundamental etiology for the majority of cases of congenital heart disease remains unknown. CHD is a multifactorial complex disease, with environmental and genetic factors playing important roles. A number of causative genes of selected congenital heart defects and genetic syndromes have been found. The molecular mechanisms of CHD may include mutations in components of the cardiac gene network, altered haemodynamics, regulatory pathway of cardiac genes , microRNA dysfunction , epignetics, adult congenital heart diseases and so on. The molecular basis of CHD is an exciting and rapidly evolving field. The continuing advances in the understanding of the molecular mechanisms of CHD will hopefully result in improved genetic counseling and care of affected individuals and their families.

5. Acknowledgements

This study was supported by the Ruikang Hospital Natural Science Foundation (code: ZKZ201001).

6. Abbreviations

ASD= atrial septal defect; VSD= ventricular septal defect; CSD= cardiac septal defect;
SRF= serum response factor (c-fos serum response element-binding transcription factor); FGF=fibroblast growth factor; BMP= bone morphogenetic protein; Nodal= nodal homolog; Wnt= wingless-type MMTV integration site family; Shh= sonic hedgehog homolog; Ihh= Indian hedgehog homolog; VEGF= vascular endothelial growth factor; NFATc1= nuclear factor of activated T-cells, cytoplasmic, calcineurin-dependent 1; ß-catenin= catenin

(cadherin-associated protein), beta 1; TGF-ß= transforming growth factor, beta 1; EGF= epidermal growth factor (beta-urogastrone) ; erbB= v-erb-b2 erythroblastic leukemia viral oncogene homolog 2, neuro/glioblastoma derived oncogene homolog; NF1= neurofibromin 1;MEF2= myocyte enhancing factor 2; Hand= transcription factor protein; RUNX2= runt-related transcription factor 2; NOTCH= Notch homolog; Hesr1/Hey1= hairy/enhancer-of-split related with YRPW motif 1; BAF60C= a subunit of chromatin-remodelling complex BAF; SMYD1= histone methyltransferase.

7. References

[1] Hoffman J I, KaplanS. The incidence of congenital heart disease, *J Am Coll Cardiol* .2002 ;39:1890-1900.

[2] V.Garg. Insights into the genetic basis of congenital heart disease,Cell. *Mol. Life Sci.* 2006; 63(10):1141–1148.

[3] Kohl HW 3rd.Rubella screening and vaccination follow-up by a hospital employee health office, *Am J Infect Control.* 1985;13(3):124-7.

[4] Singh M, Shah GL, Singh KP. Teratogenic effects of dilantin on thoraco-abdominal organs of developing chick embryos, *Indian J Exp Biol.* 2000;38(10):1026-30.

[5] Dawson BV, Johnson PD, Goldberg SJ, et al. Cardiac teratogenesis of halogenated hydrocarbon-contaminated drinking water, *J Am Coll Cardiol.* 1993 ;21(6):1466-72.

[6] Kumar SD, Dheen ST, Tay SS. Maternal diabetes induces congenital heart defects in mice by altering the expression of genes involved in cardiovascular development, *Cardiovasc Diabetol.*2007;6:34.

[7] McCart A, Latchford A, Volikos E, et al. A novel exon duplication event leading to a truncating germ-line mutation of the APC gene in a familial adenomatous polyposis family.*Fam Cancer.* 2006;5(2):205-8.

[8] Kakavas VK, Plageras P, Vlachos TA, et al. PCR-SSCP: a method for the molecular analysis of genetic diseases. *Mol Biotechnol.* 2008;38(2):155-63.

[9] Moorman AF, Christoffels VM. Cardiac chamber formation: development, genes, and evolution. *Physiol Rev.* 2003; 83 (4): 1223–1267.

[10] Michael E. Mitchell, Tara L, et al. The molecular basis of congenital heart disease. *Semin Thorac Cardiovasc Surg.*2007 ; 19 (3):228-237.

[11] Dunwoodie SL. Combinatorial signaling in the heart orchestrates cardiac induction, lineage specification and chamber formation. *Semin Cell Dev Biol.* 2007;18(1):54-66.

[12] Brand T. Heart development: molecular insights into cardiac specification and early morphogenesis. *Dev Biol.* 2003;258 (1):1–19.

[13] Gruber PJ, Epstein JA. Epstein. Development gone awry congenital heart disease. *Circ Res.* 2004;94 (3):273-283.

[14] Grego-Bessa J, Luna-Zurita L, del Monte G, et al. Notch signaling is essential for ventricular chamber development. *Dev Cell* . 2007;12:415–429.

[15] Risebro CA, Riley PR. Formation of the ventricles. *Scientific World Journal.* 2006 ;6:1862-80.

[16] Cohen ED, Tian Y, Morrisey EE. Wnt signaling: an essential regulator of cardiovascular differentiation, morphogenesis and progenitor self-renewal. *Development.* 2008;135(5):789-98.

[17] Xiao H, Zhang YY. Understanding the role of transforming growth factor-beta signalling in the heart: overview of studies using genetic mouse models. *Clin Exp Pharmacol Physiol.*2008;35(3):335-41.

[18] Moon JI, Birren SJ. Target-dependent inhibition of sympathetic neuron growth via modulation of a BMP signaling pathway. *Dev Biol.* 2008; 315(2):404-17.

[19] Mjaatvedt CH, Nakaoka T, Moreno-Rodriguez R, et al. The outflow tract of the heart is recruited from a novel heart-forming field. *Dev. Biol.* 2001; 238 (1): 97–109.

[20] Bruneau BG. The developmental genetics of congenital heart disease.*Nature.* 2008; 451(7181):943-8.

[21] High FA, Epstein JA. The multifaceted role of Notch in cardiac development and disease. *Nat Rev Genet.* 2008;9(1):49-61.

[22] Armstrong EJ, Bischoff J. Heart valve development: endothelial cell signaling and differentiation. *Circ Res.* 2004;3;95(5):459-70.

[23] Yutzey KE, Colbert M, Robbins J. Ras-related signaling pathways in valve development:ebb and flow. *Physiology* (Bethesda). 2005 ;20:390-7.

[24] Joziasse IC, van de Smagt JJ, Smith K, et al. Genes in congenital heart disease: atrioventricular valve formation. *Basic Res Cardiol.* 2008;103(3):216-27.

[25] Pierpont ME, Basson CT, Benson DW, et al. Genetic basis for congenital heart defects: current knowledge: a scientific statement from the American Heart Association Congenital Cardiac Defects Committee, Council on Cardiovascular Disease in the Young: endorsed by the American Academy of Pediatrics. *Circulation.* 2007;115:3015–3038.

[26] Ikeda Y, Hiroi Y, Hosoda T, et al. Novel point mutation in the cardiac transcription factor CSX/NKX2.5 associated with congenital heart disease. *Circ J.* 2002;66:561–563.

[27] McElhinney DB, Geiger E, Blinder J, et al. NKX2.5 mutations in patients with congenital heart disease. *J Am Coll Cardiol.* 2003;42:1650 –1655.

[28] Elliott DA, Kirk EP, Yeoh T, et al. Cardiac homeobox gene NKX2–5 mutations and congenital heart disease: associations with atrial septal defect and hypoplastic left heart syndrome. *J Am Coll Cardiol.* 2003;41:2072–2076.

[29] Schubbert S, Zenker M, Rowe SL, et al. Germline KRAS mutations cause Noonan syndrome. *Nat Genet.* 2006;38:331–336.

[30] Tartaglia M, Kalidas K, Shaw A, et al. PTPN11 mutations in Noonan syndrome: molecular spectrum, genotype-phenotype correlation, and phenotypic heterogeneity. *Am J Hum Genet.* 2002;70:1555–1563.

[31] Toko H, Zhu W, Takimoto E, et al. Csx/Nkx2-5 Is Required for Homeostasis and Survival of Cardiac Myocytes in the Adult Heart. *J Biol Chem.* 2002;277(27):24735-43.

[32] Akazawa H, Komuro I. Cardiac transcription factor Csx/Nkx2-5: Its role in cardiac development and diseases. *Pharmacol Ther.*2005;107(2):252-68.

[33] Goldmuntz E, Bamford R, Karkera JD, et al. CFC1 mutations in patients with transposition of the great arteries and double-outlet right ventricle. *Am J Hum Genet.* 2002;70(3):776-80.

[34] Davit-Spraul A, Baussan C, Hermeziu B, et al. CFC1 gene involvement in biliary atresia with polysplenia syndrome. *J Pediatr Gastroenterol Nutr.* 2008;46(1):111-2.

[35] Muncke N, Jung C, Rüdiger H, et al. Missense mutations and gene interruption in PROSIT240, a novel TRAP240-like gene, in patients with congenital heart defect (transposition of the great arteries). *Circulation.* 2003;108(23):2843-50.

[36] Finelli P, Pincelli AI, Russo S, et al. Disruption of friend of GATA 2 gene (FOG-2) by a de novo t(8;10) chromosomal translocation is associated with heart defects and gonadal dysgenesis. *Clin Genet.* 2007;71(3):195-204..

[37] Heritage ML, MacMillan JC, Anderson GJ. DHPLC mutation analysis of Jagged1 (JAG1) reveals six novel mutations in Australian alagille syndrome patients. *Hum Mutat.* 2002;20(6):481.

[38] Robinson SW, Morris CD, Goldmuntz E, et al. Missense mutations in CRELD1 are associated with cardiac atrioventricular septal defects. *Am J Hum Genet.* 2003;72(4):1047-52

[39] Tomita-Mitchell A, Maslen CL, Morris CD, et al. GATA4 sequence variants in patients with congenital heart disease. *Eur J Med Genet.* 2008;51(6):527-35.

[40] Zhu L, Zhou G, Poole S, et al. Characterization of the interactions of human ZIC3 mutants with GLI3. *Hum Mutat.* 2008;29(1):99-105.

[41] Harrison CA, Gray PC, Fischer WH, et al. An activin mutant with disrupted ALK4 binding blocks signaling via type II receptors. *J Biol Chem.* 2004;279(27):28036-44.

[42] Besser D. Expression of nodal, lefty-a, and lefty-B in undifferentiated human embryonic stem cells requires activation of Smad2/3. *J Biol Chem.* 2004;279(43):45076-84.

[43] Ferland RJ, Gaitanis JN, Apse K, et al. Periventricular nodular heterotopia and Williams syndrome. *Am J Med Genet A.* 2006;140(12):1305-11.

[44] Fan C, Liu M, Wang Q. Functional analysis of TBX5 missense mutations associated with Holt-Oram syndrome. *J Biol Chem.*2003;278(10):8780-5.

[45] Zhao F, Weismann CG, Satoda M, et al. Novel TFAP2B mutations that cause Char syndrome provide a genotype-phenotype correlation. *Am J Hum Genet.* 2001;69(4):695-703.

[46] Ko JM, Kim JM, Kim GH, et al. PTPN11, SOS1, KRAS, and RAF1 gene analysis, and genotype-phenotype correlation in Korean patients with Noonan syndrome. *J Hum Genet.* 2008;53(11-12):999-1006.

[47] Roberts AE, Araki T, Swanson KD, et al. Germline gain-of-function mutations in SOS1 cause Noonan syndrome. *Nat Genet.* 2007;39(1):70-4.

[48] Wincent J, Holmberg E, Strömland K, et al. CHD7 mutation spectrum in 28 Swedish patients diagnosed with CHARGE syndrome. *Clin Genet.* 2008;74(1):31-8.

[49] Temtamy SA, Aglan MS, Valencia M, et al. CHD7 mutation spectrum in 28 Swedish patients diagnosed with CHARGE syndrome. *Hum Mutat.* 2008;29(7):931-8.

[50] Ulucan H, Gül D, Sapp JC, et al. Extending the spectrum of Ellis van Creveld syndrome: a large family with a mild mutation in the EVC gene. *BMC Med Genet.* 2008;9:92

[51] Li D, Yu J, Gu F, et al. The roles of two novel FBN1 gene mutations in the genotype-phenotype correlations of Marfan syndrome and ectopia lentis patients with marfanoid habitus. *Genet Test.* 2008;12(2):325-30.

[52] Singh KK, Rommel K, Mishra A, et al. TGFBR1 and TGFBR2 mutations in patients with features of Marfan syndrome and Loeys-Dietz syndrome. *Hum Mutat.* 2006;27(8):770-7.

[53] Niihori T, Aoki Y, Narumi Y, et al. Germline KRAS and BRAF mutations in cardio-facio-cutaneous syndrome. *Nat Genet.* 2006;38(3):294-6.

[54] Roberts A, Allanson J, Jadico SK, et al. The cardiofaciocutaneous syndrome.*J Med Genet.* 2006 Nov;43(11):833-42.

[55] Nava C, Hanna N, Michot C, et al. Cardio-facio-cutaneous and Noonan syndromes due to mutations in the RAS/MAPK signalling pathway: genotype-phenotype relationships and overlap with Costello syndrome. *J Med Genet.* 2007;44(12):763-71.

[56] Quezada E, Gripp KW. Costello syndrome and related disorders.*Curr Opin Pediatr.* 2007;19(6):636-44.

[57] Clark EB. Mechanisms in the pathogenesis of congenital heart disease. In: Pierpont ME, Moller J, editors. The genetics of cardiovascular disease. Boston, MA' Martinus-Nijoff; 1986. p. 3 –11.

[58] Clark EB. Pathogenetic mechanisms of congenital cardiovascular malformations revisited. *Semin Perinatol* 1996;20:465– 72.

[59] Benoit G. Bruneau. The developmental genetics of congenital heart disease. *Nature.* 2008;451(7181):943-8.

[60] Hyun C, Lavulo L. Congenital heart diseases in small animals: Part I. Genetic pathways and potential candidate genes. *The Veterinary Journal;* 2006; 171 (2): 245–255.

[61] Hiroi Y, Kudoh S, Monzen K, et al. Tbx5 associates with Nkx2-5 and synergistically promotes cardiomyocyte differentiation. *Nat. Genet.* 2001;28 (3): 276–280.

[62] Goldmuntz E, Geiger E, Benson DW. NKX2.5 mutations in patients with tetralogy of fallot. *Circulation.* 2001；104 (21): 2565–2568.

[63] Stennard FA, Costa MW, Elliott DA, et al. Cardiac T-box factor Tbx20 directly interacts with Nkx2-5, GATA4, and GATA5 in regulation of gene expression in the developing heart. *Dev Biol.* 2003 ;262(2):206-24.

[64] Pashmforoush M, Lu JT, Chen H, et al. Nkx2-5 pathways and congenital heart disease: loss of ventricular myocyte lineage specification leads to progressive cardiomyopathy and complete heart block. *Cell* .2004；117 (3): 373–386.

[65] Pu WT, Ishiwata T, Juraszek AL, et al. GATA4 is a dosage-sensitive regulator of cardiac morphogenesis. *Dev. Biol.* 2004；275 (1): 235–244.

[66] Moskowitz IP, Kim JB, Moore ML, et al. A molecular pathway including Id2, Tbx5, and Nkx2-5 required for cardiac conduction system development. *Cell.* 2007;129(7):1365-76.

[67] Ching YH, Ghosh TK, Cross SJ, et al. Mutation in myosin heavy chain 6 causes atrial septal defect. *Nat. Genet.* 2005;37 (4): 423–428.

[68] Varadkar P, Kraman M, Despres D, et al. Notch2 is required for the proliferation of cardiac neural crest-derived smooth muscle cells. *Dev Dyn.* 2008;237(4):1144-52.

[69] Del Monte G, Grego-Bessa J, González-Rajal A, et al. Monitoring Notch1 activity in development: evidence for a feedback regulatory loop. *Dev Dyn.* 2007;236(9):2594-614.

[70] Kwon C, Arnold J, Hsiao EC, et al. Canonical Wnt signaling is a positive regulator of mammalian cardiac progenitors. *Proc Natl Acad Sci U S A*.2007;104(26):10894-9.
[71] Miller CT, Swartz ME, Khuu PA, et al. mef2ca is required in cranial neural crest to effect Endothelin1 signaling in zebrafish. *Dev Biol*. 2007;308(1):144-57.
[72] Ren X, Li Y, Ma X, et al. Activation of p38/MEF2C pathway by all-trans retinoic acid in cardiac myoblasts. *Life Sci*. 2007;81(2):89-96.
[73] Ueno S, Weidinger G, Osugi T, et al. Biphasic role for Wnt/beta-catenin signaling in cardiac specification in zebrafish and embryonic stem cells. *Proc Natl Acad Sci U S A*. 2007;104(23):9685-90.
[74] Groenendijk BC, Stekelenburg-de Vos S, Vennemann P, et al. The endothelin-1 pathway and the development of cardiovascular defects in the haemodynamically challenged chicken embryo. *J Vasc Res*. 2008;45(1):54-68.
[75] Couzin J. Breakthrough of The Year: Small RNAs make big splash, *Science*. 2002；298 (5602):2296-2297.
[76] Liu CG, Calin GA, Meloon B, et al. An oligonucleotide microchip for genome-wide microRNA profiling in human and mouse tissues. *Proc Natl Acad Sci U S A*. 2004;101(26):9740-4.
[77] Lee CT, Risom T, Strauss WM. MicroRNAs in mammalian development. *Birth Defects Res C Embryo Today*. 2006；78 (2):129-139.
[78] Zhang B, Wang Q, Pan X. MicroRNAs and their regulatory roles in animals and plants, *J Cell Physiol* .2007；210 (2): 279-289.
[79] Zhao Y. Ransom JF, Li A, et al. Dysregulation of cardiogenesis, cardiac conduction, and cell cycle in mice lacking miRNA-1-2. *Cell*. 2007；129 (2):303–317.
[80] Zhao Y, Samal E, Srivastava D. Serum sponse factor regulates a muscle-specific microRNA that targets Hand2 during cardiogenesis, *Nature*.2005；436 (7048):214-220.
[81] Kwon C, Han Z, Olson EN, et al. MicroRNA1 influences cardiac differentiation in Drosophila and regulates Notch signaling, *Proc Natl Acad Sci USA*. 2005；102 (52):18986–18991.
[82] Wong AH, Gottesman II, Petronis A. Phenotypic differences in genetically identical organisms: the epigenetic perspective. *Human Molecular Genetics*, 2005, 14(1):R11-R18.
[83] Armstrong L, Lako M, Dean W, et al. Epigenetic modification is central to genome reprogramming in somatic cell nuclear transfer. *Stem Cells*.2006; 24(4):805-814.
[84] Jacinto FV, Esteller M, Mutator pathways unleashed by epigenetic silencing in human cancer. *Mutagenesis*. 2007;22(4):247-53.
[85] Warnes CA. The adult with congenital heart disease: Born to be bad? *J Am Coll Cardiol*. 2005;46:1–8.
[86] Cambien F, Tiret L, Genetics of cardiovascular diseases: from single mutations to the whole genome. *Circulation*,2007;116;1714-1724 .
[87] Gatzoulis MA. Adult congenital heart disease: a cardiovascular area of growth in urgent need of additional resource allocation. *Int. J. Cardiol*. 2004； 97 (Suppl 1): 1-2.
[88] Cohen JC. Genetic approaches to coronary heart disease. *J Am Coll Cardiol*. 2006;48:A10–A14.

[89] Wallace C, Newhouse SJ, Braund P, et al. Genomewide association study identifies genes for biomarkers of cardiovascular disease: serum urate and dyslipidemia. *Am J Hum Genet.* 2008; 82:139–149.

[90] Todd AK. Bioinformatics approaches to quadruplex sequence location. *Methods* .2007;43(4):246–251.

[91] Yang W, Paschen W. Conditional gene silencing in mammalian cells mediated by a stress-inducible promoter. *Biochem Biophys Res Commun.* 2008;365(3):521-7.

6

Drosophila Model of Congenital Heart Diseases

Georg Vogler[1], Rolf Bodmer[1] and Takeshi Akasaka[1,2]
[1]*Development and Aging Program,*
Sanford-Burnham Medical Research Institute, La Jolla
[2]*Cardiology and Catheterization Laboratories,*
Shonan Kamakura General Hospital, Kanagawa
[1]*USA*
[2]*Japan*

1. Introduction

Congenital heart defects (CHD) are the most common birth defects, occurring in about 0.7% of all newborn infants. There are multiple lines of evidence that genetic components are involved in developing CHD pathogenesis. An important aspect in understanding disease mechanisms is that in addition to contributions from a single disease-causing gene (usually seen in many familial cases of CHD), a multitude of other genetically interacting loci can also influence the severity or progression of the disease, often diagnosed as idiopathic CHD. It is likely that such genetic interactions underlie a large proportion of cases of idiopathic CHD, where a direct link to known cardiogenic genes yet to be identified. Recent advances in stem cell research and in the growing field of systems biology provide a tremendous amount of new data leading to new hypotheses and to new heart disease gene candidates that may also have potential roles during heart formation and establishment of cardiac function. Usually, these hypotheses are tested in cell-based assays and eventually in the mouse model, however both systems have their own particular set of limitations. In this article we review recent advancements in using *Drosophila melanogaster* as a model organism to study basic mechanisms of heart development, cardiac function and disease.

2. Comparison between *Drosophila* and vertebrate cardiogenesis

The early development of the *Drosophila* heart shows remarkable similarities with its vertebrate counterparts, both morphologically and genetically (for review, see Bodmer, 1995; Bier and Bodmer, 2004). Our understanding of the regulation of cardiac development by a core cardiac transcription factor network (Venkatesh et al., 2000; Cripps and Olson, 2002; Olson, 2006; Bodmer and Frasch, 2010) began with the identification of the *Drosophila Nkx2.5* homologue *tinman* twenty years ago (Bodmer et al., 1990; Azpiazu and Frasch, 1993; Bodmer, 1993). One decade later, the completion of the sequencing of the *Drosophila*, mouse and human genomes has led to the identification of fly homologues of most cardiac transcription factors. The *Drosophila* model allowed the extensive genetic screening and functional analysis of Tinman (NKX2.5 Yin et al., 1997; Akasaka et al., 2006; Zaffran et al., 2006; Qian et al., 2011; Ryu et al., 2011), Hand (dHAND, eHAND, Han and Olson, 2005; Han et al., 2006; Lo et al., 2007), tailup/isl-1 (Islet, Tao et al., 2007; Mann et al., 2009), Pannier (GATA4, Alvarez et al., 2003; Fromental-Ramain et al., 2008; Qian et al., 2008; Qian and Bodmer, 2009), Neuromancer-1/-2 (TBX20, Miskolczi-McCallum et al., 2005; Qian et al., 2005a; Reim et al., 2005; Leal et al., 2009), and Dorsocross-1/-2/-3 (TBX5, Reim and Frasch, 2005) and revealed a conserved cardiac transcription factor network responsible for heart specification (Olson, 2006). *Drosophila* and vertebrates also share the same inductive and instructive signaling pathways (Wnt, FGF, BMPs, for review see Frasch, 1999; Cripps and Olson, 2002) during early heart development. This further underscores that the *Drosophila* heart, despite its evolutionary distance from vertebrates, is specified by similar, fundamental mechanisms. This remarkable degree of genetic conservation is paralleled by morphological similarities during early development: the heart originates from a lateral portion in the early mesoderm, and two bilateral regions will eventually fuse and undergo lumen formation. Such genetic and morphological similarities across phyla have led to the conclusion that the cardiovascular system of the fly and vertebrates share true homologies (Hartenstein and Mandal, 2006). Lessons learned from *Drosophila* are likely to translate into a greater understanding of vertebrate heart development and function, and thus will help to understand the pathology and improve the treatment of cardiovascular diseases, as exemplified by Neely (2010) and Qian (2011).

3. Lessons learned from studying *Drosophila* heart morphogenesis

To gain new insights into the role of the cardiac transcriptional network, different groups have begun to analyze the mechanisms underlying heart morphogenesis and heart lumen formation during *Drosophila* embryonic development. After specification, cardiomyocyte precursors (called cardioblasts) migrate towards the dorsal midline of the embryo. These cells will extend filopodia towards their contralateral counterparts to establish a dorsal cell-cell contact. They then undergo cell shape changes, thereby bending around to form a second, ventral contact and enclosing a luminal space (see Figure 1 and Rugendorff et al., 1994). By the end of embryogenesis, these cells will have differentiated into a tubular dorsal vessel, providing the circulation of hemolymph during larval and adult stages. The mechanism by which this migratory behavior is orchestrated is still poorly understood, but recent studies have established a framework of genes involved in heart morphogenesis. An important participating signal transduction pathway is the Slit/Robo pathway, which was originally identified and characterized for its role in axon guidance and in regulation of midline crossing of growing neurons (Dickson and Gilestro, 2006). Slit, an EGF-like ligand, and the Slit-receptor Roundabout (Robo) are both expressed by cardioblasts during morphogenesis and lumen formation, and ChIP data suggest that cardiac genes, such as *tinman* (Liu et al., 2009), directly regulate their expression. Mutants for *slit* or *robo* together with its paralogue *robo2* have distinct defects during these processes (Qian et al., 2005b; MacMullin and Jacobs, 2006; Santiago-Martínez et al., 2006; Medioni et al., 2008; Santiago-Martínez et al., 2008): impaired cardioblasts cell-cell adhesion, which disrupts subsequent heart morphogenesis, and impairment of cell shape changes and lumen formation. In *slit* mutants, polar (or polarly distributed) markers, including the *Drosophila* MAGUK protein Discs-large, are incorrectly localized indicating a loss of overall cardioblast polarity (Qian et al., 2005b). In addition, the cardioblasts fail to correctly change their cell shape in order to enclose a heart lumen (Medioni et al., 2008). This is accompanied by upregulation of the cell adhesion molecule Shotgun/E-Cadherin at the presumptive luminal domain, leading to increased adhesion at the luminal surfaces, which in turn is likely to prevent further lumen formation (Santiago-Martínez et al., 2008). Both, Slit and Robo are expressed during mouse heart development and expression of Slit3 and Robo2 depend on Tbx20 and Nkx2-5, respectively (Medioni et al., 2010). Functional analysis in zebrafish done by Fish et al. (2011) indicates a role for Slit/Robo signaling during zebrafish heart development. Slit/robo mutant fish hearts show a number of developmental defects, indicating a conserved requirement for this pathway during vertebrate cardiogenesis and thus a role in CHD. Again, the analysis of Slit/Robo in *Drosophila* has paved the way for the subsequent experiments done in vertebrates.

Recent work on fly heart development suggests several possible future research directions. Firstly, genetic screens in *Drosophila* should reveal additional genes involved in cell-cell signaling during development. Among them is the Netrin/Unc-5 pathway that, similar to Slit/Robo, was found to be involved in axon guidance and cell migration. In the heart, the UNC-5 ligand Netrin is also required for heart lumen formation (Albrecht et al., 2011), although with a lesser penetrance than Slit/Robo. This indicates that in fact multiple pathways are required during the formation of the heart, and it would be interesting to see if these two pathways genetically interact, which would indicate a potential cross talk between them. The *Drosophila* model therefore helps pinpoint which pathways may also interact in CHD in humans. Secondly, a more complete and detailed understanding of the signaling pathways themselves during heart development and establishment of cardiac function will be essential for understanding CHD initiation and progression. For example, co-receptors might play an important role in defining pathway sensitivity and downstream activity. In *Drosophila,* cardiac Slit/Robo signaling has been shown to require the activity of the heparan sulfate proteoglycan Syndecan (Knox et al., 2011). Since Syndecan is involved in angiogenesis (through VEGF, Chen et al., 2004) and is also upregulated during cardiac remodeling after myocardial infarction, the *Drosophila* model might help identify important components of Syndecan signaling in these disease-relevant contexts. Thirdly, the cellular machineries through which signaling pathways exert their specific function are largely unknown. Thus, we currently have no clear understanding of the intracellular mechanisms that give rise to the *slit* mutant phenotype.

4. Manipulating the heart and genome of a fly

Parallel pathways and downstream signaling cascades are thought to intersect with a number of cellular effector proteins, such as small GTPases, which in turn may influence cell migration (e.g. changes in the filopodia or lamellipodia dynamics), cell adhesion (e.g. changes in endocytosis of E-Cadherin) or cell contractions (e.g. via Rho-associated kinase activities). The activity of these genes has been studied in great detail in cell-based assays, but experimental evidence on their *in vivo* function is relatively sparse. The lack of available mutants in vertebrate model organisms often prevents such analysis, as has the shortage of tools for tissue-specific manipulations and imaging of single cells in whole animals. Therefore, very few examples of the function these proteins in the context of an entire organ or organ system exist to date (e.g. RhoDF, see Christiaen et al., 2008). In *Drosophila,* small GTPases involved in the above cellular processes have been studied by genetic manipulations during the formation of tissues other than the heart, e.g. during dorsal closure (Jacinto et al., 2002) or wound healing (Stramer et al., 2005). The embryonic *Drosophila* heart is well suited to similar experiments since it is localized just underneath the transparent cell layer of the dorsal epidermis, which allows capture of high quality fluorescent images *in vivo* (see Figure 1B). At the same time, cardiac cells can easily be manipulated using cardiac-specific Gal4-driver lines (see below) to express GFP-tagged genes, e.g. of the actin cytoskeleton, specifically in the heart. This allows the effects of specific mutations on actin dynamics to be monitored during heart formation (Medioni et al., 2008). Furthermore, a large number of fluorescently labeled genes such as actin^{GFP} that can be overexpressed are readily available from different laboratories and stock centers. Browsing through Flybase (Crosby et al., 2007; Tweedie et al., 2009), a *Drosophila* centered database, allows easy access to the records for any published construct. The power of the *Drosophila* model is the ability to combine mutant alleles of almost any gene with tissue-specific expression of fluorescently labeled markers. Thus, heart development can be studied in great detail at the organ or even the cellular level, permitting the role of individual genes to be examined in the context of a specific cellular function. This approach provides an experimental resolution that is unparalleled in any other model organism.

The technological advances in the *Drosophila* model are steadily growing. The Gal4/UAS system (Brand and Perrimon, 1993) had been groundbreaking for tissue-specific genetic manipulations, and continues to be further refined (Osterwalder et al., 2001; McGuire et al., 2004; Pfeiffer et al., 2010; Gohl et al., 2011). Gal4, a transcriptional activator from yeast and without endogenous binding sites in the *Drosophila* genome, is used to trans-activate genes that are engineered to contain Gal4-binding sites (upstream activating sequences, UAS). This heterologous system allows the expression of any UAS-fused gene in any tissue where Gal4 is expressed, which itself is driven by tissue-specific promoters. Gal4 and UAS-lines can be created either by random insertion of transposable elements into the fly's genome (Cooley et al., 1988) or targeted insertion at particular "landing sites" (Fish et al., 2007). The first method has been extensively used to create a vast amount of "enhancer trap" lines that express the Gal4 driver in many different, tissue-specific patterns including the heart. A recent technique by Gohl et al. (2011) has further increased the versatility of such Gal4-enhancer trap lines by developing a method to replace the Gal4 driver with any other reporter (e.g. GFP) or effector gene (e.g. the Gal4 repressor Gal80, which will inhibit the Gal4 activity of a different line in the intersecting cells). The Gal4/UAS system not only allows selective expression of marker genes in specific tissues (e.g. Figure 1B, expression in cardiac tissue using tinCΔ4-Gal4, Lo and Frasch, 2001), but also permits genetic manipulations by ectopic or overexpression of genes or by reducing their expression levels using RNA interference (RNAi, see below). In combination with lines that express the Gal80 repressor in a subset of Gal4-positive cells, the Gal4 expression pattern can be further spatially refined. In addition, use of a temperature-sensitive version of Gal80 (Gal80-TS, McGuire et al., 2004) gives temporal control over Gal4 expression, which then becomes active only under the permissive temperature.

One limitation of the Gal4/UAS system is that all transgenes that carry UAS sites respond at the same time. Therefore, different tissues or cells cannot be manipulated individually, although this could be a useful approach to study their interaction. The recent invention of the Q system (Potter et al., 2010) is a novel approach to circumvent this limitation. It works in a similar manner as Gal4/UAS but uses the *Neurospora* transcriptional activator QF, which recognizes its own specific binding sequence (QUAS). Just like Gal4, a fly line that expresses QF in a certain tissue or cell will drive expression of a gene that contains the QUAS binding sites. Similar to Gal80, the activity of QF can be suppressed by expression of QS (allowing further refinement of QF expression), and feeding flies quinic acid releases this suppression in a dose-dependent manner. Thus, QS gives both, spatial and temporal control over the activity of QF, just like Gal80 and Gal80^{TS} for Gal4. A combination of both the Gal4 and QF systems therefore would allow distinct expression of multiple transgenes in a precise tissue-specific and temporal-specific manner in an otherwise unchanged genetic background.

Recent advances in RNA interference (RNAi) technology, combined with the spatio-temporal control of the Gal4/UAS system, have allowed tissue-specific studies of gene function during almost any developmental stage. RNAi has therefore been useful to analyze genes that when mutated would cause early lethality or pleiotropic effects, but it is also the only method currently available to study gene function when no mutant alleles for a particular gene are available.

Systematic analysis to determine optimal hairpin formation and careful analysis of insertion sites have greatly increased the efficacy of RNAi (Ni et al., 2008; 2009; 2011). The Transgenic RNAi project (TRiP) is currently generating these optimized RNAi lines for all *Drosophila* genes, which complements other RNAi resources (like VDRC, Dietzl et al., 2007). As an alternative reverse genetic approach, the directed mutation or knockout of a particular gene of interest by homologous recombination (reviewed in Maggert et al., 2008) has also been developed further. In addition to generating a knockout allele, Huang et al. (2009) have added a recombinase-based feature that allows modification of the deleted locus by inserting virtually any sequence ("genomic engineering"). Of note, this permits modification of gene function in an otherwise unaltered genetic background. Furthermore, efforts to create genomic duplications for regions of the X chromosome have resulted in the creation of two independent sets of fly lines, one set with a duplication located on the Y chromosome (Cook et al., 2010) and one set on the 3rd chromosome (Venken et al., 2010). This will facilitate the recovery and identification of X-linked mutations and also allow assessment of the fly's susceptibility to increased gene dosages. These improved techniques of Gal4/UAS transactivation, paired with the expression of fluorescently tagged reporters and RNAi lines as well novel forward and reverse genetic techniques and resources are likely to unravel new, previously unnoticed gene functions in different tissues and under different developmental contexts.

5. Exploring fly heart function to understand CHD-related cardiomyopathies

By definition, congenital heart disease refers to the presence of structural heart and large vessel defects at the time of birth. Many of these can be repaired by surgical intervention, but depending on the severity of the defect, patients may require life-long medical follow-ups to monitor cardiac performance and to detect signs of functional decline. Furthermore, late onset complications either due to persistent impact of structural defects or related to the applied intervention are often linked to lethal arrhythmias or progressive congestive heart failure. Such secondary complications might not be caused directly by CHD genes, but due to a maladaptive response of the cardiac tissue. In the light of these considerations it is therefore necessary to understand how cardiac tissues respond to these interventions and which other genes might contribute to arrhythmias and cardiomyopathies. The *Drosophila* model has helped to identify a number of novel genes and pathways required to maintain myofibrillar organization and overall heart structure and function. Because similarities between the *Drosophila* and murine heart are found both at the molecular and functional level it is therefore likely that new risk factors of cardiac disease can be identified using *Drosophila*. The cardiac proteasomes of the mouse and the fly have been shown to be comparable with respect to their overall composition (Cammarato et al., 2011), and functional analysis revealed further evidence of the conserved cardiac characteristics of the fly heart (e.g. Ocorr et al., 2007a; Buechling et al., 2009; Choma et al., 2010). In particular, the contractile and electrical properties have been investigated in the *Drosophila* heart and found to be remarkably similar in fundamental aspects, such as the contribution of ion channels to heart contraction or the effects of mutations of genes of the myofibrillar apparatus (K. Ocorr, unpublished and Lalevée et al., 2006; Wolf et al., 2006; Ocorr et al., 2007b; Cammarato et al., 2008b; Mery et al., 2008). In addition to determining cardiac parameters in vivo and in situ (see below and Fig. 2), electrical properties can be measured using the fluorescent Ca^{2+}-sensor GCaMP (Nakai et al., 2001), where Ca^{2+}-transients are monitored *in vivo* (Lin et al., 2011).

These techniques have set the stage for using the *Drosophila* model to identify new cardiac genes involved in CHD and cardiac disease. In a recent screen for genes affecting *Drosophila* heart function under stress conditions, components of the CCR4/NOT complex, which is a regulator of gene transcription and mRNA degradation, have been shown to play a pivotal role in maintaining heart function in flies, but also in mice and possibly humans (Neely et al., 2010). In this particular study, hearts in mutant flies were functionally analyzed as semi-intact preparations (using the methods described in Ocorr et al., 2007b; 2009; Vogler and Ocorr, 2009) and subsequently analyzed for structural defects (as described in Alayari et al., 2009; Fink et al., 2009b). These methods allow the assessment of numerous fly heart parameters (such as diastolic and systolic diameters and intervals, intrinsic heart rate of the denervated heart and estimates on the degree of arrhythmias; see Fig. 2). For CCR4/NOT complex mutants, it was shown that these flies have hallmarks of dilated cardiomyopathy. Remarkably, *not3*$^{+/-}$ heterozygous mice are haploinsufficient and exhibit less resistance to cardiac stress, indicating that this pathway is required for maintaining proper heart function. Administration of HDAC inhibitors ameliorates these phenotypes, indicating that changes in chromatin remodeling are likely to play a major role. Lastly, the authors showed that a single-nucleotide polymorphism (SNP) near the human NOT3 genes is associated with prolonged long QT intervals. Together, these data show that the cardiac role of the CCR4/NOT complex is highly conserved, and that *Drosophila* indeed is useful for identifying novel genes and pathways involved in cardiac disease. Due to the broad role of the CCR4/NOT complex in regulating both, gene transcription and posttranslational modification, it remains unclear by which mechanisms and genes the cardiac phenotypes become manifest. Further analysis of the CCR4/NOT complex is therefore required, and the fly heart is likely to provide further insights. Importantly, this approach showed that RNAi-mediated genetic screening is a promising approach to identify new cardiac risk genes in humans.

In *Drosophila,* as well as in higher organisms, transheterozygous mutations can unravel a hidden link between two genes (genetic interaction). *Drosophila* is well suited for such experimental screening approaches since most genes are not duplicated, thus interactions are less likely to be masked by compensatory mechanisms. In a recent study, this particular strength of the *Drosophila* model has been successfully exploited to identify a novel link between the cardiac transcription factor *Nkx2.5*/*tinman* and the small GTPase *Cdc42* (Qian et al., 2011). In the aforementioned study, flies that were double heterozygous for *Cdc42* and *tinman* showed altered cardiac function and also showed structural defects, something not observed in the single heterozygous animals. The subsequent analysis of double heterozygous *Cdc42;Nkx2.5* mouse hearts also revealed an impaired heart function when compared to single heterozygous animals, again indicating that this genetic link between *Cdc42* and *tinman/Nkx2.5* is conserved. Such complex *in vivo* screens to unravel genetic interactions in higher eukaryotes are currently only feasible in the fly model organism. With respect to understanding the genetics of heart development and disease, *Drosophila* is the simplest genetic model with a heart (Bier and Bodmer, 2004). Moreover, from a systems biology point of view, the fly is a perfect model organism to rapidly test genetic interactions that are predicted from networks based on genetic information, bioinformatics and the integration of other data obtained from many different model organisms and patients (for the fly, such data can be accessed through DroID, the *Drosophila* interactions database, see Yu et al., 2008; Murali et al., 2010).

6. A genetic model for heart diseases

The knowledge of molecular mechanisms underlying important biological processes gained from *Drosophila* has been successfully extended to studies of human diseases especially in the field of neural degenerative diseases (Bilen and Bonini, 2005; Marsh and Thompson, 2006). Recent studies in flies have been directed towards understanding more complex and multifactorial diseases such as heart disease. In this section we specifically demonstrate how *Drosophila* can be used as a model to elucidate the molecular mechanisms of CHD and cardiomyopathies. As we mentioned above, both anatomical and molecular features of *Drosophila* heart development (as outlined in Figure 1) and aspects of adult structure and function (see Figure 2) are similar to those observed in the human heart, making *Drosophila* a useful model system with the advantage of a much simpler genetic and tissue organization.

Primary cardiomyopathies are contractile disorders of the myocardium. The majority of cases of cardiomyopathy are classified into two disease types: hypertrophic cardiomyopathy (HCM) and dilated cardiomyopathy (DCM). HCM, defined as a hypertrophic ventricle with myofibrillar disarrays, can sometimes lead to sudden death in young subjects, but many cases of HCM maintain stable hemodynamics until late stages. DCM, defined as dilated ventricle with systolic dysfunction, also shows myofibrillar disarrays and clinically exhibits refractory arrhythmias and severe heart failure. In both disease types genetic causes have been found. The first case of a male-sibling DCM with X-linked inheritance had a mutation in *dystrophin* (*dys*), a gene that plays an important role in the anchoring of muscle cells (Towbin et al., 1993). Mutations in *dys* are a cause of Duchenne-type (null function of *dys*) and Becker-type (hypomorphic function of *dys*) muscular dystrophy, whose clinical entity is characterized by progressive muscle weakness and degeneration of muscle fibers (Koenig et al., 1988). In both types late-onset cardiac dysfunction is frequently observed, and improvement of heart function is an important therapeutic target for improving life prognosis. As in humans, fly Dys is associated with the plasma membrane at the sarcomeric Z-line and is already present during early embryogenesis of the *Drosophila* heart (Taghli-Lamallem et al., 2008). In *dys* deficiency flies the myofibrillar structure of the heart cells is disorganized in that myofibrils are not tightly packed and appear sparse. This phenotype worsens with age, consistent with the late onset of cardiac dysfunction in muscular dystrophy patients. Real-time imaging of heart movements using high-speed digital video recording system allows a detailed analysis of the heart's performance and pathology, with quantitative measurements of heart period, rhythmicity, size, and fractional shortening (an index of contractility, Akasaka and Ocorr, 2009; Fink et al., 2009a). Using this methodology, it was observed that *dys* mutants exhibited a significantly wider diastolic (80-90μm) and systolic (60μm) diameter compared to laboratory wild-type strains (diastolic diameter 60μM, systolic diameter 40μm), suggesting that the *dys* mutant produces a dilated, cardiomegaly-type phenotype. In addition, fractional shortening in the mutants is reduced to 25-30% (compared to 35-40% in wild type). Those features are reminiscent of DCM in humans and a Duchenne-type mouse model (*mdx* mouse) (Quinlan et al., 2004; Wehling-Henricks et al., 2005). Interestingly, a short C-terminal form of human *dys* (Dp116, Judge et al., 2006) rescued the DCM phenotype of *dys* mutant flies (Taghli-Lamallem et al., 2008), but this micro-*dys* could not improve skeletal muscle function in the *mdx* mice model. Because this isoform is incorporated into the dystrophin glycoprotein complex (DGC) but is not capable of binding to the actin skeleton, successful DGC formation may be a critical characteristic. Failure to form this complex may then lead to the observed pathogenesis in the heart, which potentially may be due to dysfunction in force transmission and/or impairment of the signal transduction through DGC. This study is just one example of the use of *Drosophila* as a model for comprehensive human cardiac disease, and which may also allow testing the potential of therapeutic strategies such as the introduction of micro-*dys* to the heart.

Molecular and genetic examinations of cardiomyopathy populations have produced data indicating that mutations in sarcomere-related proteins are involved in the cardiomyopathy phenotype (Hershberger and Siegfried, 2011; Seidman and Seidman, 2011). Myosin is a molecular motor composed of two myosin heavy chains (MHC) and four light chains. This hexameric myosin is a major component of the thick filament and allows them to slide along the thin actin filaments in an ATP-dependent manner. Two mutant alleles of myosin, D45 (A261T) and Mhc^5 (G200D), have missense mutations occurring close to the ATP catalytic site, and it was postulated that those amino acid substitutions would affect ATPase activity (Kronert et al., 1999). In fact, ATPase activities of both D45 and Mhc^5 mutant myosin were depressed compared to wild-type myosin; however, *in vivo* motility of F-actin on a myosin coated slide showed a reduced velocity for D45 myosin to almost half of that of wild-type and an increased velocity in Mhc^5 myosin to about 115% of wild-type (Cammarato et al., 2008a). Interestingly, these myosin mutants showed different pathologies in the heart. Compared to wild-type, D45 mutant hearts are dilated exhibiting an increased systolic and diastolic diameter, whereas Mhc^5 mutants appear restricted showing a decreased diameter only during diastolic phase (Cammarato et al., 2008a). The depressed motor function and dilation in D45 myosin is evocative of DCM in humans, whereas the increased motor function and reduced diastolic function in Mhc^5 is similar to human restricted cardiomyopathy (RCM, Cammarato et al., 2008a), a rare type of cardiomyopathy in which decreased myocardium elasticity affects the ventricular blood filling during the diastolic phase. Unlike the fly D45 and Mhc^5 pathogenesis, biochemical and structural investigations in vertebrates are not always able to reveal how mutations contribute to cardiac pathologies. Instead, the role of a particular gene is primarily obtained from the phenotype and/or symptoms of a patient carrying a mutation in this gene. However, even this clinical approach requires costly and labor-intensive efforts in order to first identify these patients. In addition, clinical studies often require supplemental tests, which are sometimes difficult to perform. Reverse genetics may be able to compensate for these disadvantages of clinical studies, and especially in the fly system the availability of genetic tools for the entire genome is very useful for a systematic approach to test gene functions. For example in the fly, the *MHC* is encoded by a single gene, thus the analysis of specific mutations in this gene can inform us how alterations in myosin structure directly contribute to alterations in function and the pathophysiological consequences.

Both, dystrophin and myosin-related cardiomyopathies are caused by a dysfunction from within cardiomyocytes, and therefore are not necessarily linked to defects in heart formation, which are the basis of CHD. But can the fly model be used to investigate CHD, even though it lacks higher-order structures, such as looping, septation, and chamber formation? There are many cases of CHD where cardiomyocyte function is still far from normal, regardless of the success of corrective surgical procedures. This suggests that those cases could have primary defects within cardiomyocytes in addition to the overall morphological defects in the heart's architecture. Investigations of these questions may also benefit from the cardiomyopathy models in *Drosophila* mentioned above. Taking advantage of the *Drosophila* model we recently performed a study using data obtained from a patient with hypoplastic left heart syndrome (HLHS). HLHS is the most severe type of left-sided heart defect, and occurs in 2-4% of all infants born with congenital heart disease (Loffredo, 2000). We found that this patient had a balanced chromosomal translocation whose breakpoint is in close proximity to a member of the kinesin family (Akasaka, Grosfeld, et al., unpubl.). Heart-specific over expression of kinesin in the fly model disrupts the contractile muscle structure and reduces the quantity myofibrils. Those phenotypes resemble what is observed in micrographs of heart tissue from HLHS patients; cardiomyocytes with scant cytoplasm and myofibrillar disarray (Bohlmeyer et al., 2003). Therefore, despite the differences in the fly heart's gross anatomy this system can provide insights into CHD pathogenesis and this information can be applied to the development of both preventive and therapeutic strategies in the future.

7. Conclusions

To understand the complex etiology and genetics of congenital heart disease, synergistic efforts from all fields of medical and biological sciences are required. For many decades, the invertebrate model organism *Drosophila* has provided exciting new insights into the genetics, development and function of multi-cellular organisms. In this review, we have highlighted some of the recent advances and findings gained from a *Drosophila* model for CHD. Despite its evolutionary distance from vertebrates there is a remarkable conservation of genetics and function. The development of technologies such as time-lapse analysis of heart formation and optical techniques to study function suggest that further studies using this system will provide insights into fundamental cellular mechanisms underlying heart function and disease. The fly has been shown to be a useful model that is able to complement the shortcomings of other model systems. Its simpler genetic architecture allows researchers to dissect the basic networks involved in organ formation and by extension to gain insights into the genetics underlying CHD and cardiac diseases in the same way that the *Drosophila* model has advanced our understanding of human genetics and embryonic development.

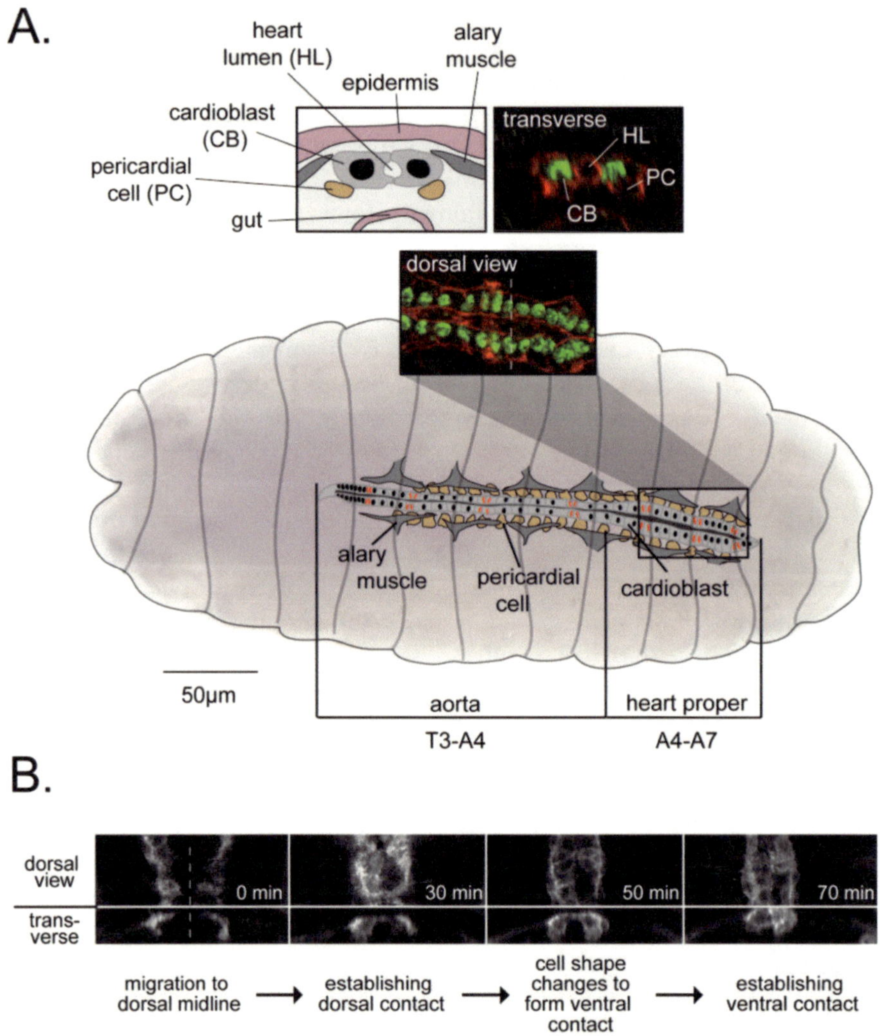

Fig. 1. **A.** Morphology of the late embryonic heart of *Drosophila*. After 17 hours of development, the cardiac precursor cells have completed migration and heart assembly. The heart is located underneath the epidermis along the dorsal midline. It consists of two morphologically different portions, the anterior aorta (spanning segments T3-A4) and the posterior heart proper (segment A4-A7), which is characterized by a much wider lumen. The two major cell types are cardioblasts (CBs), which will differentiate into cardiomyocytes, and pericardial cells (PCs), which will become nephrocyte-like cardiac support cells. The heart is also connected to specialized lateral body wall muscles, named alary muscles. The cardioblast nuclei can be specifically labeled (e.g. by anti-Nmr1 antibody, green) to assess CB alignment. Cell surfaces are stained using Dystroglycan antibody (red). The aorta and heart contain a central (HL). **B.** Heart assembly, visualized by a time-lapse movie of cardiac cells expressing actin^{GFP}. Before alignment, two lateral rows of CBs and PCs migrate towards the dorsal midline (indicated as hatched line). The CBs elongate at the dorsal side and extend filopodia towards the contralateral side to form the dorsal contact. Following this contact, the cells change in shape to contact ventrally, thereby enclosing a luminal space.

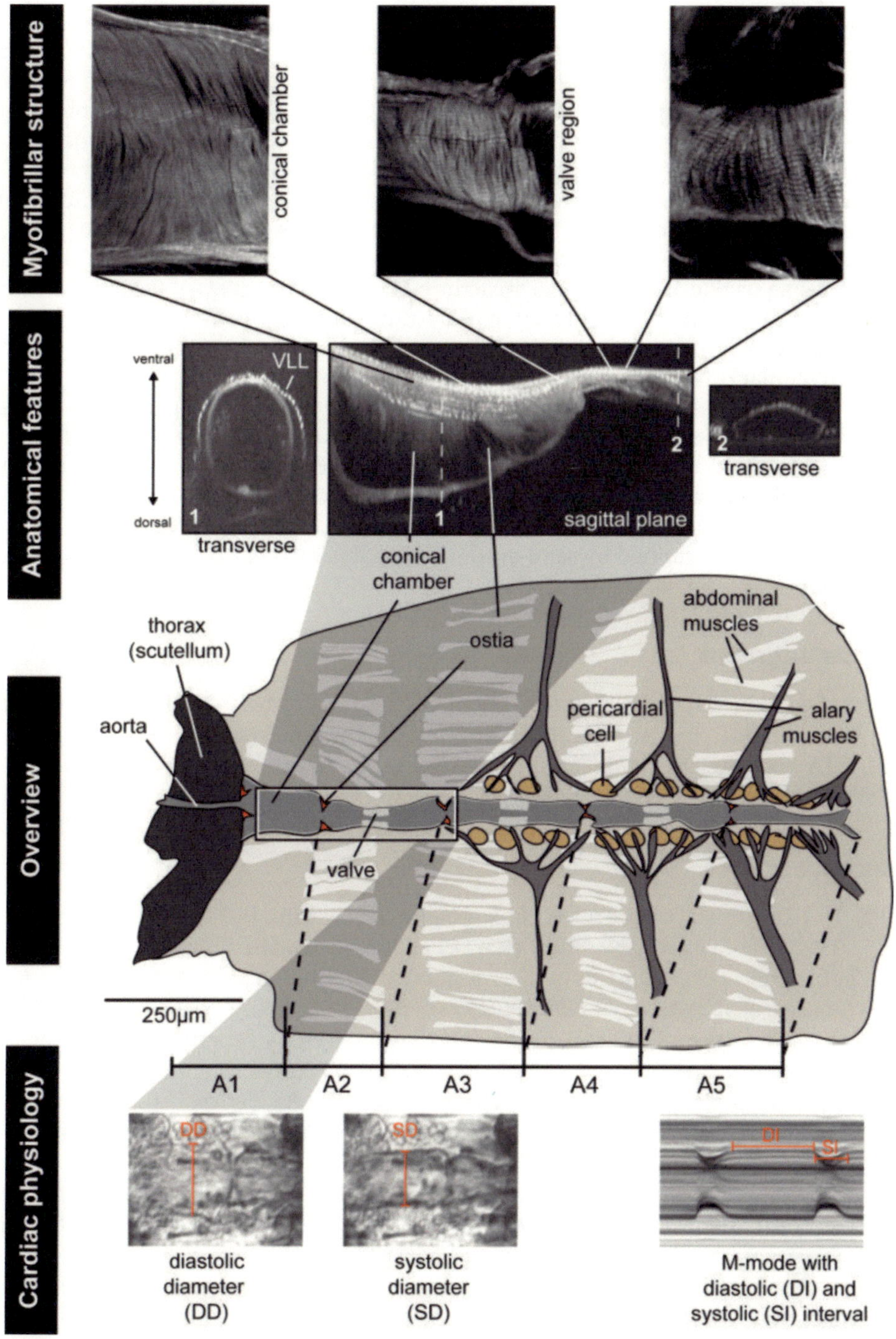

Fig. 2. Morphological features of the adult *Drosophila* heart and determination of structural and functional parameters for phenotypic analysis. Overview: The adult *Drosophila* heart is a contractile tube located at the dorsal midline of the abdomen. Along the heart, specialized cells and structures can be identified: 5 pairs of inflow valves (ostia, red) and 3 pairs of valves inside

the tube. The anterior portion of the heart shows a prominent specialization (the conical chamber, which is larger in size) and anastomoses into the aorta that runs from the posterior end of the thorax into the head capsule. Several pairs of alary muscles are attached to the heart tube, which are likely to help to maintain heart position. The pericardial cells are found alongside the heart and have a nephrocyte-like as well as other cardiac support functions. The ventral longitudinal layer consists of several multi-nucleated muscle cells that ensheath the heart from A1 to about mid-A5 (indicated as VLL in transverse section of the conical chamber). Anatomical features: The conical chamber is the largest chamber of the adult fly heart (compare transverse sections 1+2). The VLL that ventrally and laterally covers the heart can be seen in transverse section 1. Myofibrillar structure: The cardiomyocytes of the conical chamber are much larger in size and have a higher acto-myosin content compared to other regions of the heart. The cardiomyocytes of the valves show a very dense packaging of myofibrils compared to regular cardiomyocytes of the heart. Cardiac physiology: High-speed image capturing from semi-dissected fly hearts allows determination of several parameters, which are indicative for fly heart morphology and function: the diameters of the heart during diastole (DD) and systole (SD) are determined from the original movies. M-modes are generated by aligning a 1-pixel wide strip from each frame showing the location of the heart walls (Y axis) over time (X-axis) (Ocorr et al., 2007). Heart rate, durations of diastoles and systoles (DI and SI) and rhythmicity are determined by semi-automated analysis using MATlab-based software (Fink et al. 2009).

8. Acknowledgment

We are grateful to Drs. Karen Ocorr and Paul D. Grossfeld for helpful discussion and critical reading of the manuscript. This work is supported by grants from AHA to G.V., from NIH (NHLBI, NIA and NIDDK) and The Ellison Medical Foundation to R.B., and from Sanford Children's Hospital Research Center to T.A.

9. References

Akasaka, T., Klinedinst, S., Ocorr, K., Bustamante, E. L., Kim, S. K. and Bodmer, R. (2006) 'The ATP-sensitive potassium (KATP) channel-encoded dSUR gene is required for Drosophila heart function and is regulated by tinman.', *Proceedings of the National Academy of Sciences of the United States of America* 103(32): 11999-12004.

Akasaka, T. and Ocorr, K. (2009) 'Drug discovery through functional screening in the Drosophila heart', *Methods in molecular biology* 577: 235-49.

Alayari, N. N., Vogler, G., Taghli-Lamallem, O., Ocorr, K. A., Bodmer, R. and Cammarato, A. (2009) 'Fluorescent labeling of Drosophila heart structures.', *Journal of Visualized Experiments*(32).

Albrecht, S., Altenhein, B. and Paululat, A. (2011) 'The transmembrane receptor Uncoordinated5 (Unc5) is essential for heart lumen formation in Drosophila melanogaster.', *Developmental biology* 350(1): 89-100.

Alvarez, A. D., Shi, W., Wilson, B. A. and Skeath, J. B. (2003) 'pannier and pointedP2 act sequentially to regulate Drosophila heart development', *Development (Cambridge, England)* 130(13): 3015-3026.

Azpiazu, N. and Frasch, M. (1993) 'tinman and bagpipe: two homeo box genes that determine cell fates in the dorsal mesoderm of Drosophila.', *Genes & Development* 7(7B): 1325-1340.

Bier, E. and Bodmer, R. (2004) 'Drosophila, an emerging model for cardiac disease', *Gene* 342(1): 1-11.

Bilen, J. and Bonini, N. M. (2005) 'Drosophila as a model for human neurodegenerative disease', *Annual Review of Genetics* 39: 153-71.

Bodmer, R. (1993) 'The gene tinman is required for specification of the heart and visceral muscles in Drosophila', *Development (Cambridge, England)* 118(3): 719-729.

Bodmer, R. (1995) 'Heart development in Drosophila and its relationship to vertebrates', *Trends in cardiovascular medicine* 5(1): 21-28.

Bodmer, R. and Frasch, M. (2010) Heart Development and Regeneration. in R. P. Harvey and N. Rosenthal (eds.), vol. 1: Academic Press; 1 edition (June 18, 2010).

Bodmer, R., Jan, L. Y. and Jan, Y. N. (1990) 'A new homeobox-containing gene, msh-2, is transiently expressed early during mesoderm formation of Drosophila.', *Development (Cambridge, England)* 110(3): 661-669.

Bohlmeyer, T. J., Helmke, S., Ge, S., Lynch, J., Brodsky, G., Sederberg, J. H., Robertson, A. D., Minobe, W., Bristow, M. R. and Perryman, M. B. (2003) 'Hypoplastic left heart syndrome myocytes are differentiated but possess a unique phenotype', *Cardiovascular pathology : the official journal of the Society for Cardiovascular Pathology* 12(1): 23-31.

Brand, A. H. and Perrimon, N. (1993) 'Targeted gene expression as a means of altering cell fates and generating dominant phenotypes', *Development (Cambridge, England)* 118(2): 401-415.

Buechling, T., Akasaka, T., Vogler, G., Ruiz-Lozano, P., Ocorr, K. A. and Bodmer, R. (2009) 'Non-autonomous modulation of heart rhythm, contractility and morphology in adult fruit flies.', *Developmental biology* 328(2): 483-492.

Cammarato, A., Ahrens, C. H., Alayari, N. N., Qeli, E., Rucker, J., Reedy, M. C., Zmasek, C. M., Gucek, M., Cole, R. N., Van Eyk, J. E. et al. (2011) 'A Mighty Small Heart: The Cardiac Proteome of Adult Drosophila melanogaster', *PLoS ONE* 6(4): e18497.

Cammarato, A., Dambacher, C. M., Knowles, A. F., Kronert, W. A., Bodmer, R., Ocorr, K. and Bernstein, S. I. (2008a) 'Myosin transducer mutations differentially affect motor function, myofibril structure, and the performance of skeletal and cardiac muscles', *Molecular biology of the cell* 19(2): 553-62.

Cammarato, A., Dambacher, C. M., Knowles, A. F., Kronert, W. A., Bodmer, R., Ocorr, K. A. and Bernstein, S. I. (2008b) 'Myosin transducer mutations differentially affect motor function, myofibril structure, and the performance of skeletal and cardiac muscles', *Molecular biology of the cell* 19(2): 553 562.

Chen, E., Hermanson, S. and Ekker, S. C. (2004) 'Syndecan-2 is essential for angiogenic sprouting during zebrafish development.', *Blood* 103(5): 1710-1719.

Choma, M. A., Suter, M. J., Vakoc, B. J., Bouma, B. E. and Tearney, G. J. (2010) 'Physiological homology between Drosophila melanogaster and vertebrate cardiovascular systems', *Disease Models & Mechanisms*.

Christiaen, L., Davidson, B., Kawashima, T., Powell, W., Nolla, H., Vranizan, K. and Levine, M. (2008) 'The transcription/migration interface in heart precursors of Ciona intestinalis.', *Science (New York, NY)* 320(5881): 1349-1352.

Cook, R. K., Deal, M. E., Deal, J. A., Garton, R. D., Brown, C. A., Ward, M. E., Andrade, R. S., Spana, E. P., Kaufman, T. C. and Cook, K. R. (2010) 'A new resource for characterizing X-linked genes in Drosophila melanogaster: systematic coverage and subdivision of the X chromosome with nested, Y-linked duplications.', *Genetics* 186(4): 1095-1109.

Cooley, L., Kelley, R. and Spradling, A. (1988) 'Insertional mutagenesis of the Drosophila genome with single P elements.', *Science (New York, NY)* 239(4844): 1121-1128.

Cripps, R. M. and Olson, E. N. (2002) 'Control of cardiac development by an evolutionarily conserved transcriptional network.', *Developmental biology* 246(1): 14-28.

Crosby, M. A., Goodman, J. L., Strelets, V. B., Zhang, P., Gelbart, W. M. and Consortium, F. (2007) 'FlyBase: genomes by the dozen.', *Nucleic acids research* 35(Database issue): D486-91.

Dickson, B. J. and Gilestro, G. F. (2006) 'Regulation of commissural axon pathfinding by slit and its Robo receptors.', *Annual Review of Cell and Developmental Biology* 22: 651-675.

Dietzl, G., Chen, D., Schnorrer, F., Su, K.-C., Barinova, Y., Fellner, M., Gasser, B., Kinsey, K., Oppel, S., Scheiblauer, S. et al. (2007) 'A genome-wide transgenic RNAi library for conditional gene inactivation in Drosophila', *Nature* 448(7150): 151-156.

Fink, M., Callol-Massot, C., Chu, A., Ruiz-Lozano, P., Izpisua Belmonte, J. C., Giles, W., Bodmer, R. and Ocorr, K. (2009a) 'A new method for detection and quantification of heartbeat parameters in Drosophila, zebrafish, and embryonic mouse hearts', *BioTechniques* 46(2): 101-13.

Fink, M., Callol-Massot, C., Chu, A., Ruiz-Lozano, P., Izpisua Belmonte, J. C., Giles, W., Bodmer, R. and Ocorr, K. A. (2009b) 'A new method for detection and quantification of heartbeat parameters in Drosophila, zebrafish, and embryonic mouse hearts', *BioTechniques* 46(2): 101-113.

Fish, J. E., Wythe, J. D., Xiao, T., Bruneau, B. G., Stainier, D. Y. R., Srivastava, D. and Woo, S. (2011) 'A Slit/miR-218/Robo regulatory loop is required during heart tube formation in zebrafish.', *Development (Cambridge, England)* 138(7): 1409-1419.

Fish, M. P., Groth, A. C., Calos, M. P. and Nusse, R. (2007) 'Creating transgenic Drosophila by microinjecting the site-specific phiC31 integrase mRNA and a transgene-containing donor plasmid', *Nature Protocols* 2(10): 2325-2331.

Frasch, M. (1999) 'Intersecting signalling and transcriptional pathways in Drosophila heart specification', *Seminars in cell & developmental biology* 10(1): 61-71.

Fromental-Ramain, C., Vanolst, L., Delaporte, C. and Ramain, P. (2008) 'pannier encodes two structurally related isoforms that are differentially expressed during Drosophila development and display distinct functions during thorax patterning', *Mechanisms of development* 125(1-2): 43-57.

Gohl, D. M., Silies, M. A., Gao, X. J., Bhalerao, S., Luongo, F. J., Lin, C.-C., Potter, C. J. and Clandinin, T. R. (2011) 'A versatile in vivo system for directed dissection of gene expression patterns.', *Nature Methods* 8(3): 231-237.

Han, Z. and Olson, E. N. (2005) 'Hand is a direct target of Tinman and GATA factors during Drosophila cardiogenesis and hematopoiesis', *Development (Cambridge, England)* 132(15): 3525-3536.

Han, Z., Yi, P., Li, X. and Olson, E. N. (2006) 'Hand, an evolutionarily conserved bHLH transcription factor required for Drosophila cardiogenesis and hematopoiesis.', *Development (Cambridge, England)* 133(6): 1175-1182.

Hartenstein, V. and Mandal, L. (2006) 'The blood/vascular system in a phylogenetic perspective', *BioEssays: news and reviews in molecular, cellular and developmental biology* 28(12): 1203-1210.

Hershberger, R. E. and Siegfried, J. D. (2011) 'Update 2011: clinical and genetic issues in familial dilated cardiomyopathy', *Journal of the American College of Cardiology* 57(16): 1641-9.

Huang, J., Zhou, W., Dong, W., Watson, A. M. and Hong, Y. (2009) 'Directed, efficient, and versatile modifications of the Drosophila genome by genomic engineering.', *Proceedings of the National Academy of Sciences of the United States of America* 106(20): 8284-8289.

Jacinto, A., Woolner, S. and Martin, P. (2002) 'Dynamic analysis of dorsal closure in Drosophila: from genetics to cell biology', *Developmental cell* 3(1): 9-19.

Judge, L. M., Haraguchiln, M. and Chamberlain, J. S. (2006) 'Dissecting the signaling and mechanical functions of the dystrophin-glycoprotein complex', *Journal of Cell Science* 119(Pt 8): 1537-46.

Knox, J., Moyer, K., Yacoub, N., Soldaat, C., Komosa, M., Vassilieva, K., Wilk, R., Hu, J., Vasquez Pas, L. d. L., Syed, Q. et al. (2011) 'Syndecan contributes to heart cell specification and lumen formation during Drosophila cardiogenesis.', *Developmental biology*.

Koenig, M., Monaco, A. P. and Kunkel, L. M. (1988) 'The complete sequence of dystrophin predicts a rod-shaped cytoskeletal protein', *Cell* 53(2): 219-28.

Kronert, W. A., Acebes, A., Ferrus, A. and Bernstein, S. I. (1999) 'Specific myosin heavy chain mutations suppress troponin I defects in Drosophila muscles', *The Journal of Cell Biology* 144(5): 989-1000.

Lalevée, N., Monier, B., Sénatore, S., Perrin, L. and Sémériva, M. (2006) 'Control of cardiac rhythm by ORK1, a Drosophila two-pore domain potassium channel.', *Current biology : CB* 16(15): 1502-1508.

Leal, S. M., Qian, L., Lacin, H., Bodmer, R. and Skeath, J. B. (2009) 'Neuromancer1 and Neuromancer2 regulate cell fate specification in the developing embryonic CNS of Drosophila melanogaster', *Developmental biology* 325(1): 138-150.

Lin, N., Badie, N., Yu, L., Abraham, D., Cheng, H., Bursac, N., Rockman, H. A. and Wolf, M. J. (2011) 'A Method to Measure Myocardial Calcium Handling in Adult Drosophila.', *Circulation Research*.

Liu, Y.-H., Jakobsen, J. S., Valentin, G., Amarantos, I., Gilmour, D. T. and Furlong, E. E. M. (2009) 'A systematic analysis of Tinman function reveals Eya and JAK-STAT signaling as essential regulators of muscle development.', *Developmental cell* 16(2): 280-291.

Lo, P. C. H. and Frasch, M. (2001) 'A role for the COUP-TF-related gene seven-up in the diversification of cardioblast identities in the dorsal vessel of Drosophila', *Mechanisms of development* 104(1-2): 49-60.

Lo, P. C. H., Zaffran, S., Sénatore, S. and Frasch, M. (2007) 'The Drosophila Hand gene is required for remodeling of the developing adult heart and midgut during metamorphosis', *Developmental biology* 311(2): 287-296.

Loffredo, C. A. (2000) 'Epidemiology of cardiovascular malformations: prevalence and risk factors', *American journal of medical genetics* 97(4): 319-25.

MacMullin, A. and Jacobs, J. R. (2006) 'Slit coordinates cardiac morphogenesis in Drosophila.', *Developmental biology* 293(1): 154-164.

Maggert, K. A., Walker, J. M., Gong, W. J., Dahmann, C. and Golic, K. G. (2008) Methods in Molecular Biology *John M.WalkerMethods in Molecular Biology1064-37451940-6029*, vol. 420. Totowa, NJ: Humana Press.

Mann, T., Bodmer, R. and Pandur, P. (2009) 'The Drosophila homolog of vertebrate Islet1 is a key component in early cardiogenesis.', *Development (Cambridge, England)* 136(2): 317-326.

Marsh, J. L. and Thompson, L. M. (2006) 'Drosophila in the study of neurodegenerative disease', *Neuron* 52(1): 169-78.

McGuire, S. E., Mao, Z. and Davis, R. L. (2004) 'Spatiotemporal gene expression targeting with the TARGET and gene-switch systems in Drosophila', *Science's STKE* 2004(220): pl6.

Medioni, C., Astier, M., Zmojdzian, M., Jagla, K. and Semeriva, M. (2008) 'Genetic control of cell morphogenesis during Drosophila melanogaster cardiac tube formation', *The Journal of Cell Biology* 182(2): 249-261.

Medioni, C., Bertrand, N., Mesbah, K., Hudry, B., Dupays, L., Wolstein, O., Washkowitz, A. J., Papaioannou, V. E., Mohun, T. J., Harvey, R. P. et al. (2010) 'Expression of Slit and Robo genes in the developing mouse heart.', *Developmental dynamics : an official publication of the American Association of Anatomists* 239(12): 3303-3311.

Mery, A., Taghli-Lamallem, O., Clark, K. A., Beckerle, M. C., Wu, X., Ocorr, K. A. and Bodmer, R. (2008) 'The Drosophila muscle LIM protein, Mlp84B, is essential for cardiac function', *The Journal of experimental biology* 211(Pt 1): 15-23.

Miskolczi-McCallum, C. M., Scavetta, R. J., Svendsen, P. C., Soanes, K. H. and Brook, W. J. (2005) 'The Drosophila melanogaster T-box genes midline and H15 are conserved regulators of heart development', *Developmental biology* 278(2): 459-472.

Murali, T., Pacifico, S., Yu, J., Guest, S., Roberts, G. G. and Finley, R. L. (2010) 'DroID 2011: a comprehensive, integrated resource for protein, transcription factor, RNA and gene interactions for Drosophila', *Nucleic acids research* 39(Database): D736-D743.

Nakai, J., Ohkura, M. and Imoto, K. (2001) 'A high signal-to-noise Ca(2+) probe composed of a single green fluorescent protein.', *Nature biotechnology* 19(2): 137-141.

Neely, G. G., Kuba, K., Cammarato, A., Isobe, K., Amann, S., Zhang, L., Murata, M., Elmen, L., Gupta, V., Arora, S. et al. (2010) 'A global in vivo Drosophila RNAi screen identifies NOT3 as a conserved regulator of heart function.', *Cell* 141(1): 142-153.

Ni, J.-Q., Liu, L.-P., Binari, R., Hardy, R., Shim, H.-S., Cavallaro, A., Booker, M., Pfeiffer, B. D., Markstein, M., Wang, H. et al. (2009) 'A Drosophila resource of transgenic RNAi lines for neurogenetics.', *Genetics* 182(4): 1089-1100.

Ni, J.-Q., Markstein, M., Binari, R., Pfeiffer, B. D., Liu, L.-P., Villalta, C., Booker, M., Perkins, L. and Perrimon, N. (2008) 'Vector and parameters for targeted transgenic RNA interference in Drosophila melanogaster', *Nature Methods* 5(1): 49-51.

Ni, J.-Q., Zhou, R., Czech, B., Liu, L.-P., Holderbaum, L., Yang-Zhou, D., Shim, H.-S., Tao, R., Handler, D., Karpowicz, P. et al. (2011) 'A genome-scale shRNA resource for transgenic RNAi in Drosophila.', *Nature Methods*.

Ocorr, K., Fink, M., Cammarato, A., Bernstein, S. and Bodmer, R. (2009) 'Semi-automated Optical Heartbeat Analysis of small hearts', *Journal of Visualized Experiments*(31).

Ocorr, K., Perrin, L., Lim, H.-Y., Qian, L., Wu, X. and Bodmer, R. (2007a) 'Genetic control of heart function and aging in Drosophila.', *Trends in cardiovascular medicine* 17(5): 177-182.

Ocorr, K. A., Reeves, N. L., Wessells, R. J., Fink, M., Chen, H.-S. V., Akasaka, T., Yasuda, S., Metzger, J. M., Giles, W., Posakony, J. W. et al. (2007b) 'KCNQ potassium channel mutations cause cardiac arrhythmias in Drosophila that mimic the effects of aging', *Proceedings of the National Academy of Sciences of the United States of America* 104(10): 3943-3948.

Olson, E. N. (2006) 'Gene regulatory networks in the evolution and development of the heart', *Science (New York, NY)* 313(5795): 1922-1927.

Osterwalder, T., Yoon, K. S., White, B. H. and Keshishian, H. (2001) 'A conditional tissue-specific transgene expression system using inducible GAL4.', *Proceedings of the National Academy of Sciences of the United States of America* 98(22): 12596-12601.

Pfeiffer, B. D., Ngo, T.-T. B., Hibbard, K. L., Murphy, C., Jenett, A., Truman, J. W. and Rubin, G. M. (2010) 'Refinement of tools for targeted gene expression in Drosophila.', *Genetics* 186(2): 735-755.

Potter, C. J., Tasic, B., Russler, E. V., Liang, L. and Luo, L. (2010) 'The Q system: a repressible binary system for transgene expression, lineage tracing, and mosaic analysis', *Cell* 141(3): 536-548.

Qian, L. and Bodmer, R. (2009) 'Partial loss of GATA factor Pannier impairs adult heart function in Drosophila.', *Human molecular genetics* 18(17): 3153-3163.

Qian, L., Liu, J. and Bodmer, R. (2005a) 'Neuromancer Tbx20-related genes (H15/midline) promote cell fate specification and morphogenesis of the Drosophila heart', *Developmental biology* 279(2): 509-524.

Qian, L., Liu, J. and Bodmer, R. (2005b) 'Slit and Robo control cardiac cell polarity and morphogenesis.', *Current biology : CB* 15(24): 2271-2278.

Qian, L., Mohapatra, B., Akasaka, T., Liu, J., Ocorr, K., Towbin, J. A. and Bodmer, R. (2008) 'Transcription factor neuromancer/TBX20 is required for cardiac function in Drosophila with implications for human heart disease.', *Proceedings of the National Academy of Sciences of the United States of America* 105(50): 19833-19838.

Qian, L., Wythe, J. D., Liu, J., Cartry, J., Vogler, G., Mohapatra, B., Otway, R. T., Huang, Y., King, I. N., Maillet, M. et al. (2011) 'Tinman/Nkx2-5 acts via miR-1 and upstream of Cdc42 to regulate heart function across species.', *The Journal of Cell Biology*.

Quinlan, J. G., Hahn, H. S., Wong, B. L., Lorenz, J. N., Wenisch, A. S. and Levin, L. S. (2004) 'Evolution of the mdx mouse cardiomyopathy: physiological and morphological findings', *Neuromuscular disorders : NMD* 14(8-9): 491-6.

Reim, I. and Frasch, M. (2005) 'The Dorsocross T-box genes are key components of the regulatory network controlling early cardiogenesis in Drosophila', *Development (Cambridge, England)* 132(22): 4911-4925.

Reim, I., Mohler, J. P. and Frasch, M. (2005) 'Tbx20-related genes, mid and H15, are required for tinman expression, proper patterning, and normal differentiation of cardioblasts in Drosophila', *Mechanisms of development* 122(9): 1056-1069.

Rugendorff, A., Younossi-Hartenstein, A. and Hartenstein, V. (1994) 'Embryonic origin and differentiation of the Drosophila heart', ... *Genes and Evolution*.

Ryu, J.-R., Najand, N. and Brook, W. J. (2011) 'Tinman is a direct activator of midline in the Drosophila dorsal vessel.', *Developmental dynamics : an official publication of the American Association of Anatomists* 240(1): 86-95.

Santiago-Martínez, E., Soplop, N. H. and Kramer, S. G. (2006) 'Lateral positioning at the dorsal midline: Slit and Roundabout receptors guide Drosophila heart cell migration.', *Proceedings of the National Academy of Sciences of the United States of America* 103(33): 12441-12446.

Santiago-Martínez, E., Soplop, N. H., Patel, R. and Kramer, S. G. (2008) 'Repulsion by Slit and Roundabout prevents Shotgun/E-cadherin-mediated cell adhesion during Drosophila heart tube lumen formation.', *The Journal of Cell Biology* 182(2): 241-248.

Seidman, C. E. and Seidman, J. G. (2011) 'Identifying sarcomere gene mutations in hypertrophic cardiomyopathy: a personal history', *Circulation Research* 108(6): 743-50.

Stramer, B., Wood, W., Galko, M. J., Redd, M. J., Jacinto, A., Parkhurst, S. M. and Martin, P. (2005) 'Live imaging of wound inflammation in Drosophila embryos reveals key roles for small GTPases during in vivo cell migration', *The Journal of Cell Biology* 168(4): 567-573.

Taghli-Lamallem, O., Akasaka, T., Hogg, G., Nudel, U., Yaffe, D., Chamberlain, J. S., Ocorr, K. and Bodmer, R. (2008) 'Dystrophin deficiency in Drosophila reduces lifespan and causes a dilated cardiomyopathy phenotype', *Aging Cell* 7(2): 237-49.

Tao, Y., Wang, J., Tokusumi, T., Gajewski, K. and Schulz, R. A. (2007) 'Requirement of the LIM homeodomain transcription factor tailup for normal heart and hematopoietic organ formation in Drosophila melanogaster', *Molecular and Cellular Biology* 27(11): 3962-3969.

Towbin, J. A., Hejtmancik, J. F., Brink, P., Gelb, B., Zhu, X. M., Chamberlain, J. S., McCabe, E. R. and Swift, M. (1993) 'X-linked dilated cardiomyopathy. Molecular genetic evidence of linkage to the Duchenne muscular dystrophy (dystrophin) gene at the Xp21 locus', *Circulation* 87(6): 1854-65.

Tweedie, S., Ashburner, M., Falls, K., Leyland, P., McQuilton, P., Marygold, S., Millburn, G., Osumi-Sutherland, D., Schroeder, A., Seal, R. et al. (2009) 'FlyBase: enhancing Drosophila Gene Ontology annotations.', *Nucleic acids research* 37(Database issue): D555-9.

Venkatesh, T. V., Park, M., Ocorr, K. A., Nemaceck, J., Golden, K., Wemple, M. and Bodmer, R. (2000) 'Cardiac enhancer activity of the homeobox gene tinman depends on CREB consensus binding sites in Drosophila', *Time-lapse imaging of neural development: Zebrafish lead the way into the fourth dimension* 26(1): 55-66.

Venken, K. J. T., Popodi, E., Holtzman, S. L., Schulze, K. L., Park, S., Carlson, J. W., Hoskins, R. A., Bellen, H. J. and Kaufman, T. C. (2010) 'A molecularly defined duplication set for the X chromosome of Drosophila melanogaster.', *Genetics* 186(4): 1111-1125.

Vogler, G. and Ocorr, K. A. (2009) 'Visualizing the beating heart in Drosophila.', *Journal of Visualized Experiments*(31).

Wehling-Henricks, M., Jordan, M. C., Roos, K. P., Deng, B. and Tidball, J. G. (2005) 'Cardiomyopathy in dystrophin-deficient hearts is prevented by expression of a neuronal nitric oxide synthase transgene in the myocardium', *Human molecular genetics* 14(14): 1921-33.

Wolf, M. J., Amrein, H., Izatt, J. A., Choma, M. A., Reedy, M. C. and Rockman, H. A. (2006) 'Drosophila as a model for the identification of genes causing adult human heart disease', *Proceedings of the National Academy of Sciences of the United States of America* 103(5): 1394-1399.

Yin, Z., Xu, X. L. and Frasch, M. (1997) 'Regulation of the twist target gene tinman by modular cis-regulatory elements during early mesoderm development', *Development (Cambridge, England)* 124(24): 4971-4982.

Yu, J., Pacifico, S., Liu, G. and Finley, R. L. (2008) 'DroID: the Drosophila Interactions Database, a comprehensive resource for annotated gene and protein interactions.', *BMC Genomics* 9: 461.

Zaffran, S., Reim, I., Qian, L., Lo, P. C., Bodmer, R. and Frasch, M. (2006) 'Cardioblast-intrinsic Tinman activity controls proper diversification and differentiation of myocardial cells in Drosophila.', *Development (Cambridge, England)* 133(20): 4073-4083.

Part 3

Individual Heart Defects

7

Congenitally Corrected Transposition of the Great Arteries

English C. Flack and Thomas P. Graham
Vanderbilt University
USA

1. Introduction

Congenitally corrected transposition of the great arteries (ccTGA) is a rare defect combining atrioventricular discordance with ventriculoarterial discordance. The atria are connected to the opposite ventricle (left atrium to right ventricle via a tricuspid valve) and the ventricles are connected to the incorrect great artery (right ventricle to aorta). Thus oxygenated blood is circulated systemically by the morphologic right ventricle (RV) and deoxygenated blood returns to the right atrium to be pumped out the left ventricle (LV) to the lungs (Figure 1). The defect is therefore "corrected" because of the physiologic flow of blood through the body. For the purposes of this review, univentricular hearts, those with common atrioventricular (AV) valves and those with aortic atresia will not be discussed.

2. Anatomy

The most common anatomy of ccTGA is that of {S,L,L}, representing atrial and visceral situs solitus (right-sided inferior and superior vena cavae returning deoxygenated blood to a right sided atrium), L-looped ventricles (the morphologic LV with mitral valve positioned on the right), and L-transposed great arteries (aorta arising off the left-sided morphologic RV and therefore situated anterior and leftward of the pulmonary artery). The RV serves as the systemic ventricle and, in the absence of other defects, oxygen saturation is normal. The most common positions of the heart in the chest are levocardia (apex to the left) or mesocardia (midline). Patients with levo- or mesocardia and visceral situs inversus have a high likelihood of ccTGA and therefore must carefully by assessed for atrial, ventricular, and arterial concordance. Dextrocardia, in which the apex of the heart is to the right, occurs in approximately 20% of patients (Graham & Markham, 2010). In cases of dextrocardia with mirror-image anatomy the anatomic designation is {I,D,D}.

2.1 Associated defects

The most common associated defects in ccTGA are ventricular septal defects (VSDs), which occur in 60-80% of cases, pulmonary stenosis (PS) in 30-50%, and tricuspid valve (TV) anomalies in 14-56%. The VSDs are usually large, perimembranous, and subpulmonary in location. Muscular inlet defects as well as multiple VSDs may also be seen. Pulmonary stenosis, more appropriately referred to as left ventricular outflow tract obstruction

(LVOTO), may be caused by fibromuscular tissue, valvar stenosis, or aneurysmal tissue of the membranous ventricular septum. The associated combination of LVOTO and VSD represents the largest group of ccTGA patients. TV anomalies occur along a spectrum of which an Ebstein-like anomaly is often the most clinically severe. Furthermore, as the TV is subjected to systemic pressures, even normally formed valves display progressive regurgitation with age. Less common defects occurring in association with ccTGA include atrial septal defect, patent ductus arteriosus, pulmonary atresia, double-outlet RV, aortic regurgitation, mitral valve abnormalities, and subaortic stenosis (Graham & Markham, 2010; Hornung & Calder, 2010; Van Praagh et al., 1998).

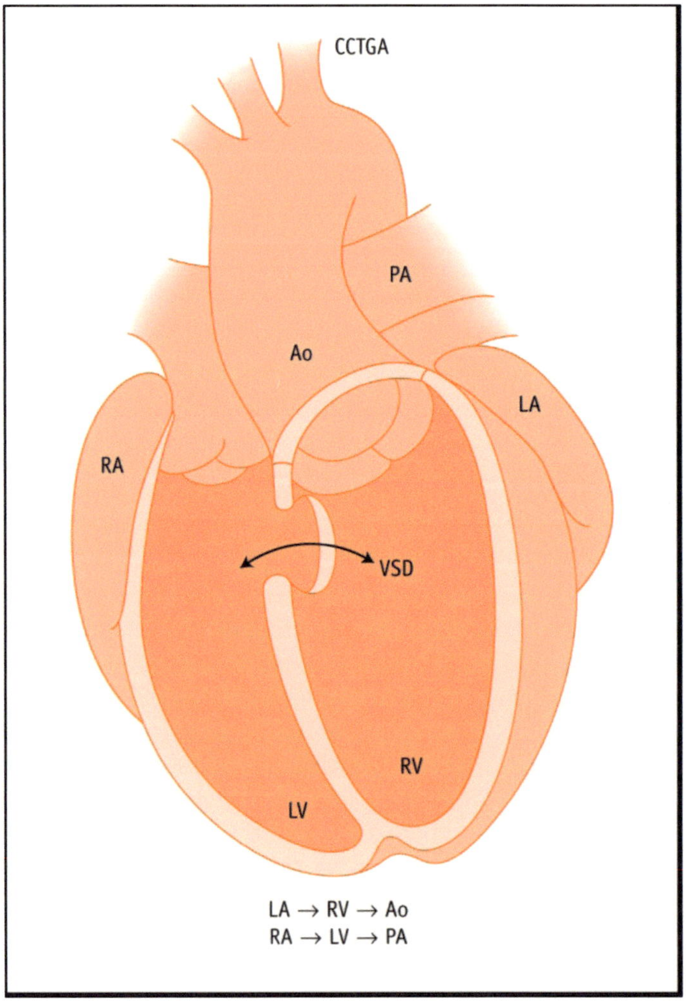

Fig. 1. Congenitally corrected transposition of the great arteries (ccTGA) with ventricular septal defect (VSD). (With permission from Springer Science + Business Media: *Current Treatment Options in Cardiovascular Medicine*, Congenitally Corrected Transposition of the Great Arteries: An Update, Vol. 9, 2007, pp. 405-413, Graham, T.P., Markham, L., Parra, D.P., & Bichell, D., Figure 1).

2.2 Coronary arteries and cardiac veins

The coronary arteries are inverted in ccTGA, as described by Ismat et al. (2002). The most common coronary positions in {S,L,L} hearts are a right coronary artery off of the left posterior aortic cusp and a left common coronary artery off the right anterior cusp. Just as the morphologic LV is situated on the right side of the heart, the morphologic left coronary artery arises off the right aortic sinus. It is this right-sided coronary that bifurcates into the anterior descending artery, which lies in the interventricular groove, and the circumflex branch that runs posterior to the heart through its course in the right AV sulcus. Additional rare anomalies have been described in which both main coronaries arise from a single ostia or one main coronary gives rise to the other (i.e., anterior descending off the right coronary artery) (Hornung & Calder, 2010; Ismat et al., 2002). The cardiac veins seem to correspond to ventricular and coronary anatomy as described in a pathological series by Bottega et al (2009). Although the coronary sinus emptied as normal into the right atrium, dilated Thebesian veins and large collaterals were commonly noted on ccTGA specimens. Venous collateralization was noted between the two ventricles, allowing the morphologic LV to drain via Thebesian veins or collaterals to the coronary sinus. These venous anomalies are thought to be of benefit in providing access to both ventricles in some percutaneous procedures (Bottega et al, 2009).

2.3 Conduction system

The conduction system often consists of dual AV nodes and inversion of AV bundles. An increasing incidence of AV block, at a rate of approximately 2% per year, occurs even in the absence of surgical repair and is more likely in the presence of an intact ventricular septum (Daliento et al., 1986; Huhta et al., 1983). Anderson et al. (1974) consistently demonstrated the finding of an anterior and right-sided AV node that was situated anterolateral to the mitral-pulmonary valve junction. This node connects to the morphologic (right-sided) LV by a descending bundle of conducting tissue that travels anterior and lateral to the pulmonary outflow tract. The bundle branches are inverted, each typical of the morphologic ventricle they serve. In the presence of a subpulmonary VSD the descending AV bundle is located on the anterosuperior and anteroinferior borders of the defect. This is in contrast to concordant hearts {S,D,S} in which the conduction bundle travels along the posteroinferior margin of the VSD. Many ccTGA patients also have a posteriorly-situated AV node, which is often hypoplastic, in addition to a functional anterior node. Depending on the alignment of the interatrial and interventricular septae this posterior node may or may not have connections to the ventricles. Patients with appropriate alignment of the atrial and ventricular septae may be more likely to have two AV nodes with corresponding conduction bundles present. Invading fibrosis of the proximal AV node bundle as well as distal conduction bundles has been described on pathological specimens from older patients with correlating electrocardiogram (ECG) findings of complete heart block, suggesting fibrotic invasion is involved in the development of AV block (Anderson et al., 1974; Daliento et al., 1986).

3. Incidence and genetics

The incidence of ccTGA in patients with congenital heart disease (CHD) is approximately 0.5% with a slight male predominance (Graham & Markham, 2010; Piacentini et al., 2005). Although a specific genetic defect is yet to be defined for ccTGA, the recurrence risk of d-

TGA for siblings of ccTGA patients is 2.6% with an overall recurrence risk of 5.2% for ccTGA siblings to have some type of congenital heart defect (Piacentini et al., 2005). A recurrence risk of >5% is higher than expected, as the risk is typically thought to be 1-3% for unaffected parents to have an additional child with congenital heart disease (Van der Bom et al., 2011).

4. Natural history and outcome

The natural history of ccTGA depends largely on the presence of associated defects. Patients under 5 years old who also have VSD, LVOTO, and/or TV abnormalities represent the highest frequency of non-surgical deaths. However patients with isolated ccTGA (no associated lesions) may survive into their 4th and 5th decades (Hoffman, 2009; Presbitero et al., 1995). Many patients will demonstrate one or more complications including heart block, tricuspid regurgitation (TR), and congestive heart failure (CHF). Approximately 2-4% of ccTGA patients have ventricular pre-excitation (Wolff-Parkinson-White syndrome) and should undergo radiofrequency ablation of accessory pathways in cases of symptomatic reentrant tachycardia. Atrial tachycardia such as atrial fibrillation and flutter often occur with increasing age, atrial enlargement, and after surgical repair where suture lines and scars may support focal reentrant circuits. By 45 years of age 67% of ccTGA patients with associated defects will have developed CHF, as shown in Figure 2, whereas only 25% of ccTGA patients without associated lesions will have progressed to CHF by this age (Graham et al., 2000). Prieto et al suggests that outcome is dependent on morphology of the TV (the systemic AV valve), as this was the only predictor of severe regurgitation and RV dysfunction in a cohort of ccTGA patients described after mean follow-up of 20 years.

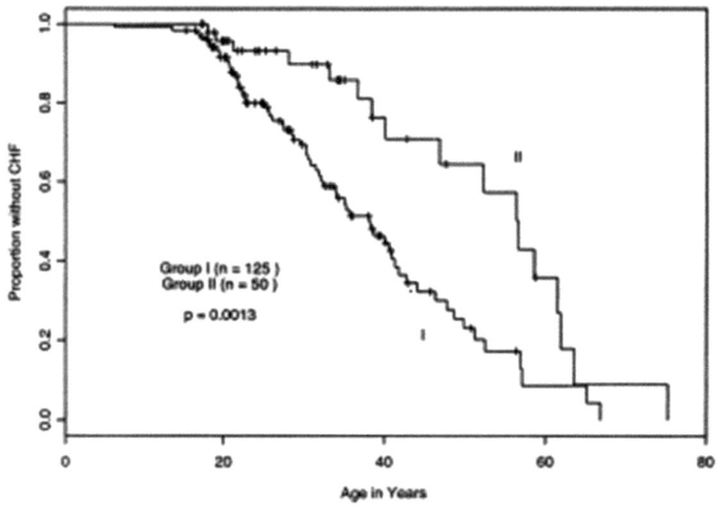

Fig. 2. Freedom from CHF in group I (associated lesions, n=125) and group II (no significant associated lesions, n=50) as a function of increasing age. (Reprinted from *Journal of the American College of Cardiology*, Vol. 36, No. 1, Long-term outcome in congenitally corrected transposition of the great arteries: A multi-institutional study, pp. 255-261, Copyright 2000 with permission from Elsevier).

The authors concluded that severe TV insufficiency leading to RV dysfunction has the greatest impact on long-term survival in both operated and unoperated patients. In patients who underwent surgical intervention for ccTGA, 20-year survival rate was 90% for patients with competent TVs, whereas survival was only 35% for patients with severe TV insufficiency. Furthermore, patients who were diagnosed with severe TV insufficiency demonstrated a rapid deterioration in clinical status with RV failure occurring on average 5 years after onset of insufficiency (Prieto et al., 1998). Overall natural history in the ccTGA patient without associated defects is promising, as patients may remain relatively asymptomatic through early and mid-adulthood. However the frequent development of complications in the 4th and 5th decades often culminates in the progressive development of RV (systemic) dysfunction and heart failure, requiring aggressive medical management and possible surgical intervention (Presbitero et al., 1995).

5. Diagnosis

Just as the natural history is largely dependent on defects associated with ccTGA, so is timing of presentation and diagnoses.

5.1 Prenatal diagnosis

Fetal diagnosis of many forms of CHD continues to improve. However the fetus with ccTGA and mild or no additional intracardiac anomalies may be overlooked by routine ultrasound screening. Distinct features notable on prenatal ultrasound that may improve detection of ccTGA are parallel course of the great arteries in combination with dextrocardia, abnormal insertion of the papillary muscles, and/or an abnormal TV (McEwing & Chaoui, 2004; Paladini et al., 2006; Shima et al., 2009). A retrospective review by Wan et al. found no difference in the number of cardiac interventions, timing of surgery, or survival between a cohort of ccTGA patients diagnosed prenatally (n = 14) and postnatally (n = 26). However, because 70% of this cohort required cardiac intervention prior to 3 years of age, the authors suggest prenatal diagnosis is important for preparation and counseling of the family (2009). A recent review of 11 cases of fetal ccTGA diagnoses describes the use of four-dimensional echocardiography and spatiotemporal image correlation (STIC), in which the relationship of the great arteries can be assessed in several different orthogonal planes by placement of a reference dot on images reconstructed from acquired volume data sets (Zhang et al., 2011).

5.2 Early presentation and diagnosis

Diagnoses of infants and children may occur after murmur evaluation, as VSDs are commonly associated lesions. In cases of large VSDs or severe TV regurgitation, some infants may present in CHF with diaphoresis, pallor, tachypnea, inability to gain weight, hepatomegaly, and a gallop on exam. Auscultation of the ccTGA patient may also reveal a loud, single second heart sound (S2) at the left 2nd intercostal space, with absence of S2 over the right 2nd intercostal space (Friedberg & Nadas, 1970). The presence of VSD combined with LVOTO may lead to a cyanotic presentation from decreased pulmonary blood flow. However, some degree of LVOTO may be protective of the lung bed in patients with large VSDs, and may delay a CHF presentation despite the normal decrease in pulmonary vascular resistance.

5.3 Late presentation and diagnosis

Interestingly, if there are no additional associated defects ccTGA may go unnoticed until adolescence or adulthood. Case reports have even cited incidental findings and late diagnoses of ccTGA in adults in the fifth to eighth decades of life (Chang et al., 2009; Jennings et al., 1984; Orchard et al., 2010; Scardi et al., 1999). A cohort of patients with ccTGA over 18 years of age who presented to an adult CHD clinic over a 15 year period is described by Beauchesne et al (2002). Sixty-six percent of these patients were over 18 years of age when diagnosed, and 17% of the cohort was over 60 years old at the time of diagnosis. Common reasons for referral in such patients range from abnormal ECGs and cardiomegaly on chest radiographs to complete heart block and murmurs (Presberito et al., 1995).

6. Evaluation

6.1 Chest radiograph

The CXR in ccTGA patients with mesocardia or levocardia typically demonstrates a straightened upper-left cardiac border from the leftward-positioned ascending aorta. Dextrocardia usually occurs with normal situs and, as stated previously, occurs in 20% of ccTGA patients (Figure 3). The presence of abdominal situs solitus and dextrocardia should raise suspicion of ccTGA. In the patient without any associated defects, an atypical cardiac position in an otherwise normal CXR may be the only indication of ccTGA.

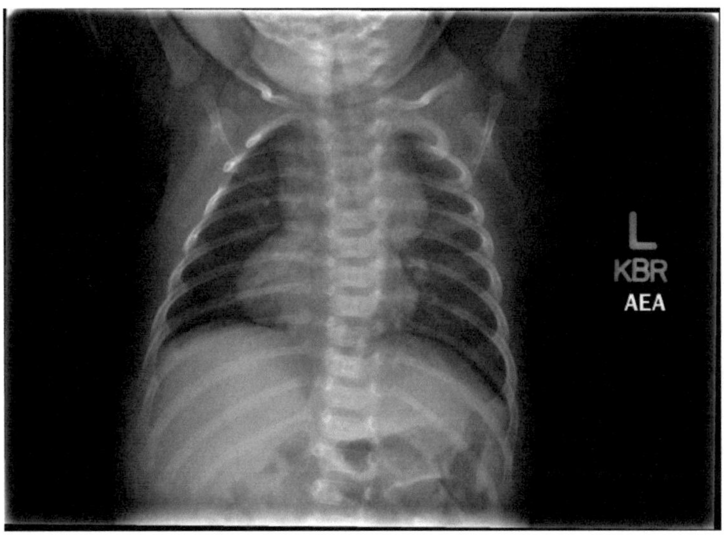

Fig. 3. CXR of infant with dextrocardia, abdominal situs solitus, and ccTGA. Note the position of the cardiac apex pointed to the right. The left heart border demonstrates the prominent left-sided ascending aorta. The thymic shadow is seen over the right mediastinum.

However marked cardiomegaly, left atrial enlargement, and an increase in pulmonary vasculature may be present in patients with a large VSD and significant left to right shunt. A CXR with impressive cardiomegaly and left atrial enlargement may also be indicative of an Ebstein-like malformation of the TV. The presence of pulmonary stenosis or atresia will demonstrate darkened lung fields from attenuated pulmonary blood flow. Overall, the degree of cardiomegaly and amount of visible pulmonary vascularity is dependent on the presence and direction of shunting, as well as the severity of LVOTO (Carey & Ruttenberg, 1964).

6.2 Electrocardiogram

The ECG in patients with ccTGA is most significant for a superior QRS axis and atypical septal activation. As discussed previously, the conduction system in ccTGA consists of inverted AV bundles. Therefore the septum is activated from right to left, demonstrating presence of septal Q waves in the right precordial leads (QR pattern in leads V4R and V1) and absence of Q waves in the left precordial leads (rS pattern in lead V6). In fact, undiagnosed ccTGA patients with such a pattern on ECG have been diagnosed with remote inferior infarcts (Jennings et al., 1984; Warnes, 2006). Preexcitation may be observed in those patients with ccTGA and Wolff-Parkinson-White. Finally, varying degrees of AV block may be present, as well as patterns of right or left-sided chamber enlargement.

6.3 Echocardiography

Transthoracic echocardiography (TTE) as an imaging modality is relatively inexpensive, widely available, and noninvasive. As with many types of CHD, TTE is the first line and most useful modality in the diagnosis of ccTGA. The anatomical designation (most commonly {S,L,L} as discussed previously), is first assigned by demonstrating atrial position, ventricular looping, and arterial looping. Morphology of the RV is seen on TTE by the presence of coarse trabeculations and a moderator band, whereas the LV has a smooth-walled endocardium and a funnel-shaped appearance. The level of the TV is inferior to the MV, which may also give a clue to ventricular inversion. In evaluation of the outflow tracts, the aorta in ccTGA is usually anterior and to the left of the PA. Once the diagnosis of ccTGA is made through demonstration of discordance between atria and ventricles as well as ventricles and great arteries, several anatomic objectives should be defined in the TTE evaluation. Semilunar and AV valve morphology as well as presence and severity of regurgitation warrant full description. Coronary origins should be identified and their proximal courses described. The degree of LVOTO is important as well as any additional defects present, as these will impact whether and what type of surgical repair is necessary (Oechslin, 2009). Transesophageal echocardiography (TEE) has been shown to have greater accuracy over TTE in correctly defining atrial situs and chordal AV valve attachments in adult patients with ccTGA (Caso et al., 1998). TEE is also more useful for investigation of intracardiac vegetations in cases of suspected endocarditis and in evaluation of thrombus in the atrial appendages, which may be applicable to the ccTGA patient with sustained atrial arrhythmias.

6.4 Cardiac catheterization

Rather than a modality for diagnosis, cardiac catheterization (Figure 4) is typically reserved for the post-surgical patient who would benefit from an intervention such as LV to pulmonary artery (PA) conduit dilation or stent placement. For patients undergoing surgical palliation for single-ventricle ccTGA anatomy, catheterization is performed to assess pressure, function, and valve regurgitation prior to surgery. Most interesting, however, is the adult patient who presents with ischemic heart disease and is discovered on cardiac catheterization to have ccTGA after abnormal catheter passes or inversion of coronary arteries on angiography (Jennings et al., 1984).

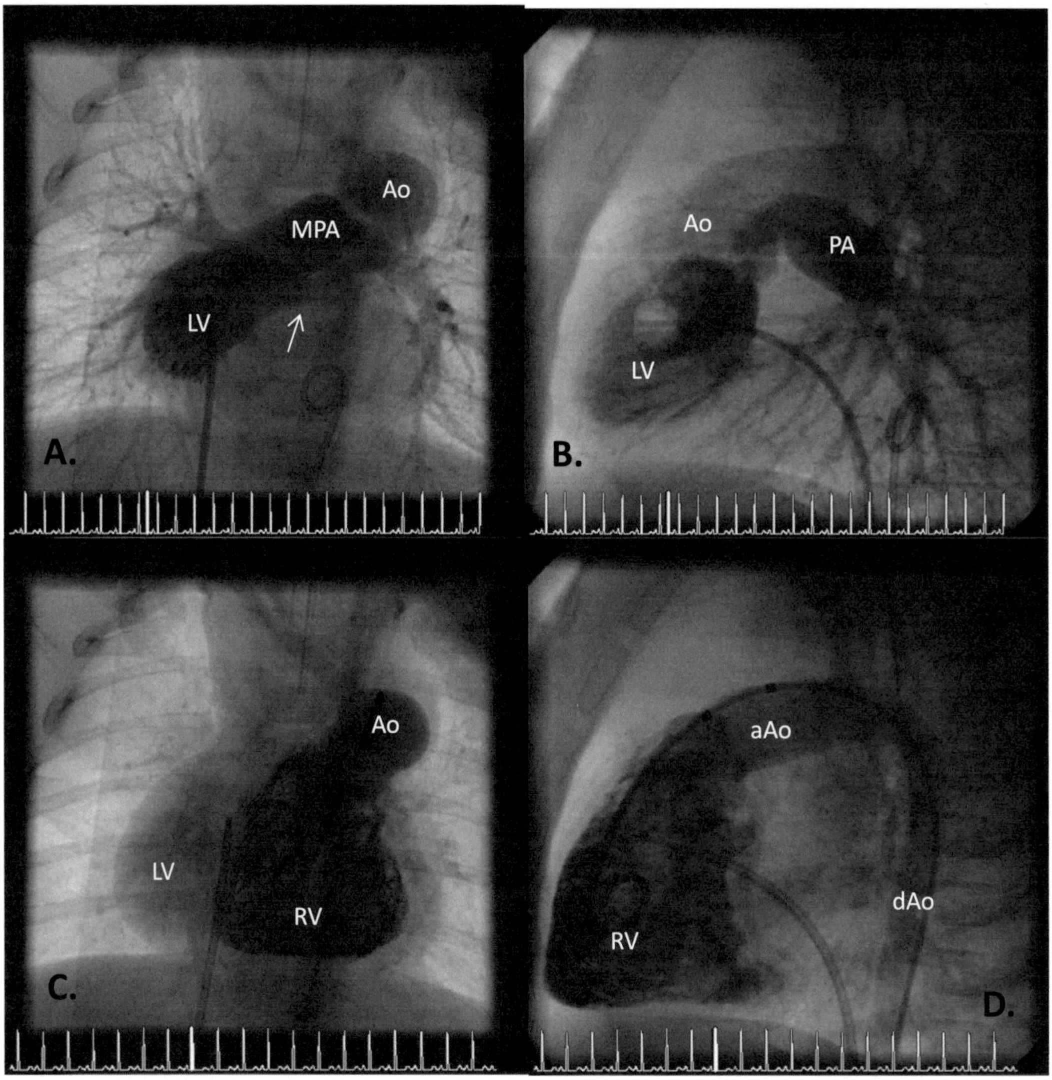

Fig. 4. Cardiac catheterization of ccTGA infant with dextrocardia, pulmonary stenosis, and VSD (same infant as in Fig. 3). (A.) Anterior-posterior projection. A catheter is positioned in the right-sided morphologic left ventricle (LV). Contrast fill the LV, pulmonary trunk, and pulmonary arteries. Contrast flows right to left across the VSD (arrow) and fills the aorta. (B.) Lateral projection. Contrast from the LV flows through the LV outflow tract, across the pulmonary valve, and fills the pulmonary arteries. The aorta fills by right to left shunting through the VSD. Note the aorta is anterior to the pulmonary artery. (C.) Anterior-posterior projection. A catheter is positioned retrograde into the left-sided morphologic right ventricle (RV). Contrast fills the trabeculated RV and the leftward aorta. (D.) Lateral projection. Contrast fills the large RV, ascending, and descending aorta. LV, left ventricle; RV right ventricle; Ao, Aorta; aAo, ascending aorta; dAo, descending aorta; MPA, Main pulmonary artery; PA, Pulmonary artery.

6.5 Cardiac Magnetic Resonance Imaging (cMRI)

Cardiac MRI is now used in many types of CHD to further define anatomy and to quantify ventricular function and volume (Figure 5). For initial diagnosis, cMRI may be helpful in patients with restricted TTE windows, to define visceroatrial situs, and to delineate complex associated defects. In patients with interruption of the inferior vena cavae, systemic return from the lower body can be difficult to delineate by echocardiography, but is well defined by cMRI. Because echocardiographic evaluation of RV function in ccTGA patients is limited by geometric assumptions, cMRI has become the gold standard for RV function and volume assessment. TV morphology as well as degree of regurgitation can also be determined through cMRI. Prior to performing anatomic surgical repair in a ccTGA patient beyond infancy, cMRI may be useful in evaluation of LV mass, volume, and ejection fraction. Furthermore, if there are concerns about degree of LV dysfunction, perfusion studies with delayed enhancement MRI may be performed to directly investigate scarring of the LV myocardium prior to committing this ventricle to systemic workload. Cardiac MRI may therefore be a useful modality for evaluation of ccTGA patients not only as an adjunct to TTE for initial diagnosis, but also for assessment prior to surgical repair and serial follow-up of the systemic RV. If the presence of MRI-incompatible pacemaker or prosthetic valve precludes assessment by MRI, computed tomography (CT) scans can depict anatomy but cannot yield functional data as does MRI (Schmidt et al., 2000; Teo & Hia, 2011).

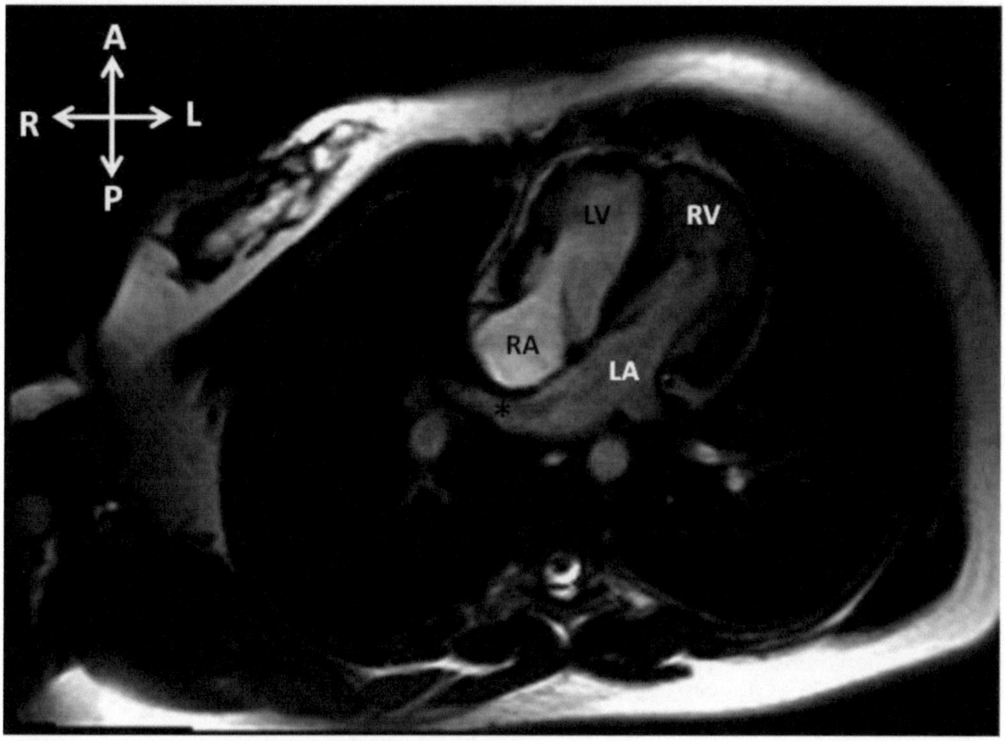

Fig. 5. Oblique cut T2-weighted MRI image of 4-chamber cardiac view of ccTGA patient with levocardia. The RA empties into a right-sided, smooth-walled, morphologic LV. A star (*) labels the entrance of a right pulmonary vein into the left atrium, which empties into a trabeculated, left-sided, morphologic RV. RA, right atrium; LV, left ventricle; LA, left atrium; RV, right ventricle.

6.6 Exercise and stress testing

Cardiopulmonary exercise testing by treadmill is an important adjunct for ccTGA patient evaluation and management. In those patients able to perform treadmill tests, exercise capacity is determined through minute ventilation, carbon dioxide production, and oxygen consumption. Impaired exercise capacity in ccTGA patients has been shown to correlate with diastolic dysfunction in the form of increased RV filling pressures as measured by tissue Doppler imaging (Tay et al., 2011). Cardiopulmonary exercise testing in combination with gadolinium-enhanced MRI has been utilized to demonstrate RV myocardial fibrosis hypothesized to be responsible for RV dysfunction (Giardini et al., 2006). Systemic RV function can also be evaluated by dobutamine stress testing, in which MRI is performed at baseline and with dobutamine infusion. Objectively defining the capacity of the systemic RV to respond to stress may guide treatment on both initial and follow-up evaluations (Dodge-Khatami et al., 2002; Fratz et al., 2008). Sequential testing, performed either by exercise testing or by dobutamine stress test, is useful to assess overall cardiopulmonary function and response to medical or surgical therapy.

7. Management

7.1 Medical management

CHF medical management for the ccTGA patient with systemic RV has been extrapolated from CHF therapy for LV failure. This primarily includes β-adrenergic receptor blockade (β-blockers), diuretics and afterload-reducing agents with an angiotensin-converting enzyme (ACE) inhibitor (Winter et al., 2009). Digoxin may also be useful for its inotropic and antiarrhythmic effects. Angiotensin receptor blockade with losartan was evaluated in a multicenter, randomized, placebo-controlled clinical trial by Dore and colleagues (2005) but found to have no improvement on exercise capacity and no reduction in neurohormonal levels in patients with systemic right ventricles. Overall, evidence-based therapy for optimal CHF treatment in patients with systemic RV is lacking. Beyond medication, cardiac resynchronization has emerged as a therapy for patients with impaired systemic RV function and widened QRS morphology on ECG. Increased QRS duration as a result of bundle branch block or conventional pacemaker is typically greater than 120-140 ms with some patients having QRS duration >200 ms. Such electromechanical dyssynchrony creates inefficiency in ventricular ejection, whereas restoring synchrony has been shown to decrease QRS duration with improvement in RV filling time, ejection fraction, and overall CHF symptoms (Diller et al., 2006; Janousek et al., 2004; Kordybach et al., 2009). Takemoto et al. (2010) reports the use of transvenous permanent para-Hisian pacing in an 8 year old with ccTGA. Restoration of cardiac synchrony decreased the QRS duration from 198 ms to 94 ms, decreased interventricular conduction delay from 137 ms to 37 ms, and improved the patient's CHF symptoms from NYHA (New York Heart Association) class III to NYHA class II over a period of 6 months. Limitations in cardiac resynchronization therapy include difficulty in percutaneous lead delivery, although this has successfully been accomplished even in ccTGA cases of dextrocardia (Malecka et al., 2010).

7.2 Surgical management

Indications for surgical management in ccTGA patients of all ages continue to evolve and most often are determined on a case-by-case basis. Beauchanese et al. (2002) described a cohort of 44 unrepaired adult ccTGA patients. Of these, the 30 patients who required surgical intervention had significantly larger pre-operative cardiothoracic ratios on chest radiographs, and had moderate to severe or severe systemic AV valve regurgitation. The ejection fraction of the systemic ventricle between the operated and unoperated groups was not statistically significant (Beauchesne et al., 2002). As discussed previously and depicted in Figure 2, nearly 2/3 of unrepaired ccTGA patients with associated defects will have developed CHF by the age of 45 years. Even asymptomatic adults with ccTGA have been shown by echocardiography to have RV dysfunction through the use of tissue Doppler quantification techniques (Bos et al. 2006). Thus the natural evolution of ccTGA for the majority of patients is eventual RV dysfunction and TV regurgitation. It is postulated that progression to failure in a systemic RV is unavoidable because the RV and TV are not anatomically suited to withstand the systemic pressure for which the LV and MV are intended. One mechanism thought to contribute to progressive RV decompensation is worsening TR from annular dilation and/or displacement of the septal leaflet of the TV as the RV remodels to accommodate systemic afterload.

ccTGA {S,L,L} Surgical Repair and Palliation			
Classic / Physiologic Repair		**Anatomic Repair**	
Associated Defect	Repair	Associated Defect	Double Switch Repair
VSD	VSD closure	VSD + normal PV	•VSD closure •Atrial switch (Senning / Mustard) •Arterial switch
VSD + PS	VSD closure + PS relief	PS / Atresia + VSD	•VSD closure + RV-PA conduit •Atrial switch + Arterial switch
VSD + PS/Atresia	Biventricular Repair: •VSD closure + LV-PA conduit	PS / Atresia + routable VSD	•RV-PA conduit • Atrial switch + Rastelli
	Univentricular Repair: • Systemic to PA shunt • Bidirectional Glenn • Fontan	Severe RV dysfunction Small RV Abnormal atrial anatomy	•Hemi-Mustard with bidirectional Glenn (modified atrial switch) •Arterial switch or Rastelli procedure
TR	Tricuspid valve repair or replacement	TR	PA banding to decrease TR or tricuspid valve repair / replacement

Table 1. ccTGA {S,L,L} Surgical Repair and Palliation. VSD, ventricular septal defect; PS, pulmonary stenosis; PA, pulmonary artery; PV, pulmonary valve; RV, right ventricle; TR, tricuspid regurgitation; BDG, Bidirectional Glenn

Depending on the age of presentation and extent of associated lesions, surgical repair may include one or more of several approaches (Table 1). In patients with a VSD and no LVOTO, "classic" or "physiologic" repair may include VSD closure only. Specific techniques must be employed in ccTGA patients to avoid damage to the conduction system during VSD closure. Because the AV conduction bundle descends along the anterior rim of the VSD and travels along the septal side of the right-sided morphologic LV, it is recommended to suture the VSD patch along the morphological right ventricular aspect of the septum. The surgical approach should be via right atriotomy and right-sided mitral valve. Ideally the VSD patch will lie partially on the morphologic LV septal aspect (to avoid damage to the TV superiorly) and partially on the morphologic RV aspect of the septum inferiorly (to avoid damage to the main conduction bundle) (Jonas, 2004). Physiologic repair may also include relief of pulmonary stenosis (PS) and/or LV to PA conduit placement. There is, however, the possibility that decreasing LV pressure by VSD closure and/or PS relief may allow the ventricular septum to realign towards the LV, resulting in displacement of the TV septal leaflet and increasing TR (Kral Kollars et al. 2010; Said et al. 2011). In a cohort of 123 patients with ccTGA presenting for classic biventricular repair over 33 years, the surgical group undergoing repair of VSD + PS demonstrated the greatest survival whereas patients requiring TV replacement at their initial operation exhibited the shortest survival. Risk factors for death in the VSD +/- PS relief groups included pre-operative RV end diastolic pressure greater than 17mmHg and complete heart block. Survival rates at 1-, 5-, 10-, and 15-years for patients who underwent classic repair were 84%, 75%, 68%, and 61%, respectively, although 17 of the 113 patients in this subgroup underwent Fontan and achieved 100% survival in short-term follow-up (Figure 6). The univentricular pathway with Fontan was assigned to ccTGA patients for which biventricular repair was contraindicated, as in patients with straddling AV valve tissue, inaccessible or multiple VSDs, or unbalanced complete AV canals (Hraska et al. 2005). More recently Bogers et al. (2010) confirmed that classic repair in which the RV remains the systemic ventricle results in significant incidence of reoperation and overall suboptimal survival.

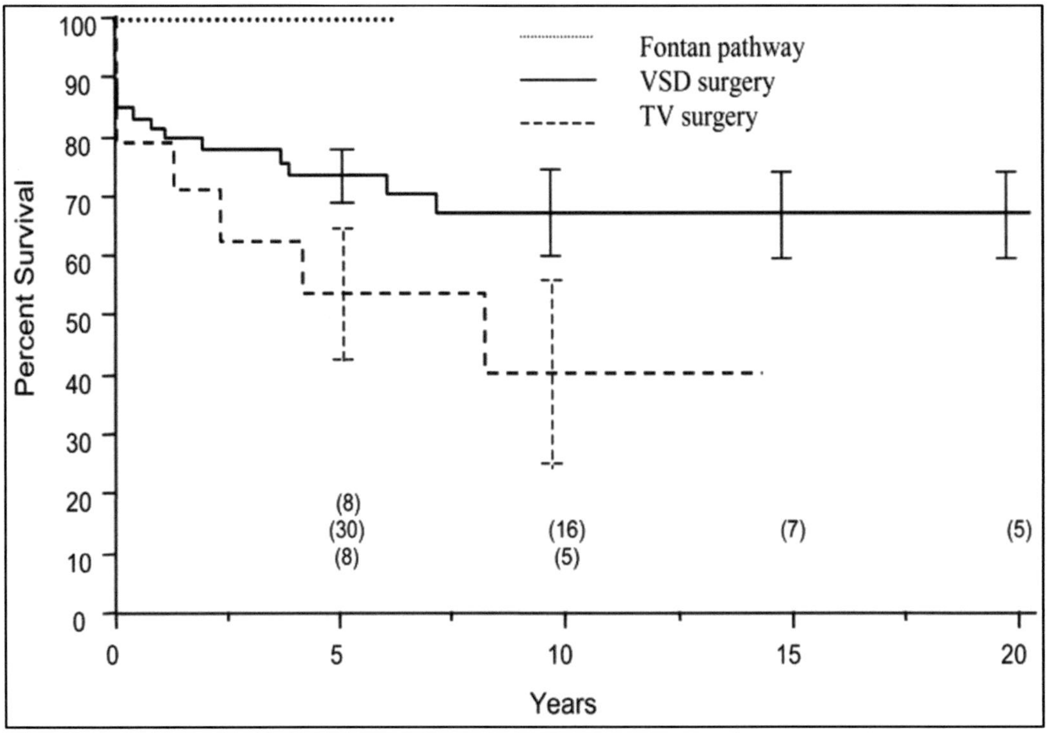

Fig. 6. Operative survival in ccTGA patients undergoing Fontan pathway (*dotted line*; n = 17), VSD surgery (*solid line*; n = 76), and TV surgery (*dashed line*; n = 14). Numbers of patients at risk are in parentheses. Error bars indicate 70% confidence limits. VSD, ventricular septal defect; TV, tricuspid valve. (Reprinted from *The Journal of Thoracic and Cardiovascular Surgery*, Vol. 129, No. 1, Long-term outcome of surgically treated patients with corrected transposition of the great arteries, pp. 182-191, Copyright 2005 with permission from Elsevier).

The "anatomic" or "Double Switch" (DS) operation was developed in response to unsatisfactory outcomes after the classic repair. Components of the DS (Figure 7A) include arterial switch with coronary artery transfer, VSD closure if necessary, and interatrial baffle by Senning or Mustard procedure. The Senning and Mustard operations, referred to as an "atrial switch," serve to direct systemic venous flow to the TV and RV and pulmonary venous flow to the mitral valve and LV. The purpose of the DS is to improve long term outcome by restoring the LV and MV to the systemic circulation. Requirements for this repair before committing the LV to the systemic workload include pre-operative LV pressure that is 80-100% systemic and normal LV wall thickness and function for a systemic LV (Duncan & Mee, 2005; Poirier et al., 2004). In the absence of LVOTO, pulmonary hypertension, or an unrestrictive VSD, the morphologic LV requires training prior to committing it to the systemic ventricle in the DS. LV training has been performed by placement of a pulmonary artery band (PAB) which is then serially tightened to introduce a greater pressure load nearing that of systemic pressure to the naïve LV. Median banding time for the purpose of LV retraining has been reported on average to be 13-14 months (Ly et al., 2009; Poirier et al., 2004; Winlaw et al., 2005). Morphologic LV reconditioning with PAB in patients with systemic RV after atrial switch for dextrotransposition of the great arteries (dTGA) has been described by Poirier et al (2004). PAB was performed in this population prior to anatomic correction or as bridge to transplant, and the success rate of completing adequate LV retraining was significantly less in patients beyond 12 years of age (20% of patients over 12 years completed the protocol, whereas 62% of patients less than 12 years were able to complete the PAB protocol, $p = 0.02$). Although a well defined standard for age of PAB placement in this setting is yet to be realized, it is apparent that candidacy for LV training with PAB beyond adolescence is questionable. Also concerning is report of late LV dysfunction in ccTGA patients who underwent DS operation after successful LV retraining by PAB placement (Quinn et al., 2008).

Rather than performing pulmonary artery banding in symptomatic ccTGA patients with intention of anatomic repair, Metton and associates (2010) advocate the use of PAB in asymptomatic ccTGA neonates and infants with intact ventricular septum to maintain rather than train the LV. In Metton's group the TV was not repaired at PAB placement, as it was thought that PAB placement may improve TR that was present prior to banding (Ly et al., 2009). This mechanism is described by Kral Kollars et al. (2010) in 14 patients who underwent PAB for LV retraining (median age 1.1 years, range 0 to 12 years). Eleven of the 14 patients had an increase in LV pressure of ≥2/3 systolic RV pressure with PAB and demonstrated significantly decreased TR as the LV geometry became more spherical and the interventricular septum shifted toward the morphologic RV. Patients who underwent classic ccTGA repair with procedures that reduced LV pressure below that of the RV, such as VSD closure with LV to PA conduit placement, demonstrated significantly increased TR postoperatively.

Although it is reasonable to medically manage mild TR with anticongestive therapy and afterload reduction, surgical intervention is indicated in cases of moderate or moderate to severe TR. TV repair for ccTGA patients is rarely successful, and most patients require valve replacement, which can be problematic in young children because of the relatively large prosthesis needed to allow for growth. Palliation with PAB may therefore be reasonable in infants and young children, since it has been shown that severe TV insufficiency leading to RV dysfunction has the greatest impact on long-term survival (Kral Kollars et al., 2010;

Prieto et al., 1998). Several groups have concluded that TV replacement should be considered at the earliest sign of RV dysfunction, with recommendations to consider operation before systemic ventricular ejection fraction (EF) decreases below 40 and 44% (Mongeon et al., 2011; Van Son et al., 1995).

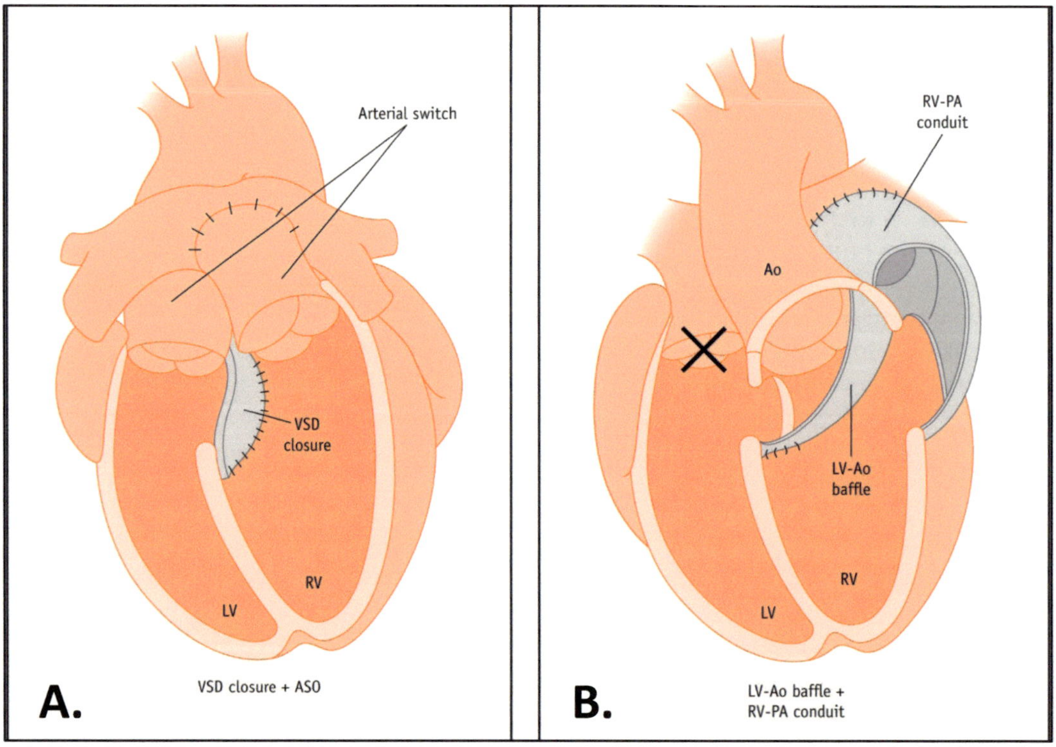

Fig. 7. The Double Switch operation for ccTGA. (A.) The double-switch anatomic surgical repair for ccTGA with VSD consists of an arterial switch, VSD closure, and atrial venous switch (not shown) by intra-atrial baffle operation (i.e., Senning or Mustard repair). (B.) The double-switch for ccTGA with left ventricle (LV) outflow tract obstruction includes an anatomical LV - aorta (Ao) baffle (i.e., Rastelli repair) and anatomical right ventricle (RV) - pulmonary artery (PA) conduit. Although not pictured, the baffle and conduit repair are also in combination with an atrial switch. (With permission from Springer Science + Business Media: *Current Treatment Options in Cardiovascular Medicine*, Congenitally Corrected Transposition of the Great Arteries: An Update, Vol. 9, 2007, pp. 405-413, Graham, T.P., Markham, L., Parra, D.P., & Bichell, D., Figure 1).

The combination of progressive systemic RV dysfunction and TR has lead to the consideration of a variation in DS operation for patients with LVOTO. Rather than combining the atrial and arterial switches, the Senning or Mustard atrial switch procedure is combined with a Rastelli operation, in which the LV outflow is channeled from the LV through a large VSD to the aorta and an RV to PA conduit is placed (Figure 7B). This operation is technically challenging and subject to the need for conduit replacements as well as possible reoperation for interatrial or interventricular baffle obstructions. Specific to the Senning / Rastelli operation, risk factors associated with death include longer cardiopulmonary bypass and aortic cross-clamp times, and there is an increased risk of complete heart block and ventricular dysfunction if the existing VSD requires enlargement (Gaies et al., 2009; Shin'oka et al., 2007). Nevertheless, intermediate results in a small group of ccTGA patients with VSD and LVOTO who underwent this form of anatomic repair suggest good biventricular function and mild or no AV valve insufficiency up to 17 years post-operatively (Hörer et al., 2007).

An additional variation in the DS for patients with severe RV dysfunction, hypoplasia of the RV, or abnormal right atrial anatomy includes a modified atrial switch termed the "hemi-Mustard/bidirectional Glenn," which is performed in combination with either an arterial switch or a Rastelli procedure. In this operation the interatrial baffle only includes the IVC return, as the SVC is reimplanted into the pulmonary artery to create a cavo-pulmonary Glenn shunt, and the SVC portion of the RA is oversewn. Midterm outcomes from the hemi-Mustard/Glenn as reported by Malhotra et al. (2011) are favorable and hold several advantages over the traditional Senning or Mustard atrial switch. The authors report a prolonged lifespan of the RV to PA conduit due to volume-unloading the RV, increased intra-atrial space for pulmonary venous return (and therefore less risk of pulmonary venous obstruction), and less risk for arrhythmia with the reduction in intra-atrial suture lines. It remains to be seen if the hemi-Mustard / bidirectional Glenn variant of the DS will prove favorable in long-term studies.

8. Outcomes: Physiologic vs. anatomic repair

Alghamdi and associates (2006) published a meta-analysis of 11 nonrandomized studies totalling 124 ccTGA patients and compared in-hospital mortality between physiologic and anatomic repair. Patient age at time of repair ranged from 3 months to 55 years with 41% of patients undergoing definitive repair prior to 1995. Thirty patients underwent physiologic repair, 69 underwent Rastelli-type anatomic repair, and 25 received anatomic repair with arterial switch. The Rastelli-type anatomic repair had significantly lower hospital mortality while era of operation before 1995 demonstrated an increased mortality risk. A large risk analysis performed by Shin'oka et al. (2007) combined ccTGA patients with a group of systemic RV patients with discordant AV connections, (n=189) and compared long-term results of definitive surgical repair with respect to hospitalization, late mortality, and reoperation. Risk factors for hospital death included preoperative moderate TR and intraoperative cardiopulmonary bypass time of over 240 minutes. The presence of TR was also a risk factor for late mortality. Reoperation risks included preoperative cardiomegaly (cardiothoracic ratio of >0.6) and presence of TR, operative need for VSD enlargement, and patient size of <10 kg. Although survival of classic repair in patients without TR was satisfactory in comparison to anatomic repair, patients with ccTGA and discordant AV connections with TR demonstrated improved survival with anatomic repair. More recently Lim and colleagues (2010) report results from a multicenter study including 167 patients who underwent biventricular ccTGA repair. Of the patients studied, 123 underwent physiologic repair (ASD or VSD closure, TV surgery, and/or pulmonary ventricle to PA conduit placement), and 44 underwent anatomic repair (atrial + arterial switch or atrial + interventricular re-routing procedure) over the years 1983 - 2009. Long-term results of biventricular repair revealed an estimated survival of 83.3% ± 0.05% at 25 years. The incidence of complete heart block was lower for the anatomic repair group, and there was a late mortality of 5.9% after physiologic repair in comparison to 0% after anatomic repair.

Freedom from systemic AV valve regurgitation and ventricular dysfunction was significantly higher after anatomic repair. The authors concluded that anatomic is superior to physiologic repair in patients with two adequately sized ventricles. However high risk groups such as those patients with RV dysfunction or the need for LV training warrant careful selection prior to undergoing anatomic repair. Taken together, these outcomes favor anatomic over classic / physiologic repair with careful preoperative assessment of TR for the purpose of risk stratification.

9. Follow-up and special considerations

Patients with ccTGA require outpatient follow-up every 1-2 years by a pediatric or adult congenital cardiologist. Symptomatology, ventricular function, and valvar insufficiency should further guide frequency of follow-up. It is recommended an ECG be performed at each visit to monitor for AV block with periodic consideration of Holter monitor. Cardiopulmonary exercise testing is performed to assess overall function as well as response to medical or surgical therapy. RV function in the unrepaired or physiologically repaired ccTGA patient must be closely monitored with serial echocardiography even in asymptomatic patients (Bos et al., 2006). Cardiac MRI with cine data used to quantify RV volume, mass, and ejection fraction is the best modality to serially quantify RV function, and should be performed every 3-5 years.

9.1 Pregnancy

Pregnancy in the ccTGA patient is generally well tolerated except in the presence of maternal NYHA class III-IV symptoms, moderate or severe AV valve regurgitation, or poor ventricular function (EF<40%). Evaluation of pregnancy outcome in 22 women with ccTGA revealed 50 live births in 60 total pregnancies (83%). However, the rate of miscarriage in the ccTGA mothers was higher than the general population (Connolly et al., 1999). A recent cohort of patients by Gelson and colleagues (2011) revealed high maternal and neonatal morbidity in women with systemic right ventricles with a significant number of babies born small for gestational age. Although cyanosis in women with ccTGA has been shown to be a risk factor for miscarriage, the women in the cohort of Gelson et al. were normally saturated (Gelson et al., 2011; Thierrien et al. 1999). The risk of congenital heart defects in the offspring of mothers with ccTGA has not been defined.

9.2 Heart transplant

Patients for which heart transplantation may be considered are those with end-stage RV failure, significant LV dysfunction and pulmonary valve abnormalities precluding successful DS operation, or uncontrollable arrhythmia (Duncan & Mee, 2005). For patients undergoing surgical intervention, poor preoperative EF of the systemic ventricle has been shown to predict the eventual need for transplantation (Beauchesne et al., 2002).

10. Conclusions and special considerations

Although debate continues over efficacy and long-term follow-up of physiologic vs. anatomic repair for ccTGA, recent outcomes data favor anatomic correction in which systemic function is restored to the LV. Management considerations specific to this population of complicated patients include type and timing of surgical intervention to pursue. The age and eligibility of pulmonary artery banding for LV retraining is yet to be standardized, and as pulmonary banding for maintenance of LV function in the asymptomatic infant is further evaluated, individualized decisions such as these are sure to produce much debate.

11. References

Alghamdi, A.A., McCrindle, B.W., & Van Arsdell, G.S. (2006). Physiologic Versus Anatomic Repair of Congenitally Corrected Transposition of the Great Arteries: Meta-Analysis of Individual Patient Data. *Annals of Thoracic Surgery*, Vol. 81, No. 4, (April 2006), pp. 1529-1535, ISSN 0003-4975.

Anderson, R.H., Becker, A.E., Arnold, R., & Wilkinson, J.L. (1974). The Conducting Tissues in Congenitally Corrected Transposition. *Circulation*, Vol 50, (1974), pp. 911-923, ISSN 1524-4539.

Beauchesne, L.M., Warnes, C.A., Connolly, H.M., Ammash, N.M., Tajik, A.J., & Danielson, G.K. (2002). Outcome of the Unoperated Adult Who Presents With Congenitally Corrected Transposition of the Great Arteries. *Journal of the American College of Cardiology*, Vol. 40, No. 2, (July 2002), pp. 285-290, ISSN 1558-3597.

Bogers, A.J., Head, S.J., de Jong, P.L., Witsenburg, M., & Kappetein, A.P. (2010). Long term follow up after surgery in congenitally corrected transposition of the great arteries with a right ventricle in the systemic circulation. *Journal of Cardiothoracic Surgery*, Vol. 5, Article No. 74, (September 2010), ISSN 1749-8090.

Bos, J.M., Hagler, D.J., Silvilairat, S., Cabalka, A., O'Leary, P., Daniels, O., Miller, F.A., & Abraham, T.P. (2006). Right Ventricular Function in Asymptomatic Individuals with a Systemic Right Ventricle. *Journal of the American Society of Echocardiography*, Vol. 19, No. 8, (August 2006), pp. 1033-1037, ISSN 0894-7317.

Bottega, N.A., Kapa, S., Edwards, W.D., Connolly, H.M., Munger, T.M., Warnes, C.A., & Asirvatham, S.J. The cardiac veins in congenitally corrected transposition of the great arteries: Delivery options for cardiac devices. *Heart Rhythm*, Vol. 6, No. 10, (October 2009), pp. 1450-1456, ISSN 1547-5271.

Carey, L.S. & Ruttenberg, H.D. (1964). Roentgenographic features of congenital corrected transposition of the great vessels: A comparative study of 33 cases with a roentgenographic classification based on the associated malformations and hemodynamic states. *American Journal of Roentgenology, Radium Therapy, and Nuclear Medicine*, Vol. 92, No. 3, (September 1964), pp. 623-651, ISSN 0002-9580.

Caso, P., Ascione, L., Lange, A., Palka, P., Mininni, N., & Sutherland, G.R. (1998). Diagnostic value of transesophageal echocardiography in the assessment of congenitally corrected transposition of the great arteries in adult patients. *American Heart Journal*, Vol. 135, No. 1, (January 1998), pp. 43-50, ISSN 0002-8703.

Chang, H-Y., Yin, W-H., Hsiung, M-C., & Young, M-S. (2009). A Heart Reversed Triply: Situs Inversus Totalis with Congenitally Corrected Transposition of the Great Arteries in a Middle-Aged Woman. *Echocardiography: A Journal of Cardiovascular Ultrasound and Allied Techniques*, Vol. 26, No. 5, (May 2009), pp. 617-621, ISSN 1540-8175.

Connolly, H.M., Grogan, M., & Warnes, C.A. (1999). Pregnancy among women with congenitally corrected transposition of the great arteries. *Journal of the American College of Cardiology*, Vol. 33., No. 6, (May 1999), pp. 1692-1695, ISSN 1558-3597.

Daliento, L., Corrado, D., Buja, G., John, N., Nava, A., & Thiene, G. (1986). Rhythm and Conduction Disturbances in Isolated, Congenitally Corrected Transposition of the Great Arteries. *The American Journal of Cardiology*, Vol. 58, No. 3, (August 1986), pp. 314-318, ISSN 0002-9149.

Diller, G. P., Okonko, D., Uebing, A., Ho, S. Y., & Gatzoulis, M. A. (2006). Cardiac resynchronization therapy for adult congenital heart disease patients with a systemic right ventricle: analysis of feasibility and review of early experience. *Europace*, Vol. 8, No. 4, (April 2006), pp. 267-272, ISSN 1099-5129.

Dodge-Khatami, A., Tulevski, I.I., Bennink, G.B., Hitchcock, J.F., de Mol, B.A., van der Wall, E.E., & Mulder, B.J. (2002). Comparable Systemic Ventricular Function in Healthy Adults and Patients With Unoperated Congenitally Corrected Transposition Using MRI Dobutamine Stress Testing. *Annals of Thoracic Surgery*, Vol. 73, No. 6, (June 2002), pp. 1759-1764, ISSN 0003-4975.

Dore, A., Houde, C., Chan, K-L., Ducharme, A., Khairy, P., Juneau, M., Marcotte, F., & Mercier, L-A. (2005). Angiotensin Receptor Blockade and Exercise Capacity in Adults with Systemic Right Ventricles: A Multicenter, Randomized, Placebo-Controlled Clinical Trial. *Circulation*, Vol. 112, No. 16, (October 2005), pp. 2411-2416, ISSN 1524-4539.

Duncan, B.W. & Mee, R.B. (2005). Management of the failing systemic right ventricle. *Seminars in Thoracic and Cardiovascular Surgery: Pediatric Cardiac Surgery Annual*, Vol. 17, No. 2, (Summer 2005), pp. 160-169, ISSN 1092-9126.

Fratz, S., Hager, A., Busch, R., Kaemmerer, H., Schwaiger, M., Lange, R., Hess, J., & Stern, H.C. (2008). Patients After Atrial Switch Operation for Transposition of the Great Arteries Can Not Increase Stroke Volume Under Dobutamine Stress as Opposed to Patients with Congenitally Corrected Transposition. *Circulation Journal*, Vol. 72, No. 7, (July 2008), pp. 1130-1135, ISSN 1347-4820.

Friedberg, D.Z. & Nadas, A.S. (1970). Clinical profile of patients with congenital corrected transposition of the great arteries: A study of 60 cases. *The New England Journal of Medicine*, Vol. 282, No. 19, (May 1970), pp. 1053-1059, ISSN 1533-4406.

Gaies, M.G., Goldberg, C.S., Ohye, R.G., Devaney, E.J., Hirsch, J.C., & Bove, E.L. (2009). Early and Intermediate Outcome After Anatomic Repair of Congenitally Corrected Transposition of the Great Arteries. *Annals of Thoracic Surgery*, Vol. 88, No. 6, (December 2009), pp. 1952-1960, ISSN 0003-4975.

Gelson, E., Curry, R., Gatzoulis, M.A., Swan, L., Lupton, M., Durbridge, J., Deans, C., Steer, P., & Johnson, M.R. (2011). Pregnancy in women with a systemic right ventricle after surgically and congenitally corrected transposition of the great arteries. *European Journal of Obstetrics and Gynecology and Reproductive Biology*, Vol. 155, No. 2, (April 2011), pp. 146-149, ISSN 0301-2115.

Giardini, A., Lovato, L., Donti, A,. Formigari, R., Oppido, G., Gargiulo, G., Picchio, F.M., & Fattori, R. (2006). Relation Between Right Ventricular Structural Alterations and Markers of Adverse Clinical Outcome in Adults with Systemic Right Ventricle and Either Congenital Complete (After Senning Operation) or Congenitally Corrected Transposition of the Great Arteries. *The American Journal of Cardiology*, Vol. 98, No. 9, (November 2006), pp. 1277-1282, ISSN 0002-9149.

Graham, T.P., Bernard, Y.D., Mellen, B.G., Celermajer, D., Baumgartner, H., Cetta, F., Connolly, H.M., Davidson, W.R., Dellborg, M., Foster, E., Gersony, W.M., Gessner, I.H., Hurwitz, R.A., Kaemmerer, H., Kugler, J.D., Murphy, D.J., Noonan, J.A.,

Morris, C., Perloff, J.K., Sanders, S.P., & Sutherland, J.L. (2000). Long-Term Outcome in Congenitally Corrected Transposition of the Great Arteries: A Multi-Institutional Study. *Journal of the American College of Cardiology*, Vol. 36, No. 1, (July 2000), pp. 255-261, ISSN 1558-3597.

Graham, T.P. & Markham, L.W. (2010). Congenitally corrected transposition of the great arteries, In: *Diagnosis and Management of Adult Congenital Heart Disease*, M.D. Gatzoulis & G.D. Webb (Eds.), pp. 371-377, Churchill Livingstone, ISBN 978-0-7020-3426-8, Edinburgh.

Graham, T.P., Markham, L., Parra, D.P., & Bichell, D. (2007). Congenitally Corrected Transposition of the Great Arteries: An Update. *Current Treatment Options in Cardiovascular Medicine*, Vol. 9, No. 5, (October 2007), pp. 405-413, ISBN 1092-8464.

Hoffman, J.I.E. (2009). Congenitally Corrected Transposition of the Great Arteries, In: *The Natural and Unnatural History of Congenital Heart Disease*, Julien I.E. Hoffman (Ed.), pp. 206-217, Wiley-Blackwell, ISBN 978-1-4051-7927-0, Oxford.

Hörer, J., Schreiber, C., Krane, S., Prodan, Z., Cleuziou, J., Vogt, M., Holper, K., & Lange, R. (2008). Outcome after Surgical Repair/Palliation of Congenitally Corrected Transposition of the Great Arteries. *The Thoracic and Cardiovascular Surgeon*, Vol. 56, No. 7, (October 2008), pp. 391-397, ISSN 1439-1902.

Hörer, J., Haas, F., Cleuziou, J., Schreiber, C., Kostolny, M., Vogt, M., Holper, K., & Lange, R. (2007). Intermediate-term results of the Senning or Mustard procedures combined with the Rastelli operation for patients with discordant atrioventricular connections associated with discordant ventriculoarterial connections or double outlet right ventricle. *Cardiology in the Young*, Vol. 17, No. 2, (April 2007), pp. 158-165, ISSN 1047-9511.

Hornung, T.S. & Calder, L. (2010). Congenitally corrected transposition of the great arteries. *Heart*, Vol. 96, No. 14, (July 2010), pp. 1154-1161, ISSN 1468-201X.

Hraska, V., Duncan, B.W., Mayer, J.E., Freed, M., del Nido, P.J., & Jonas RA. (2005). Long-term outcome of surgically treated patients with corrected transposition of the great arteries. *The Journal of Thoracic and Cardiovascular Surgery*, Vol. 129, No. 1, (January 2005), pp. 182-191, ISSN 0022-5223.

Huhta, J.C., Maloney, J.D., Ritter, D.G., Ilstrup, D.M., & Feldt, R.H. (1983). Complete atrioventricular block in patients with atrioventricular discordance. *Circulation*, Vole. 67, No. 6, (June 1983), pp. 1374–1377, ISSN 1524-4539.

Ismat, F.A., Baldwin, H.S., Karl, T.R., & Weinberg, P.M. (2002). Coronary anatomy in congenitally corrected transposition of the great arteries. *International Journal of Cardiology*, Vol. 86, No. 2-3, (December 2002), pp. 207-216, ISSN 0167-5273.

Janousek, J., Tomek, V., Chaloupecky, V. A., Reich, O., Gebauer, R. A., Kautzner, J., & Hucin, B. (November 2004). Cardiac resynchronization therapy: a novel adjunct to the treatment and prevention of systemic right ventricular failure. *Journal of the American College of Cardiology*, Vol. 44, No. 9, (November 2004), pp. 1927-1931, ISSN 1558-3597.

Jennings, H.S., Primm, R.K., Parrish, M.D., Prager, R.L., & Graham, T.P. (1984). Coronary arterial revascularization in an adult with congenitally corrected transposition. *American Heart Journal*, Vol. 108, (September 1984), pp. 598-600, ISSN 0002-8703.

Jonas, R.A. (2004). Congenitally corrected transposition of the great arteries, In: *Comprehensive Surgical Management of Congenital Heart Disease*, Richard. A. Jonas (Ed.), pp. 483-496, Hodder Arnold, ISBN 978-0-3408-0807-8, London.

Kordybach, M., Kowalski, M., & Hoffman, P. (2009). Heart failure in a patient with corrected transposition of the great arteries. When is biventricular pacing indicated? *Acta Cardiologica*, Vol. 64., No 5., (October 2009), pp. 673-676, ISSN 0001-5385.

Kral Kollars, C.A., Gelehrter, S., Bove, E.L., & Ensing, G. (2010). Effects of Morphologic Left Ventricular Pressure on Right Ventricular Geometry and Tricuspid Valve Regurgitation in Patients with Congenitally Corrected Transposition of the Great Arteries. *The American Journal of Cardiology*, Vol. 105, No. 5, (March 2010), pp. 735-739, ISSN 0002-9149.

Lim, H-G., Lee, J.R., Kim, Y.J., Park, Y-H., Jun, T-G., Kim, W-H., Lee, C-H., Park, H.K., Yang, J-H., Park, C-S., & Kwak, J.G. (2010). Outcomes of Biventricular Repair for Congenitally Corrected Transposition of the Great Arteries. *Annals of Thoracic Surgery*, Vol. 89, No. 1, (January 2010), pp. 159-167, ISSN 0003-4975.

Ly, M., Belli, E., Leobon, B., Kortas, C., Grollmüss, O.E., Piot, D., Planché, C., & Serraf, A. (2009). Results of the double switch operation for congenitally corrected transposition of the great arteries. *European Journal of Cardio-thoracic Surgery*, Vol. 35, No. 5, (May 2009), pp.879-884 , ISSN 1010-7940.

Malecka, B., Bednarek, J., Tomkiewicz-Pajak, L., Klimeczek, P., Zabek, A., Pasowicz, M., & Lelakowski, J. (2010). Resynchronization therapy transvenous approach in dextrocardia and congenitally corrected transposition of great arteries. *Cardiology Journal*, Vol. 17, No. 5, (2010), pp. 503-508, ISSN 1897-5593.

Malhotra, S.P., Reddy, V.M., Qui, M., Pirolli, T.J., Barboza, L., Reinhartz, O., & Hanley, F.L. (2011). The hemi-Mustard/bidirectional Glenn atrial switch procedure in the double-switch operation for congenitally corrected transposition of great arteries: Rationale and midterm results. *The Journal of Thoracic and Cardiovascular Surgery*, Vol. 141, No. 1, (Janurary 2011), pp. 162-170, ISSN 0022-5223.

McEwing, R.L. & Chaoui, R. (2004). Congenitally corrected transposition of the great arteries: clues for prenatal diagnosis. *Ultrasound in Obstetrics and Gynecology*, Vol. 23, No. 1, (January 2004), pp. 68-72, ISSN 1469-0705.

Metton, O., Gaudin, R., Ou, P., Gerelli, S., Mussa, S., Sidi, D., Vouhé, P., & Raisky, O. (2010). Early prophylactic pulmonary artery banding in isolated congenitally corrected transposition of the great arteries. *European Journal of Cardio-thoracic Surgery*, Vol. 38, No. 6, (December 2010), pp. 728-735, ISSN 1010-7940.

Mongeon, F-P., Connolly H.M., Dearani, J.A., Li, Z., & Warnes, C.A. (2011). Congenitally Corrected Transposition of the Great Arteries: Ventricular Function at the Time of Systemic Atrioventricular Valve Replacement Predicts Long-Term Ventricular Function. *Journal of the American College of Cardiology*, Vol. 57, No. 20, (May 2011), pp. 2008-2017, ISSN 1558-3597.

Oechslin, E. (2009). Physiologically "Corrected" Transposition of the Great Arteries, In *Echocardiography in Pediatric and Congenital Heart Disease: From Fetus to Adult*, W.W. Lai, L.L. Mertens, M.S. Cohen & T. Geva, (Eds.), pp. 439-455, Wiley-Blackwell, ISBN 978-1-4051-7401-5, Oxford.

Orchard, E.A., Ormerod, O., Myerson, S., & Westaby, S. (2010). Congenitally Corrected Transposition of the Great Arteries Presenting in a Nonagenarian. *Circulation*, Vol. 122, No. 9, (August 2010), pp. e441-444, ISSN 1524-4539.

Paladini, D., Volpe, P., Marasini, M., Russo, M.G., Vassallo, M., Gentile, M., & Calabro, R. (2006). Diagnosis, characterization and outcome of congenitally corrected transposition of the great arteries in the fetus: a multicenter series of 30 cases.

Ultrasound in Obstetrics and Gynecology, Vol. 27, No. 3, (March 2006), pp. 281-285, ISSN 1469-0705.

Piacentini, G., Digilio M.C., Capolino, R., De Zorzi, A., Toscano, A., Sarkozy, A., D'Agostino, R., Marasini, M., Russo, M.G., Dallapiccola, B., & Marino, B. (2005). Familial Recurrence of Heart Defects in Subjects with Congenitally Corrected Transposition of the Great Arteries. *American Journal of Medical Genetics*, Vol. 137, No. 2, (August 2005), pp. 176-180, ISSN 1552-4833.

Poirier, N.C., Yu, J.H., Brizard, C.P., & Mee, R.B. (2004). Long-term results of left ventricular reconditioning and anatomic correction for systemic right ventricular dysfunction after atrial switch procedures. *The Journal of Thoracic and Cardiovascular Surgery*, Vol. 127, No. 4, (April 2004), pp. 975-981, ISSN 0022-5223.

Presbitero, P., Somerville, J., Rabajoli, F., Stone, S., & Conte, M.R. (1995). Corrected transposition of the great arteries without associated defects in adult patients: clinical profile and follow up. *British Heart Journal*, Vol. 74, No. 1, (July 1995), pp. 57-59, ISSN 0007-0769.

Prieto, L.R., Hordof, A.J., Secic, M., Rosenbaum, M.S., & Gersony, W.M. (1998). Progressive Tricuspid Valve Disease in Patients With Congenitally Corrected Transposition of the Great Arteries. *Circulation*, Vol. 98, No. 10, (September 1998), pp. 997-1005, ISSN 1524-4539.

Quinn, D.W., McGuirk, S.P., Metha, C., Nightingale, P., de Giovanni, J.V., Dhillon, R., Miller, P., Stumper, O., Wright, J.G., Barron, D.J., & Brawn, W.J. (2008). The morphologic left ventricle that requires training by means of pulmonary artery banding before the double-switch procedure for congenitally corrected transposition of the great arteries is at risk of late dysfunction. *The Journal of Thoracic and Cardiovascular Surgery*, Vol. 135, No. 5, (May 2008), pp. 1137-1144, ISSN 0022-5223.

Said, S.M., Burkhardt, H.M., Schaff, H.V., & Dearani, J.A. (2011). Congenitally Corrected Transposition of Great Arteries: Surgical Options for the Failing Ventricle and/or Severe Tricuspid Regurgitation. *World Journal for Pediatric and Congenital Heart Surgery*, Vol. 2, No. 1, (January 2011), pp. 64-79, ISSN 2150-1351.

Scardi, S., Knoll, P., & Pandullo, C. (1999). Corrected Transposition of the Great Vessels and Situs Inversus Viscerum in a 65-Year-Old Oligosymptomatic Woman. *Circulation*, Vol. 100, No. 7, (August 1999), pp. 777, ISSN 1524-4539.

Schmidt, M., Theissen, P, Deutsch, H.J., Dederichs, B., Franzen, D., Erdmann, E., & Schicha, H. (2000). Congenitally corrected transposition of the great arteries (L TGA) with situs inversus totalis in adulthood: findings with magnetic resonance imaging. *Magnetic Resonance Imaging*, Vol. 18, No. 4, (May 2000), pp. 417-422, ISSN 0730-725X.

Shima, Y., Nakajima, M., Kumasaka, S., & Migita, M. (2009). Prenatal diagnosis of isolated congenitally corrected transposition of the great arteries. *Archives of Gynecology and Obstetrics*, Vol. 279, No. 4, (April 2009), pp. 557-559, ISSN 1432-0711.

Shin'oka, T., Kurosawa, H., Imai, Y., Aoki, M., Ishiyama, M., Sakamoto, T., Miyamoto, S., Hobo, K., & Ichihara, Y. (2007). Outcomes of definitive surgical repair for congenitally corrected transposition of the great arteries or double outlet right ventricle with discordant atrioventricular connections: risk analyses in 189 patients. The Journal of thoracic and cardiovascular surgery, Vol. 133, No. 5, (May 2007), pp. 1318-28, ISSN 0022-5223.

Takemoto, M., Nakashima, A., Muneuchi, J., Yamamura, K-I., Shiokawa, Y., Sunagawa, K., & Tominaga, R. (2010). Para-Hisian Pacing for a Pediatric Patient with a

Congenitally Corrected Transposition of the Great Arteries (SLL). *Pacing and Clinical Electrophysiology*, Vol. 33, No. 1, (January 2010), pp. e4-7, ISSN 1540-8159.

Tay, E.L., Frogoudaki, A., Inuzuka, R., Giannakoulas, G., Prapa, M., Li, W., Pantley, G., Dimopoulos, K., & Gatzoulis, M.A. (2011). Exercise intolerance in patients with congenitally corrected transposition of the great arteries relates to right ventricular filling pressures. *International Journal of Cardiology*, Vol. 147, No. 2, (March 2011), pp. 219-223, ISSN 0167-5273.

Teo, L.L. & Hia, C.P. (2011). Advanced cardiovascular imaging in congenital heart disease. *International Journal of Clinical Practice*, Vol. 65, Suppl. 171, (April 2011), pp. 17-21, ISSN 1742-1241.

Thierrien, J., Barnes, I., & Somerville, J. (1999). Outcome of Pregnancy in Patients with Congenitally Corrected Transposition of the Great Arteries. *The American Journal of Cardiology*, Vol. 84, No.7, (October 1999), pp. 820-824, ISSN 0002-9149.

Van der Bom, T., Zomer, A.C., Zwinderman, A.H., Meijboom, F.J., Bouma, B.J., & Mulder, B.J. (2011). The changing epidemiology of congenital heart disease. *Nature Reviews Cardiology*, Vol. 8, No. 1, (January 2011), pp. 50-60, ISSN 1759-5002.

Van Praagh, R., Papagiannis, J., Grunenfelder, J., Bartram, U., & Martanovic, P. (1998) Pathologic anatomy of corrected transposition of the great arteries and surgical implications. *American Heart Journal*, Vol 135, No. 5, (May 1998), pp. 772-785, ISSN 0002-8703.

Van Son, J.A, Danielson, G. K., Huhta, J. C., Warnes, C. A., Edwards, W. D., Schaff, H. V., Puga, F. J., & Ilstrup, D. M. (1995). Late results of systemic atrioventricular valve replacement in corrected transposition. *The Journal of Thoracic and Cardiovascular Surgery*, Vol. 109, No. 4, (April 1995), pp. 642-653, ISSN 0022-5223.

Wan, A.W., Jevremovic, A., Tierney, E.S., McCrindle, B.W., Dunn, E., Manlhiot, C., Wald, R.M., Kingdom, J.P., Jaeggi, E.T., & Nield L.E. (2009). Comparison of Impact of Prenatal Versus Postnatal Diagnosis of Congenitally Corrected Transposition of the Great Arteries. *The American Journal of Cardiology*, Vol. 104, No. 9, (November 2009), pp. 1276-1279, ISSN 0002-9149.

Warnes, C.A. (2006). Transposition of the Great Arteries. *Circulation*, Vol. 114, No. 24, (December 2006), pp. 2699-2709, ISSN 1524-4539.

Winlaw, D.S., McGuirk, S.P., Balmer, C., Langley, S.M., Griselli, M., Stümper, O., De Giovanni, J.V., Wright, J.G., Thorne, S., Barron, D.J., Brawn, W.J. (2005). Intention-to-Treat Analysis of Pulmonary Artery Banding in Conditions With a Morphologic Right Ventricle in the Systemic Circulation With a View to Anatomic Biventricular Repair. *Circulation*, Vol. 111, No. 4, (February 2005), pp. 405-411, ISSN 1524-4539.

Winter, M.M., Bouma, B.J., Groenink, M., Konings, T.C., Tijssen, J.G., van Veldhuisen, D.J., & Mulder, BJ. (2009). Latest insights in therapeutic options for systemic right ventricular failure: a comparison with left ventricular failure. *Heart*, Vol. 5, No. 1, (June 2009), pp. 960-963, ISSN 1468-201X.

Zhang, Y., Cai, A., Sun, W., & Zhao, Y. (2011). Prenatal diagnosis of fetal congenitally corrected transposition of the great arteries. *Prenatal Diagnosis*, Vol. 31, No. 6, (June 2011), pp. 529-535, ISSN 1097-0223.

8

Proximal Anomalous Connections of Coronary Arteries in Adults

Pierre Aubry[1], Xavier Halna du Fretay[2], Patrick A. Calvert[1,3], Patrick Dupouy[4], Fabien Hyafil[5], Jean-Pierre Laissy[6] and Jean-Michel Juliard[1]
[1]*Department of Cardiology, Bichat Hospital, Paris*
[2]*Department of Cardiology, Foch Hospital, Suresnes*
[3]*Department of Cardiology, Papworth Hospital NHS Foundation Trust, Cambridge,*
[4]*Department of Interventional Cardiology and Cardiovascular Imaging, Hôpital Privé d'Antony, Antony*
[5]*Department of Nuclear Medicine, Bichat Hospital, Paris*
[6] *Department of Radiology, Bichat Hospital, Paris,*
[1,2,4,5,6]*France*
[3]*United Kingdom*

1. Introduction

Isolated proximal **ANO**malous connections of **COR**onary arteries (ANOCOR) are not rare with an angiographic prevalence and tomographic prevalence of 0.5% and 1.3% respectively, in adult populations. The diagnosis of ANOCOR is sometimes fortuitous in adults undergoing a coronary angiography to detect a coronary artery disease (CAD). The absence of diagnosis in young people may have severe consequences with sudden death occurring frequently during intensive exertion. The prognosis depends mainly on the initial course of the ectopic coronary vessel. Preaortic course with intramural segment is recognized as high risk for sudden death in children or young adults. Management of ANOCOR with intramural course may be difficult in patients >35 years of age and with no evidence of myocardial ischemia. The mechanisms of life-threatening cardiac events are still not well understood even if anatomical risk factors are identified. Fortunately, most cases of ANOCOR are simply incidental anatomical findings. Multidetector computed tomography (CT) is recognized as the best imaging technique for identifying ANOCOR. Intravascular ultrasonography (IVUS) may help to quantify the severity of high-risk ANOCOR. In the ACC/AHA 2008 guidelines for the management of adults with congenital heart disease, surgical repair is the treatment of choice for high-risk ANOCOR (Warnes et al. 2008). However, this therapeutic management is based on little solid data with limited long-term follow-up. Percutaneous coronary intervention (PCI) has been proposed in some ANOCOR. The limited experience of most angiographers in detection of ANOCOR may explain non infrequent misdiagnoses with erroneous interpretations of ANOCOR. Large-scale prospective multicenter studies are needed to improve screening and imaging strategies and to better define the treatment of these potentially lethal congenital coronary abnormalities.

Today, prospective registries are ongoing in France and North and South America with the goal of assessing the natural history of ANOCOR, as well as the long-term impact of surgical repair or PCI. The present review will focus on recent imaging modalities allowing us to revisit previous concepts and definitions.

2. Embryology and normal anatomy

The basics of cardiac development are needed to understand congenital coronary malformations and to avoid incorrect interpretation leading sometimes to erroneous diagnoses (Gittenberger-de Groot et al. 2005).

2.1 Embryology

The looping of the heart and the completion of the great vessels occur before the connection of coronary arteries to the aorta. Neural crest cells play an essential role in the outflow tract septation and coronary artery development. An additional element is the contribution of extracardiac cell populations like epicardium-derived cells. Coronary vascular formation occurs relatively late in development after covering of the myocardium by the epicardium. A plexus of epicardially derived vessels connects to the aortic root. It is generally considered that the initial segment of the coronary arteries develops by endothelial ingrowth from the peritruncal ring rather than by endothelial outgrowth from the aorta (Bogers et al., 1989). That is why the expression *anomalous connection* will often be used in this review. Otherwise, the concept of ingrowth permits a better understanding of the numerous ANOCOR patterns. Proximal left and right coronary arteries connect to the left posterior and anterior sinuses which are closest to the right ventricular outflow tract and pulmonary trunk. In the normal heart, the left posterior sinus is also known as the left sinus, and the anterior sinus, the right sinus. Recent experimental insights suggest that multiple endothelial strands penetrate the three sinuses at the onset of the proximal coronary vascular formation (Ando et al., 2004). Then, the left and the right stems develop by fusion of endothelial strands, and the strands connecting the right posterior sinus disappear. Therefore, the right posterior sinus is also known as the non-coronary sinus. Anomalous origin of coronary arteries may occur in isolation without abnormal myocardial outflow tract development. Inconsistencies exist with regard to the exact mode of development of these congenital abnormalities in otherwise normal hearts.

2.2 Normal anatomy

On an axial cross-sectional CT view, the origin of the left coronary arises at the 3- to 5-o'clock position and the right coronary at the 10- to 12-o'clock position (figure 1). Knowledge of the position of the heart within the mediastinum is essential for appropriate analysis of imaging tools (Anderson & Loukas, 2009). Due to the orientation of the aorta, the origin of the coronary arteries is not well visualised simultaneously on the same axial image. The left ostium is more cranial in comparison with the right ostium. Shortly after their origin, the coronary arteries run across the epicardial surface of the heart surrounded by fat. The proximal segment of the right coronary artery (RCA) courses directly in the right atrioventricular groove, whereas the left coronary artery (LCA) courses initially between the pulmonary trunk and the left appendage.

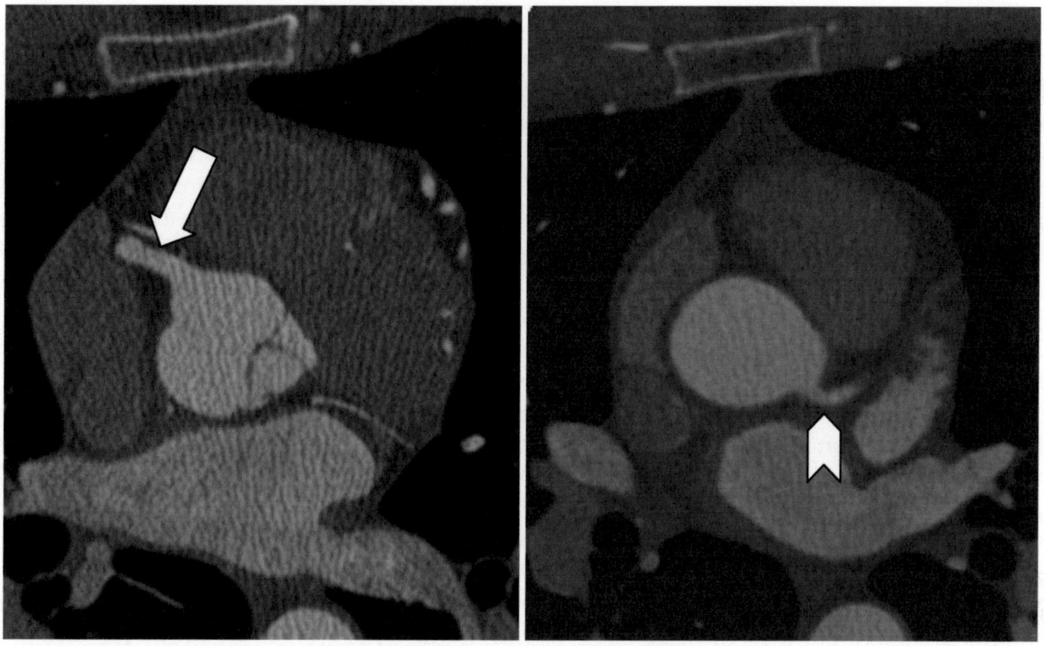

Fig. 1. Axial cross-sectional computed tomography views showing normal origin of the right coronary artery (arrow) and left coronary artery (arrow head).

Cardiologists and radiologists should be aware of the normal origin and anatomical variants (Angelini, 2007) of the coronary arteries (table 1) in order to make an accurate diagnosis of ANOCOR.

Normal connections	
Left coronary	Left main dividing into LAD and CX coronary arteries
Right artery	Single ostium
Site of left connection	In mid-left sinus
Site of right connection	In mid-right sinus
Level of connection	Upper half of sinus
Ostium shape	Circular
Angulation with aorta	45 to 90°
Initial course to aorta	Extramural
Anatomical variants	
Left coronary	Separate origin of LAD and CX coronary arteries in left sinus
Right coronary	Separate origin of conus artery in right sinus
Site of left connection	Close to the right sinus
Site of right connection	Close to the non-coronary sinus
Level of connection	Up to 10 mm above the level of the sinotubular junction
Ostium shape	Ovoid
Angulation with aorta	90 to 135°

Table 1. Normal connections and anatomical variants of the coronary arteries. CX: circumflex, LAD: left anterior descending.

In the normal heart, the coronary arteries arise from the upper half of sinuses, close to the sinotubular junction in most of cases (Muriago et al., 1997). A connection above the level of the sinotubular junction is possible. The coronary orifices are not always located in the centre of aortic sinuses. The left coronary ostium may lie near the junction between the left and right aortic sinuses, whereas the right ostium may lie near the junction between the right and the non-coronary aortic sinuses (Muriago et al., 1997). The discrimination between a common variant and an anomalous origin from an unusual site within the appropriate sinus is often difficult. It is inappropriate to use the notation of left and right aortic sinuses when there is an anomalous aortic origin of one of the coronary arteries. The categorisation proposed by the working group of Leiden (Gittenberger-de Groot et al., 1983) is based on the view by an observer positioned in the sinus farthest from the pulmonary trunk. The sinus at the right hand of the observer is named sinus 1 and gives rise to the right coronary artery in the normal heart, whereas the sinus at the left hand is named sinus 2 and normally gives rise to the left coronary artery. Another classification is used in this review with the two sinuses adjacent to the pulmonary trunk called respectively appropriate sinus and opposite sinus. The origin of mistakes that occur in the literature is often due to the confused interpretation describing the relationships of the ectopic coronary arteries with the adjacent structures, mainly the great vessels. The schematic representation, often cited, with a cross-section view of the aortic and pulmonary valves is erroneous. Indeed, the aortic and pulmonary annuluses are not in the same plane and the latter is more superior. Therefore, it is easy to understand that the initial path of the RCA is facing the subpulmonary infundibulum and not the pulmonary trunk (figure 2). According to the position and the

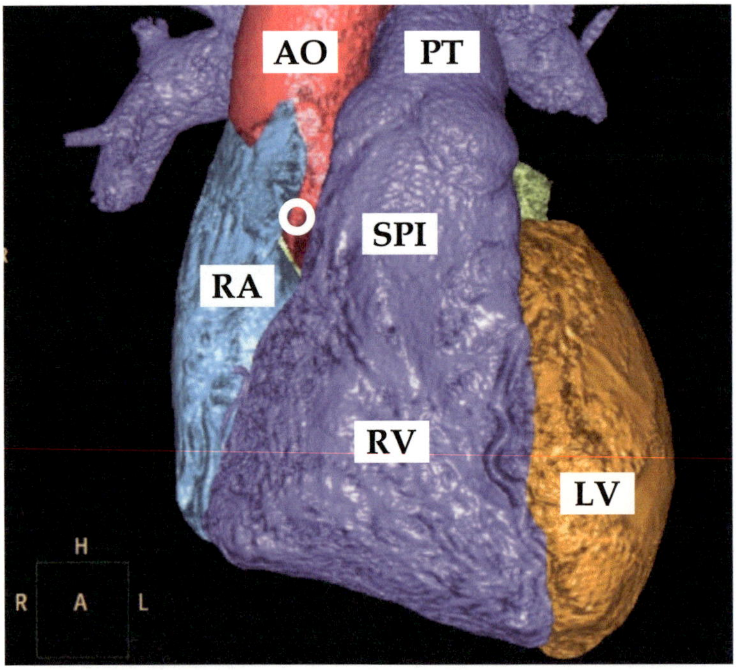

Fig. 2. Volume-rendered computed tomography image of the heart with the normal origin of the right coronary artery (white circle) marked. AO: aorta, LV: left ventricle, PT: pulmonary trunk, RA: right atrium, RV: right ventricle, SPI: subpulmonary infundibulum.

orientation of the initial pulmonary trunk, the origin of the LCA is hidden by the pulmonary trunk. Consequently, it is crucial to accept that the initial preaortic course of an ectopic coronary artery may be in contact with the subpulmonary infundibulum or pulmonary trunk or both. Thus, the definition of the so-called interarterial course is too simplistic in our opinion. Another major pitfall in this field is the confused anatomical interpretation of the space between the aortic and pulmonary roots. In fact, there is no muscular septum between the origins of the great vessels (Loukas et al., 2009). Therefore, the visualization of an ectopic coronary artery coursing between the subpulmonary infundibulum and the interventricular septum does not necessarily imply an intramyocardial course. The ectopic vessel passes rather on the myocardial septum and close to the subpulmonic infundibulum. Thus, for the reasons discussed above, we chose to identify 4 ectopic courses regarding their relationships with the great vessels: preinfundibular, retroinfundibular, preaortic and retroaortic courses, in opposition to the usual definition with 4 ectopic courses: prepulmonary, intraseptal, interarterial and retroaortic courses (Roberts & Shirani, 1992).

At the level of the aortic and pulmonary valves, the aortic and pulmonary walls are in close contact surrounded by large fatty tissues. The adjacent area between the great vessels may vary according to age, intrathoracic deformations, and acquired heart diseases. A clockwise or counter-clockwise rotation of the aortic root can modify the relationship of a normal coronary origin with the pulmonary trunk or subpulmonary infundibulum.

3. Classification

So far, no consensus exists to define and classify easily the wide spectrum of the congenital coronary artery abnormalities (Angelini, 2002). Numerous, sometimes long or complex, descriptions have been presented in the literature (Angelini 2007, Dodge-Khatami et al., 2000, Jacobs & Mavroudis, 2010, Rigatelli et al., 2009, Roberts, 1986). We propose, in this review focused on the proximal anomalous connections of the coronary arteries, a simplified classification with 8 types (table 2). This classification is based on an anatomical view with the contribution of postmortem data (Frescura et al., 1998) and recent imaging modalities. By definition, the abnormalities involve the orifices of the LCA and RCA, and their branches. Different types of ANOCOR may be observed in the same patient. Diagnosis of ANOCOR is sometimes uncertain, especially in cases of an incomplete or poor-quality imaging. We consider that an accurate anatomical diagnosis should be the first step when an ANOCOR is suspected.

type I	anomalous connection with the opposite sinus
type II	anomalous connection with the contralateral artery
type III	anomalous connection with the appropriate sinus
type IV	anomalous connection with the non-coronary sinus
type V	anomalous connection above the sinotubular junction
type VI	single coronary artery
type VII	anomalous connection with the pulmonary artery
type VIII	other abnormalities

Table 2. Simplified classification of proximal anomalous connections of the coronary arteries.

3.1 Anomalous connection with the opposite sinus (type I)

The ectopic orifice may be in contact with the ostium in right location or close to the latter (figure 3). The main anomalies involve a RCA arising from the opposite sinus, a left main coronary artery (LMCA), or a left anterior descending (LAD) coronary artery and/or circumflex (CX) coronary artery arising from the opposite sinus.

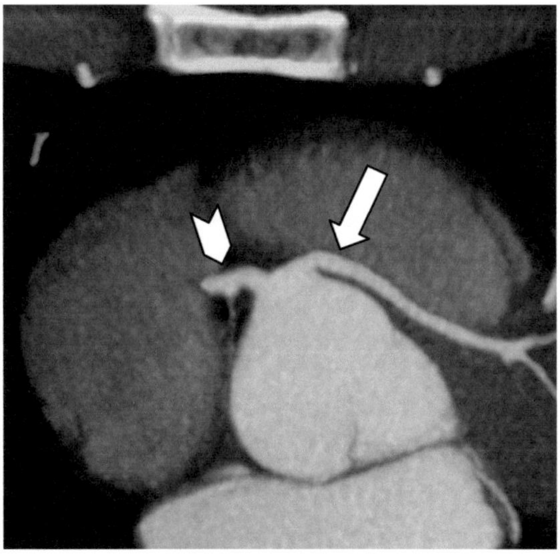

Fig. 3. Axial computed tomography image showing an anomalous connection of the left main coronary artery (arrow) with the opposite sinus close to the normal origin of the right coronary artery (arrow head).

3.2 Anomalous connection with the contralateral artery (type II)

By definition, the RCA is the contralateral artery of the LCA, and the LCA the contralateral artery of the RCA. In most cases, an anomalous connection in the contralateral artery results in a unique coronary ostium (figure 4).

Generally, this abnormality is not separated from the anomalous connection with the opposite sinus. In our opinion, it seems interesting to make a difference between these abnormalities. Firstly, a connection of the ectopic coronary artery with the proximal segment of the contralateral involves, almost without exception, the LCA or their branches. Secondly, in theory, the risk of intramural course can be excluded. Finally, this classification may include an anomalous origin distant from the aorta. In theses uncommon cases, the classification used in this study implies that an anomalous connection can exist between two coronary arteries whatever the level of the connection from the origin to the distal segment. The anomalous connections of the LCA with the opposite sinus or contralateral artery are generally associated with an absent LMCA in the appropriate sinus. However, rare cases of atresia of the LMCA originated from the left coronary sinus have been described (Levisman et al., 2009) with an embryonic small vessel often solely visible by CT.

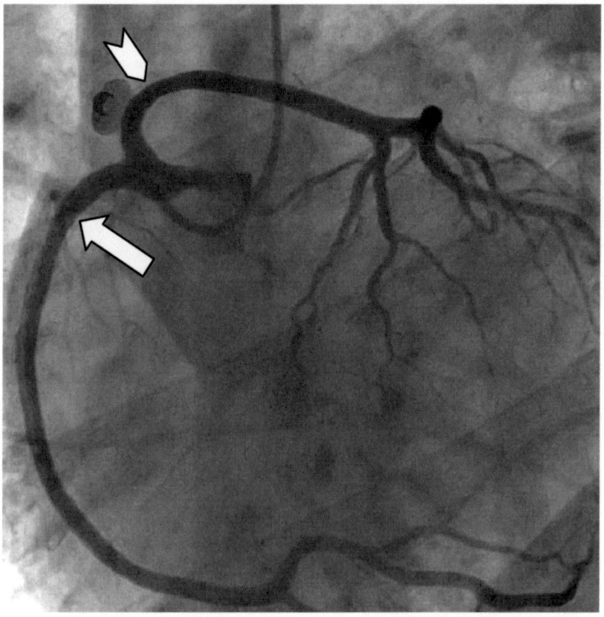

Fig. 4. Angiographic view showing an anomalous connection of the left main coronary artery (arrow head) with the proximal right coronary artery (arrow).

3.3 Anomalous connection with the appropriate sinus (type III)

An anomalous orifice of a coronary artery is usually linked with an ectopic ostium. Nevertheless, in rare postmortem observations (Frescura et al., 1998), a valve-like stenosis has been described with a ridge, consequence of an aortic wall fold that is in contact with an ostium in right position. Recently, a LMCA originated from the left sinus in the usual site, but with a slit-like orifice due to a tangential initial course associated with a short intramural segment, has been described (Angelini et al., 2010). An ectopic origin of a coronary artery in the appropriate sinus remains possible, but the limit between a true abnormality and a common variant may be tenuous, such as a connection in the lower half of the sinus, or near the commissural junction between the left and right cusps.

3.4 Anomalous connection with the non-coronary sinus (type IV)

ANOCOR from the non-coronary sinus proved by surgical or postmortem examination were previously described as exceptional. Nevertheless, a higher frequency of the latter is noticed in recent studies using tomographic imaging.

3.5 Anomalous connection above the sinotubular junction (type V)

A high take-off from the aorta at least 10 mm above the sinotubular junction is generally considered as an anomalous connection (Hlavacek et al., 2010). However, the height of take-off judged to represent the abnormality is based on few solid data. Indeed, a level of 4 mm has been reported in a postmortem study (Frescura et al., 1998). Therefore, the criteria to determine an anomalous aortic origin above the sinotubular junction should be redefined with the contribution of non-invasive imaging. Usually, the ectopic vessel continues to arise above the appropriate sinus (figure 5).

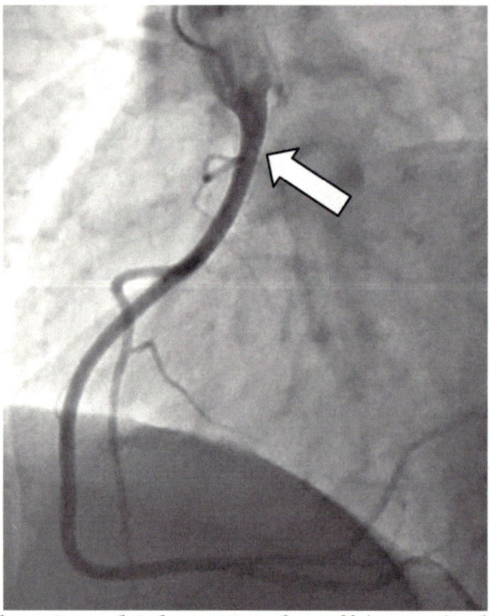

Fig. 5. Angiographic view showing a high aortic take-off (arrow) of the right coronary artery.

3.6 Single coronary artery (type VI)

The definition of a single coronary artery is often ambiguous in the literature. In our view, a single coronary should be clearly differenced from an ANOCOR with a single ostium, as described on figure 5. In both cases, the solitary vessel supplies the entire coronary circulation. Nevertheless, the flow is always antegrade beyond a single ostium, while a single artery supplies the coronary circulation of a part of the myocardium by a retrograde filling (figure 6). Moreover, with our definition, a single coronary artery is never associated with an abnormal proximal course.

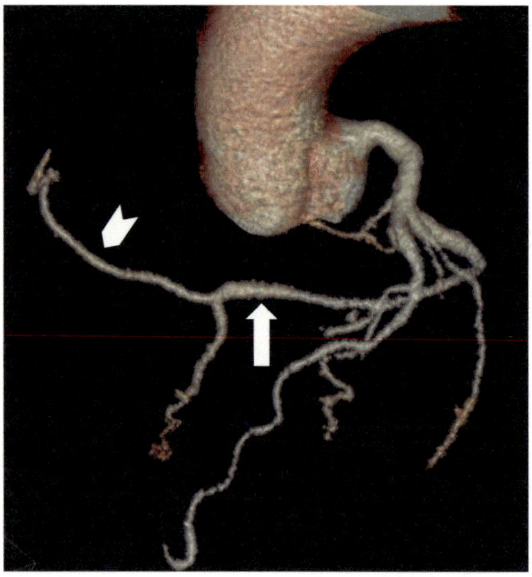

Fig. 6. Volume-rendered computed tomography image showing a single coronary artery with a normal left ostium, and a circumflex coronary artery (arrow) supplying the myocardium usually fed by the right coronary artery (arrow head).

3.7 Anomalous connection with the pulmonary artery (type VII)

In patients with anomalous connection with the pulmonary artery, the most commonly artery is the LMCA. Usually, the latter is connected with the left posterior pulmonary sinus, facing the left posterior aortic sinus. Numerous epicardial collateral vessels are observed between the anomalous coronary artery that arises from the pulmonary artery and the normal contralateral coronary artery that arises from the aorta (fig 7). An origin of the RCA from the pulmonary artery is less frequently than the LCA.

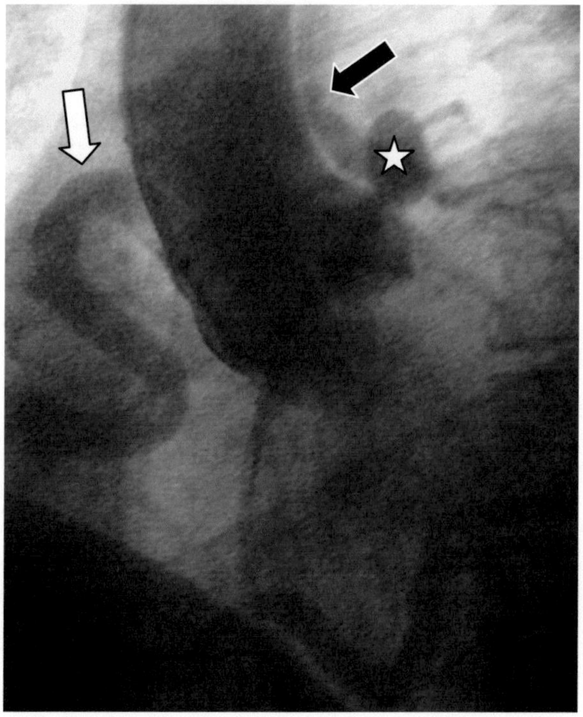

Fig. 7. Aortic angiography view showing an anomalous connection of the left main (white star) with the pulmonary trunk (black arrow) with an enlarged right coronary artery (white arrow) filling by a retrograde flow the left coronary circulation.

3.8 Other abnormalities (type VIII)

Numerous other ANOCOR have been reported in the literature, but with a very low incidence. Beside anomalous connections in the aorta or the pulmonary artery, an ectopic origin from a brachiocephalic artery, bronchial artery or internal mammary artery is possible, but anecdotal. A rotation of the aortic root may modify the position of normal coronary origin regarding the pulmonary trunk or subpulmonary infundibulum. The latter is on the border between a true ANOCOR and an acquired anomaly.

4. Prevalence

Data are numerous in literature about the angiographic prevalence of congenital coronary abnormalities. The latter are found in >1% including abnormalities of origin and distribution, anomalies of coronary termination, and often some anatomical variants. If any anatomical pattern observed in >1% of an unselected population is considered as normal or variant of normal, then an anomalous origin of the coronary arteries is not exceptional. Indeed, the angiographic prevalence is around 0.5% in a cohort pooling several studies published since 1990 (Angelini et al., 1999, Aydinlar et al., 2005, Cieslinski et al., 1993, Garg et al., 2000, Kardos et al., 1997, Ouali et al., 2009, Rigatelli et al., 2003, Tuncer et al., 2006, Yamanaka et al., 1990) and with the possibility to individualise clearly the following ANOCOR: anomalous connection with the opposite sinus or non-coronary sinus, anomalous connection with the contralateral coronary artery, single coronary artery, and anomalous connection with the pulmonary artery. The latter was excluded in one study (Ouali, 2009). In this large (n=236,694) and relatively homogeneous cohort of adults with no structural congenital defect, 1 067 anomalous origins were identified, therefore a mean prevalence of 0.45% (table 3). The latter is ranged between 0.2 and 1.7%. The highest prevalence is observed in the sole prospective study, rather performed by a well-renowned team, recognized as an expert in the field of ANOCOR (Angelini et al., 1999). Otherwise, a misdiagnosis (as in most cases of "missing" coronary arteries) may explain some differences of prevalence, especially in the old retrospective studies. The high take-off from the aorta and the anomalous connection with an unusual site of the appropriate sinus were not included in this cohort.

Authors	Coronary angiograms n	Anomalous connections n	Anomalous connections %
Angelini, 1999	1,950	34	1.7
Aydinlar, 2005	12,059	39	0.3
Cieslinski, 1993	4,016	22	0.5
Garg, 2000	4,100	35	0.9
Kardos, 1997	7,694	39	0.5
Ouali, 2009	7,330	20	0.3
Rigatelli, 2003	5,100	34	0.7
Tuncer, 2006	70,850	110	0.2
Yamanaka, 1990	126,595	734	0.6
Total	236,694	1,067	0.45

Table 3. Angiographic prevalence of proximal anomalous connections of the coronary arteries in adult populations.

The prevalence of ANOCOR varies according to the type of coronary artery and connection (table 4). The most frequent anomaly involves the CX coronary artery with a prevalence of 3/1 000, while the anomalous connection with the pulmonary artery is the less frequent abnormality with a prevalence of 8/100 000. Both anomalous connections of the LMCA and of the LAD coronary artery are observed with a prevalence of 2/10 000. The prevalence of an ectopic origin of the RCA is of 1/1 000. The related frequency (4/10 000) of a single artery is certainly overestimated in the cohort. Indeed, contrary to the classification used in our review, most previous studies categorized a single ostium with an abnormal proximal course, as a single artery. Some patterns, generally not counted, are identified with difficulty by angiography. That is the case of an abnormal origin above the sinotubular junction. Two-hundred-and four (0.2%) high take-off from the aorta, most commonly the RCA, were reported in a large study (Yamanaka et al., 1997). In only one study (Angelini et al., 1999), an anomalous connection with an unusual site of the appropriate sinus was noticed, regarding the RCA without exception, with a prevalence of 1.1%. Few studies distinguished origin from the opposite sinus and from the contralateral artery. In the CASS study, among 71 anomalous origins, 52 (73%) arose from the opposite sinus and 19 (27%) from the contralateral artery (Click et al., 1988).

Type of anomaly	Number	%
Anomalous aortic connection of the left main coronary artery	49	0.02
Anomalous aortic connection of the left anterior descending coronary artery	55	0.02
Anomalous aortic connection of the circumflex coronary artery	636	0.3
Anomalous aortic connection of the right coronary artery	226	0.1
Anomalous connection with the pulmonary artery	18	0.008
Single artery	83	0.04

Table 4. Angiographic prevalence of abnormalities of the coronary arteries according to the type of coronary artery and connection in a population of 236,694 adults.

A more accurate analysis of ANOCOR needs other imaging modalities. The diagnosis of some ANOCOR suspected during conventional angiography should be confirmed by cardiac CT scan. The studies (Fujimoto et al., 2011, Rodriguez-Granillo et al. 2009, Schmitt et al., 2005) assessing the prevalence of ANOCOR with CT scan reported a higher rate of abnormalities, even if the patients referred for CT following selective coronary angiography were excluded (table 5). This fact is due on several reasons. On the one hand, a more accurate diagnosis of ANOCOR is performed with CT scan in comparison with conventional coronary angiography. On the other hand, some patterns of ANOCOR are easily discovered only by CT scan, such as anomalous connection with an unusual site of the appropriate sinus, high take-off form the aorta or orthotropic origins from the clockwise or counter-clockwise rotated aortic root (Schmitt 2005). With these additional abnormalities, the CT prevalence of ANOCOR, in a cohort pooling 8,184 adults from 3 studies (table 5), is of 1.3%.

Authors	Computed tomography n	Anomalous connections n	Anomalous connections %
Fujimoto, 2011	5,869	74	1.3
Rodriguez-Granillo, 2009	577	6	1.0
Schmitt, 2005	1,738	24	1.4
Total	8,184	104	1.3

Table 5. Computed tomography prevalence of anomalous connections of the coronary arteries in adult populations.

The prevalence of ANOCOR in a general population, for example at birth, remains unknown. Large studies based on an autopsy population without methodological biases are lacking. Otherwise, the aforementioned angiographic prevalence involves, almost without exception, adult populations.

5. Orifices, initial and ectopic courses

An exact analysis of the orifices and courses of ANOCOR is of crucial importance, while the pathophysiological mechanisms of cardiac adverse events are mainly based on anatomical findings.

5.1 Orifices

A normal coronary orifice is more or less round, or slightly ovoid. Our knowledge about orifices of ANOCOR is mostly taken from postmortem (Frescura et al., 1998, Kragel et al., 1988) and individual peroperative examinations. The invasive coronary arteriography has understandable limitations for the visualization of the orifice shape. More recently, qualitative and quantitative assessment of the orifices and initial paths of ANOCOR has been documented by IVUS during conventional coronary angiography (Angelini et al., 2003). It is important to consider that an anomalous origin of a coronary artery does not imply systematically an abnormal shape of its orifice. The ANOCOR connected with the contralateral artery must have, in theory, a normal coronary orifice. Indeed, the initial segment, the first millimetres at least, of the ectopic coronary has a normal angulation (>45°) with the contralateral artery. On the contrary, the anomalous origins from the inappropriate sinus with an initial course tangential to aorta are most often associated with an abnormal orifice. A slit-like ostium is generally described in the postmortem descriptions. A similar feature is found by surgeons through an intra aortic view (figure 8). Rare selective coronary angiograms suggest the presence of a membrane-like ostial stenosis (Angelini et al., 2006). As mentioned above, an abnormal orifice of a coronary artery connected with the usual site of the appropriate sinus has been described, but rarely (Frescura et al., 1998).

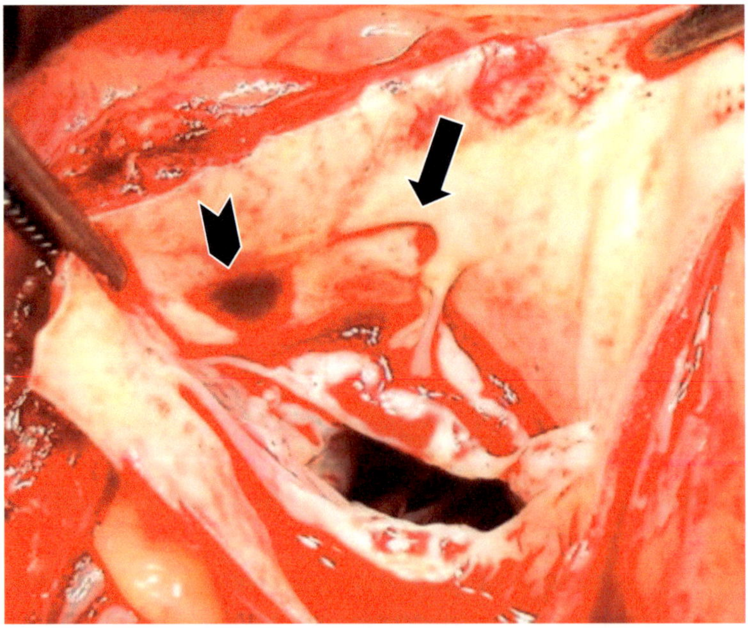

Fig. 8. Peroperative view showing an ectopic origin of the right coronary artery (arrow) from the left sinus close to the origin of the left coronary artery (arrowhead).

5.2 Initial courses

It is admitted that a slit-like orifice, almost without exception, is associated with an intramural course. The latter means a course of the first millimetres of the ectopic vessel in the aortic media. Therefore, no adventitia exists between the coronary media and aortic media. The length of the intramural path is ranged from 5 to 25 mm, much longer for the left ANOCOR (Angelini & Flamm, 2007). An intramural course is not synonymous with a preaortic course, and inversely (Houyel & Planché, 2008). The ANOCOR arising from the opposite sinus, and without a preaortic or retroaortic course, have generally a normal orifice, while they move quickly from the aorta, and their initial courses are therefore extramural. The ANOCOR with a retroaortic course have in most cases a juxtamural course regarding the aorta, although rare observations with abnormal orifice and/or intramural course have been reported. The ANOCOR with a high take-off above the sinotubular junction may have an abnormal orifice with a vertical intramural initial course. Generally, the orifice of the anomalous connections with the pulmonary artery is circular with an extramural or juxtamural initial course. Coronary IVUS, now easily available, gives important quantitative parameters regarding the orifices and initial courses of ANOCOR (Angelini & Flamm 2007). The ellipsoid shape of an ectopic orifice is well visualized. Also important, coronary IVUS highlighted systematically a hypoplasia of the intramural segment in comparison with the more distal, extramural segment.

5.3 Ectopic courses

The ectopic course of an ANOCOR may be defined as the coronary path between the orifice and the point where the ectopic artery meet up with an appropriate myocardial area. The length of the ectopic course varies considerably regarding the site of ectopic ostium and relationships with the adjacent structures. The definitions of different ectopic courses are still used in an ambiguous fashion. Usually, 4 subgroups of anomalous origin of the LCA from the opposite sinus are described: anterior to pulmonary trunk, between aorta and pulmonary trunk, in ventricular septum, and posterior to aorta courses (Roberts & Shirani, 1992). For the purpose of being close to the anatomical descriptions and recent imaging contributions, we classify the ANOCOR into 7 courses relating to their links with the great vessels and/or ventricles (table 6). We chose to define each course according to the closest adjacent cardiac structure (figure 9).

type A	preinfundibular course
type B	retroinfundibular course
type C	preaortic course with intramural path
type D	preaortic course without intramural path
type E	retroaortic course
type F	absent proximal ectopic course
type G	other ectopic courses

Table 6. Different courses of anomalous origins of the coronary arteries.

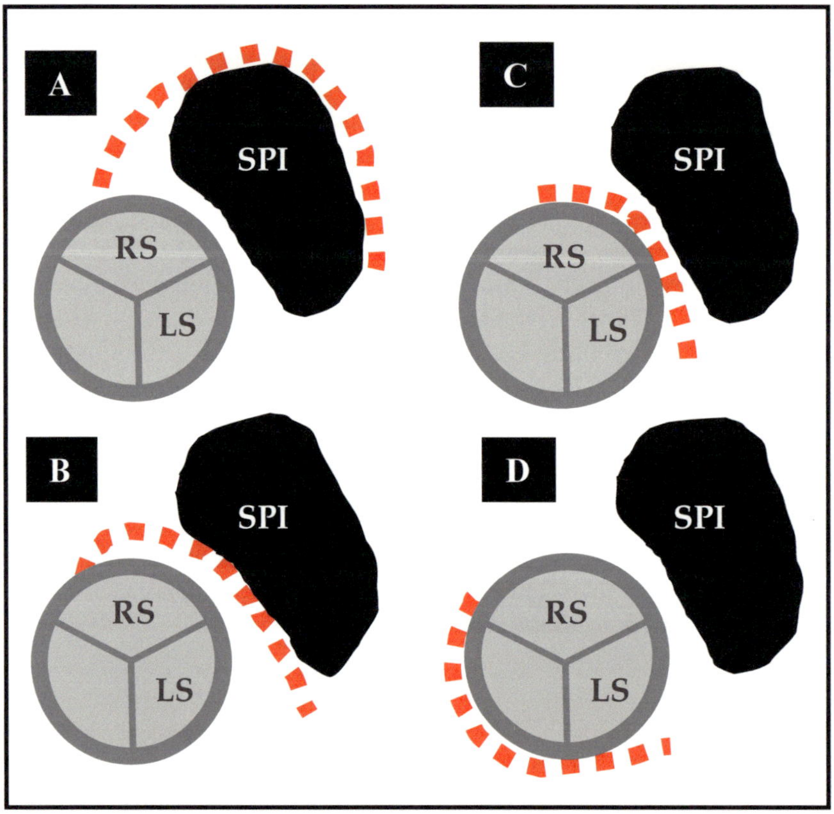

Fig. 9. Anatomic representation of the courses of an anomalous left coronary artery arising from the right sinus. A: preinfundibular course, B: retroinfundibular course, C: preaortic course, D: retroaortic course. LS: left sinus, RS: right sinus.

5.3.1 Preinfundibular course (type A)

The prepulmonary course involves the ectopic paths coursing on the surface of the pulmonary trunk or subpulmonary infundibulum. The latter is mostly concerned. In case of a long and sinuous course, both pulmonary trunk and subpulmonary infundibulum may be in contact with the ectopic vessel. The vessel coursing with a prepulmonary path, almost without exception, is the left coronary artery (LMCA or LAD or septal branch arising from the opposite sinus or the RCA).

5.3.2 Retroinfundibular course (type B)

A clear understanding of the retroinfundibular course remains difficult. Due to a low risk of lethal cardiac events, examinations of heart specimens with a retroinfundibular course are rare. However, tomographic imaging allowed a better analysis of their relationships with the adjacent structures (figure 10). The retroinfundibular course, without exception, involves the LCA and their branches. The ectopic vessel first courses behind the subpulmonary infundibulum, then crosses between the latter and the ventricular septum, and finally emerges from the interventricular space to join the left ventricle on the epicardial surface at the mid LAD level. In the literature, the retroinfundibular course is also known as subpulmonic or intraseptal or intraconal course. The nomenclature used in this review appears more appropriate regarding the cardiac anatomy. The left coronary artery (LMCA or LAD) with retroinfundibular course provide always one or more septal branches in the floor of the right ventricular outflow tract.

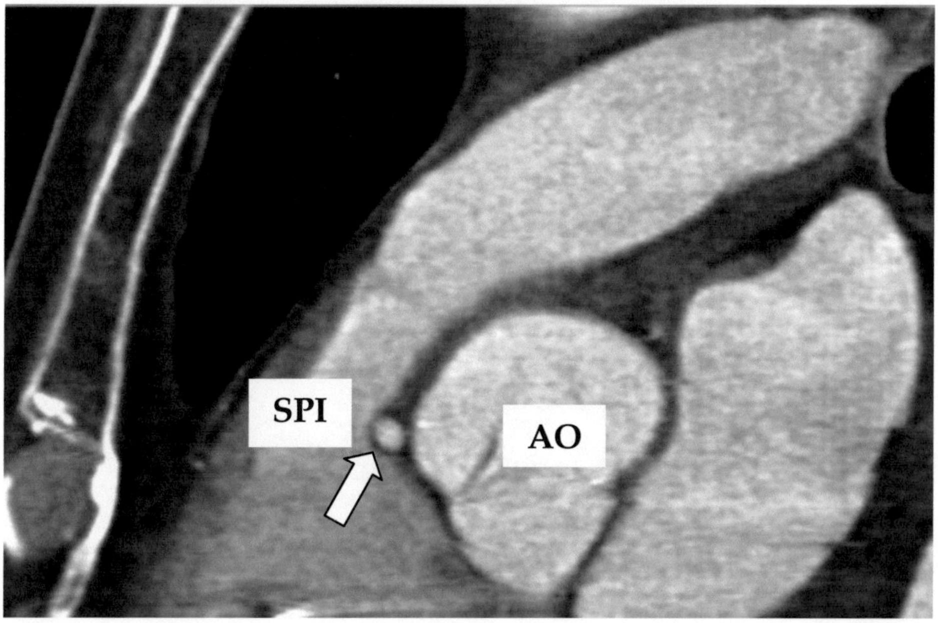

Fig. 10. Computed tomography imaging of an ectopic left main coronary artery (arrow) arising from the right sinus with a retroinfundibular course. AO: aorta, SPI: subpulmonary infundibulum.

5.3.3 Preaortic course with intramural segment (type C)

The typical preaortic course is tangential to the aorta through the fibroadipose tissue separating the arterial roots, (figure 11). Nomenclatures using the so-called interarterial course, in other words between the aorta and the pulmonary artery, may be ambiguous. In fact, a LCA connected in the opposite sinus or contralateral artery, and coursing anterior to the aorta, is in contact first with the subpulmonary infundibulum. A close contact with the pulmonary trunk is also possible because a LCA arising from the opposite sinus with a preaortic path, courses distally near the usual origin of the vessel before to join the interventricular groove. Conversely, an ectopic RCA is in contact first with the pulmonary trunk and then with the subpulmonary infundibulum before to join the atrioventricular groove. ANOCOR with high take-off from the aorta above the sinuses have, by definition, a preaortic course. The presence of an intramural segment, as defined above, must be systematically looked for in order to stratify the risk.

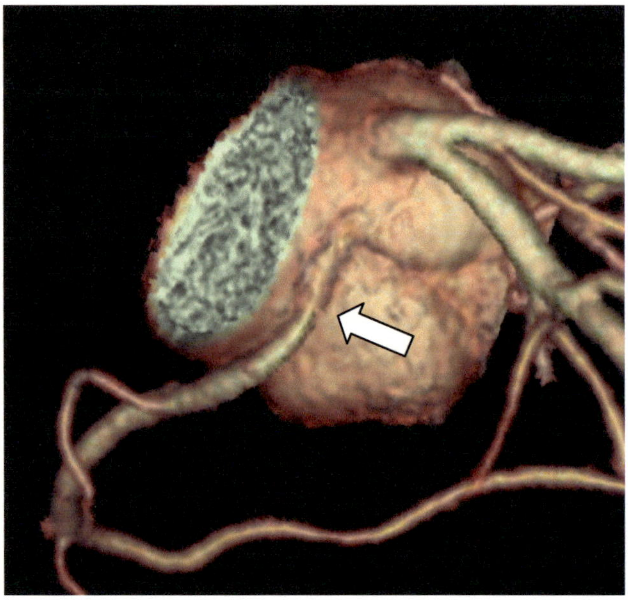

Fig. 11. Volume-rendered computed tomography images of an ectopic right coronary artery (arrow) arising from the left sinus with a preaortic course tangential to the aorta.

5.3.4 Preaortic course without intramural segment (type D)

As mentioned before, a preaortic course without intramural segment is possible, for example an ectopic vessel with an orthogonal take-off from the contralateral or a high origin from the aorta. The ectopic course is juxtamural with the aorta. Making a distinction between preaortic course without intramural segment and preaortic course with intramural course is essential, while the latter has a recognized higher risk of life-threatening symptoms.

5.3.5 Retroaortic course (type E)

The retroaortic course, the most commonly encountered ectopic course, is also the easier to diagnose. This course involves, almost without exception, the LCA. Unlike other coronary arteries, the CX coronary artery is associated, to the exclusion of uncommon patterns, with the same ectopic course, i.e. a retroaortic course. The ectopic vessel courses first behind or more precisely below the aorta, then crosses between the aortic root and the left atrium with a juxtamural course, and finally emerges into the left atrioventricular groove between the left atrial appendage and the left atrium (figure 12).

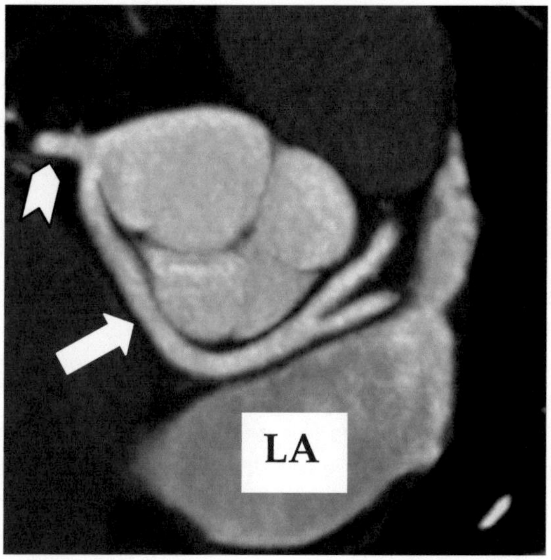

Fig. 12. Computed tomography imaging of anomalous connection of the left main coronary artery (arrow) with the right sinus close to the right coronary artery (arrowhead). LA : left atrium.

5.3.6 Absent proximal ectopic course (type F)

As mentioned above, a single coronary artery is never associated with an abnormal proximal course. The myocardium usually dependant on the absent coronary artery is fed by a retrograde flow using a coronary network, near normal. Besides, a coronary artery, connected with the contralateral artery far from the proximal segment of the latter, may have normal relationships with the cardiac structures.

5.3.7 Other ectopic courses (type G)

Rare ANOCOR, such as abnormal origin from the aortic arch, may have another ectopic course, often complex, in contact with several structures. A LMCA with an anomalous connection with the pulmonary trunk courses usually facing the left side of the latter.

6. Angiographic diagnosis of ectopic vessels and courses

6.1 Angiographic diagnosis of ectopic vessels

The diagnosis of ANOCOR in adult patients is usually suspected or achieved during a selective coronary angiography scheduled to evaluate or to rule out a CAD. The invasive coronary angiography is no longer considered the method of choice, in other terms *the gold standard*, for an accurate diagnosis of ANOCOR. Studies have described the correlations between invasive angiography and CT angiography but always in small populations. Correct identification of the ectopic vessel was achieved by conventional angiography in 69% (9/13) of ANOCOR (Shi et al., 2004). Selective catheterization and precise vessel determination was possible in only 53% (8/15) of ANOCOR (Schmitt et al., 2005). The coronary abnormality was accurately depicted in 44% (4/9) of ANOCOR (de Jonge et al., 2008). Several shortcomings of the conventional angiography are obvious, such as a difficult canulation of the abnormal orifice, a two-dimensional interpretation of the ectopic course, or an incomplete visualization of the ectopic vessel, leading to an erroneous diagnosis, particularly if the angiographer is not aware with the congenital coronary abnormalities. In addition, the selective coronary angiography is not able to analyse the shape of the ectopic orifice, to quantify a hypoplasic segment exactly, or to identify an intramural course. Despite these limitations, often some angiographic views typically make an interpretation easier.

6.1.1 Angiographic diagnosis of anomalous connection with the opposite sinus (type I)

Selective angiography of some ANOCOR arising from the opposite sinus may be a challenge, especially with the RCA. The origin of the latter is often characteristic with an orifice at the level of the sinotubular junction and close to the commissural zone between the right and the left coronary cusps. The two ostia are generally non adjacent, which explains why the catheter used for the LCA does not generally find the ectopic right orifice. Other catheters (Judkins right, Amplatz left) are required. Nevertheless, the ellipsoid shape of the orifice and the lack of orthogonal take-off, explain the non rare failures of satisfactory angiography. Instead of an additional aortography, usually not very contributory, a tomographic imaging will allow the diagnosis of ANOCOR to be confirmed or not. When selective angiography is possible, the views of an ectopic RCA originated from the left sinus are typical, with a normal or slightly enlarged ostial lumen in the 30° left anterior oblique (LAO) projection, while a narrowing of the first segment is visible in the 30° right anterior oblique (RAO) projection, expressing the ellipsoid shape of the orifice and the initial intramural course (figure 13).

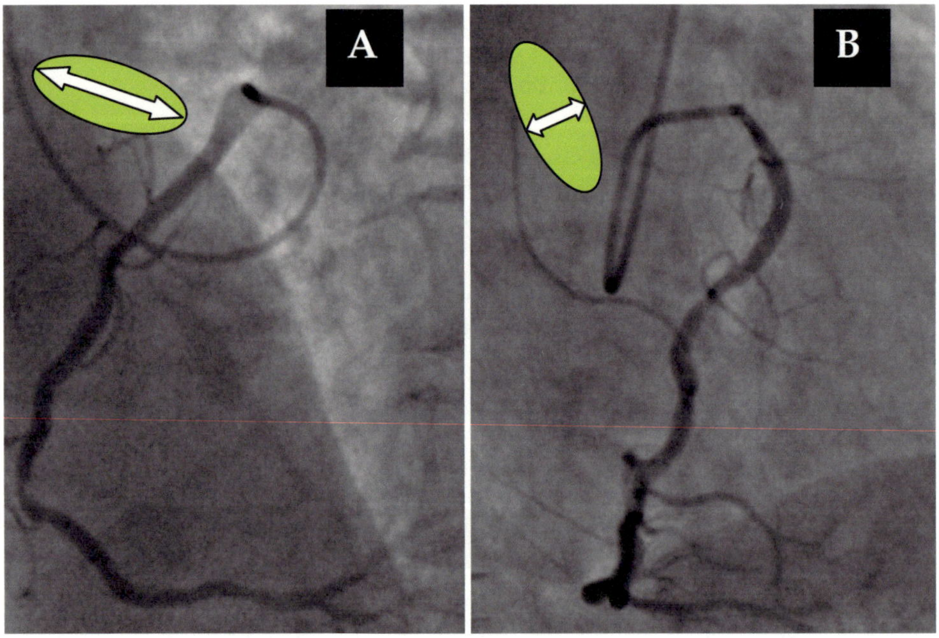

Fig. 13. Selective angiogram of an anomalous connection of the right coronary artery with the left sinus in 20° left anterior oblique projection (A) and left 30° right anterior oblique projection (B) with a schematic representation of X-ray plane (arrow).

The ectopic orifice of the left coronary artery (LMCA, LAD coronary artery or CX coronary artery) is in most cases very close to the right coronary orifice, and sometimes contiguous. Thus, a selective angiography is generally easier using Judkins right catheter or Amplatz left or right catheters. A multipurpose catheter may be useful to catheterize the orifice of an aberrant circumflex coronary artery.

6.1.2 Angiographic diagnosis of anomalous connection with the contralateral artery (type II)

Obviously, angiographic diagnosis of anomalous connection with the contralateral artery is usually easy, with the exception of a too selective angiography leading to a misdiagnosis, for example an ectopic CX coronary artery originated from the proximal segment of the RCA.

6.1.3 Angiographic diagnosis of anomalous connection with the appropriate sinus (type III)

A lack of identification remains possible. Diagnosis of anomalous connection with the appropriate sinus is usually only suspected with X-ray coronary angiography, and contribution of tomographic imaging is essential.

6.1.4 Angiographic diagnosis of anomalous connection with the non-coronary sinus (type IV)

Angiographic diagnosis of anomalous origin from the non-coronary sinus is always challenging with frequent difficulties of a selective canulation. Moreover, the interpretation of angiographic views is often ambiguous and needs complementary imaging.

6.1.5 Angiographic diagnosis of anomalous connection above the sinotubular junction (type V)

Difficulties in identifying a high take-off from the aorta by conventional angiography are non unusual. Many catheters, similar to these used for saphenous vein grafts, are often required. Moreover, an initial intramural course may make selective injections more difficult. Finally, the distinction between a normal variant of origin and a high take-off at least 10 mm above the sinotubular junction is ambiguous in most cases. Once again, the coronary CT angiography will be able to delineate accurately the level of the coronary ostia.

6.1.6 Angiographic diagnosis of single coronary artery (type VI)

The diagnosis of a single coronary artery is easy with a single orifice in the appropriate sinus and the lack of ectopic proximal course. All major coronary arteries course the atrioventricular and interventricular grooves. Coronary angiography needs large fields to visualize the whole coronary circulation.

6.1.7 Angiographic diagnosis of anomalous connection with the pulmonary artery (type VII)

Conventional angiography of anomalous connection with the pulmonary artery is not always easy. Indeed, the contralateral artery, mostly the RCA, is considerably enlarged with an ostial diameter around 10 mm and a diffused dilation of the artery, making a selective intubation and an adequate opacification with regular coronary catheters difficult. An aortography in LAO projection is useful allowing simultaneous visualization of the aorta and the pulmonary trunk. The most common site of drainage is the pulmonary trunk. Multiple collateral vessels coursing the subpulmonary infundibulum and the right ventricle are present, as well as a large collateral circulation through the interventricular septum, between the RCA and the LCA.

6.1.8 Angiographic diagnosis of other anomalies (type VIII)

Rare abnormal origins, apart from aorta, contralateral coronary artery and pulmonary artery, are generally never identified by conventional angiography.

6.2 Angiographic diagnosis of ectopic courses

As mentioned above, the rate of an accurate diagnosis of ANOCOR is relatively low (<70%) with conventional angiography. Correct angiographic identification of the different possible courses followed by an ectopic vessel is achievable, but requires special training. Numerous examples of misinterpretation of the ectopic course in the literature imply that the rate of erroneous delineation is certainly high in the real life. Before the wide growth of non-invasive imaging, some authors have proposed interesting methods to identify the different anomalous courses of ANOCOR quickly and correctly (Ishikawa & Brandt, 1985, Serota et al., 1990). As the ectopic course of RCA and CX, almost without exception, is typical with a preaortic course and a retroaortic course respectively, these methods are only dedicated to the LCA (LCMA or LAD coronary artery) originated from the opposite sinus or the contralateral artery. The LCA may follow 1 of 4 previously described paths: preinfundibular, retroinfundibular, preaortic and retroaortic. The angiographic criteria used by Serota et al. are based on selective coronary angiograms in the RAO and LAO projections. The method suggested by Ishikawa et al. use angiographic features derived from a selective coronary angiogram in RAO projection and from a 30° RAO ventriculography. The lateral projection may be helpful in some cases. The main features are summarized in table 7. Despite of a meticulous analysis, these methods are sometimes incorrect.

6.2.1 Angiographic diagnosis of preinfundibular course

The LCA courses on the surface of the subpulmonary infundibulum and sometimes the root of the pulmonary artery, and reaches the interventricular septum at the mid LAD level. Therefore, the LAD coronary artery is relatively short. In RAO and LAO projections, the initial course of the LCA passes anteriorly and upward. The LMCA and the proximal segment of the CX coronary artery form an "eye" with the LMCA as the superior edge and the CX coronary artery as the inferior edge (figure 14).

6.2.2 Angiographic diagnosis of retroinfundibular course

The LCA courses behind the subpulmonary infundibulum, then in contact with the left ventricular septum, and finally emerges at mid LAD level. Thus, the LAD coronary artery is relatively short. In RAO and LAO projections, the initial course of the LCA passes anteriorly and downward. The upward loop of the CX coronary artery and the LMCA form an "eye". Septal branches arising from the LMCA are an additional clue (figure 15).

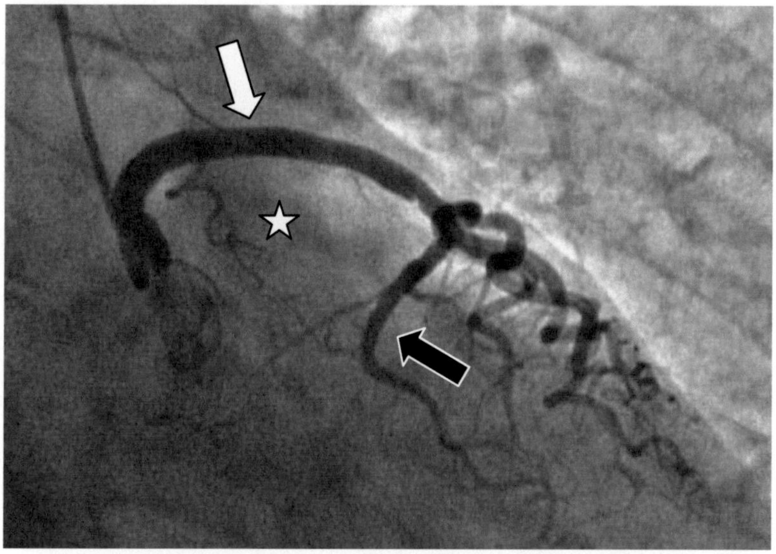

Fig. 14. Angiographic view (right anterior oblique projection) showing a preinfundibular course of a left main coronary artery (white arrow) forming an "eye" (star) with the circumflex coronary artery (black arrow).

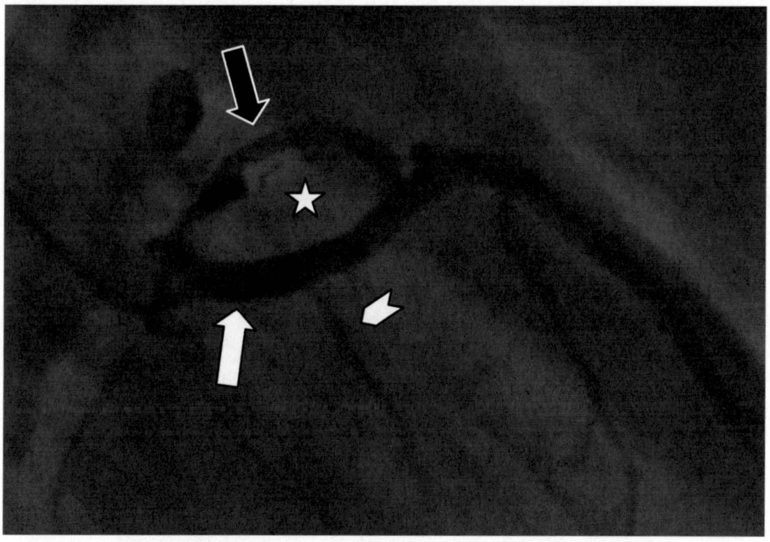

Fig. 15. Angiographic view (right anterior oblique projection) showing a retroinfundibular course of a left main coronary artery (white arrow) forming an "eye" (star) with the circumflex coronary artery (black arrow). Note a septal branch (arrow head) originated from the left main coronary artery.

6.2.3 Angiographic diagnosis of preaortic course

The LCA courses initially between the aorta and subpulmonary infundibulum, and behind the pulmonary trunk at left coronary sinus level. Then, the LMCA follows a normal course to its bifurcation. Therefore, all segments of the LAD coronary artery are visualized, and the orientation of the CX coronary artery is normal. The initial course of the LMCA is upward and slightly posterior in RAO and LAO projections (figure 16). During 30° RAO ventriculography, the distal LMCA appears as a radiopaque "dot", anterior to the aorta.

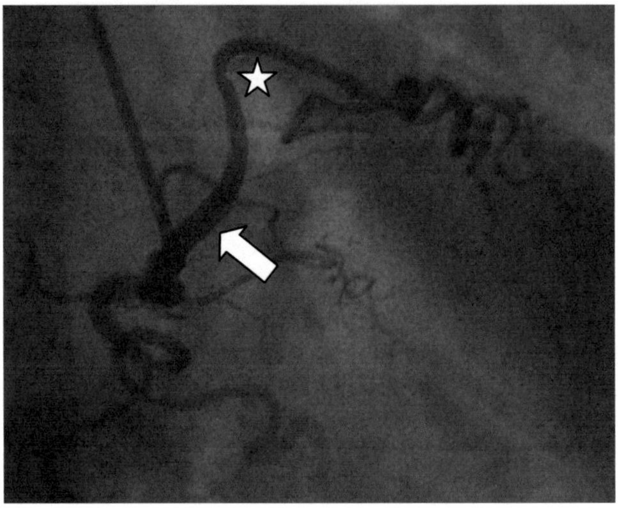

Fig. 16. Angiographic view (right anterior oblique projection) showing a preaortic course of a left main coronary artery (white arrow) arising from the right sinus with a posterior and upward loop (star).

6.2.4 Angiographic diagnosis of retroaortic course

The LCA courses behind or beneath the aorta and emerges at the left atrioventricular groove. In RAO and LAO projections, the LCA passes posteriorly and downward (figure 17). During 30° RAO ventriculography, the mid LCA appears as a radiopaque "dot", posterior to the aorta.

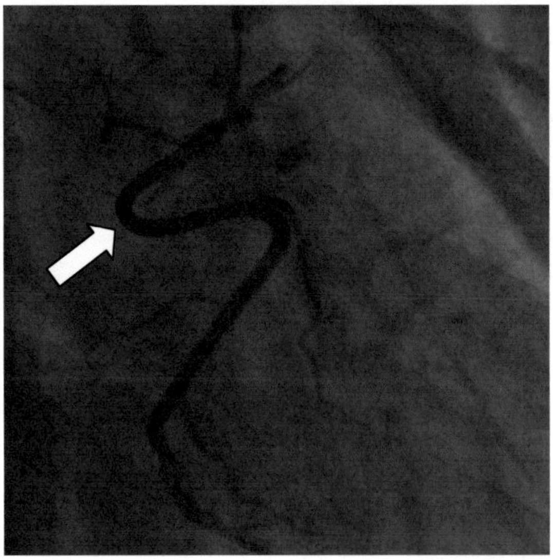

Fig 17. Angiographic (right anterior oblique projection) view showing a retroaortic course of an ectopic circumflex coronary artery (arrow) arising from the right sinus.

	ectopic course	initial loop	eye sign	dot sign	LAD length	septal branches
type A	preinfundibular	anterior and upward	yes	no	short	no
type B	retroinfundibular	anterior and downward	yes	no	short	yes
types C and D	preaortic	posterior and upward	no	yes	normal	no
type E	retroaortic	posterior and downward	no	yes	normal	no

Table 7. Main angiographic characteristics of ectopic courses of anomalous connections of the left coronary artery with the opposite sinus or contralateral artery. LAD: left anterior descending coronary artery.

7. Intravascular ultrasonography (IVUS)

IVUS is an intracoronary imaging technique which provides qualitative and quantifiable features of the coronary anatomy in ANOCOR. Its high spatial resolution about 0.15 mm achieves a good anatomic visualization of the coronary artery wall. Other imaging modalities are not too competitive to analyse the shape and area of the ectopic orifice, and to identify an intramural segment. In this field, the contribution of the group of Angelini has been essential with a routinely use of IVUS in ANOCOR with a suspected intramural course (Angelini et al., 2003, Angelini et al., 2006, Angelini, 2007, Angelini & Flamm, 2007). In ANOCOR with intramural segment, IVUS imaging often visualizes the aortic wall at the level of the ectopic orifice. Several features, similar to histological and anatomical characteristics of ANOCOR with an intramural course, are well depicted by IVUS. Pharmacologic provocative tests may be associated during IVUS procedure. IVUS use is mentioned in ACC/AHA 2008 guidelines for adults with congenital heart disease, with a recommendation of class IIa and a level of evidence C, in order to delineate potential mechanisms of flow restriction (Warnes et al., 2008). Angelini et al. have defined several consistent IVUS characteristics regarding to ANOCOR with intramural segment (Angelini & Flamm, 2007).

7.1 Abnormal orifice

The orifice is never circular with an ovoid or ellipsoidal shape. The area of the slit-like ostium is not necessary significantly reduced, like during selective coronary angiography. It is the fact that the longest diameter of the orifice may be as long as the diameter of the distal segment. Importantly, the IVUS shows a normal intima tunica without atherosclerotic plaque.

7.2 Intramural hypoplasia

An IVUS hypoplasia of the intramural segment is demonstrated with a ratio <1.0 between the intramural minimal circumference and the distal reference circumference. The length of the intramural segment, generally ranged from 5 to 15 mm, may vary depending of the site of the ectopic orifice. The narrowing diameters and surfaces must be compared with the distal reference parameters. The baseline area of stenosis is the ratio between the distal area (mm^2) minus the intramural area (mm^2), and the distal area (mm^2). The degree of area obstruction varies between 30 and 70%.

7.3 Lateral compression

The intramural segment of the ectopic has an abnormal shape (figure 18), resulting from a shared media with the aorta and a probably incomplete growth of the ectopic vessel in the aortic wall. The cross section is more or less oblong. The lateral compression is defined as a smaller area than that possessed by a circle of the same circumference. This parameter is quantified with the asymmetric ratio of the smallest to the largest diameter <1.0.

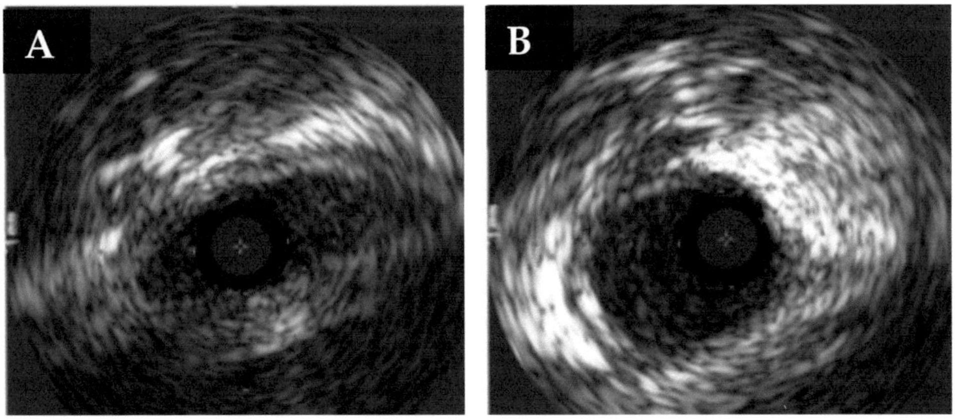

Fig. 18. Intravascular ultrasound images showing the intramural segment (A) and the extramural segment (B) of an ectopic right coronary artery connected with the left sinus.

Despite first promising results, the IVUS imaging tool has several limits. Non selective canulation of the vessel may disrupt the procedure. The possibility of artefacts has been pointed out, as well as the decreasing in the precision of measurements, due to the tangential orientation of the vessel (Angelini & Flamm, 2007). Moreover, ST-T changes and angina may occur during IVUS manoeuvres.

8. Non-invasive imaging modalities

Selective coronary angiography does not always assure the diagnosis of ANOCOR, particularly to identify accurately the origin of the RCA from the left sinus, or to delineate the initial course of an ectopic vessel. Over the last decade, the multislice tomographic imaging made dramatically breakthroughs, so much that the electrocardiography-gated multidetector coronary CT angiography has become the method of choice for evaluation of known or suspected ANOCOR (Sundaram et al., 2010). Tomographic reconstructed images provide useful supplemental information with volumetric views allowing an analysis of ANOCOR in 3-D spatial orientation (Gharib et al., 2008, Manghat et al., 2005). However, other non-invasive methods have been used to diagnose or evaluate ANOCOR.

8.1 Echocardiography

Transthoracic echocardiography (TTE) is not commonly used to examine the coronary arteries. The parasternal short-axis plane, with the help of the colour flow mapping, is the best view for an echographic visualization of the coronary origins (Frommelt et al., 2003). Nevertheless, the ability of the TTE to identify the coronary origins with confidence becomes less easy with age and increase in the body mass. Transoesophageal echocardiography (TEE) may improve the imaging quality (figure 19) but not necessarily the diagnostic ability. Several studies have reported the echocardiographic prevalence of ANOCOR particularly in paediatric populations or young adults. An anomalous connection with the opposite sinus was found in 4 cases (0.2%) in a series of 2388 children or adolescents referred for innocent murmurs or functional assessments (Davis et al., 2001), and in 3 cases (0.09%) in 3504 (mean age, 30 years) asymptomatic athletes (Zeppilli et al., 1998). In the latter study a clear visualization of both ostia was obtained in 90% of cases. Therefore, the echographic prevalence is lower than those reported with selective coronary angiography and tomographic imaging techniques. The limited discriminating power of TTE to distinguish some ANOCOR may explain this discrepancy. TTE lacks reliability to identify a small RCA or CX coronary artery with an ectopic origin. Besides, an ectopic vessel with preaortic course crosses very closely the appropriate sinus, and thus may pretend a normal origin. Nevertheless, in young adults or in patients with a satisfactory acoustic window, several echographic characteristics must be known (Cohen et al., 2010). An abnormal diastolic colour flow between the aorta and the pulmonary trunk is often the first identification of an ANOCOR with a preaortic course. However, only the first millimetres of the ectopic vessel are visualized, and, often, the TTE is inconclusive in ruling out some ectopic paths. Thus, a suspected retroinfundibular or preaortic course with TTE should be always confirmed with other imaging modalities. In addition, TTE is not able to describe the shape of an ectopic orifice and to measure a possible ostial narrowing. TEE may identify some high take-off above the sinotubular junction with the long-axis view. Echographic diagnosis of anomalous origin of the LCA from the pulmonary trunk is mainly based on indirect features with a dilation of the RCA and a multiple collateral flow through the interventricular septum. In practice, the management of an ANOCOR should never be discussed with only echocardiographic imaging in adult patient.

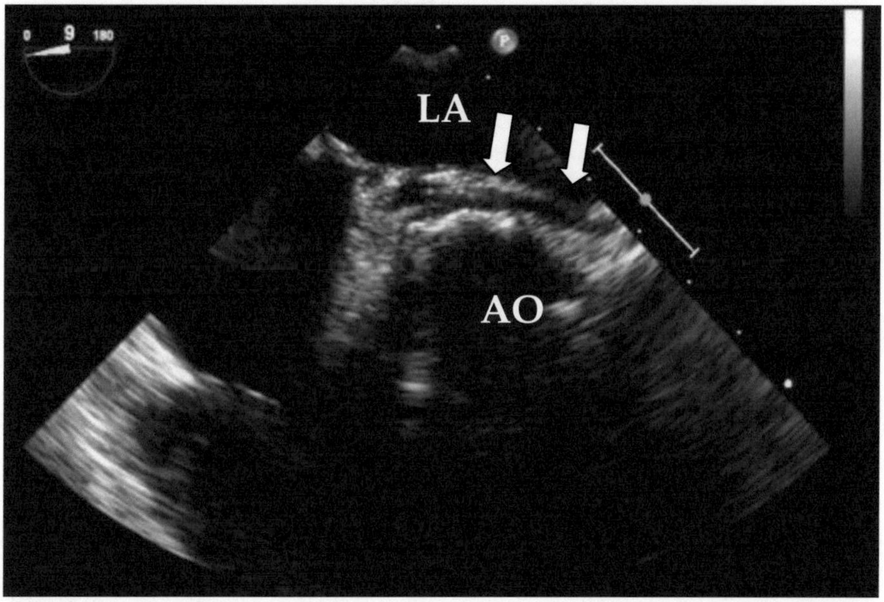

Fig. 19. Short-axis transoesphageal echocardiographic view showing an ectopic circumflex coronary artery (arrows) coursing between the aorta (AO) and the left atrium (LA) with a retroaortic course.

8.2 Magnetic resonance angiography

Magnetic resonance (MR) angiography is a non invasive imaging technique that does not expose to ionizing radiation and to potentially nephrotoxic contrast media. Cardiac MR angiography allows 3-D reconstruction of the heart and can identify the origin of coronary arteries (figure 20). The relationships with neighbouring structures are well visualized. Nonetheless, due to insufficient spatial resolution and cardiac movements, this imaging technique fails sometimes to describe accurately the anatomy of the ectopic course of the ANOCOR, especially the orifice and the visualization of a lateral compression in the aortic wall. Otherwise, MR angiography is a less available technique in comparison to the CT angiography, and identifies not as good the degree of atherosclerotic associated lesions. Nevertheless, coronary MR angiography remains an attractive option in young population to avoid ionizing radiation. Several studies have shown the feasibility of coronary MR angiography to identify ANOCOR. In a selected population of 19 patients with known ANOCOR by a previous selective coronary angiography, sensitivity and sensibility for detecting anomalous origins and ectopic courses were 100% with MR angiography (Post et al., 1995). Delineation of the ectopic course was erroneous in 3 of 19 patients (16%) with the conventional coronary angiography. The hypothesis that MR angiography may be useful in the identification of ANOCOR was confirmed in 12 of 14 patients (86%) with a known anomaly (Mc Connell et al., 1995). A series of 21 patients with known or suspected ANOCOR (9 LMCA or LAD coronary arteries, 6 CX coronary arteries and 6 RCA) underwent a MR angiography (Bunce et al., 2003). All patients had undergone a selective coronary angiography but in 11 patients (52%) the proximal course was uncertain.

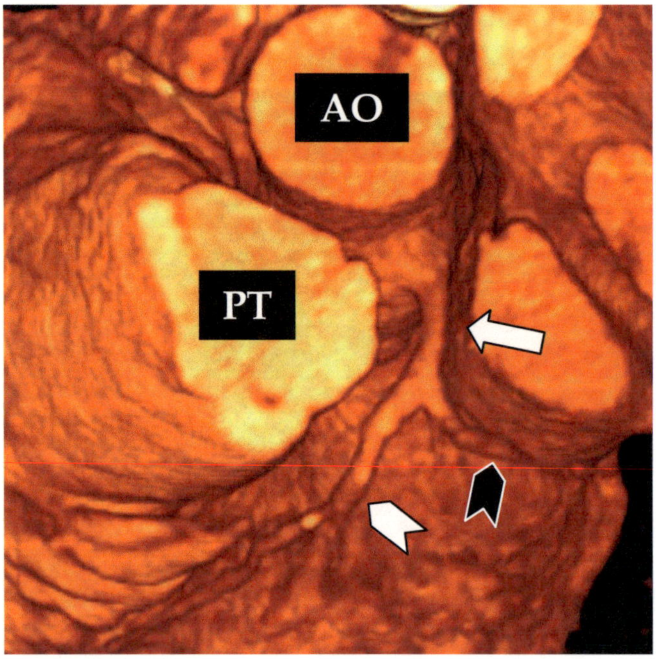

Fig. 20. Volume-rendered magnetic resonance angiography showing a normal origin of the left main coronary artery (arrow) dividing into left anterior descending coronary artery (white arrow head) and circumflex coronary artery (black arrow head). AO: aorta, PT: pulmonary trunk.

In addition, selective canulation of ectopic vessel was not possible in 3 cases, and the ectopic artery was not identified in 1 case. MR angiography depicted correctly all ANOCOR, and in 13 patients (62%) a preaortic course, which passes between the aorta and right ventricular outflow tract, was affirmed. MR angiography seems to be an accurate tool as primary investigation in symptomatic young patients. In older population, due to a higher prevalence of the coronary artery disease, the CT angiography is generally preferred.

8.3 Multidetector computed tomography angiography

In comparison with aforementioned non-invasive tools imaging, multidetector CT angiography has the major advantage of a better spatial resolution. Despite, the need of administration of contrast media and the use of ionizing radiation, the CT angiography is becoming for most practioners the preferred test in adult patients with known or suspected ANOCOR. The impressive 3-D ability of CT angiography to identify unambiguously the origin and the ectopic course of an ANOCOR (figure 21) explain easily its wide use. However, it must be remembered that the production of consistent and reliable imaging is one thing, and that the correct interpretation of the latter is another thing. In ACC/AHA 2008 guidelines for adults with congenital heart disease, CT and MR angiography are recognized useful as the initial screening method in centers with expertise in such imaging (Warnes et al. 2008).

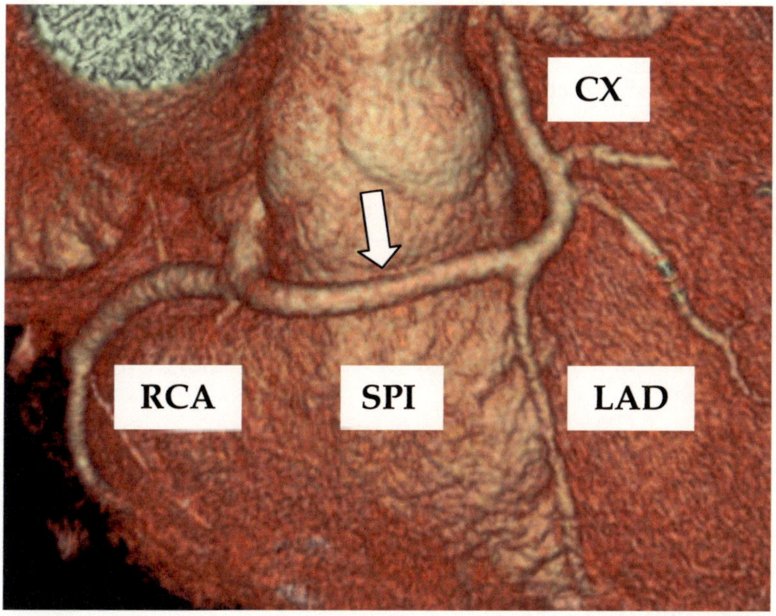

Fig. 21. Three-dimensional volume-rendered reconstruction of computed tomography showing an ectopic origin of the left main coronary artery (white arrow) arising from the right coronary artery with an ectopic course coursing on the subpulmonary infundibulum. CX: circumflex coronary artery, LAD: left anterior descending coronary artery, RCA: right coronary artery, SPI: subpulmonary infundibulum.

Numerous studies, often with small populations, have described the interest of CT angiography in the ANOCOR field. Some of them have been already mentioned above

(Fujimoto et al, 2011, Schmitt et al. 2005, Rodriguez-Granillo et al, 2009). In a series of 28 patients with known ANOCOR (4 LMCA, 15 CX coronary arteries and 9 RCA), the origin and ectopic course was correctly identified in all patients (Ropers et al., 2001). All patients had had previously an X-ray coronary arteriography. A correct analysis was achieved in only 3 patients (11%) with the latter. Nine-teen ANOCOR in 12 patients were correctly analysed with CT angiography in another small series (Datta et al., 2004). Twelve ANOCOR (1 LMCA, 1 LAD coronary artery, 4 CX coronary arteries, 5 RCA and 1 single artery) in adults patients (mean age 63 years) were analysed retrospectively with invasive (11 patients) and non-invasive tests (Leddet et al., 2008). All ANOCOR were well identified with CT angiography. However, the interpretation of one photo is ambiguous in the paper with a listed preinfundibular course instead of a retroinfundibular course. Selective coronary angiography identified accurately the origin and the ectopic course of ANOCOR in 8 of 10 cases (80%) and in 2 of 10 cases (20%), respectively. The position of CT angiography cannot be ignored either before or after invasive coronary angiography. The latter and the CT imaging are complementary in most cases of ANOCOR in adult patients (Kim et al., 2006). The main characteristics of invasive and non-invasive imaging techniques are summarized in the table 8.

Characteristics	TTE	MRA	CTA	SCA	IVUS
Invasive	no	no	no	yes	yes
Ionizing radiation	no	no	yes	yes	yes
Iodine contrast media use	no	no	yes	yes	no
Spatial resolution (mm)	0.8	1.2 x 1.8	0.5	0.3	0.15 (axial)
Visualization of adjacent structures	++	+++	+++	no	no
3-D reconstruction	no	yes	yes	no	no
Visualization of orifice	no	+	+	+	+++
Identification of intramural segment	+	+	+	+	+++
Identification of ectopic course	+	+++	+++	++	no
Identification of CAD	no	+	++	+++	+++ (limited)

Table 8. Comparison of imaging techniques in adult populations. 3-D: three-dimensional, CAD: coronary artery disease, CTA: computed tomography angiography, IVUS: intravascular ultrasonography, MRA: magnetic resonance angiography, SCA: selective coronary angiography.

Regarding to tomographic studies, the analysis of the literature shows non rare erroneous interpretations of ectopic courses of some ANOCOR, especially anomalous origins of LMCA or LAD coronary artery arising from the opposite sinus, with a misinterpretation between the preaortic course and retroinfundibular course.

9. Clinical presentations

ANOCOR are rarely recognized in infancy, except for anomalous connections with the pulmonary artery (Richard et al., 2005). Numerous clinical presentations are possible leading to the diagnosis of ANOCOR in young people and adults, but the situation seems different between < 30-year old and ≥ 30-year old. In populations with a known high prevalence of coronary artery and valvular diseases, the ANOCOR is usually diagnosed fortuitously during a selective coronary angiography. The clinical presentations are similar to those observed with symptomatic acquired heart diseases, and the association of an

ANOCOR with a significant CAD is common. Sudden ANOCOR-related death is rare in such patients. Some ANOCOR may also be identified late in patients referred for evaluation of various atypical symptoms. In young populations, the latter can lead also to the diagnosis of ANOCOR. Nevertheless, serious symptoms usually related to exertion, are possible. Last but not least, a sudden death related to a high risk ANOCOR may be the first event in the life of a young patient. Fortunately, only a small subgroup of ANOCOR, including mainly anomalies with an intramural segment and anomalous connections with the pulmonary artery, may entail life-threatening adverse events. In patients with significant acquired heart disease, relationships between the coronary abnormality and clinical status should be made clear as far as possible. The clinical presentations of anomalous origins from the pulmonary artery differ from that of anomalous origins form the aorta.

9.1 Sudden deaths

Analysis of necropsy cases has been crucial to highlight the lethal risk of some ANOCOR (Frescura et al. 1998, Kragel & Williams, 1988). In a postmortem series of 242 congenital abnormalities of coronary arteries, 49 anomalous connections of the LCA and 52 anomalous connections of the RCA with the opposite sinus were identified (Virmani et al., 2001). Sudden death was observed in 57% of LCA abnormalities and 25% of RCA abnormalities. Most of them had a preaortic course. The profile of the patients suffered from sudden death is often typical: young age, frequent intensive exercise, and non systematic premonitory symptoms. In a necropsy study of 150 consecutive sudden deaths occurring in a population ≤ 35-year old, 16 sudden deaths related to non-atherosclerotic coronary disease were identified (Corrado et al., 1992). Three (19%) of them were ANOCOR (11, 22 and 29 year-old patients). Sudden death occurred during effort. In a series of 27 ANOCOR (23 LMCA and 4 RCA from the opposite sinus) identified at autopsy in young athletes, sudden death occurred during intense exertion in 25 cases or immediately after in 2 cases (Basso, et al. 2000). In 126 nontraumatic sudden deaths collected during a 25-year autopsy study of military recruits, there were 21 (17%) ANOCOR, all LCA originated from the opposite sinus, with a preaortic course (Eckart et al. 2004). Thus, sudden death, especially during exercise, is a fairly common mode of revealing high-risk ANOCOR in young populations. Some sudden cardiac arrests may survive up to hospitalization with public education and emergency care systems. The individual incidence of sudden death in asymptomatic patients with high risk ANOCOR remains unknown.

9.2 Other symptoms

All usual cardiac symptoms are possible, i.e. angina, chest pain, dyspnea, syncopes, palpitations. In autopsy studies mentioned above, prodromal symptoms before sudden death were noted in up to 56% of patients (Eckart et al., 2004) but often underestimated or hidden owning to the patient profile (athlete or military). In another study, only 55% of patients had no cardiac history (Basso et al., 2000). Syncope and chest pain, exercise-related almost without exception, are the most frequent symptoms However, it must be remembered that the population studied was subjected to extreme exercise, unusual for a general population. In the latter, symptoms leading to the diagnosis of ANOCOR are variable and sometimes no such typical with chest discomfort or palpitations. Obviously, stable angina and acute coronary syndromes are possible if a significant CAD is associated. In a retrospective study, 301 anomalous origin from the opposite sinus were identified among

210,700 adult patients underwent selective coronary angiography (Krasuski et al., 2011). The mean age (58 ± 14 years) was relatively high in the ANOCOR cohort. As presenting symptoms, chest pain and dyspnea were common (66% and 58% of patients, respectively), as well as a myocardial infarction (24% of patients). However, the prevalence of significant CAD was of 68% in this population. Clinical presentations similar to CAD-related presentations are possible in ≥ 50-year old patients free of significant CAD (Angelini et al., 2006).

9.3 Anomalous connection with the pulmonary artery

The clinical presentation of anomalous connections with the pulmonary artery is different in children and adult populations. The mortality rate is high in infancy. In anomalous connection of the LCA with the pulmonary artery, an intermediate survival is possible with a major enlargement of the RCA and multiple intercoronary collaterals. In patients who survive into childhood, left ventricular enlargement and/or dysfunction, mitral valve incompetence, heart failure, myocardial infarction, or ventricular arrhythmias are reported, usually before 35 years age. Dyspnea and/or angina on exertion are the most frequent presenting symptoms (Kottayil et al., 2011). However, sudden death due to malignant ventricular arrhythmias may be the first cardiac event (Frapier et al., 1999). Fortuitous discovery is rare in asymptomatic patients with a continuous murmur due to interventricular collateral flow.

10. Screening and risk identification

Screening of ANOCOR in young populations and risk identification of known ANOCOR are both, two great challenges in order to impact on the incidence of life-threatening cardiac events.

10.1 Screening

In view of the fairly rare nature of ANOCOR it would be inappropriate to screen an unselected population. Moreover, the economic impact of screening in large populations should always be taken in consideration. Major obstacle of large-scale screening is the substantial number of young athletes eligible for evaluation (Maron et al. 2005). The subgroup of young athletes is certainly an interesting population in which to develop screening strategies. In a review of 387 sudden death in young athletes <35 years of age (Maron, 2003), the third most frequent cause is congenital anomalies of coronary arteries (13.7%) after hypertrophic cardiomyopathy (26.4%) and commotio cordis (19.9%). Among athletes suffering from an ANOCOR-related sudden death, a considerable number of anomalies were clinically silent. Although an intense exertion remains sometimes difficult to quantify, it would be reasonable to select among the young athletes those who will be exposed to competitive and high-intensity sports. However, time and content of such screening remain debatable. In the absence of specific European guidelines, the Study Group on Sports Cardiology of the Working Group on Cardiac Rehabilitation and Exercise Physiology of the European Society of Cardiology proposed recently, through a consensus statement, a screening project of young competitive athletes for prevention of sudden death (Corrado et al. 2005). The latter, based mainly on the large Italian experience, includes medical history, physical examination and 12-lead ECG. The screening should start at the beginning of competitive activity, which usually corresponds to an age of 12-14 years. This strategy seems useful in diagnosing an early hypertrophic cardiomyopathy. Otherwise, a resting ECG is unable to identify young people with ANOCOR except some anomalous connections in pulmonary artery (Cohen & Berger, 2010). Exercise stress test, with a known low sensibility in symptomatic high risk ANOCOR, is clearly inadequate for screening of an asymptomatic population. Among non-invasive imaging tools, ETT has the potential to identify some ANOCOR. Nevertheless, capacity for ETT should be dramatically increased and cardiologist should be trained to visualize coronary ostia. Meanwhile, better information among young athletes of frightening cardiac symptoms, i.e. chest pain or syncope in exertion, appears probably as a useful preventive measure to reduce the calamitous impact on the well-know sport benefits of each exercise-related sudden death. In addition, the visualization (or at least a meticulous search for) of origins of coronary arteries should be a routine part of any echocardiographic procedure in young population referred for functional assessments. Recently, the first series of familial ANOCOR was published with identification of 5 families in which a child or a young person <30-year old was diagnosed with preaortic ANOCOR generally symptomatic and another family member was identified with a preaortic ANOCOR through echocardiographic screening (Brothers et al., 2008). A systematic TTE screening for children and young people in families with a history of a major cardiac ANOCOR-related event (sudden death or aborted sudden death) may be discussed.

10.2 Risk identification

It is insufficient to note an abnormal origin of a coronary artery. A complete diagnosis with the orifice and the course of the ANOCOR will allow an accurate prognostic stratification. Risk identification is a major stage after a diagnosis of ANOCOR, because important therapeutic decisions and restrictive recommendations on lifestyle may follow from the final classification of the coronary abnormality. Usually, ANOCOR are identified at low-risk or high-risk with a strong evaluation criterion (sudden death). Nevertheless, one have to keep in mind that low-risk does not signify no risk. This classification is based first on postmortem examinations, because many of the patients with high-risk ANOCOR were previously diagnosed at autopsy. Now, with a better knowledge of these abnormalities and the development of imaging tools allowing an early diagnosis, it is mandatory that cardiologists and radiologists be familiar with the spectrum of congenital coronary abnormalities and their potential clinical relevance. However, the angiographers may be faced with difficult decisions for example a symptomatic patient with a low-risk ANOCOR or an asymptomatic patient with a high-risk ANOCOR. So far, no solid data are available on the natural history of ANOCOR with abnormal origin from the aorta. Several characteristics and parameters allow evaluation of sudden-death risk in most ANOCOR. However, in some cases, the classification may be difficult, and without enough information, it seems preferable to avoid too strict therapeutic rules. Indeed, it is always intriguing and not clear that among patients with the same high-risk ANOCOR, some will suffer from early sudden death, while others will die later in life of unrelated cause .

10.2.1 Type of coronary abnormality

Despite its rare frequency, the natural history of anomalous connections with the pulmonary artery is better known, and the latter are classified as high-risk. The risk of sudden death is related to malignant arrhythmias or acute myocardial infarction. Progressive left ventricular dilatation and dysfunction secondary to chronic myocardial ischemia is the trigger for rhythmic disturbances occurring usually before 35 years of age. The main subgroup of high-risk ANOCOR includes abnormalities with a preaortic course associated with an intramural segment, especially anomalous connections of LCA and RCA from the opposite sinus. If initially, the LCA with preaortic course has been recognized as the most frequent sudden death-related ANOCOR, it is clear that the RCA arising from the opposite sinus may also be a cause of sudden death (Frescura et al, 1998, Kragel & Roberts, 1988, Taylor et al., 1992). As previously discussed, almost without exception, the RCA originating from the left sinus has a preaortic course and thus a high-risk profile. The smaller myocardial territory at risk in right versus left ANOCOR is hypothesized to explain the lower incidence of sudden death in right ANOCOR despite it being more frequent than left ANOCOR. Universally, anomalous connection of the CX coronary artery, with an almost exclusive retroaortic course, is classified as low-risk ANOCOR. The subgroup of ectopic LMCA or LAD coronary artery represents certainly the greatest challenge for angiographers to accurately identify the ectopic course. As mentioned above, ANOCOR with preaortic course and ANOCOR with retroinfundibular course were previously often confused. The latter are recognized as low-risk in contrast to the ANOCOR with preaortic course. In the young population, a misdiagnosis may lead to dramatic consequences. Currently, the widely used tomographic tools allow an easy and flexible image interpretation, which should limit the risk of mistake. Other courses of LMCA or LAD coronary artery, i.e. preinfundibular and retroaortic courses are classified as low-risk. Surprisingly, anomalous origins in the opposite sinus and anomalous origins in the contralateral artery are rarely distinguished. As aforementioned, frequency of an intramural segment may be different between an abnormal connection near the orifice of the contralateral artery and an abnormal connection in the contralateral artery.

10.2.2 Symptoms and induced-myocardial ischemia

The numerous ANOCOR-related sudden deaths reported in the literature suggest that they are in most cases unpredictable. However, a more accurate analysis of the data shows that in more than half of patients suffering from sudden death, premonitory symptoms were identified after the fatal event, especially chest pain and syncope on exertion. These deaths are always to be deplored but some characteristics of the exposed population can explain an absence of diagnosis. On the one hand, young athletes may hide or underestimate symptoms, and they do not systematically interfere with usual intensive and repetitive efforts. On the other hand, medical teams can misinterpret some clinical presentations in a young and healthy population with a low prevalence of CAD, as unimportant. In addition, exercise stress tests are usually reassuring. Difficulties in inducing myocardial ischemia with the usual tools are well-described, even in symptomatic high-risk ANOCOR. In as series of 27 sudden deaths in young athletes, due to ANOCOR, all maximal exercise stress tests (6/6) were judged within normal limits (Basso et al. 2000). In addition, intermittent ischemia was described in rare cases (Brothers et al., 2010). The experience of fractional flow reserve (FFR) assessment with a pressure-wire during coronary catheterization remains limited. Angelini and coworkers speculated that functional tests suggested usually in patients with CAD are probably not appropriate for risk evaluation in patients with ANOCOR, and proposed pharmacologic tests simulating extreme exercise efforts (Angelini et al. 2003). In order to increase dramatically cardiac output and stroke left ventricular volume, concomitant administration of saline, atropine and dobutamine may lead to a significant systolic expansion of aorta. IVUS can identify the impact of this on the degree of lateral compression in the intramural segment, with sometimes a visualization of >50% area stenosis.

10.2.3 Age

Age at the time of anomaly discovery is an important parameter in risk identification. In anomalous connections with the pulmonary artery, the risk of major adverse cardiac events exists probably during the entire life, even if this risk is more pronounced in early childhood. In contrast, for anomalous origins from the aorta, most sudden deaths occur between 10 and 35 years of age. Clinicopathologic presentations of 142 cardiac deaths in patients with congenital coronary anomalies were reviewed (Taylor et al., 1992). Sudden death occurred in 78 patients (32%). Younger patients (≤ 30-year old) died suddenly more frequently in comparison with older patients, 62% versus 12%, p=0.001, respectively, despite a lower frequency of CAD, 1% versus 40%, p = 0.00001, respectively. In a series of 690 sudden deaths occurred between 14 and 40 years of age, prevalence of ANOCOR identified as sole cause of death was of 8% between 14 and 20 years of age, of 4% between 21 and 30 years of age, and of 0.5% between 31 an 40 years of age (Virmani et al., 2001). Risk of sudden death in the absence of CAD seems very low after the age of 50 years, including so-called interarterial high-risk ANOCOR. However, some ANOCOR with intramural segment may be symptomatic late requiring interventional and/or surgical treatment (Angelini et al., 2006).

10.2.4 Associated coronary artery disease

Obviously, the presence of CAD will interfere with the management of ANOCOR. A significant ostial or juxtaostial narrowing due to an intramural segment should not be confused with a fixed atherosclerotic stenosis. Sites of significant atherosclerotic lesions should be clearly distinguished, especially between ectopic segment and normal path. Association of CAD with ectopic segment of ANOCOR with a single ostium or with proximal path of a single coronary increases the risk. A higher prevalence of CAD has been suggested in CX coronary arteries but the location of atherosclerotic lesions is not always defined accurately in studies. However, most of them seem concordant with a higher incidence of atherosclerotic lesions in CX coronary arteries (Click et al., 1989, Wilkins et al. 1988). Table 9 summarizes the main characteristics of low-risk and high-risk ANOCOR in young and adult populations.

	Low-risk	High-risk
Anomalous connection with the pulmonary artery	-	+
Preaortic course with intramural segment	-	+
Other courses with intramural segment	-	+
Other courses without intramural segment	+	-
Valve-like ostial stenosis	-	+
Other anomalous connections	+	-
History of aborted sudden death	-	+
History of chest pain related to exertion	-	+
History of syncope related to exertion	-	+
History of severe ventricular arrhythmias	-	+
Induced-myocardial ischemia	-	+
Any anomaly above age of 50 years*	+	-
Ectopic segment with significant atherosclerotic lesion	-	+

* Except anomalous connections with the pulmonary artery.

Table 9. Main characteristics of low-risk and high-risk proximal anomalous connections of the coronary arteries.

11. Pathophysiological mechanisms

The degree of understanding of the pathophysiological mechanisms differs between the different types of ANOCOR.

11.1 Anomalous connections with the pulmonary artery

For the first clinical description of an anomalous connection with the pulmonary artery (Bland et al., 1933), pathophysiological mechanisms were established and well understood (Edwards, 1964). In anomalous connections of the LCA with the pulmonary trunk, the most frequent abnormality, the left ventricular myocardium is initially fed by less saturated blood under high pulmonary vascular resistances. Then, the antegrade flow to the LCA decreases with an eventual reversal of flow due to the decrease in pulmonary vascular resistances, leading to a coronary steal phenomenon. A long asymptomatic period until adulthood is possible in patients with dominant RCA and multiple large intercoronary collaterals between RCA and LCA. However, permanent myocardial hypoperfusion progressively impairs left ventricular function with occurrence of dyspnea and/or heart failure in young age. Mitral insufficiency, generally mild or moderate, is frequent, due to papillary muscle ischemia. Hibernating myocardium is possible requiring myocardial viability studies in order to rule out idiopathic dilated cardiomyopathy. As aforementioned, low ventricular function and/or myocardial infarction sequelae may be the trigger for malignant ventricular arrhythmias revealing the coronary abnormality.

11.2 Anomalous connections with the aorta

In subgroups of anomalous origins from the aorta, mechanisms of life-threatening cardiac events are less clear. Even if most sudden deaths are almost due to ventricular fibrillation, the accurate sequence leading to lethal arrhythmic disturbance often remains unknown or debated. Hypotension and extreme bradycardia seem to occur before the malignant ventricular arrhythmia. Experimental studies are lacking in the field of ANOCOR. Numerous hypotheses have been speculated. The oldest of them, still often widely held, is the compression of the ectopic vessel between the aorta and the pulmonary artery. However, such mechanism has never been demonstrated. Extrinsic compression of the LCA in normal location, from a markedly dilated pulmonary artery trunk has been described (Caldera et al., 2009, de Jesus Perez et al., 2009, Lyndsey et al., 2008). Nevertheless, relationships between an ANOCOR with preaortic course and a non dilated pulmonary artery are different. As previously discussed, RCA or LCA with preaortic course are not necessary close to the pulmonary artery. Therefore, anatomical characteristics of ANOCOR with preaortic course and intramural segment are probably more interesting for comprehension of induced-myocardial ischemia (Angelini, 2007). It is important to consider that myocardial ischemia is not necessarily the result of significant differences between supply and demand of myocardial oxygen. In the absence of fixed atherosclerotic stenosis, the determinants of myocardial ischemia are not truly reproducible in patients with ANOCOR. Most young athletes are able to perform intensive and repetitive efforts which do not interfere with their performances until the occurrence of a life-threatening cardiac event. Thus, the subject continues to intrigue pathologists and physiologists. Invasive approach with IVUS advocated by Angelini et al. permitted a better comprehension between anatomical features of ectopic vessel and pathophysiological mechanisms of ischemia. If symptoms are a suggestive of a compressive etiology, one must consider IVUS as it is the gold standard anatomical technique. A slit-like orifice may have a large area, but can collapse with a valve-like manner, during an abrupt increase in pressure and/or volume in the aorta. Vessel hypoplasia is another potential cause of decrease in blood supply under extreme conditions. CT imaging and IVUS are useful to demonstrate a non atherosclerotic reduction of the lumen vessel in the initial ectopic path (figure 22). Another abnormality contributing to myocardial ischemia is the intramural segment of the ectopic vessel. Histology and ultrasonography demonstrated the non circular shape of intramural segment thoroughly. The oblong area of the latter may be more exposed to the dynamic changes of the aortic wall.

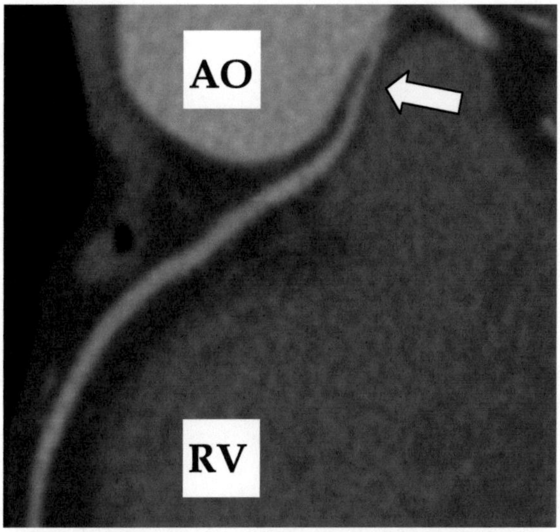

Fig. 22. Multiplanar reconstruction of computed tomography showing an hypoplasia of the initial path (arrow) of a right coronary artery arising from the left sinus. AO: aorta, RV: right ventricle.

If numerous anatomical risk factors were identified, the relative contribution of each factor is not clear. In a study, no significant differences were found in length of intramural segment, coronary ostial size, or angle of coronary take-off between right or left ANOCOR arising from the opposite sinus, with (n=12) and without (n=18) sudden death (Taylor et al., 1997). Age ≥ 30 years was the only factor with a lower incidence of sudden death. Apart from the fact that intensive exercises are preferably performed during the young age, the dramatic reduction of sudden death risk after the age of 30 years remains surprising. The progressive hardening of the aortic wall has been suggested as a pathophysiological mechanism, with less dynamic changes of the aortic media during exertion. Otherwise, clotting and spasm have often been suspected but rarely proven as further mechanisms leading to acute coronary events. Furthermore, large sequelae of transmural myocardial infarction are rare in necropsy cases. Nevertheless, chronic myocardial ischemic damage may occur and lead to fatal arrhythmias. Histologic examination of heart specimens of young athletes suffering from sudden death may show patchy replacement-type fibrosis (Basso et al., 2000) or scattered foci of contraction band necrosis (Corrado et al., 1992). CX coronary artery arising from the opposite sinus or the RAC is a well-known abnormality deemed benign. Nevertheless, suspicion exists about an earlier atherosclerotic formation in the proximal path of ectopic CX coronary arteries. Angiographic demonstration of a reduction of the lumen is not rare. However, besides atherosclerotic narrowing, a distortion of CX coronary artery may also be suspected in case of enlarged aortic root due to their close relationships. The mechanism of a potentially higher incidence of CAD of ectopic CX coronary artery in the retroaortic segment remains unclear.

12. Management, recommendations, and treatments

If most of ANOCOR are benign and require no specific investigation or treatment, other abnormalities such ANOCOR classified as high-risk or symptomatic ANOCOR require a meticulous and accurate analysis in order to offer the best management in the present state of our knowledge.

12.1 Management

First of all, the coronary abnormality should be clearly defined with a correct interpretation of ectopic origin, initial course regarding to aortic wall, and ectopic course regarding to adjacent structures. Uncertain diagnosis or high-risk ANOCOR need always complementary imaging investigation allowing a useful confrontation. All cardiologists and radiologists are not familiar with the large spectrum of congenital coronary abnormalities, and the opinion of a practitioner experienced in the field of ANOCOR should be mandatory before decision-making. Recent investigation conducted by the Anomalous Coronary Artery Working Group of the Congenital Heart Surgeon's Society showed a heterogeneous management of young adults with ANOCOR associated with a preaortic course (Brothers et al., 2009). In 36th Bethesda Conference focused on trained athlete with an identified cardiovascular abnormality, detection of coronary anomalies of wrong sinus origin in which a coronary artery passes between the aorta and pulmonary artery should result in exclusion from all participations in competitive sport (Graham et al., 2005). Participation in all sport 3 months after successful operation would be permitted for an athlete without ischemia, ventricular or tachyarrhythmia, or dysfunction during maximal exercise testing was another recommendation of the 36th Bethesda Conference. As previously mentioned, presence of symptoms, high-risk anatomical features and young age are the main criteria requiring a special attention in order to prevent a sudden cardiac death. Even if false-negative cases are frequent, stress exercise tests with nuclear imaging are necessary in this population exposed. More aggressive investigations, such pharmacological tests simulating extreme exercise have been suggested but are not without dangers (Angelini et al., 2003). According to current understanding, only an intramural segment seems to be clearly related with a high-risk of sudden death, and the best means in identifying intramural segment is IVUS. The definition of a cut-off age in deciding a population as high-risk remains difficult in practice. If the literature gives relatively clear information in < 30-year old and > 50-year old patients, the management of patients between 30 and 50 years of age is often problematic. Restriction of activity, particularly competitive sport and intensive exertion, is often recommended if a surgical repair is not indicated. Medical treatment with essentially beta-blockers is sometimes associated. Due to possible but rare late deaths or subclinical myocardial ischemia after surgical repair of ANOCOR, long-term follow-up with regular cardiovascular evaluation is needed (Brothers et al., 2007, Brothers et al., 2009). Presence of significant atherosclerotic coronary disease or valvular disease requiring cardiac surgery permits sometimes a concomitant treatment of a high-risk ANOCOR. Furthermore, identification of

ANOCOR is crucial before aortic surgery in order to avoid an injury of the ectopic vessel or to compress along its course by a valvular prosthesis.

12.2 Recommendations

ACC/AHA 2008 guidelines for the management of adults with congenital heart disease (Warnes et al., 2008) give recommendations for congenital coronary abnormalities of ectopic aortic origin and for anomalous left coronary artery from the pulmonary artery (table 10).

Recommendations for congenital coronary anomalies of ectopic aortic origin		
	Class	Level of evidence
Surgical coronary revascularization should be performed in patients with any of the following indications:		
a. Anomalous left main coronary artery coursing between the aorta and pulmonary artery.	1	B
b. Documented coronary ischemia due to coronary compression (when coursing between the great vessels or in intramural fashion).	1	B
c. Anomalous origin of the right coronary artery between aorta and pulmonary artery with evidence of ischemia.	1	B
Surgical coronary revascularization can be beneficial in the setting of documented vascular wall hypoplasia, coronary compression, or documented obstruction to coronary flow, regardless of inability to document coronary ischemia.	IIa	C
Surgical coronary revascularization may be reasonable in patients with anomalous left anterior descending coronary artery coursing between the aorta and pulmonary artery.	IIb	C
Recommendations for anomalous left coronary artery from the pulmonary artery		
	Class	Level of evidence
In patients with an anomalous left coronary artery from the pulmonary artery, reconstruction of a dual coronary artery supply should be performed. The surgery should be performed by surgeons with training and expertise in congenital heart disease at centers with expertise in the management of anomalous coronary artery origins.	1	C

Table 10. ACC/AHA 2008 recommendations for anomalous connections with aorta and pulmonary artery.

Surgical repair is indicated for LMCA with preaortic course regardless of symptoms. Surgical repair is also indicated for RCA with preaortic course in association with symptoms and/or inducible ischemia. A conservative approach is recommended in asymptomatic in patients with ectopic RCA in association with preaortic course. Position of PCI with limited experience and without long-term follow-up is not established in the ACC/AHA guidelines. Furthermore, the risk stratification with age is not clearly exposed. Only, a young patient is defined as a patient with an age less than 50 years. Despite of absence of randomized studies and limited information about long term follow-up in high risk patients, current guidelines are fairly directive in favor of large surgical indications in high–risk ANOCOR with ectopic origin from the aorta. In accordance with its well-described natural history, an anomalous LCA connected with pulmonary artery should be repaired surgically regardless of age. Surprisingly, congenital coronary abnormalities do not appear on the list of specific congenital heart defects in the recent European 2010 guidelines (Baumgartner et al., 2010).

12.3 Treatments of anomalous connections with the pulmonary artery

Correction of anomalous connections with the pulmonary artery should always be proposed regardless symptoms and age, with as possible establishment of a dual coronary system. The restitution of an antegrade flow in the LCA is associated with an improvement of the left ventricular function and a reduction of the ischemic mitral regurgitation. At mid-term, regression of the intercoronary collateral network and decrease in size of dilated RCA are observed. Numerous surgical methods have been attempted to repair coronary abnormality, including Takeuchi tunnel procedure, venous or arterial bypass grafts, or direct aortic reimplantation. The latter, although technically more challenging, appears today as the method of choice in patients with favorable anatomy (Kottayil et al., 2011). The implantation of the LMCA into the aorta is a more physiological correction and avoids the late risks of venous grafts. Takeuchi procedure is a technique of repair with the creation of a baffle within the pulmonary artery to divert the blood from the origin of the ectopic LMCA to the aorta (Takeuchi et al., 1979). Due to a high rate of reoperations for supravalvular pulmonary stenosis, baffle leak or obstruction of the intrapulmonary channel, the Takeuchi procedure is almost no longer used. Ectopic LCA usually originates from the left posterior pulmonary sinus facing the left side of the aorta. The excised ectopic coronary is directly implanted just above the sinotubular junction. The site of pulmonary excision is repaired with autologous pericardium. Sometimes, strategies to lengthen the anomalous coronary artery are necessary. Mitral repair or replacement is recommended in patients with severe mitral regurgitation. Establishment of a satisfactory left myocardial perfusion may resolve mild and some moderate mitral insufficiencies (Fehrenbacher et al., 2010). Mechanical circulatory support should be considered in patients with intractable left ventricular failure in postoperative setting (Dodge-Khatami et al., 2002). With increased experience with direct aortic implantation technique and better postoperative management, the perioperative mortality rate, initially up to 20%, decreased dramatically of about 10%. Due to the rare frequency of patients with a coronary artery arising from pulmonary artery who survive into childhood, large prospective studies in adults who underwent surgical repair are lacking. Studies, pooling generally children and adult populations, reported a 10-year survival rate between 85 and 95% (Ben Ali et al., 2009, Brown et al., 2008, Fehrenbacher et al., 2010). Close long-term follow-up after surgical repair is recommended to detect residual ischemia.

12.4 Treatments of anomalous connections with the aorta

12.4.1 Surgical treatment

Surgical treatment is recommended in patients with high-risk anomalous connections with the aorta (Warnes et al, 2008). However, an inhomogeneous management of high-risk ANOCOR is observed in practice (Brothers et al., 2009). Surgical repair techniques are numerous and current therapeutic strategies may vary among clinicians due to marked heterogeneity in physician opinions. Obviously, the left high-risk ANOCOR are easier entrusted to surgeon. Nevertheless, surgical repair of right high-risk ANOCOR has been reported (Garcia-Rinaldi et al., 2004). In contrast to anomalous connections with pulmonary artery, direct aortic reimplantation is rarely possible due to an, almost without exception, intramural segment. Several techniques have been proposed (Said et al. 2010): unroofing of the coronary artery, creation of a neo-ostium, reimplantation of the coronary artery, translocation of the pulmonary artery with patch angioplasty of the coronary artery and coronary bypass grafting. Unroofing consists to a longitudinal excision of the common wall between the aorta and the ectopic coronary artery coursing tangentially with an intramural segment (figure 23). Excision starts at the anomalous ostium and continues into the appropriate sinus. To create a neo-ostium, a probe passed through the intramural segment and the coronary artery is opened at the location at which the probe exits the aortic wall (figure 23). In the absence of intramural segment, reimplantation of the coronary artery is possible. The ectopic ostium is excised and implanted in the appropriate sinus above the sinotubular junction. Another technique may be used in the absence of intramural segment, with a translocation of the pulmonary trunk anteriorly and leftward to avoid a compression of the ectopic artery. This technique may be associated with patch angioplasty of the ectopic coronary artery (Karl et al., 2010). The coronary artery is open well beyond the intramural segment and a patch of autologous pericardium creates a large neo-ostium. Finally, coronary artery bypass grafting with saphenous vein or internal mammary artery is another possibility. Thus, correction of intramural segment is not systematically. The choice of the technique depends of surgeon's preference, anatomical pattern of ANOCOR, and existence of CAD requiring myocardial revascularization. Coronary artery bypass grafting is proposed in older adults with concomitant CAD. The use of venous or arterial conduits in young people exposes to a long-term patency concern, because of competitive flow. For most operators, the creation of a neo-ostium is the more physiological treatment without the risk of take-down of the commissural junction between the right and left coronary sinuses observed sometimes with the unroofing technique. No comparative data exist about these different surgical methods. Surgical practice has evolved in the time from coronary artery bypass grafting to direct surgical repair. To date, unroofing technique seems the more used in young people (Davies et al., 2009, Frommelt et al., 2011, Mainwaring et al. 2011). The rate of perioperative death is near to zero in small series of children and young people (Davies et al., 2009, Erez et al., 2006, Karl et al., 2010). Recently, Krasuski et al. reported the impact of surgery in patients with ANOCOR from the opposite sinus (Krasuski, et al., 2011). A cohort of 301 adults from 210,700 cardiac catherizations performed over a 35-year period was retrospectively analysed. The incidence of anomalous connections with the opposite sinus was of 0.14%, and in 54 of 301 patients (18%) an interarterial course between the aorta and pulmonary artery was identified, thus an incidence of 3/10.000 of high-risk ANOCOR with 18 left ANOCOR (33%) and 36 right ANOCOR (67%). Surgical management was chosen in 28 of 54 patients (52%), and in 8 of 18 left ANOCOR (44%) and 20 of 36 right ANOCOR (56%). Coronary artery bypass grafting was used as treatment in most of cases (71%). At 10 years, no difference in survival was observed between interarterial ANOCOR managed surgically or medically. Some characteristics of the cohort studied may explain the lack of benefit associated with surgical repair. As aforementioned, the study population consisted of relatively old patients with a mean age of 58 years and with a high prevalence of CAD.

The latter was present in 86% of ANOCOR managed surgically and in 50% of ANOCOR managed medically. Abnormal stress tests were more frequent in surgical patients (90%) versus 43% in patients with medical management. Moreover, whether the primary indication for surgery was CAD or coronary abnormality was not clarified. The authors concluded that the results of their study must not be applied to younger patients because the mortality risk is not the same. Mainwaring et al. reported medium-term results after surgical repair of ANOCOR in 50 patients with a mean age of 14 years (Mainwaring, et al., 2011). Congenital cardiac abnormalities were associated in 14 patients. Interarterial and intramural courses were present in 100% and 70% of patients, respectively. An unroofing procedure was performed in 36 of 50 patients (72%). All patients (n=9) with single coronary ostium and without an intramural path underwent pulmonary artery translocation. With a mean follow-up of 5.3 years, satisfactory follow-up was obtained in 47 patients, and all have remained free of cardiac symptoms. Functional results of modern surgical methods are recognized as good in young people with most of patients free of symptoms at a medium-term follow-up (Erez et al., 2006, Karl, et al. 2010). However, Brothers et al. reported that subclinical ischemia may occur after surgical repair of anomalous aortic origin of a coronary artery (Brothers et al., 2007). In this study, 9 asymptomatic children or adolescents (5 to 18 years) had post operative evaluations (range 2 to 48 months) suggestive of silent ischemia. This data highlight the need of long-term follow-up in young people undergoing surgical repair of ANOCOR.

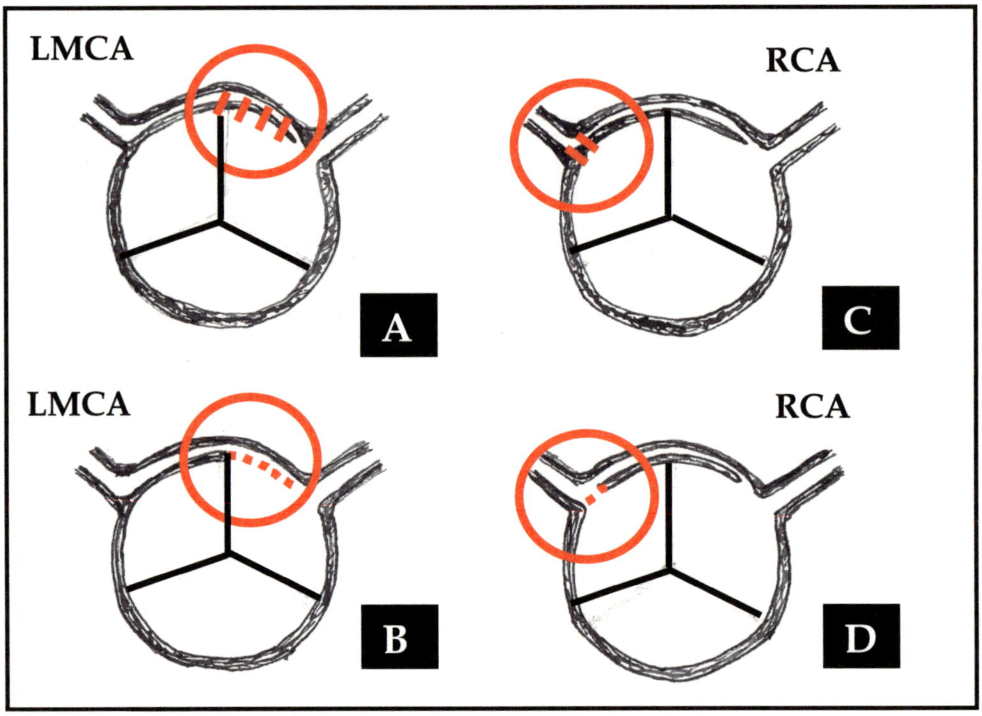

Fig. 23. Diagram representation of surgical repair of an anomalous left main coronary artery (LMCA) arising from the right sinus and associated with an intramural segment. A and B: unroofing technique. C and D: creation of a neo-ostium. RCA: right coronary artery.

12.4.2 Interventional treatment

Coronary angioplasty with stenting is a more recent therapeutic method in the field of ANOCOR. So far, only cases report or small groups of ANOCOR have been reported. Percutaneous coronary intervention (PCI) in ANOCOR with and without associated CAD must be distinguished. In fact, most of PCI are performed in ANOCOR with significant atherosclerotic lesions within or distal to ectopic course, and sometimes during acute coronary syndrome (Jaffe et al., 2009). PCI may be attractive as an alternative to surgical repair in young patients without CAD. Nevertheless, the capacities of a stent to adapt to anatomical characteristics of an ANOCOR with an intramural segment should be accurately analyzed before its use can be recommended. Hariharan et al. displayed potential concerns with canulation difficult, incomplete coverage of ostium without protruding into the aorta, uncertainly regarding the true diameter, risk of aortic dissection, and unknown restenosis risk (Hariharan et al. 2002). Angelini et al. suggest the use of PCI in patients with symptomatic right ANOCOR associated with ischemia induced by a nuclear stress test (Angelini et al., 2007). During cardiac catheterization, IVUS is crucial to evaluate the minimal lumen area, length of intramural segment, arterial diameters and results after stent deployment. However, evaluation data of interventional treatment of right ANOCOR are currently too poor to envisage on extension of this technique to left ANOCOR. In AHA/ACC 2008 guidelines, PCI is not recommended in therapeutic management (Warnes et al., 2008).

13. Perspectives

Among the wide spectrum of congenital abnormalities of coronary arteries, proximal anomalous connections of coronary arteries (ANOCOR) represent a significant subgroup, which continues to promote debate. A more simple classification, and recognized by all, would have the advantage to avoid confusions. A non insignificant prevalence of about 1% in the general population and, in particular, the presence of anatomical patterns associated with a risk of sudden death require that the current research supplies data sufficiently robust in order to improve the management of ANOCOR. Young competitive athletes are a well-known population which pays a heavy toll to high-risk ANOCOR. Cooperation between physicians is necessary in order to prevent sport-related fatalities and to determine the modalities of cost-effective screening. From a diagnostic point of view, tomographic techniques, especially CT angiography, represent today an unrivaled tool by their ability to supply multiple volumetric reconstructions. Therefore, accurate diagnosis of the ectopic origin and non-ambiguous interpretation of the ectopic course are possible in most of cases. However, ANOCOR are still often discovered fortuitously in adult populations during selective coronary angiography by angiographers with sometimes a limited experience in the field of ANOCOR. It seems that the knowledge of angiographers should be improved in order to limit the risk of misinterpretation. Systematic usage of tomographic imaging solves this problem, while at the same time educating angiographers. Currently, high-risk ANOCOR are identified well, however the management of them is heterogeneous, specially the timing and mode of treatment. There clearly remains a gap between the practices and the recommendations, sometimes due to misunderstanding, but also relating to physician opinion. The absence of long-term follow-up after surgical repair and the difficulties of undertaking randomized studies, and as the unknown natural history of ANOCOR all may explain the divergence between clinical practice and current guidelines. Surgical treatment demonstrates a preference for the unroofing technique in ANOCOR arising from the aorta and direct aortic implantation for ANOCOR connected with the pulmonary artery. Perioperative risks are low, except in some anomalous connections with the pulmonary artery, but the long-term evaluation is lacking. To date, the role of PCI remains undetermined. The low incidence of ANOCOR requiring a percutaneous or a surgical repair would justify that these congenital abnormalities being taken care off in a center specialized in the management of ANOCOR. Several attempts have been made to set up observational registries to determine the outcome of different strategies in the field of ANOCOR (Angelini 2007, Aubry et al., 2008, Brothers et al., 2007, Pelliccia, 2001). To date, two registries are ongoing, one in North and South America, and one in France. The registry of anomalous aortic origin of the coronary artery of The Congenital Heart Surgeons' Society (www.chssdc.com) has been set up to determine the outcome of children or young adults (≤ 30-year old) with high-risk ANOCOR. This registry includes those managed conservatively and with surgical intervention. The ANOCOR with interarterial, intramural, and/or intraseptal courses are classified as high-risk. The registry consists of a retrospective cohort of patients diagnosed between 1 January, 1998 and 20 January, 2009 and a prospective cohort of patients newly diagnosed from 21 January, 2009. The registry of proximal anomalous connections of coronary arteries (ANOCOR Registry) of the French Society of Cardiology (www.sfcardio.fr) is a prospective observational study of patients (≥ 15-year old) diagnosed with an ANOCOR. The main objective of this registry is to describe the chosen therapeutic strategies according to the type of ANOCOR. The secondary objectives are to describe the cardiac morbidity and mortality and to estimate the impact of different therapeutic strategies at a 5-year follow-up. The ANOCOR registry started 31 January, 2010 with an inclusion period of 3 years. With such multicenter registries dedicated to ANOCOR, evidence-based guidelines will probably be easier to establish in an attempt to achieve a better understanding of the clinical profile and the impact of interventional correction on the natural history of these congenital coronary abnormalities.

14. References

Anderson, R. & Loukas, M. (2009). The importance of attitudinally appropriate description of cardiac anatomy. *Clin Anat,* Vol. 22, pp. 47-51

Ando, K.; Nakajima, Y.; Yamagishi, T.; Yamamoto, S. & Nakamura, H. (2004). Development of proximal coronary arteries in quail embryonic heart. Multicapillaries penetrating the aortic sinuses fuse to form main coronary trunk. *Circ Res,* Vol. 94, pp. 346-352.

Angelini P. (2007). Coronary artery anomalies: an entity in search of an identity. *Circulation,* Vol. 115, pp. 1296-305.

Angelini, P. & Flamm, S. (2007). Newer concepts for imaging anomalous aortic origin of the coronary arteries in adults. *Cathet Cardiovasc Interv,* Vol. 69, pp. 942-954.

Angelini, P. (2002). Coronary artery anomalies - current clinical issues: definitions, classification, incidence, clinical relevance, and treatment guidelines. *Tex Heart Inst,* Vol. 29, pp. 271–278.

Angelini, P.; Velasco, J.; Ott, D. & Khoshnevis, G. (2003). Anomalous coronary artery arising from the opposite sinus: descriptive features and pathophysiological mechanisms, as documented by intravascular ultrasonography. *J Invasive Cardiol,* Vol. 15, pp. 507-514.

Angelini, P.; Villason, S.; Chan, C. & Diez, J. (1999). Normal and anomalous coronary arteries in humans. In: *Coronary artery anomalies: a comprehensive approach*. Angelini, P. Philadelphia: Lippincott Williams & Wilkins, pp. 27-150.

Angelini, P.; Walmsley, R.; Cheong, B, & Ott, A. (2010). Coronary artery originating from the normal sinus but with acute angulation and intramural course, leading to critical stenosis. *Tex Heart Inst J*, Vol. 37, pp. 221-225.

Angelini, P.; Walmsley, R.; Libreros, A. & Ott, D. (2006). Symptomatic anomalous origination of the left coronary artery from the opposite sinus of Valsalva. Clinical presentations, diagnosis, and surgical repair. *Tex Heart Inst J*, Vol. 33, pp. 171-179.

Aubry, P.; Joudinaud, T. & Hyafil, F. (2008). Anomalous origin of coronary arteries in adults. *Ann Cardiol Angeiol*, Vol. 57, pp. 327-334.

Aydinlar, A.; Cicek, D.; Sentruk, T.; Gemici, K.; Serdar, O.; Kazazoglu, A.; Kumbay, E. & Cordan, J. Primary congenital anomalies of the coronary arteries. A coronary arteriographic study in western Turkey. (2005). *Int Heart J*, Vol. 46, pp. 97-103.

Basso, C; Maron ,B; Corrado, D. & Thiene, G. (2000). Clinical profile of congenital coronary artery anomalies with origin from the wrong aortic sinus leading to sudden death in young competitive athletes. *J Am Coll Cardiol*; Vol. 35, pp. 1493–1501.

Baumgartner, H.; Bonhoeffer, P.; De Groot, N.; de Haan, F.; Deanfield, J.; Galie, N.; Gatzoulis, M.; Gohleke-Barewolf C.; Kaemmerer, H.; Kilner, P.; Meijboom, F.; Mulder, B.; Oechsli, E.; Oliver, J.; Serraf, A.; Szatmari, A.; Thaulow, E.; Vouhe, P. & Walma, E. (2010). ESC Guidelines for the management of grow-up congenital heart disease (new version 2010). The Task Force on the Management of Grow-up Congenital Heart Disease of the European Society of Cardiology (ESC). *Eur Heart J*, Vol. 31, pp. 2915-2957.

Ben Ali, W.; Metton, O.; Roubertie, F.; Pouard, P.; Sidi, D.; Raisky, O. & Vouhé P. (2009). Anomalous origin of the left coronary artery from the pulmonary artery: late results with special attention to the mitral valve. *Eur J Cardiothorac Surg*, Vol. 36, pp. 244-248.

Bland, E.; White, P. & Garland, J. (1933). Congenital anomalies of the coronary arteries: report of an unusual case associated with cardiac hypertrophy. *Am Heart J*, Vol. 8, pp. 787-801.

Bogers, A.; Gittenberger-de Groot, A.; Poelman, R.; Péault, B. & Huysmans, H. (1989). Development of the origin of the coronary arteries, a matter of ingrowth or outgrowth? *Anat Embryol*, Vol. 180, pp. 437-441.

Brothers, J.; Carter, C.; McBride, M.; Spry, T. & Paridon, S. (2010). Anomalous left coronary artery origin from the opposite sinus of Valsalva: evidence of intermittent ischemia. *J Thorac Cardiovasc Surg*, Vol. 140, pp. e27-e29.

Brothers, J.; Gaynor, J.; Jacobs, J.; Caldarone, C.; Jegatheeswaran, A. & Jacobs, M. (2010). The registry of anomalous aortic origin of the coronary artery of The Congenital Heart Surgeons' Society. *Cardio Young*, Vol. 20 (Suppl. 3), pp. 50-58.

Brothers, J.; Gaynor, J.; Paridon, S.; Lorber, R. & Jacobs, M. (2009). Anomalous aortic origin of a coronary artery with an interatrial course: understanging current management strategies in children and young adults. *Pediatr Cardiol*, Vol. 30, pp. 911-921.

Brothers, J.; McBride, M.; Seliem, M.; Marino, B.; Tomlinson, R.; Pampaloni, M.; Gaynor,J.; Spray, T. & Paridon, S. (2007). Evaluation of myocardial ischemia following surgical repair of anomalous aortic origin of a coronary artery in a series of pediatric patients. *J Am Coll Cardiol*, Vol 50, pp. 2078-2082.

Brothers, J.; Stephens, P.; Gaynor, W.; Lorber, R.; Vricella, L. & Paridon, S. (2008). Anomalous aortic origin of ac coronary artery with an interarterial course. Should family screening be routinely? *J Am Coll Cardiol*, Vol. 51, pp. 2062-2064.

Brown, J.; Ruzmetov, M.; Parent, J.; Rodefeld, M. Turrentine, M. (2008). Does the degree of preoperative mitral regurgitation predict survival of the need for mitral valve repair or replacement in patients with anomalous origin of the left coronary artery from the pulmonary artery? *J Thorac Cardiovasc Surg*, Vol. 136, pp. 743-748.

Bunce, N.; Lorenz, C.; Keegan, J.; Lesser, J.; Reyes, E.; Firmin, D. & Pennell, D. (2003). Coronary artery anomalies: assessment with free-breathing three-dimensional coronary MR angiography. *Radiology*, Vol. 227, pp. 201-208.

Caldera, A.; Cruz-Gonzales, I.; Bezerra, H.; Cury, R.; Palacios, I.; Cockrill, B. & Inlessis-Azuaje, I. (2009). Endovascular therapy for left main compression syndrome. Case report and literature review. *Chest*, Vol. 135, pp. 1648-1650.

Cielslinski, G.; Rapprich, B. & Kober, G. (1993). Coronary anomalies: incidence and importance. *Clin Cardiol*, Vol. 16, pp. 711-715.

Click, R.; Holmes, D.; Vliestra, R.; Kosinski, A.; Kronmal, R. & the participants of the Coronary Artery Surgery Study (CASS). *J Am Coll Cardiol*, Vol. 13, pp. 531-537.

Cohen, M. & Berger, S. (2010). The electrocardiogram as an adjunct in diagnosing congenital coronary arterial anomalies. *Cardiol Young*, Vol. 20 (Suppl. 3), pp. 59-67.

Cohen, M.; Herlong, R. & Silverman, N. (2010). Echographic imaging of anomalous origin of the coronary arteries. *Cardiol Young*, Vol. 20 (Suppl. 3), pp. 26-34.

Corrado, D.; Pelliccia, A.; Bjornstad, H.; Vanhees, L.; Biffi, A.; Borjesson, M.; Panhuyzen-Goedkoop, N.; Deligiannis, A.; Solberg, E.; Dugmore, D.; Mellvig, K.; Assanelli, D.; Delise, P.; van-Buuren, F.; Anastasakis, A.; Heidbuchel, H.; Hoffman, E.; Fagard, R.; Priori, S.; Basso, C.; Arbustini, E.; Blomstrom-Lunqvist, C.; McKenna, W. & Thiene, G. (2005). Cardiovascular pre-participation screening of young competitive athletes for prevention of sudden death: proposal for a common European protocol. Consensus statement of the Study Group on Sports Cardiology of the Working Group on Cardiac Rehabilitation and Exercise Physiology and the Working Group of Myocardial and Pericardial Diseases of the European Society of Cardiology. *Eur Heart J*, Vol. 26, pp. 516-524.

Corrado, D.; Thiene, G.; Cocco, P. & Frescura, C. (1992). Non-atherosclerotic coronary artery disease and sudden death in the young. *Br Heart J*, Vol. 68, pp. 601-607.

Datta, J.; White, C.; Gilkeson, R.; Meyer, C.; Kansal, S.; Jani, S.; Arildsen, R. & Read, K. (2005). Anomalous coronary arteries in adults: depiction at multi-detector row CT angiography. *Radiology*, Vol. 235, pp. 812-818.

Davies, J.; Burkhart, H.; Dearani, J.; Suri, R.; Phillips, S.; Warnes, C. & Sundt, T. (2009). Surgical of anomalous aortic origin of a coronary artery. *Ann Thorac Surg*, Vol. 88, pp. 844-847.

Davis, J.; Cecchin, F.; Jones, T. & Portman, M. (2001). Major coronary artery anomalies in a pediatric population. Incidence and clinical importance. *J Am Coll Cardiol*, Vol. 37, pp. 593-597.

de Jesus Perez, V.; Haddad, F.; Vagelos, R.; Fearon, W.; Feinstein, J. & Zamanian, R. (2009). Angina associated with left main coronary artery compression in pulmonary hypertension. *J Heart Lung Transplant*, Vol. 28, pp. 527-530.

de Jonge, G.; van Ooijen, P.; Pirs, L.; Dikkers, R.; Tio, R.; Willems, T.; van den Heuvel, A.; Zijlstra, F. & Oudkerk, M. (2008). Visualization of anomalous coronary arteries on-dual source computed tomography. *Eur Radiol*, Vol. 18, pp. 2425-32.

Dode-Khatami, A.; Mavroudis, C. & Backer, C. (2002). Anomalous origin of the left coronary artery from the pulmonary artery: collective review of surgical therapy. *Ann Thorac Surg*, Vol. 74, pp. 946-955.

Dodge-Khatami, A.; Mavroudis, C. & Backer C. (2000). Congenital heart surgery nomenclature and database project: anomalies of the coronary arteries. *Ann Thorac Surg*, Vol. 69 (Suppl. 4), pp. S270-S297.

Eckart, R.; Scoville, S.; Campbell, C.; Shry, E. Stajduhar, K.; Opper, R.; Pearse, L. & Virmani, R. (2004). Sudden-death in young adults: a 25-year review of autopsies in military recruits. *Ann Intern Med*, Vol. 141, pp. 829-834.

Edwards, J. (1964). The direction of blood flow in coronary arteries arising from the pulmonary trunk. *Circulation*, Vol. 29, pp. 163-166.

Erez, E.; Tam, V.; Doublin, N. & Stakes, J. (2006). Anomalous coonary artery with aortic origin and course between the great arteries: improved diagnosis, anatomic findings, and surgical treatment. *Ann Thorac Surg*, Vol. 82, pp. 973-977.

Fehrenbacher, T.; Mitchell, M.; Ghanayem, N. & Tweddell, J. (2010). Surgery and critical care for anomalous coronary artery from the pulmonary artery. *Cardiol Young*, Vol. 20 (Suppl. 3), pp. 35-43.

Frapier JM.; Leclercq, F.; Bodino, M. & Chaptal PA. (1999). Malignant ventricular arrhythmias revealing anomalous origin of the left coronary artery from the pulmonary artery in two adults. *Eur J Cardio-thorac Surg*, Vol. 15, pp. 539-541.

Frescura, C.; Basso, C.; Thiene G.; Corrado, D.; Pennelli, T.; Angelina, A. & Daliento, L. (1998). Anomalous origin of coronary arteries and risk of sudden death: a study based on an autopsy population of congenital heart disease. *Hum Pathol*, Vol. 29, pp. 689-695.

Frommelt, P.; Frommelt, M.; Tweddell, J. & Jaquiss, R. (2003). Propective echocardiographic diagnosis and surgical repair of anomalous origin of a coronary artery from the opposite sinus with an interatrial course. *J Am Coll Cardiol*, Vol. 42, pp. 148-154.

Frommelt, P.; Sheridan, D.; Berger, S.; Frommelt, M. & Tweddell, J. (2011). Ten-year experience with surgical unroofing of anomalous aortic origin of a coronary artery from the opposite sinus with an interarterial course. *J Thorac Cardiovasc Surg*, in press.

Fujimoto, S.; Kondo, T.; Orihara, T.; Sugiyama, J.; Kondo.; Kodama, T.; Fukazawa, H.; Nagaoka, H.; Oida, A.; Yamazaki, J. & Takase, S. (2011). Prevalence of anomalous origin of coronary artery detected by multi-detector computed tomography at one center. *J Cardiol*, Vol. 57, pp. 69-76.

Garcia-Rinaldi, R.; Sosa, J.; Olmeda, S.; Cruz, H.; Carballido, J. & Quintana, C. (2004). Surgical treatment of right coronaries arteries with anomalous origin and slit ostium. *Ann Thorac Surg*, Vol. 77, pp. 1525-1529.

Garg, N.; Tewari, S.; Kapoor, A.; Gupta, D. & Sinha, N. (2000). Primary congenital anomalies of the coronary arteries: a coronary arteriographic study. *Int J Cardiol*, Vol. 74, pp. 39-46.

Gharib, A.; Ho, V.; Rosing, D.; Herzka, D.; Stuber, M.; Arai, A. & Pettigrew, R. (2008). Coronary artery anomalies and variants: technical feasibility of assessment with coronary MR angiography at 3T. Radiology, Vol. 247, pp. 220-227.

Gittenberger-de Groot, A.; Barteklings, M.; Deruiter, M. & Poelmann R. (2005). Basics of cardiac development for the understanding of congenital heart malformations. *Pediatr Res,* Vol. 57, pp. 169-176.

Gittenberger-de Groot, A.; Saeur A.; Oppenheimer-Dekker, A. & Quaegebeur J. (1983). Coronary arterial anatomy in transposition of the great arteries. A morphologic study. *Ped Cardiol,* Vol. 4, pp. 15-24.

Graham, T.; Driscoll, D.; Gersony, W.; Newburger, J.; Rocchini, A. & Towbin, J. (2005). Task force 2: congenital heart disease. *J Am Coll Cardiol,* Vol. 45, pp. 1326-1333.

Hariharan, R.; Kacere, R. & Angelini, P. (2002). Can stent-angioplasty be a valid alternative to surgery. When revascularization is indicated for anomalous origination of a coronary artery form the opposite sinus ? *Tex Heart J,* Vol. 29, pp. 308-313.

Hlavaceck, A.; Loukas, M.; Spicer, D. & Anderson R. (2010). Anomalous origin and course of the coronary arteries. *Cardiol Young,* Vol. 20 (Suppl. 3), pp. 20-25.

Ishikawa, T. & Brandt, P. (1985). Anomalous origins of the left main coronary artery from the right anterior aortic sinus: angiographic definition of anomalous course. *Am J Cardiol,* Vol. 55, pp. 770-776.

Jacobs, M. & Mavroudis C. (2010). Anomalies of the coronary arteries: nomenclature and classification. *Cardiol Young,* Vol. 20 (Suppl. 3), pp. 15-19.

Jaffe, R.; Shiran, A.; Gaspar, T.; Lewis, B. & Halon, D. (2009). Primary stenting of an anomalous left main coronary artery with an interatrial course during cardiac arrest. Imaging with CT angiography. *Circ Cardiovasc Imaging.,* Vol. 2, pp. 351-352.

Karl, T.; Provenzano, S. & Nunn, G. (2010). Anomalous aortic origin of a coronary artery: a universally applicable surgical surgery. *Cardiol Young,* Vol. 20 (suppl. 3), pp. 44-49.

Kim, S.; Seo, J.; Do, K.; Heo, J.; Lee, J.; Song, J.; Choe, Y.; Kim, T.; Yong, H.; Choi, S.; Song, K. & Lim, T. (2006). Coronary artery anomalies: classification and ECG-gated multi-detector row CT findings with angiographic correlation. *Radiographics,* Vol. 26, pp. 317-334.

Kordos, A.; Babai, L.; Rudas, L.; Gaal, T.; Horvath, T.; Talosi, L.; Toth, K.; Sarvary, L. & Szasz, K. (1997). Epidemiology of congenital coronary artery anomalies: a coronary arteriography study on a central European population. *Cathet Cardiovasc Diagn,* Vol. 42, pp. 270-275.

Kottayil, B.; Jayakumar, K.; Dharan, B.; Pillai, V.; Ajitkumar, V.; Menon, S. & Sanjay, G. (2011). Anomalous origin of left coronary artery from pulmonary artery in older children and adults: direct aortic implantation. *Ann Thorac Surg,* Vol. 91, pp. 549-554.

Kragel, A. & Roberts, W. (1988). Anomalous origin of either the right or left main coronary artery form the aorta with subsequent coursing between aorta and pulmonary trunk: analysis of 32 necropsy cases. *Am J Cardiol,* Vol. 62, pp. 771-777.

Krasuski, R.; Magyar D.; Hart, S.; Kalahasti, V.; Lorber, R.; Hobbs, R.; Pettersson, G. & Blackstone, E. (2011). Long-term outcome and impact of surgery on adults with coronary arteries originating from the opposite coronary cusp. *Circulation,* Vol. 123, pp. 154-162.

Leddet, P.; Couppie, P.; Burget, J.; Reeb, T.; De Poli, F. & Hanssen, M. (2008). Identification of anomalous coronary arteries and their anatomic course by multidetector computed tomography coronarography. A retrospective registry. *Ann Cardio Angéiol,* Vol. 57, pp.256-267.

Levisman, J.; Budoff, M. & Karlsberg, R. (2009). Congenital atresia of the left main coronary artery. *Cathet Cardiovasc Interv,* Vol. 74, pp. 465-467.

Lindsey, J.; Brilarkis, E. & Banerjee, S. (2008). Acute coronary syndrome due to extrinsic compression of the left main coronary artery in a patient with severe pulmonary hypertension: successful treatment with percutaneous coronary intervention. *Cardiovasc Revasc Med,* Vol. 9, pp. 47-51.

Loukas, M.; Groat, C.; Khangura R.; Owens D. & Anderson R. (2009). The normal and abnormal anatomy of the coronary arteries. *Clin Anat,* Vol. 22, pp. 114-128.

Louyel, L. & Planché, C. (2008). Interarterial and intramural coronary trajectories: anatomical aspects and surgical implications. *Arch Mal Coeur,* Vol. 95, pp. 500-506.

Mainwaring, R.; Reddy, M.; Reinhartz, O.; Petrossian, E.; MacDonald, M.; Nasirov, T.; Miyake, C. & Hanley, F. (2011). Anomalous aortic origin of a coronary artery: medium-term results after surgical repair in 50 patients. *Ann Thorac Surg,* Vol. 92, pp. 691-697.

Manghat, N.; Morgon-Hugues, G.; Marshall, A. & Roobottom, C. (2005). Multidetector row computed tomography: imaging congenital coronary artery anomalies in adults. *Heart,* Vol. 91, pp. 1515-1522.

Maron, B. (2003). Sudden death in young athletes. *N Engl J Med,* Vol. 349, pp. 1064-1075.

Maron, B.; Douglas, P.; Graham, T.; Nishimura, R. & Thomson, P. (2005). Task force 1: preparticipation screening and diagnosis of cardiovascular disease in athletes. *J Am Coll Cardiol,* Vol. 45, pp. 1322-1326.

McConnell, M.; Ganz, P.; Selwyn, Li, W.; A.; Edelman, R. & Manning, W. (1995). Identification of anomalous coronary arteries and their anatomic course by magnetic resonance coronary angiography. *Circulation,* Vol. 92, pp. 3158-3162.

Muriago, M.; Sheppard, M.; Ho S. & Anderson R. (1997). Location of the coronary arterial orifices in the normal heart. *Clin Anat,* Vol. 10, pp. 297-302.

Ouali, S.; Neffeti, E.; Sendid, K.; Elghoul, K.; Remedi, F. & Boughzela, E. (2009). Congenital anomalous aortic origins of the coronary arteries in adults: a Tunisian coronary arteriography study. *Arch Cardio Diseas,* Vol. 102, pp. 201-208.

Pelliccia, A. (2001). Congenital coronary artery anomalies in young patients. New perspectives for timely identification. *J Am Coll Cardiol,* Vol 37, pp. 598-599.

Post, J.; van Rossum, A.; Bronzwaer, J.; de Cock, C.; Hofman, M.; Valk, J. & Visser, C. Magnetic resonance angiography of anomalous coronary arteries. A new gold standard for delineating the proximal course? *Circulation,* Vol. 92, pp. 3163-3171.

Richard, A.; Godart, F.; Brevière, G.; Francart, R.; Foucher, C. & Rey, C. (2007). Abnormal origin of the left coronary artery from the pulmonary artery: a retrospective study of 36 cases. *Arch Mal Coeur,* Vol. 100, PP. 433-438.

Rigatelli, G.; Docali, G.; Rossi, P.; Bovolon, D.; Rossi, D.; Bandello, A.; Lonardi, G. & Rigatelli, G. (2003). Congenital coronary artery anomalies angiographic classification revisited. *Int J Cardiovasc Imaging,* Vol. 19, pp.361-369.

Roberts, W. & Shirani, J. (1992). The four subtypes of anomalous origin of the left main coronary artery from the right aortic sinus (or from the right coronary artery). *Am J Cardiol,* Vol. 70, pp. 119-121.

Roberts, W. (1986). Major anomalies of coronary arterial origin seen in adulthood. *Am Heart J,* Vol. 111, pp. 941-963.

Rodriguez-Granillo, G.; Rosales, M.; Pugliese, F.; Fernadez-Pereira, C. & Rodriguez, A. (2009). Prevalence and characteristics of major and minor coronary artery anomalies in an adult population assessed by computed tomography coronary angiography. *EuroInterv*, Vol. 4, pp.641-647.

Ropers, D.; Moshage, W.; Daniel, W.; Jessl, J.; Gottwik, M. & Achenbach, S. (2001). Visualization of coronary artery anomalies and their anatomic course by contrast-enhanced electron beam tomography and three-dimensional reconstruction. *Am J Cardio*, Vol. 87, pp. 193-197.

Said, A.; Dearani, J.; Burkhart, H. & Schaff, H. (2010). Surgical management of congenital coronary arterial anomalies in adults. *Cardiol Young*, Vol. 20 (suppl. 3), pp. 68-85.

Schmitt, R.; Froehner, S.; Brunn, J.; Wagner, M.; Brunner, H.; Cherevatyy, O.; Gietzen, F.; Christopoulos, G.; Kerber, S. & Fellner, F. (2005). Congenital anomalies of the coronary arteries: imaging with contrast-enhanced, multidetector computed tomography. *Eur Radiol*, Vol. 15, pp. 1110–1121.

Serota, H.; Barth, III, C.; Seuc, C.; Vandormael, M.; Aguirre, F. & Kern, M. (1990). Rapid identification of the anomalous coronary arteries in adults: the "dot" and the "eye" method. *Am J Cardiol*, Vol. 65, pp. 891-898.

Shi, H.; Aschoff, A.; Brambs, H. & Hoffmann, M. (2004). Multislice CT imaging of anomalous coronary arteries. *Eur Radiol*, Vol. 14, pp. 2172-2181.

Sundaram, B.; Kreml, R. & Patel, S. (2010). Imaging of coronary artery anomalies. *Radiol Clin N Am*, Vol. 48, pp. 711-727.

Takeuchi, S.; Imamura, H.; Katsumoto, K.; Hayashi, I.; Katohgi, T.; Yozu, R.; Ohkura, M. & Inoue, T. (1979). New surgical method for repair of anomalous left coronary artery from pulmonary artery. *J Thorac Cardiovasc Surg*, Vol. 78, pp. 7-11.

Taylor, A.; Byers, J.; Cheitlin, M. & Virmani, R. (1997). Anomalous right and left coronary artery from the contralateral coronary sinus: "high-risk" abnormalities in the initial coronary artery course and heterogeneous clinical outcomes. *Am Heart J*, Vol. 133, pp. 428-435.

Taylor, A.; Rogan, K. & Virmani, R. (1992). Sudden cardiac death associated with isolated coronary artery anomalies. *J Am Coll Cardiol*, Vol. 20, pp. 640-647.

Tuncer, C.; Batyraliev, T.; Yilmaz, R.; Gokce, M.; Eryonucu, B. & Koroglu, S. (2006). Origin and distribution anomalies of the left anterior descending artery in 70,850 adult patients: multicenter data collection. *Cathet Cardiovasc Interv*, Vol. 68, pp. 574-585.

Virmani, R.; Burke, A. & Farb, A. (2001). Sudden cardiac death. *Cardiovasc Pathol*, Vol. 10, pp. 211-218.

Warnes, C.; Williams, R.; Bashore, T.; Child, J.; Connolly, H.; Dearani, J.; del Nido, P.; Fasules, J.; Graham, T.; Hijazi, Z.; Hunt, S.; King, M.; Landzberg, M.; Miner, P.; Radford, M.; Walsh, E. & Webb, G. (2008). ACC/AHA 2008 guidelines for the management of adults with congenital heart disease. *J Am Coll Cardiol*, Vol. 52, pp. e143-e263.

Wilkins, C.; Betancourt, B.; Mathur, V.; Massumi, A.; De Castro, M.; Garcia, E. & Hall, R. (1988). Coronary artery anomalies. A review of more than 10,000 patients from the Clayton cardiovascular laboratories. *Tex Heart J*, Vol. 15, pp. 166-173.

Yamanaka, O. & Hobbs, R. Coronary artery anomalies in 126,596 patients undergoing coronary arteriography. *Cathet Cardiovasc Diagn*, Vol. 21, pp. 28-40.

Zeppilli, P.; dello Russo, A.; Santini, C.; Plamieri, V.; Natale, L.; Giordano, A. & Frustaci, A. (1998). In vivo detection of coronary artery anomalies in asymptomatic athletes by echocardiographic screening. *Chest*, Vol. 114, pp. 89-93.

Part 4

Management of Congenital Heart Disease

Evaluation and Emergency Treatment of Criticlly Ill Neonate with Cyanosis and Respiratory Distress

Emina Hadzimuratovic[1] and Admir Hadzimuratovic[2]
[1]*Department of Neonatology, Pediatric Clinic, University Medical Center Sarajevo,*
[2]*Department of Nephrology, Pediatric Clinic, University Medical Center Sarajevo*
Bosnia and Herzegovina

1. Introduction

A severely ill neonate with cyanosis and respiratory distress is a diagnostic challenge. The clinician must perform a rapid evaluation to determine whether congenital heart disease is a cause so that potentially lifesaving measures can be instituted.

2. Differential diagnosis

The causes of cyanosis can be classified as respiratory, cardic, central nervous system (CNS) or other disorders.

3. Evaluation

During a physical examination if an infant appears blue, the following questions need immediate answer:

3.1 Does the infant have respiratory distress?

If the infant has increased respiratory effort with increased rate, retractions and nasal flaring, respiratory disease should be high on the list of differential diagnosis. Cyanotic heart disease usually presents without respiratory symptoms but can have effotless tachypnea (rapid respiratory rate without retractions).

3.2 Does the infant have murmor?

A murmor usually implies heart disease. Transposition of great vessels can present without a murmor.

3.3 Is the cyanosis continous, intermittent, sudden in oncet or occuring only with feeding?

Intermittent cyanosis is more common with neurologic disorders, as these infants may have apneic spells alternating with periods of normal breathing. Continuous cyanosis is usually associated with intrinsic lung disease or heart disease. Cyanosis with feeding may occur with esophageal atresia and severe esophageal reflux. Cyanosis that disappears with crying may signify choanal atresia.

a. **Respiratory diseases**
   1. Lung diseases
      a. Hyaline membrane disease
      b. Transiet tachypnea of the newborn
      c. Pneumonia
      d. Meconium aspiration
   2. Air leak syndrome
   3. Congenital defects (eg. Diaphragmatic hernia, hypoplastic lungs, lobar emphysema, cystic adenomatoid malformation, diaphragmal abnormality)

b. **Cardiac diseases**
   1. All cyanotic heart diseases includin transposition of great arteries, total anomalous pulmonary venous return, Ebstein's anomaly, tricuspid atresia, pulmonary atresia, pulmonary stenosis, tetralogy of Fallot, patent ductus arteriosus and ventricular septal defect
   2. Persistent pulmonary hypertension
   3. Severe congestive heart failure

c. **CNS diseases**
   Periventricular-intraventricular hemorrhage, meningitis and primary seizure disorder can all cause cyanosis. Neuromuscular disorders such as Werdnong-Hoffmanndisease and congenital myotonic dystrophy can cause cyanosis.

d. **Other disorders**
   1. Methemoglobinemia
   2. Polycythemia/hyperviscostiy syndrome
   3. Hypothermia
   4. Hypoglycemia
   5. Sepsis
   6. Pseudocyanosis caused by fluorescent lighting
   7. Respiratory depression secondary to maternal medications (eg. magnesium sulfate and narcotics)
   8. Shock
   9. Upper airway obstruction. Choanal atresia is nasal passage obstruction caused most commonly by a bony abnormality. Other causes are laryngeal web, tracheal stenosis, goiter and Pierre Robin syndrome.

Table 1. Differential diagnosis of cyanosis in the newborn

3.4 Is there differential cyanosis?

If there is cyanosis of upper or lower part of the body only, this usually signifies serious heart disease. The more common pattern is cyanosis restricted to the lower part of the body, which is seen in patients with patent ductus arteriosus with left-to right shunt. Cyanosis restricted to the upper half of the body is seen occasionally in patients with pulmonary hypertension, patent ductus arteriosus, coarctation of aorta and D-transposition of great arteries.

3.5 What is the prenatal and delivery history?

An infant of a diabetic mother has increased risk of hypoglycemia, polycytemia, respiratory distress syndrome and heart disease. Infection, which can occur with premature rupture of membranes, may cause shock and hypotension with resultant cyanosis. Amniotic fluiod abnormalities, such as oligohydramnios (associated with hypoplastic lungs) or polyhydramnios (associated with esophageal atresia), may suggest a cause for cyanosis. Cesarean section is associated with increased respiratory distress.

4. Cardiac disease

Congenital heart disease produces cyanosis when obstruction to right ventricular outflow causes intracardiac right-to-left shunting or when complex anatomic defects, unassociated with pulmonary stenosis, cause an admixture of pulmonary and systemic venous return in the heart. Cynosis from pulmonary edema may also develop in patients with heart failure caused by left-to-right shunts, although the degree is usually less severe. Cyanosis may be caused by persistence of fetal pathways, for example, right-to-left shunting across the foramen ovale and ductus arterious in the presence of persistent pulmonary hypertension of the newborn (PPHN).

5. Cardiac evaluation of newborn infant

In the cardiac evaluation of the newborn infant, understanding the circulatory status at birth is very important. As the result of fetal circulation, newborn infants have right ventricular (RV) dominance associated with a thick RV wall, elevated pulmonary vascular resistance (PVR), and a thick medial layer of the pulmonary arterioles. The thick pulmonary artery smooth muscle gradually becomes thinner, and it resembles that of the adult by the time the baby is age 6 to 8 weeks. Most perinatal changes in hemodynamics are related to the thinning of the pulmonary vascular smooth muscle, resulting in a gradual fall in the PVR and a loss of RV dominance of the neonate. Premature infants in general have lessRV dominance than full-term infants, and the PVR is not as high in the full-term neonate, which adds variability to the process. Because of these unique aspects of the perinatal circulatory system, the basic tools in the initial cardiac evaluation discussed are less reliable and the findings may be different in the newborn infant. Therefore echo studies are commonly performed in the neonatal cardiac evaluation. Some important aspects of normal and abnormal findings in physical examination, electrocardiograpgy (ECG), and chest x-ray films of the neonate are briefly reviewed in this chapter.

5.1 Physical examination

1. Normal physical findings that are unique in normal newborn infants
   a. Heart rate is generally faster (usually over 100 beats/min, with normal ranges from 70 to 180 beats/min) than that of older children and adults.
   b. A varying degree of acrocyanosis is the rule rather than the exception.
   c. Mild arterial desaturation with arterial Po2 as low as 60 mmHg is not unusual in an otherwise normal neonate. This may be caused by an intrapulmonary shunt through an as yet unexpanded portion of the lungs or by a right-to-left arterial shunt through the patent foramen ovale (PFO).

  d. There is relative hyperactivity of the RV, with the point of maximal impuls (PMI)at the lower left sternal border (LLSB) rather than at the apex.
  e. The second heart sound (S2) may be single in the first days of life, and occasionally an ejection click (reflecting pulmonary hypertension) is audible.
  f. An innocent heart murmur may be present. The most common one in this age group is the pulmonary flow murmur of the newborn infant.
  g. Peripheral pulses are easily palpable in all extremities, including the foot, in every normal infant.
2. Additional important features of premature infants
  a. The pulmonary flow murmur of the newborn infant is more frequent and louder in premature than in full-term infants.
  b. The likelihood of a patent ductus arteriosus (PDA) murmur is greater in premature infants.
  c. The peripheral pulses normally appear bounding because of the lack of a normal amount of subcutaneous tissue.
3. Abnormal phycical findings
  The following abnormal physical findings cardiac pathology.
  a. Cyanosis, particularly when it does not improve with oxygen administration, requires further evaluation.
  b. Decreased or absent peripheral pulses in the lower extremities suggest coarctation of aorta (COA). Generalized weak peripheral pulses suggest hypoplastic left heart syndrome (HLHS) or circulatory shock. Bounding peripheral pulses suggest an aortic run-off lesion such as PDA or persistent truncus arterious.
  c. Tachypnea of greater than 60 breaths/min with or without retraction is abnormal.
  d. Hepatomegaly may suggest a heart defect manifesting with congestive heart failure (CHF). A midline liver suggests asplenia or polysplenia syndrome.
  e. A heart murmur may be a presenting sign of congenital heart disease (CHD). However, innocent murmurs are more common than pathologic murmurs.
  f. An irregular rhythm or abnormal heart rate may suggest cardiac arrhythmias.
  g. Blood pressure readings in the lower extremities 6 to 7 mm Hg lower than those in the arm require further evaluation for COA.

5.2 Blood gases

Normal 1-day-old infant may have P02 as low as 60 mmHg, but transcutaneous oxygen saturation is higher than 90%.

5.3 Electrocardiographraphy

1. The normal ECG of a newborn infant is different from that of a child or an adult as follows:
  a. Sinus tachycardia with a rate as high as 180 beats/min.
  b. A rightward QRS axis with a mean of +125 degrees and a maximum of +180 degrees.
  c. Relatively small voltages for the QRS complex and the T wave.
  d. RV dominance with tall R waves in the RPLs (V4R, V1, and V2).
  e. Occasional q waves in V1(seen in about 10% of normal neonates)
  f. Benign arrhythmias

2. An abnormal ECG may be in the form of an abnormal P axis, abnormal QRS axis, hypertrophy of the ventricles or atria, vantricular conduction disturbances, or arrhythmias. Because of the wide ranges of normal values, many newborn infants with significant CHDs may show a normal ECG for their age. Arrhythmias in neonates are discussed later in this chapter.
   a. P axis
      1. A P axis in the right lower quadrant (+90 to + 180 degrees) suggests atrial situs inversus, asplenia syndrome, or incorrectly placed ECG electrodes.
      2. A superor P axis suggests an ectopic atrial rhythm, as seen in polysplenia syndrome.
   b. QRS axis
      1. A superiorly oriented QRS axis between 0 and -150 degrees (left anterior hemiblock) suggests partial or complete ECD, including splenic syndromes, or tricuspid atresia.
      2. A QRS axis less than + 30 degrees is abnormal and indicates left axis deviation (LAD) in the neonate. The QRSetween + 30 and +60 degrees is unusual and indicates relative LAD.
      3. A QRS axis greater than +180 degrees (in the range of -150 to -180 degrees) may indicate RAD.
   c. Left ventricular hypertrophy (LVH) is suggested in the newborn infant when the following are present:
      1. Left atrial hypertrophy (LAD) or relative LAD (less than +60 degrees) for the neonate.
      2. An R/S progression in the precordial leads that resembles the adult R/S progression.
      3. QRS voltages demonstrating abnormal leftward and posterior forces or abnormal inferior forces for age
   d. Right ventricular hypertrophy (RVH) is difficult to diagnose because of the normal dominance of the RV at this age. However, the following are helpful clues to RVH in the newborn infant.
      1. S waves in lead I 12 mm or greater
      2. Pure R waves with no S waves in V1 greater than 10 mm.
      3. R waves in V1 greater than 25 mm or R waves in aVR greater than 8 mm.
      4. A qR pattern in V1 (this is also seen in 10% of normal neonates).
      5. Upright T waves in V1 after 3 days of age.
      6. Right axis deviation (RAD) with the QRS axis greater than + 180 degrees.
   e. Atrial hypertrophy
      1. Right atrial hypertrophy (RAH) is present when the P wave amplitude is greater than 3 mm in any lead.
      2. Left atrial hypertrophy (LAH) iswhen the P wave duration is 0.08 sec or greater (usually with notched P waves in the limb leads and biphasic P waves in V1).
   f. Ventricular conduction disturbances (i.e , right bundle branch block (RBBB),left bundle branch block (LBBB), Wolff-Parkinson-Wite (WPW) syndrome, and intraventricular block)are present when the QRS duration is 0.07 sec or more (not 0.1 sec or greater as in the adult)

1. RBBB may be associated with Ebstein anomaly and COA in the newborn. It is sometimes seen in otherwise normal neonates.
2. LBBB is extremely rare in the newborn infant.
3. Intraventricular block (with a widening of the QRS complex throughout the QRS duration) is more significant than RBBB because it is often associated with significant metabolic abnormalities (e.g., hypoxia, acidosis, hyperkalemia) and diffuse myocardial diseases.
4. WPW syndrome may be an isolated finding or may be associated with CHDs such as Ebstein anomaly or L-TGA. It is a frequent cause of SVT.

5.4 Chest roentgenography

1. Normal CXR findings
   a. The cardiothoracic (CT) ratio of normal newborn infants may be greater than 0.5 because of inadequate inspiration and a large thymic shadow.
   b. The thymic shadow may have any of several shapes, including a classic sail sign, or may have undulant or smooth borders, either unilateral or bilateral, on the upper mediastinum.
   c. Cardiac silhouette is not always as well defined in neonates as in older children.
   d. Evaluation of pulmonary vascular markings in the neonate poses a special problem. Although a reduced PBF is usually easier to detect (and indicates serious cyanotic CHD), increased vascularity is not always apparent even when the pulmonary blood flow is large. The distinction between increased PBF and pulmonary venous congestion is often difficult.
2. Abnormal chest x-ray findings: A cardiac problem is suggested by an abnormal size, position, or silhouette of the heart, by an abnormal shape or position of the liver, and by increased or decreased pulmonary vascularity on CXR films.
   a. Heart size
   The CT ratio is of limited value, since that of normal neonates is usually greater than 0.5. Many serious CHDs that eventually result in cardiomegaly show a normal heart size in neonates. Unequivocal cardiomegaly may be due to CHD (such as ventricular septal defect (VSD), PDA, transposition of the great arteries (TGA), Ebstein anomaly, hypoplastic left heart syndrome (HLHS), and other), myocarditis or cardiomyopathy, pericardial effusion, metabolic disturbance (e.g., hypoglycemia, severe hypoxemia, and acidosis), and overhydration or overtransfusion.

   In the newborn infant who is intubated and on a ventilator, the heart size is greatly influenced by the ventilator setting. For example, a premature infant with a large-shunt PDA may have a normal-sized heart on chest x-ray film if the ventilator settings are high, especially the positive end-expiratory pressure.
   b. Abnormal cardiac silhouettes may be of considerable help in suggesting the correct diagnosis.
      1. A boot-shaped heart (coeur en sabot) is seen in tetralogy of Fallot (TOF) and in tricuspid atresia.
      2. An egg-shaped heart with narrow waist may be seen in TGA.
      3. A large, globular heart is seen in Ebstein anomaly.

c. Dextrocardia or mesocardia
   The presence of dextrocardia or mesocardia does not always indicate a serious heart defect. The segmental approach should be used for further evaluation. Four common situations seen in dextrocardia or mesocardia are situs inversus totalis with a normal heart, a rightward displacement of a normallyformed heart due to hypoplasia of the right lung, a complex cyanotic CHD, and asplenia or polysplenia syndrome.
d. The situs of abdominal viscera: A left-sided liver with the heart in the right side of the chest is seen in situs inversus totalis with normal heart. The liver and the cardiac apex on the same side suggest a complex cyanotic CHD. A midline liver suggests asplenia or polysplenia syndrome.
e. Pulmonary vascular markings
   1. Increased pulmonary vascular marking (PVM) in a cyanotic infant suggest TGA, persistent truncus arteriosus, or single ventricle. In an acyanotic infant, increased PVMs suggest VSD, PDA, or endocardial cushion defect (ECD).
   2. Decreased PVMs suggest a critical cyanotic CHD with decreased pulmonary blood flow(PBF), such as pulmonary atresia, tricuspid atresia, mor TOF with severe pulmonary stenosis or atresia.
   3. A ground-glass appearance or a reticulated pattern of the lung fields is characteristic of pulmonary venous obstruction.

6. Suggested approach to neonates with central cyanosis

a. Although a significant heart murmur usually suggests a cardiac basis for the cyanosis, several of the more severe cardiac defects (transposition of the great vessels) may not initially be associated with a murmur.
   Heart murmurs.
   1. Innocent heart murmurs: More than 50% of full-term newborn infants (and a higher percentage of premature infants) have an innocent systolic murmur at some time during the first week of life. Infants with innocent heart murmurs have normal ECG and chest x-ray findings. The four most common innocent murmurs in the newborn period are as follows:
      a. Pulmonary flow murmur is most common. It is more often found in premature and small-for-gestational-age infants than in full-term infants. A soft systolic murmur (grade 1 to 2/6), heard best at the upper left sternal border (ULSB), transmits well to bozh sides of the chest, axillae, and the back.
      b. Transient systolic murmur of PDA is soft (grade 1 to 2/6), audible at the ULSB and in the left infraclavicular area on the first day. It usually disappears shortly thereafter.
      c. Transient systolic murmur of tricuspid regurgitation is indistinguishable from that of VSD and is most common in infants who had fetal distress or neonatal asphyxia.
      d. Vibratory systolic innocent murmur is a counterpart of Still's murmur in older children. It is audible at the LLSB, apex, or midprecordium.
   2. Pathologic heart murmurs: Most pathologic murmurs except atrial septal defect (ASD) are audible during the first month of life. The time of appearance of a murmur depends on the nature of the defect.

a. Heart murmurs of stenotic lesions (e.g., aortal stenosis (AS), pulmonary stenosis (PS)) are audible immediately after birth and persist, because they are independent of the level of the PVR.
b. Heart murmurs of L-R shunt lesions, especially those of a large VSD, may appear later, when the PVR decreases. The murmur of ASD appears late in infancy or in childhood.
c. The continuous murmur of a large PDA may not appear for 2 to 3 weeks. Instead, it is a crescendo systolic murmur with a slight or no diastolic component.

Even in the absence of a murmur, a newborn infant may have a serious heart defect that requires immediate attention, e.g., severe cyanotic heart disease such as TGA or pulmonary atresia with a closing PDA. Infants who are in severe CHF may not have a loud murmur until the myocardial function is improved with anticongestive measures.

b. Chest x-ray films may reveal pulmonary causes of cyanosis and urgency of the problem.They will also hint at the presence and the type of any cardiac defects.
c. Arterial blood gases on room air will confirm or rule out central cyanosis. Elevated Pco2 suggests pulmonary or central nervous system (CNS) problems. Low pH may be seen in sepsis, circulatory shock, or severe hypoxemia.
d. Hyperoxia test is one method of distinguishing cyanotic congenital heart disease from pulmonary disease. Neonates with cyanotic congenital heart disease usually do not have significantly raised arterial Pao2 during administration of 100% oxygen. If the Pao2 rises above 150 mmHg during 100% oxygen administration, an intracardiac shunt can usually be excluded, although the Pao2 of some patients with cyanotic congenital heart lesions may be transiently increased to greater than 150 mm Hg because of intracardiac streaming patterns. The Pao2 in patiens with pulmonary disease generally increases significantly as ventilation - perfusion inequalities are overcome by oxygen administration. In infants with a CNS disorder, the Pao2 completely normalizes during artificial ventilation. Hypoxia in many heart lesions is profound and constant, whereas in respiratory disorders and in primary hypertension of the neonate (PPHN), arterial oxygen tension is not as low and often varies with time or changes in ventilator management. Hyperventilation may improve the hypoxia in neonates with PPHN and only occasionally in those with cyanotic heart disease.
e. An ECG should be obtained if a cardiac origin of cyanosis is suspected.
f. Two-dimensional echocardiography is the definitive noninvasive test to determine the presence of congenital heart disease. The information obtained is essential in avoiding unnecessary cardiac catheterization and angiography in the absence of a cardiac defect, as well as in making a specific diagnosis.
g. Umbilical artery line: A Po2 value in a preductal artery (such as right radial artery) higher than that in a postductal artery (umbilical artery line) by 10 to 15 mm Hg suggests an R-L shunt through a PDA. Such a differential Po2 level may result from persistent pulmonary hypertension of the newborn (PPHN), critical AS, interrupted aortic arch, or coarctation of the aorta. An echo study will clarify the cause of the differential Po2 levels.
h. Cardiology consultation is called for if a cardiac origin of cyanosis is suspected.

7. Heart failure in the newborn infant

The clinical picture of CHF in the neonate may simulate another disorder such as meningitis, sepsis, pneumonia, or bronchiolitis. Tachypnea, tachycardia, pulmonary crackles or rhonchi, hepatomegaly, and weak peripheral pulses are common presenting signs. Heart murmur is either faint or absent. Cardiomegaly on chest x-ray film is always present, with or without increased PVMs or pulmonary edema. Causes of CHF in the neonate are listed in Table 2.

a. **Structural heart defects**

At birth
- Hypoplastic left heart syndrome (HLHS)
- Severe tricuspid or pulmonary regurgitation
- Large systemic AV fistula

Week 1
- TGA
- Large PDA in premature infant
- Total anomalous pulmonary venous return (TAPVR) below diaphragm

Week 1-4
- Critical AS or PS
- Preductal COA

b. **Noncardiac causes**
1. Birth asphyxia (resulting in transient myocardial ischemia)
2. Metabolic: hypoglycemia, hypocalcemia
3. Severe anemia (as seen in hydrops fetalis)
4. Neonatal sepsis
5. Overtransfusion or overhydration

c. **Myocardial disease**
1. Myocarditis
2. Transient myocardial ischemia (with or without birth asphyxia)
3. Catdiomyopathy (seen in infants of diabetic mothers)

d. **Disturbances in heart rate**
1. Supravetricular tachycardia (supraventricular tachycardia (SVT) or paroxysmal atrial tachycardia(PAT))
2. Atrial flutter or fibrillation
3. Congenital heart block (when associated with CHD)

The time of onset of CHF varies rather predictably with the type of CHD.

Table 2. Cause of heart failure in the neonate

Two important CHDs that present with CHF in the newborn period are hypoplastic left heart syndrome (HLHS) and large PDA in premature infants. Transient myocardial ischemia and infants of diabetic mothers are other causes of CHF in the neonate.

8. Hypoplastic left heart syndrome

a. Prevalence:HLHS occurs in 1% of all CHDs and is the most common cause of death from CHD during the first month of life.
b. Pathology and pathophysiology

1. HLHS includes a group of closely related anomalies characterized by hypoplasia of the left ventricul (LV) (from atresia or severe stenosis of the aortic and/or mitral valves) and hypoplasia of the ascending aorta and aortic arch. The LA is small, and the atrial septum is frequently intact other than the PFO.
2. During fetal life the pulmonary vascular resistance (PVR) is higher than the systemic vascular resistance (SVR), and the dominant RV maintains normal perfusing pressure in the descending aorta through the ductal R-L shunt, even in the presence of the nonfunctioning hypoplastic LV. However, difficulties arise after birth, primarily from two factors: (1) reversal of the vascular resistance in the two circuits with the SVR higher than the PVR, and (2) closure of the PDA. The end result is a marked decrease in systemic cardiac output and aortic pressure, resulting in circulatory shock and metabolic acidosis. An increase in PBF in the presence of the nonfunctioning LV results in an elevated LA pressure and pulmonary edema.

c. Clinical manifestations
   1. The neonate is critically ill in the first few hourse to days of life, with mild cyanosis, tachycardia, tachypnea, and pulmonary crackles.
   2. Poor peripheral pulses and vasoconstricted extremities are characteristic. The S2 is loud and single. Heart murmur is usually absent, but a grade 1 to 3/6 ejection systolic murmur may be present over the precordium.
   3. The ECG shows RVH. Rarely, left ventricular hypertrophy (LVH) pattern is present because V5 and V6 electrodes are placed over the dilated RV.
   4. Chest x-ray films show pulmonary venous congestion or pulmonary edema. The heart is only mildly enlarged.
   5. The arterial blood gas determination reveals severe metabolic acidosis in the presence of a slightly decreased Po2, a characteristic finding of this condition.
   6. Echo findings are diagnosticand usually obviate cardiac catheterization. Severe hypoplasia of the aorta and aortic annulus and the absent or distorted mitral valve are usually imaged. The LV cavity is diminutive. The RV cavity is markedly dilated, and the tricuspid valve is large.A partially constricted PDA may be imaged.
   7. Progressive hypoxemia and acidosis result in death, usually in the first month of life.

d. Management
   1. Preoperatively the goal is to achieve adequate systemic oxygen delivery. Patency of the ductus arteriosus is critical for survival until surgery. Blood flow to the pulmonary and systemic circulations should be nearly balanced (goal p/s ratio of 1). The immediate therapy for all infants with HLHS is an intravenous infusion of prostaglandin E1 (PGE1) in order to pharmacologically manipulate the ductus arteriosus (DA) and maintain ductal patency. A continuous infusion of the prostaglandin is initiated, preferably through a central catheter, at a rate of 0.05 to 0.1 μg/kg per minute. However, numerous side effects are associated with PGE1 infusion such as respiratory depression, fever, lethargy, irritability, myoclonic jerks, flushing, edema, pyloric stenosis, hyperostosis, necrotizing enetrocolitis, as well as structural remodeling of the DA and the pulmonary vessels, with a reported incidence of these complications ranging from 10 to 40%. (7,8) In the future

Sildenafil could be a reasonable alternative to PGE1 for maintaining DA patency, since it can also prevent and reverse DA closure through a mechanism that is distinct, and eventually safer, from the PGE1 mechanism. (9) An audible murmur and adequate peripheral perfusion provide evidence of ductal patency; however, Doppler echocardiography is needed to confirm flow. Once the ductus is open, the rate of infusion may be reduced to decrease the risk for potential adverse effects. Unrestricted blood flow through the ductus arteriosus is necessary for systemic perfusion. Sometimes even a temporary discontinuation of the prostaglandin infusion is possible, with careful monitoring of blood pressure and urine volume as well as frequent echocardiographic examinations, in order to enable maintenance of balance between systemic and pulmonary blood flow. (4)

The pulmonary/systemic (p/s) ratio preoperatively is dictated by the adequacy of the interatrial communication. An infant with a mildly restrictive interatrial communication may have balanced circulation and remain in a clinically stable condition as long as the ductus arteriosus remains open. Oxygen saturations of 75% to 85% by pulse oximetry suggest adequate balance between systemic and pulmonary blood flow. Ventilatory support may be needed for apneic episodes or tenacious secretions, both common adverse effects of treatment with prostaglandin E1. Judicious use of inotropic support is initiated if evidence of low cardiac output is detected. Infusion of dopamine at a rate of 3 to 5 μg/kg per minute usually results in improved ventricular function. High-dose inotropic support should be used with caution because it can result in increased SVR and cause a shift in the p/s ratio to greater than 1. In our institution we do not recommend the use of dopamine as a "standard" since we consider it a "dirty" drug with a lot of potential unexpected effects. Diuretics may be necessary to help alleviate the increased volume load on the right ventricle.

Infants with an unrestrictive inter-atrial communication may be in a stable condition initially, but signs of congestive heart failure may develop as the PVR (pulmonary vascular resistance) decreases. When oxygen saturations are approximately 90%, systemic blood flow may be reduced, resulting in tissue hypoperfusion, metabolic acidosis, and a low cardiac output state. In infants with high oxygen saturation and evidence of tissue hypoperfusion, controlled mechanical ventilation is often initiated to improve the p/s ratio and systemic cardiac output.

Severe tricuspid regurgitation (TR) could be another issue that complicates the life of the intensivist dealing with a newborn with HLHS. Good preoperative management with mechanical ventilation in order to lower the degree of TR results in a better short-term prognosis of stage 1 Norwood operation. (4)

The goal of respiratory management is to increase pulmonary vascular resistance and decrease systemic vascular resistance. The p/s ratio can be manipulated by increasing PVR by increasing the PaCO2. PaCO2 can be increased by adding supplemental inspired carbon dioxide, a potent pulmonary vasoconstrictor, to the ventilator circuit. This approach for increasing PaCO2 is preferred over hypoventilation, which may lead to atelectasis. PVR can also be increased by decreasing the concentration of inspired oxygen by adding supplemental nitrogen gas to attain a fraction of inspired oxygen of 0.17 to 0.19. PVR can also be increased by maintaining the hematocrit at greater than 0.40, a state that optimizes oxygen-carrying capacity and increases the viscosity of the blood. Although these medical management strategies may provide temporary palliation, infants with marked pulmonary overcirculation and systemic hypoperfusion benefit from early surgical correction, because the methods to reverse this situation have limited effectiveness. Infants with HLHS who are born with a severely restricted or no inter-atrial communication, a rare occurrence, have profound hypoxemia. In fact, morbidity and mortality remain high in the subset of patients with an intact or very restrictive atrial septum. (10) The severe restriction of blood flow across the atrial septum results in a life-threatening situation and these patients, which present with severe cyanosis and hemodynamic instability, require urgent postnatal cardiac catheterization to relieve the septal obstruction and improve oxygenation. (11) Relief of the obstruction can be achieved by a balloon atrial septostomy or blade septostomy at the time of cardiac catheterization or a surgical atrial septectomy. The tenuous condition of these infants makes each of these interventions high risk. The choice of intervention depends on the severity of the obstruction, the infant's cardiac anatomy and physiology, and the experience of the available medical and surgical team.

2. Surgical: Three options are available in the management of these infants:do nothing or choose one of two surgical options. The surgical options are the Norwood operation (followed by a Fontan operation) and cardiac transplantation. The surgical procedure of choice remains controversial.
    1. Norwood operation
        a. The first-stage Norwood operation is performed on the neonate. This operation consists of (1) division of the MPA and closure of the distal stump, (2) a right-sided Gore-Tex shunt (usually a 4-mm tube) to provide PBF, (3) excision of the atrial septum (for adequate interatrial mixing), and (4) construction of a new aortic arch between the proximal main pulmonary artery (MPA) and the hypoplastic ascending aorta and aortic archm using an aortic or pulmonary artery allograft. The surgical mortality rate is 35% or higher.
        b. A cavopulmonary shunt (or bidirectional Glenn operation) is carried out at 6 months of age. Mortality is less than 5%.
        c. A modified Fontan operation is carried out when the patient is a year and a half old. Overall survival after the Fontan operation is about 50% at 4 years.
    2. Cardiac transplantation is considered to be the procedure of choice in some centers. The transplantation is not a cure for the defect but creates a lifelong medical problem, the threat of infection and rejection.

9. Premature neonates with a large PDA

a. Prevalence.

Significant PDA with CHF occurs in 15% of prematures with a birth weight of less than 1,750 g and in 40% to 50% of those with a birth weight of less than 1,500 g.

b. Pathophysiology

This is a special problem in premature infants who have been recovering from hyaline membrane disease. With improvement in oxygenation the PVR drops rapidly, but the ductus remains patent because its responsiveness to oxygen is immature in the premature newborn infant. The resulting large L-R ductal shunt makes the lungs stiff, and weaning the infant from ventilator and oxygen therapy becomes difficult. Infants who remain on ventilators for a long time develop bronchopulmonary dysplasia with resulting pulmonary hypertension (cor pulmonale) and right-sided heart failure.

c. Clinical manifestations

1. The history usually reveals that a premature infant with hyaline membrane disease has made some improvement during the first few days after birth, but this is followed by inability to wean the infant from the ventilator or a need to increase ventilator settings or oxygen requirement in 4-to 7-day-old premature infants. Apneic spells or episodes of bradycardia may be initial signs in infants who are not on ventilators.
2. Bounding peripheral pulses and a hyperactive precordium are usually present. The classic continuous murmur of PDA at the ULSB is diagnostic, but the murmur is sometimes systolic only at the middle and upper LSB. Premature infants who are fluid overloaded or retaining fluid may also present with the hyperdynamic precordium, an ejection systolic murmur, bounding pulse, and wide pulse pressure.
3. The ECG is usually normal.
4. Chest x-ray films show cardiomegaly and evidence of pulmonary edema or pulmonary venous congestion in addition to varying degrees of the lung disease.
5. 2D echo study confirms the diagnosis. It provides anatomic information about the diameter, length, and shape of the ductus. The Doppler study of the ductus (with the sample volume placed at the pulmonary end of the ductus) provides important functional information such as ductal shunt patterns (pure L-R, bidirectional, or predominant R-L shunt), pressure in the PA, and magnitude of the ductal shunt or pulmonary perfusion status. An indirect estimate of the magnitude of the shunt can be made by the LA and LV dimensions.

d. Management: For symptomatic infants, either pharmacologic (indomethacin) or surgical closure of the ductus is indicates. A small PDA that is not causing CHF should be followed up medically for 6 months without surgical ligation because of the possibility of spontaneous closure.

1. Indomethacin (a prostaglandin synthetase inhibitor), 0.2 mg/kg IV every 12 hours for up to three doses, may be used on selected cases. A second course is occasionally necessary for adequate ductal closure. Contraindications to the use of indomethacin include (1) BUN over 25 mg/dL or creatinine levels over 1.8 mg/dL, (2) a platelet count below 80,000/mm^3, (3) a bleeding tendency (including intracranial hemorrhage), (4) necrotizing enterocolitis, and (5) hyperbilirubinemia.
2. A European study showed that ibuprofen given IV (10 mg/kg followed by 5 mg/kg every 24 hours, two times), starting on the 3rd day of life, was as effective as indomethacin (0.2 mg/kg IV every 12 hours, three times), with a lower incidence of oliguria and a less deleterious effect on the cerebral blood flow than indomethacin. However, ibuprofen is not approved for use in premature PDA in this country.

3. If the medical treatment is unsuccessful or if the use of indomethacin is contraindicated, a surgical ligation of the ductus is indicated. The standard operative approach to the PDA has been through a posterolateral thoracotomy. The safety, effectiveness, and minimally invasive nature of video-assisted thoracoscopic surgery (VATS) have been reported for premature PDA. Advantages of the technique may include no need to cut the muscle and to spread ribs, thus a reduced compromise of respiratory mechanics and of chest wall deformity.

10. Persistent pulmonary hypertension of the newborn

(Persistent Fetal Circulation)

PPHN occurs in term and post-term infants. Predisposing factors include birth asphyxia, meconium aspiration pneumonia, early-onset sepsis, hypoglycemia, polycythemia, maternal use of nonsteroidal anti-inflammatory drugs with in utero constriction of the ductus arterious, and pulmonary hypoplasia as a result of diaphragmatic hernia, amniotic fluid leak, oligohydramnions, or pleural effusions. PPHN is often idiopathic. Some patients with PPHN have low plasma arginine and nitric oxide metabolite concentrationsand polymorphisms of the carbamoyl phosphate synthase gene, findings suggestive of a possible subtle defect in nitric oxide production. The incidence is 1/500-1,500 live births with a wide variation between different clinical centers.

a. Pathophysiology: Persistence of the fetal circulatory pattern of right-to-left shunting through the PDA and foramen ovale after birth is due to excessively high pulmonary vascular resistance. Fetal pulmonary vascular resistance is usually elevated relative to fetal systemic or postnatal pulmonary pressure. This fetal state permits shunting of oxygenated umbilical venous blood to the left atrium (and brain) through the foramen ovale and bypasses the lungs through the ductus arterious to the descending aorta. After birth, pulmonary vascular resistance normally declines rapidly as a consequence of vasodilation secondary to gas filling the lungs, a rise in postnatal Pao2, a reduction in Pco2, increased pH, and release of vasoactive substances. Increased neonatal pulmonary vascular resistance may (1) be maladaptive from an acute injury (e.g., not demonstrating normal vasodilation in response to increased oxygen and other changes after birth); (2) be the result of increased pulmonary artery medial muscle thickness and extension of smooth muscle layers into the usually nonmuscular, more peripheral pulmonary arterioles in response to chronic fetal hypoxia; (3) be due to pulmonary hypoplasia (diaphragmatic hernia, Potter syndrome); (4) be obstructive as a result of polycythemia or total anomalous pulmonary venous return; or (5) be due to alveolar capillary dysplasia, a lethal, possibly familial disorder characterized by a thickened alveolar septum and a reduced number of small pulmonary arteries and capillaries. Apart from the etiology, profound hypoxia from right-to-left shunting and normal or elevated Pco2 are present.
b. Clinical Manifestations: Infants become ill in the delivery room or within the first 12 hr of life. PPHN related to polycythemia, idiopathic causes, hypoglycemia, or asphyxia may result in severe cyanosis with tachypnea, although initially, signs of respiratory distress may be minimal. Infants who have PPHN associated with meconium aspiration, group B streptococcal pneumonia, diagphragmatic hernia, or pulmonary hypoplasia usually exhibit cyanosis, grunting, flaring, retractions, tachycardia, and

shock. Multiorgan involvement may be present. Myocardial ischemia, papillary muscle dysfunction with mitral and tricuspid regurgitation, and cardiac stunning produce cardiogenic shock with decreased pulmonary blood flow, tissue perfusion, and oxygen delivery. The hypoxia is quite labile and often out of proportion to the findings on chest roentgenograms.

c. Diagnosis: PPHN should be suspected in all term infants who have cyanosis with or without fetal distress, intrauterine growth restriction, meconium-stained amniotic fluid, hypoglycemia, polycythemia, diaphragmatic hernia, pleural effusions, and birth asphyxia. Hypoxia is universal and is unresponsive to 100% oxygen given by oxygen hood, but it may respond transiently to hyperoxic hyperventilation administered after endotracheal intubation or to the application of a bag and mask. A Pao2 gradient between a preductal (right radial artery) and a postductal (umbilical artery) site of blood sampling greater than 20 mm Hg suggest right-to-left shunting through the ductus arteriosus. Real-time echocardiography combined with Doppler flow studies demonstrates right-to-left shunting across a patent foramen ovale and a ductus arteriosus. Deviation of the intraatrial septum into the left atrium is seen in severe PPHN. Tricuspid or mitral insufficiency may be noted on auscultation as a holosystolic murmur and can be visualized echocardiographically together with poor contractility when PPHN is associated with myocardial ischemia. The degree of tricuspid regurgitation can be used to estime pulmonary artery pressure. The 2nd heart sound is accentuated and not split. In asphyxia-associated and idiopathic PPHN , the chest roentgenogram is normal, whereas in PPHN associated with pneumonia and diaphragmatic hernia, it shows the specific lesions of parenchymal opacification and bowel in the chest, respectively. The differential diagnosis of PPHN includes cyanotic heart disease (especially obstructed total anomalous pulmonary venous return) and the associated etiologic entities that predispose to PPHN (e.g., hypoglycemia, polycythemia, sepsis).

d. Treatment: Therapy is directed toward correcting any predisposing disease (hypoglycemia, polycithemia) and improving poor tissue oxygenation. The response to therapy is often unpredictable, transient, and complicated by the adverse effects of drugs or mechanical ventilation. Initial management includes oxygen administration and correction of acidosis, hypotension, and hypercapnia. Persistent hypoxia should be managed with intubation and mechanical ventilation.

   Treatment with inhaled nitric oxide (iNO) is indicated for newborns with an oxygen index (OI) of less than 25. Nitric oxide (NO) is an endothelially derived gas signaling molecule that relaxes vascular smooth muscle and that can be delivered to the lung by means of an inhalation device . In 2 large, randomized trials, NO reduced the need for extracorporeal membrane oxygenation (ECMO) by approximately 40%. Although these trials led to the US Food and Drug Administration (FDA) approving iNO as a therapy for persistent pulmonary hypertension of the newborn (PPHN), iNO did not reduce mortality, the length of hospitalization, or the risk of neurodevelopmental impairment. A randomized study confirmed that beginning iNO at a milder or earlier point in the disease course (for an oxygenation index of 15-25) did not decrease the incidence of ECMO and/or death or improve other patient outcomes, including the incidence of neurodevelopmental impairment.The use of iNO has not been demonstrated to reduce the need for ECMO in newborns with congenital diaphragmatic hernia. In these newborns, iNO should be used in non-ECMO centers to allow for acute stabilization, followed by immediate transfer to a center that can provide extracorporeal membrane oxygenation (ECMO).Contraindications to iNO include congenital heart disease characterized by left ventricular outflow tract obstruction (eg, interrupted aortic arch, critical aortic stenosis, hypoplastic left heart syndrome) and severe left ventricular dysfunction.The appropriate starting dose is 20 ppm. Doses higher than this have not been shown to be more effective and have been associated with adverse effects, including methemoglobinemia and increased levels of nitrogen dioxide (NO_2).Appropriate lung recruitment and expansion are essential to achieve the best response. If a newborn has severe parenchymal lung disease and PPHN, strategies such as HFV may be required.Most newborns require iNO for less than 5 days. In general, the dose can be weaned to 5 ppm after 6-24 hours of therapy. The dose is then slowly weaned and discontinued when the FiO_2 is less than 0.4-0.6 and the iNO dose is 1 ppm. Abrupt discontinuation at higher doses should be avoided because it may cause abrupt rebound pulmonary hypertension. In centers that do not have immediate availability of ECMO support, use of iNO must be approached with caution. Because iNO cannot be abruptly discontinued, transport with iNO is usually needed if a subsequent referral for ECMO is necessary. This capability should be determined in collaboration with the ECMO center before treatment is started. The use of iNO with high frequency ventilation (HFV) creates particular problems for transport, and this should be considered before these therapies are combined in a non-ECMO center.

ECMO, an adaptation of cardiopulmonary bypass, is used when optimal support fails to maintain acceptable oxygenation and perfusion . The introduction of ECMO and other new therapies has had a major effect on reducing the mortality rate associated with PPHN. ECMO support can now be provided using a double-lumen catheter in the internal jugular vein; thus, ligation of the right common carotid artery can be avoided. Although iNO is an effective pulmonary vasodilator, ECMO remains the only therapy that has been proven to be life-saving for PPHN. Therefore, timely transfer to an ECMO center is vital for newborns with severe PPHN.However, it is often difficult to determine the proper timing of a referral to an ECMO center. Referral and transfer should occur before refractory hypoxemia develops. Early consultation and discussion with clinicians at the ECMO center is strongly recommended. Continuous delivery of NO is required during transport. Baseline criteria for newborns considered for ECMO are generally as follows:

- Gestation of more than 34 week
- Weight more than 2000 g
- No major intracranial hemorrhage on cranial sonograms (ie, larger than a grade II hemorrhage)
- Reversible lung disease or mechanical ventilation for 7-14 days
- No evidence of lethal congenital anomalies or inoperable cardiac disease

11. Transient myocardial ischemia

a. Prevalence

Transient myocardial ischemia is a rarely recognized condition; the prevalence is unknown.

b. Pathology and pathophysiology
   1. Subendocardial ischemia or necrosis (possibly secondary to hypoxic pulmonary vasoconstriction) occurs in the papillary muscles and other areas of the ventricles in the newborn infant who had prenatal or perinatal hypoxia and distress. Evidence of pulmonary hypertension, bidirectional shunts at the atrial and/or ductal levels, and TR are usually present. Variable degrees of LV dysfunction are demonstrable by echocardiography.
   2. Three levels of severity have been recognized.
      a. Transient tachypnea of the newborn is the mildest form of the condition. Mild LV dysfunction leads to fluid retention, pulmonary edema, and reduced lung compliance producing tachypnea.
      b. Transient tricuspid (or mitral) regurgitation results from papillary muscle infarction (evidenced by elevated serum levels of creatine phosphokinase MB fraction).
      c. Severe CHF with cardiogenic shock is the most severe form of myocardial dysfunction seen in the newborn infant.

c. Clinical manifestations
   1. Tachypnea develops usually in full-term neonates with a low Apgar score. Mild cyanosis may also be present.
   2. A systolic murmur of TR or MR is commonly present. Rarely, CHF with gallop rhythm, hypotension, and vascular collapse result.
   3. The ECG may show generalized flat T waves and minor ST segment depression. Abnormal Q waves suggestive of anterior or inferior infarction may be seen.
   4. CXR films show varying degrees, sometimes marked, of cardiomegaly. PVMs may be increased due to pulmonary venous congestion (described as wet lung) in severely affected neonates.
   5. Echo study reveals varying degrees of myocardial dysfunction, including an enlarged LA and /or LV, decreased contractility of the LV, and mitral regurgitation (MR).
   6. Laboratory studies may reveal mild reduction of Po2 and pH (but usually without CO2 retention), hypoglycemia, and elevated CPK MB fraction in patients with significant TR. A myocardial perfusion scan may show a diffuse impairment of thallium-201 uptake (different from myocarditis, in which myocardial perfusion is normal).
   7. Infants with transient myocardial ischemia usually recover unless it is associated with severe acidosis, CNS damages, or advanced sepsis.

d. Management
   1. Supportive measures with administration of oxygen, correction of acidosis, and treatment of hypogycemia are all that are required for mild cases.
   2. For severely affected infants, ventilatory assistance, short-acting inotropic agents (such as dopamine), a vasodilator agent, and fluid restriction and diuretic(s) may be indicated.

12. Emergency treatment if cyanotic CHD is suspected

If a cyanotic CHD is suspected, PGE1 should be started or made available. The starting dose is 0.05 to 0.1 μg/kg/min, administered in a continuous IV drip. When the desired effects

(increased Po2, increased systemic blood pressure, and improved pH) are achieved, the dose should be reduced step-by-step to 0.01μg/kg/min. When there is no effect with the initial starting dose, it may be increased to 0.4 μg/kg/min.
If echocardiography is not immediately available, the clinician caring for a newborn with possible cyanotic heart disease should not hesitate to start a prostaglandin infusion (for a possible ductal-dependent lesion). Because of the risk of hypoventilation associated with prostaglandins, a practitioner skilled in neonatal endotracheal intubation must be available. Three common side effects of Prostaglandin E1 IV infusion are apnea (12%), fever (14%), and flushing (10%).

13. Summary

The evaluation of the cyanotic neonate should be done in an algorithmic manner that focuses on evaluation and management of the most life-threatening disease processes first.The hyperoxia test should be utilized early in the evaluation of these patients to assist in the differentiation and categorization of the cyanotic event. Be careful to obtain a detailed history of the prenatal, birth, and postnatal periods, as physicians will often be able to narrow the differential by the history alone. Neonates may decompensate very quickly, and preparations for a life-saving emergency should be made as soon as possible.

14. References

[1] Baba K, Ohtsuki S, Kamada M, Kataoka K, Ohno N, Okamoto Y, et al. Preoperative management for tricuspid regurgitation in hypoplastic left heart syndrome. Ped Internat 2009;51:399-404.
[2] Fricker FJ. Hypoplastic Left Heart Syndrome - Diagnosis and early management. NeoReviews 2008;9:253.
[3] Hoffmann GM, Ghanayem NS, Kampine JM, Berger S, Mussatto KA, Litwin SB, et al. Venous saturation and the anaerobic threshold in neonates after the Norwood procedure for hypoplastic left heart syndrome. Ann Thorac Surg 2000;70:1515-21.
[4] Singh GH, Fong LV, Salmon AP, Keeton BR. Study of low dosage prostaglandin – usages and complication. Eur Heart J 1994;15:377-81.
[5] Lewis AB, Freed MD, Heymann MA, Roehl SL, Kensey RC. Side effects of therapy with prostaglandin E1 in infants with critical congenital heart disease. Circulation 1981;64: 893-8.
[6] Thiebaud B, Michelakis E, Wu XC, Harry G, Hashimoto K, Archer SL. Sildenafil Reverses O2 constriction of the rabbit Ductus Arteriosus by inhibiting Type 5 phosphodisesterase and activating BK Ca Channels. Ped Res 2002;52:19-24.
[7] Rychik J, Rome JJ, Collins MH, DeCampli WM, Spray TL. The hypoplastic left heart syndrome with intact atrial septum: atrial morphology, pulmonary vascular histopathology and outcome. J Am Coll Cardiol 1999;34:554-60.
[8] Atz AM, Feinstein JA, Jonas RA. Preoperative management of pulmonary venous hypertension in hypoplastic left heart syndrome with restrictive atrial septal defect. Am J Cardiol 1999;83:1224-8.

[9] Newburger JW, Jonas RA, Wernovsky G. A comparison of the preoperative neurologic effects of hypothermic circulatory arrest versus low-flow cardiopulmonary bypass in infant heart surgery. N Engl J Med 1993;329:1057-64.
[10] Miller SP, McQuillen PS, Hamrick S, Xu D, Glidden DV, Charlton N. Abnormal brain development in newborns with congenital heart disease. N Engl J Med. 2007;357:1928-38.
[11] Tabbutt S, Nord AS, Jarvik GP. Neurodevelopmental outcomes after staged palliation for hypoplastic left heart syndrome. Pediatrics 2008;121:476-83.
[12] Dorfman AT, Marino BS, Wernovsky G, Tabbutt S, Ravishankar C, Godinez RI, et al. Critical heart disease in the neonate: Presentation and outcome at a tertiary care center. Pediatr Crit Care Med 2008;9:193-202
[13] Behrman RE, Kliegman RM, Jenson HB. Nelson Textbook of Pediatrics (17th edition). Philadelphia: W.B.Sauders, 2004
[14] Senka Mesihović- Dinarević. Dječija kardiologija: od fetusa do adolescenta. Medicinski fakultet ,Sarajevo; 2000
[15] Gomella TL. Neonatology: Management, Procedures, On-Call Problems. Diseases, and Drugs (4th edition). Appleton & Lange; 1999
[16] Chambers CD, Hernandez-Diaz S, Van Marter LJ, Werler MM, Louik C, Jones KL, et al. Selective serotonin-reuptake inhibitors and risk of persistent pulmonary hypertension of the newborn. *N Engl J Med*. Feb 9 2006;354(6):579-87. [Medline].
[17] Steinhorn RH, Kinsella JP, Pierce C, Butrous G, Dilleen M, Oakes M, et al. Intravenous sildenafil in the treatment of neonates with persistent pulmonary hypertension. *J Pediatr*. Dec 2009;155(6):841-847.e1. [Medline].
[18] Bahrami KR, Van Meurs KP. ECMO for neonatal respiratory failure. *Semin Perinatol*. Feb 2005;29(1):15-23. [Medline].
[19] Farrow KN, Fliman P, Steinhorn RH. The diseases treated with ECMO: focus on PPHN. *Semin Perinatol*. Feb 2005;29(1):8-14.[Medline].
[20] UK collaborative randomised trial of neonatal extracorporeal membrane oxygenation. UK Collaborative ECMO Trail Group. *Lancet*. Jul 13 1996;348(9020):75-82. [Medline].
[21] Shah PS, Ohlsson A. Sildenafil for pulmonary hypertension in neonates. *Cochrane Database Syst Rev*. Aug 10 2011;CD005494.[Medline].
[22] Walsh-Sukys MC, Tyson JE, Wright LL, Bauer CR, Korones SB, Stevenson DK, et al. Persistent pulmonary hypertension of the newborn in the era before nitric oxide: practice variation and outcomes. *Pediatrics*. Jan 2000;105(1 Pt 1):14-20. [Medline].
[23] Wung JT, James LS, Kilchevsky E, James E. Management of infants with severe respiratory failure and persistence of the fetal circulation, without hyperventilation. *Pediatrics*. Oct 1985;76(4):488-94. [Medline].
[24] Konduri GG, Solimano A, Sokol GM, Singer J, Ehrenkranz RA, Singhal N, et al. A randomized trial of early versus standard inhaled nitric oxide therapy in term and near-term newborn infants with hypoxic respiratory failure. *Pediatrics*. Mar 2004;113(3 Pt 1):559-64.[Medline].
[25] Steinhorn RH. Nitric oxide and beyond: new insights and therapies for pulmonary hypertension. *J Perinatol*. Dec 2008;28 Suppl 3:S67-71. [Medline]. [Full Text].

[26] Pawlik TD, Porta NF, Steinhorn RH, Ogata E, deRegnier RA. Medical and financial impact of a neonatal extracorporeal membrane oxygenation referral center in the nitric oxide era. *Pediatrics*. Jan 2009;123(1):e17-24. [Medline].

[27] Metra M, Giubbini R, Nodari S, et al. Differential effects of beta-blockers in patients with heart failure: A prospective, randomized, double-blind comparison of the long-term effects of metoprolol versus carvedilol. *Circulation*. Aug 1 2000;102(5):546-51. [Medline]. [Full Text].

[28] Rosenthal D, Chrisant MR, Edens E, et al. International Society for Heart and Lung Transplantation: Practice guidelines for management of heart failure in children. *J Heart Lung Transplant*. Dec 2004;23(12):1313-33. [Medline].

[29] Shaddy RE. Optimizing treatment for chronic congestive heart failure in children. *Crit Care Med*. Oct 2001;29(10 Suppl):S237-40.[Medline].

[30] Shaddy RE, Tani LY, Gidding SS, et al. Beta-blocker treatment of dilated cardiomyopathy with congestive heart failure in children: a multi-institutional experience. *J Heart Lung Transplant*. 1999;18:269-74. [Medline].

[31] Taketomo CK, Hurlburt-Hodding J, Kraus DM. *Pediatric drug handbook*. 1997-1998.

10

Fontan Surgery: Experience of One Cardiovacular Center

Monica Guzman, Juan Marcos Guzman and Miguel Ruz
Cardiovascular Clinic
Colombia

1. Introduction

In order to establish a normal, in-series circulation physiologically, very different from the circulation in parallel which the children are born with single ventricle, doctors Fontan and Baudet (2) and Kreutzer (3) concurrently developed surgical treatment of patients with tricuspid atresia to achieve a passive flow through the pulmonary vascular bed (1).
Management strategies for patients with functional single ventricle required a staged group of procedures where the ultimate goal is to have a single ventricle with a working pressure and volume close to normal as well as normal systemic oxygen saturation (1). It is known that both vascular development and lung maturation are essential for achieving benefits of cavopulmonary connection; the time of surgery has been defined arbitrarily and even more time to transition between partial to total cavopulmonary connection (1).
Single ventricle or univentricular heart anatomically or physiologically characterized by:

- Both atrioventricular valves attached to a single systemic ventricular chamber
- Severe stenosis or atresia of the atrioventricular valves
- There is no separation between the ventricles
- One of the ventricles is hypoplastic or absent

The essential characteristics of hypoplastic left heart syndrome syndrome are:

1. Stenosis or atresia of the mitral valve
2. Underdeveloped severely hypoplastic left ventricular
3. Stenosis or aortic valve atresia
4. Small aortic root
5. Ductal dependent for systemic blood flow

Thus, patients with these syndromes will have a parallel circulation in which the systemic and pulmonary circulations will be supplied by "mixed" blood.
The following are the physiological characteristics of hypoplastic left heart syndrome:

- Non-functional left ventricle
- Pulmonary venous return directed to the right atrium through a patent foramen ovale, atrial septal defect or rarely, total anomalous pulmonary venous drainage
- Mixed systemic and pulmonary venous return in right atrium
- The right ventricle supplies the systemic and pulmonary circulation in parallel
- Retrograde blood flow from the ductus arteriosus to the coronary arteries
- In these patients, ductal closure would result an inadequate systemic perfusion and metabolic acidosis with progressive coronary ischemia, and death.

In these patients one treatment option is repair in three stages, as follows:
The first stage repair (Norwood operation: Classic or Sano) seeks to:

- Provide systemic circulation: the right ventricle is used to support the systemic circulation
- Ensure non-restrictive egress of the pulmonary venous return to "bypass" the left ventricle, the atrial septal defect is enlarged or created in the absence of (in case it did not exist)
- Create an outflow tract obstruction-free system: the aorta is reconstructed
- Provide a controlled pulmonary blood supply, creating a shunt between the systemic and pulmonary circulations

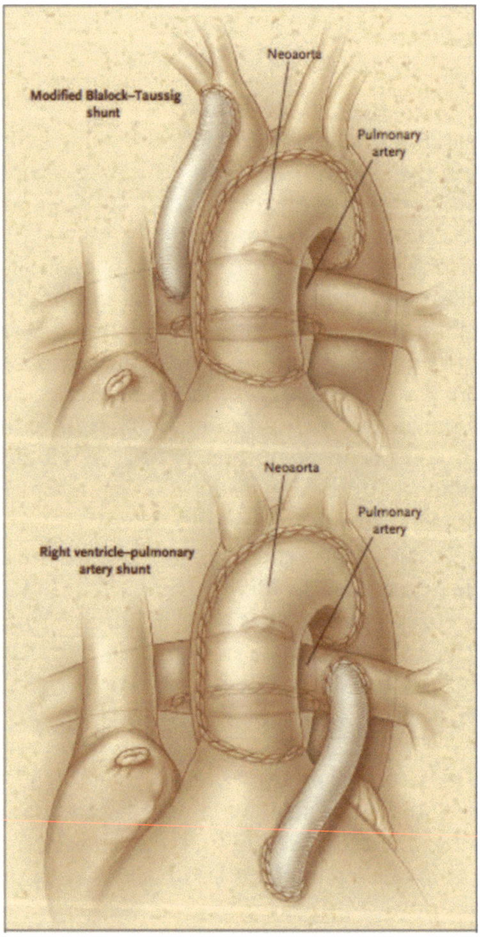

Fig. 1. First Stage: The Norwood procedure with a Modified Blalock-Taussig shunt or a right ventricle - pulmonary artery shunt (Sano)

The second stage repair (Glenn operation), which Takes place 6 to 8 months after-the Norwood is looking for:
anastomosing the superior cava to the pulmonary artery, thus direct systemic venous return to the pulmonary artery, begin to create a circulation in series. Fig 2.

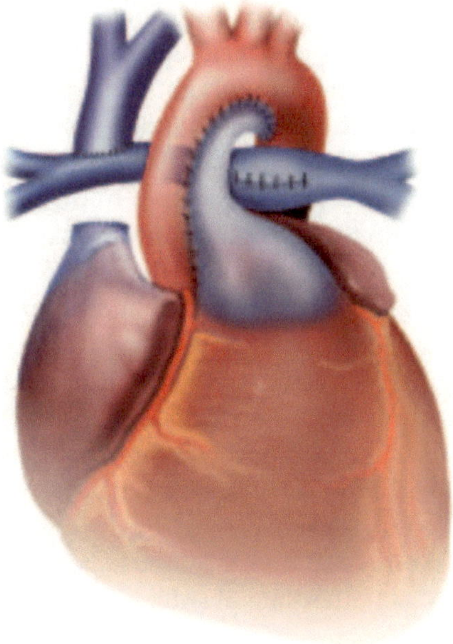

Fig. 2. Second Stage: BT shunt has been replaced with bidirectional Glenn procedure.

The third stage repair (Fontan operation), which is performed in children 12 kg or 4 years old, looking for:

anastomosing the inferior cava vein to the pulmonary artery and thus reduces the volume load of the single ventricle and complete the creation of a series circulation (4,5,6). Fig. 3.

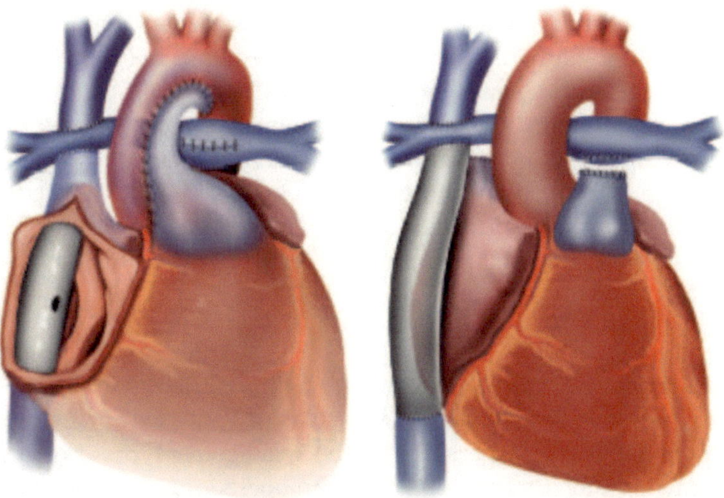

Fig. 3. Third Stage: (a) Fenestrated Fontan with lateral tunnel or (b) Fontan extra-cardiac conduit.

2. Surgical technique

All patients were operated through a median sternotomy with extracorporeal circulation and moderate hypothermia. We used two techniques of total cavopulmonary anastomosis, according to anatomical characteristics of each patient. The technique I corresponds to the construction of an intracardiac lateral tunnel constructed with a patch of polytetrafluoroethylene (PTFE) sutured to the lateral aspect of the right atrium, thereby building a tunnel that diverts intracardiac blood from the inferior cava to the right pulmonary artery, thus completing total cavo-pulmonary connection. For these patients we routinely use aortic clamping and cardioplegia with blood. The technique II is interposition of a PTFE tube between the transected inferior cava and pulmonary artery, ipsilateral to the inferior cava vein, also completing total cavo-pulmonary connection. This is known as extracardiac Fontan. Use of aortic clamping and cardioplegia is optional according to surgeon's preference. Both techniques are performed with almost routine fenestration of 4 to 5 mm. In the technique I, a circular punch incision in the PTFE patch is made, so to communicate intracardiac lateral tunnel with atrial mass receiving the pulmonary venous return. In technique II, the fenestration is created by a similar punch incision in the lateral PTFE inner tube and a similar incision on the lateral aspect of the right atrium, proceeding to be anastomosed both holes as Luther-lateral (7.8).

3. Type of study

Analytical study of cross-sectional, cohort analysis.

4. Population and sample

We included all patients with univentricular hearts who underwent Fontan operation. We reviewed the records of the patients included in the univentricular heart protocol and database service Congenital Cardiac Surgery Cardiovascular Clinic of Santa Maria de Medellin (Colombia), identifying all patients undergoing the Fontan operation with technique total cavopulmonary anastomosis between 1994 and 2010.

We reviewed the medical records, operative reports and echocardiograms.

Monitoring. All patients who survived the Fontan surgery underwent clinical and echocardiographic follow-up. We also obtained information about procedures performed after surgery, medication use and functional ability (classified according to New York Heart Association guidelines), interviewing parents and cardiologists caring for for each patient.

5. Results

Management strategies in cases of functional single ventricle have come to a group of procedures where the goal is to obtain a ventricular pressure and volume close to normal. Our study demonstrated our experience in the management protocol of univentricular patients in total cavopulmonary connection (Fontan operation). As in other centers, the most commonly used technique has been the fenestrated, extra-cardiac Fontan, which in our study represent 58.9% of the total sample (30 patients) - Table No.1. The hospital stay was 13.6 days on average.

	Frecuency	Porcentage	Cumulative Percentage
Fenestrated Atriopulmonary	2	3.6	3.6
Atriopulmonary not fenestrated	1	1.8	5.4
Fenestrated Extracardiac	30	53.6	58.9
Not Fenestrated extracardiac	16	28.6	87.5
Fenestrated intracardiac	4	7.1	94.6
Not fenestrated intracardiac	3	5.4	100.0
Total	56	100,0	

Table 1. Fontan type

	Frecuency	Percentage	Cumulative Percentage
No	48	85.7	85,7
Yes	8	14.3	100,0
Total	56	100.0	

Table 2. Death

The number of patients who failed was a total of 8; the cause in 4 of them (50% of total deaths) was low output syndrome which was present in the first 72 hours postoperatively, and the remaining 4 patients died after 72 hours after Fontan. These patients had a progressive deterioration associated with symptoms and signs of heart failure, protein-losing enteropathy, persistent chylothorax, affecting directly their functional status and no response to medical management. These data are shown in Table No. 3.

	Frecuency	Percentage	Cumulative Percentage
	48	85.7	85.7
Low Output	4	7.1	92.9
Fontan failed	4	7.1	100.0
Total	56	100.0	

Table 3. Cause of death

The end result is shown in Table No. 4, where 47 of them (84%) were discharged and continued in a functional stage I 9n 82.1% of them (Table No. 5). One patient (1.8%) sample was transferred from the Cardiovascular Clinic to another facility outside the country.

	Frecuency	Percentage	Cumulative Percentage
Discharge	47	84	84
Death	8	14.2	14.2
Transfer	1	1.8	100.0
Total	56	100.0	

Table 4. Cause of discharge

	Frecuency	Percentage	Cumulative Percentage
I	48	85.7	96.4
II	1	1.8	98.2
not evaluated	7	12.5	100.0
Total	56	100.0	

Table 5. Current functional class

Based on this study we conclude that the Fontan operation is a safe with a mortality rate comparable to that reported in previously published large series (Our series 14.3%), which is shown in the table No. 2. The Mayo Clinic experience, shows a overall mortality after Fontan, of 16%, but Many factors may have contributed to decreased early mortality after Fontan. Improved patient selection, younger age at time of operation, refinements in surgical techniques and postoperative management may all have had important roles.

6. Discussion

The evolution in the medium and long term outcome of patients operated with the original technique described by Fontan in the 70s demonstrated problems with the incorporation of all the systemic venous atrium in the circuit, characterized primarily by supraventricular arrhythmias and formation of thrombi (9,10,11). This is explained by atrial dilatation and inefficient circulation through this atrium which progressively becomes larger. But, changes in surgical techniques have been made to minimize these problems and improve long-term outcome (9).

At present there are different techniques for completion of the total cavopulmonary diversion: the intracardiac lateral tunnel (technique I) and extracardiac conduit (Technician II), which are the most widely used worldwide and are just two ways that we have employed. We have most often used the intracardiac lateral tunnel and extracardiac conduit including for those patients with abnormal systemic venous return and/or lung disease, which is usually seen in patients with heterotaxy syndrome. Regarding the use or non use of fenestration, this has also been the subject of much discussion, there are groups of surgeons that use the fenestration routinely and others who use it selectively (12,13). We are using this routinely in all our patients because pulmonary vascular resistance is a dynamic phenomenon and therefore it is not always easy to predict its behavior during the postoperative period. It seems safer for the patient having a fenestration that allows you to maintain adequate cardiac output during periods of high pulmonary vascular resistance, plus helps reduce the incidence of prolonged pleural effusions, resulting in decreased hospital length of stay (12,13)

With the passage of time have defined a number of criteria considered important for success in the performance of a Fontan-type surgery. These have included age, single ventricle morphology, anatomy of the pulmonary arteries, the atrioventricular valve function among others (14,15).

Kirklin and colleagues (15) reported 102 patients who had Fontan between 1975 and 1985. They found that age less than 4 years was a risk factor for mortality. Subsequently, the Children`s Hospital Boston reviewed 500 patients between 1973 and 1991 and found similar results in relation to age (16). As for the type of functional single ventricle, these techniques have been implemented for patients classically diagnosed with tricuspid atresia, but now with the increased survival of patients diagnosed with hypoplastic left heart syndrome, the question arises about the reduced ability of right ventricle to be able in time to support adequately the work of a single ventricle physiology to complete the process to the Fontan (3,17,18). This perception has not been recently supported (19.20). Mosca and colleagues show their results in 100 patients with Fontan performed between 1992 and 1998. They found no significant difference in the outcome compared to other types of single ventricle (21). Pizarro subsequently concluded that the Fontan can be performed safely in patients with SHIV making some modifications in surgical technique according to ventricular morphology, the mass ratio - volume and hemodynamic parameters, further suggests that Fontan surgery can be successful at earlier ages avoiding long exposure to hypoxia and risk of paradoxical embolism (1).

Our results regarding operative mortality and mid-term survival are comparable to those reported by other groups. In these studies, the mortality rate varied between 0 and 27% with an average of 10.5% and the 5-year survival varied between 81% and 93%, with an average of 87.5% (9,10,22, 23).

In relation to our surgical protocol in stages, 73.9% of patients had a bidirectional Glenn operation around 6 months of age, preparatory for the Fontan operation. The advantages of this strategy have been previously described (24,25,26).

Regarding the use of anticoagulation, we decided to keep our patients with oral anticoagulation for about 6 months with the objective of preventing thrombosis at the site of fenestration, after this period of time, we defined the need to close the fenestration.

This study determined that the average hospital stay was 13.9 days.

7. Conclusions

Management strategies in cases of functional single ventricle have come to a group of procedures where the goal is to obtain a ventricular pressure and volume close to normal. This analytical cross-sectional, cohort analysis is meant to show expertise in the management protocol of univentricular patients by total cavopulmonary connection (Fontan operation.) in Cardiovascular Clinic Santa Maria in the city of Medellin. Based on this study we conclude that the Fontan operation is safe with a mortality rate comparable to previously published large series (14.3%); the results are independent of the type of ventricle and the hospital length of stay is short (average hospital stay of 13.9 days). Postoperatively, is that over 90% of patients were in functional class I - II.

8. References

[1] Pizarro Ch, Mroczek T, Gidding S, Murphy J, and Norwood W. Fontan Completion in Infants. Ann Thorac Surg 2006; 81:2243–9.
[2] Fontan F, Baudet E. Surgical repair of tricuspid atresia. Thorax 1971;26:240–8.
[3] Kreutzer G, Galindez E, Bono H, de Palma C, Laura JP. An operation for the correction of tricuspid atresia. J Thorac Cardiovasc Surg 1973; 66: 613–21.
[4] Andropoulus D, Stayer S, Russell I. Anesthesia for congenital heart disease 2010.
[5] Anderson R, Pozzi M, Hutchinson S. Hypoplastic left heart syndrome 2005.
[6] Lake C. Pediatric cardiac anesthesia 2005.
[7] Jonas R. Comprehensive surgical management of congenital heart disease 2004.
[8] Nichols D. Critical heart disease in infants and children 2006.

[9] Becker R, Frangini P, Urcelay G, Castillo E, Heusser E, Arnaiz P et al. Fontan procedure: early and mid-term results with total cavopulmonary anastomosis. Rev MÈd Chile 2002; 130: 1217-1226.

[10] Driscoll D, Offord K, Feldt R, Schaff H, Puga F, Danielson G. Five to fifteen years follow-up after Fontan operation. Circulation 1992; 85: 469-96.

[11] Gelatt M, Hamilton R, Mc Crindle B, Gow R, Williams W, Trusler G et al. Risk factors for atrial tachyarrythmias after the Fontan operation. J Am Coll Cardiol 1994; 24: 1735-41.

[12] 12. Bridges N, Mayer J, Lock J, Jonas R, Hanley F, Keane J et al. Effect of baffle fenestration on outcome of the modified Fontan operation. Circulation 1992; 86: 1762-9.††††

[13] Airan B, Sharma R, Kumar Chowudari S, Mohanty S, Bhan A, Kumar Chowdhari U. Univentricular repair: is routine fenestration justified? Ann Thorac Surg 2000; 69: 1900-6.

[14] Choussat A, Fontan F, Besse P, Vallot F, Chauve A, Bricand H. Selection criteria for Fontan's procedure. In: Anderson RH, Shine-bourne EA, eds. Pediatric cardiology 1977. Edinburgh: Churchill Livingstone, 1978:559-66.

[15] Kirklin JK, Blackstone EH, Kirklin JW, Pacifico AD, Bargeron LM. The Fontan operation: ventricular hypertrophy, age, and date of operation as risk factors. J Thorac Cardiovasc Surg 1986;92:1049–64.

[16] Gentles TL, Mayer JE, Gauvreau K, et al. Fontan operation in five hundred consecutive patients: factors influencing early and late outcome. J Thorac Cardiovasc Surg 1997; 114:376 -91.

[17] Gaynor JW, Bridges ND, Cohen MI, et al. Predictors of outcome after the Fontan operation: is hypoplastic left heart syndrome still a risk factor? J Thorac Cardiovasc Surg 2002; 123:237- 45.

[18] Stamm C, Friehs I, Mayer J, et al. Long-term results of the lateral tunnel Fontan operation. J Thorac Cardiovasc Surg 2001; 121:28–41.

[19] Uemura H, Yagihara T, Kawashima Y, et al. What factors affect ventricular performance after a Fontan-type operation? J Thorac Cardiovasc Surg 1995;110:405–15.

[20] Julsrud PR, Weigel TJ, Van Son JA, et al. Influence of ventricular morphology on outcome after the Fontan procedure. Am J Cardiol 2000; 86:319 -23.

[21] Mosca RS, Kulik TJ, Goldberger CS, et al. Early results of the Fontan procedure in one hundred consecutive patients with hypoplastic left heart syndrome. J Thorac Cardiovasc Surg 2000;119:1110–8.

[22] Cetta F, Feldt R, O'leary P, Mair D, Warnes C, Driscoll D et al. Improved early morbidity and mortality after Fontan operation: the Mayo Clinic experience, 1987 to 1992. J Am Coll Cardiol 1996; 28: 480-6.††

[23] Laschinger J, Redmond M, Cameron D, Kan J, Ringel R. Intermediate results of the extracardiac Fontan procedure. Ann Thorac Surg 1996; 62: 1261-7.

[24] Knott-Craig C, Danielson G, Schaff H, Puga F, Weaver A, Driscoll D. The modified fontan operation. An analysis of risk factors for early postoperative death or takedown in 702 consecutive patients from one institution. J Thorac Cardiovasc Surg 1995; 109: 1237-43.

[25] Bridges N, Jonas R, Mayer J, Flanagan M, Keane J, CastaÒeda A. Bidirectional cavopulmonary anastomosis as interim palliation for high-risk Fontan candidates early results. Circulation 1990; 82: IV170-6.†††

[26] Jacobs M, Rychik J, Rome J, Apostolopoulou S, Pizarro C, Murphy J et al. Early reduction of the volume work of the single ventricle: the hemo-Fontan operation. Ann Thorac Surg 1996; 62: 456-62.††

Part 5

International Issues

11

Challenges in the Management of Congenital Heart Disease in Developing Countries

Fidelia Bode-Thomas
University of Jos
Nigeria

1. Introduction

The 2011 World Bank classification of nations and their economies based on 2010 per capita Gross National Incomes (GNI) lists 35 countries as low income (GNI 1005 US Dollars or less), 56 as lower middle income (1006 - 3975 USD), 54 upper middle income (3976 - 12275 USD) and 70 as high income (12,276 USD or more). Low and middle income countries are often conveniently referred to as developing countries (World Bank, 2011) but vary greatly in their levels of economic, infra-structural and health care development. The challenges of managing congenital heart disease in many low income and lower middle income countries are overwhelming, with very few or in some cases no treatment and prevention strategies in place at all. On the other hand, many upper middle income countries and a few lower middle income ones having been able to establish successful programmes for the treatment of congenital heart disease, albeit not without challenges, are striving to extend these services to the under-served parts of their populations while still confronted with challenges of prevention.

Congenital heart disease (CHD) refers to the presence of a structural abnormality of the heart and / or great vessels that is present at birth and is of actual or potential functional significance. The term usually excludes congenital arrhythmias and cardiomyopathies even though these may be based on genetic or other abnormalities that are present at birth (Hoffman & Kaplan, 2002). In recent decades, the management of congenital malformations of the heart has improved remarkably in the developed world such that even very complicated lesions are now amenable to treatment. The situation in many of the least developed countries / regions is the direct opposite - only very few children born with congenital heart disease ever receive the appropriate treatment or care. This is the result of several factors that may be considered obstacles or challenges to congenital heart disease management in these regions. Thus, hundreds of thousands of children die each year from congenital heart disease, while millions more remain in desperate need of treatment in the developing world. Alleviating the sufferings of such children is a major challenge to practitioners and perhaps even more so to the families of affected children. Several strategies have been advocated and used in attempts to help some of the affected children access the necessary care. These strategies vary from transporting a few affected children to other countries for treatment, to short-term visits by teams of experts from advanced countries to perform surgical procedures on a few children, to establishing regional centres of excellence for training and treatment in some developing countries (Stolf 2007, Pezzella 2010). These strategies however are also not without their own inherent challenges. This chapter will highlight some of the peculiarities of management and the practical problems often encountered in the diagnosis, treatment and prevention of congenital heart diseases in the developing world.

2. Burden of congenital heart disease in developing countries

There is a paucity of data on the incidence or birth prevalence of congenital heart disease in most developing countries. A few studies from developing countries coupled with a review of several studies from developed countries suggest similar range from country to country and across different time periods (Subramanyan et al., 2000; Khalil et al., 1994; Hoffman & Kaplan, 2002). However, the reported incidence in developed countries has steadily increased from about 4 to 5 per 1000 live births in the 1950's to as much as 50 to 75 per 1000 live births more recently – largely due to improved diagnosis using echocardiography which enables the diagnosis of many more trivial lesions than had hitherto been the case (Hoffman & Kaplan, 2002). The number of children born with congenital heart disease in developing countries have generally been extrapolated (based on the assumption of similar worldwide incidence) by applying rates obtained from older studies in developed countries to estimated numbers of live births in the developing countries and thus the actual figures may be much higher. Indeed, there generally is a paucity of data on the birth prevalence of all congenital malformations from developing countries, so that the impacts of these defects have been systematically underestimated in the past (Howson et al., 2004). These authors have also emphasized the huge public health importance of these disorders and provided more comprehensive extrapolated data than had hitherto been available. They have further highlighted the role of factors such as constrained diagnostic capabilities, poor health-related statistics, lack of birth defect surveillance and registries, and over-reliance on hospital-based rather than population-based studies as factors that have contributed to the underestimation of the toll of congenital anomalies in developing countries, where 94% of birth defects and 95% of their associated deaths occur. Other factors that have contributed both to the higher proportion of birth defects and their absolute numbers in these countries include their higher birth rates and higher prevalence of risk factors such as higher proportion of older mothers, exposure to environmental teratogens and poverty, which is very often associated with maternal malnutrition and more frequent infections. Congenital cardiac malformations constitute at least one quarter of all birth defects and are among the most severe and life-threatening. It is estimated that 960,000 of the slightly over 1 million children born with CHD worldwide annually are born in low and middle income countries – Table 1 (March of Dimes, 2006).

Because of the paucity of treatment facilities in developing regions and the known fact that without treatment 60% of congenital heart diseases are lethal within the first two years of life (Adams, 1959), it is also widely recognized that many more children die from congenital heart disease in developing countries compared with the developed. In addition to the deaths that may be directly attributable to heart disease, many children with congenital heart disease also die from some of the infectious diseases of childhood that are so prevalent in the less developed regions of the world. For these reasons, prevalence studies though more readily available in developing countries than incidence studies, tend to underestimate the burden of congenital heart disease (Saxena, 2005), since prevalence is a function both of incidence and mortality or survival rates. The disability-adjusted life years (DALYs) lost may give a more accurate picture of the disease burden since this measure takes into account the incidence, mortality as well as the quality of life of those who survive. However, there is a paucity of all these categories of data from developing countries, making it difficult to estimate the true burden of congenital heart disease. What is undisputable is that congenital heart disease in developing countries is associated with a very high mortality rate and that in spite of this, hundreds of thousands more children are added every year to the growing pool of affected children requiring intervention. Estimates of the actual numbers of these children however vary widely. This absence of accurate data constitutes one of the major obstacles to efforts to tackle the problem of congenital heart disease in developing countries as it underrates the problem, hinders planning and undermines arguments for more resource allocation in the face of the many other competing health care needs.

Country	estimated affected births per year
Bangladesh	33,844
Brazil	26,568
China	148,844
DRC*	19,805
Ethiopia	22,499
India	198,385
Indonesia	35,076
Nigeria	37,146
Pakistan	42,166

** Democratic Republic of the Congo*
Adapted from: March of Dimes Global Report on Birth Defects, 2006

Table 1. Estimated number of congenital heart disease live births in selected developing countries

3. Peculiarities and challenges of CHD diagnosis and treatment in developing regions

Because of the stage of their socio-economic and infrastructural development and the fact that the treatment of congenital heart disease requires specialized centres that are expensive to establish and to maintain, the management of congenital heart disease in developing regions differs in many significant and challenging aspects from what obtains in the developed world. A major contributing factor is that congenital heart disease is usually not considered a priority for resource allocation by policy makers in developing countries (Saxena, 2005). Many such countries and also international donor agencies have been pre-occupied by infectious diseases and lack policies on congenital heart disease control and treatment even if under the umbrella of paediatric cardiac diseases and / or congenital malformations (Children's HeartLink, 2007). Some of the major peculiarities of congenital heart disease patients and programmes in developing regions therefore include:

3.1 Late diagnosis

Late diagnosis - unlike in developed countries where prenatal diagnosis and neonatal corrective surgery are now the norm, CHD in developing countries are typically diagnosed late (Bannerman & Mahalu, 1998; Saxena, 2005; Mocumbi et al., 2011). The mean age at diagnosis or treatment varies depending on whether the data are from a purely paediatric service or include adults as well and can range from the first day of life to almost 80 years (Bode-Thomas et al., 2003, Mocumbi et al., 2011; Ibadin et al., 2005). As a result, most of the cases seen are those with more 'favourable' lesions that have been 'naturally selected' (Rao, 2007). Some of the reasons for this pattern of late diagnosis have been identified as:

3.1.1 Late presentation

Late presentation due to high level of illiteracy in many of these populations, coupled with lack of awareness about health issues generally, but especially about CHD. This is compounded by poverty and lack of access to basic medical care (Children's HeartLink, 2007). Thus the first presentation to hospital or to a specialist may be because of complications.

3.1.2 Ignorance about CHD even among health workers

Ignorance about CHD even among health workers, leading to frequent non-diagnosis or mis-diagnosis with wrong treatment and /or inappropriate counseling (LeBlanc, 2009). Heart disease is often wrongly assumed to be rare or very unlikely in children, so that its index of suspicion among health workers is very low. It is therefore not uncommon for children with CHD to have been treated for various other conditions such as tuberculosis or asthma before being eventually referred to a specialist that makes the correct diagnosis. The parents of a child with tetralogy of Fallot who were both health workers for example, had resigned themselves to his early demise as they were told no definitive treatment existed. He presented to a tertiary centre with endocarditis at 10 years of age and after a turbulent admission eventually had his heart lesion repaired in another country. Though his heart is 'healed', he now suffers from a seizure disorder.

3.2 Paucity of personnel and facilities for diagnosis and treatment

These are persistent problems that have been highlighted by many authors. They not only contribute to late diagnosis but also to late treatment if at all diagnosed, or no treatment at all and eventual loss to follow-up. Some of the patients receive palliative medical treatment e.g. for heart failure or propranolol to help reduce the frequency of hypercyanotic attacks in patients tetralogy of Fallot or similar physiology. However, with the absence of health insurance in many countries, the direct and indirect healthcare costs both of routine hospital visits (transportation, medication and loss of man hours) and repeated hospitalizations often result in 'catastrophic health care expenditure' for the families (Sadoh, 2011). As a result, many go into debt, sink further into poverty and/or default from follow-up.

3.3 High prevalence of complications

Due to late presentation and lack of treatment coupled with the high prevalence of infections and nutritional deficiencies in many developing communities, patients with congenital heart disease frequently present with such complications as chronic congestive heart failure, severe polycythemia, frequent and severe hypercyanotic attacks, cerebro-vascular accidents, malnutrition and infective endocarditis – or develop them in the course of follow-up. These frequently necessitate hospital admissions to treat the complications and are a further drain on family and health system resources. Thus paradoxically, although congenital heart diseases are often not considered to be of priority and their treatment usually not budgeted for, they still constitute a huge drain on limited health care resources. The same factors also predispose patients to high rates of surgical complications and mortality in the few available surgical treatment facilities (Rao, 2007; Mocumbi et al., 2011). Channeling these more or less wasted resources into planned care for these children will obviously yield more fruitful results.

3.4 Emphasis on palliative and closed heart procedures and on "curable" congenital heart lesions

In some parts of the developing world it is a luxury even to have rudimentary cardiac surgery services. When present these are often plagued by scarce resources including funds, personnel, expertise, equipment and consumables. In some places shortage of electricity and water supplies compound the problems. It is usually necessary to prioritize care and triage patients so that as many children as possible can benefit from the available resources without also undertaking procedures that may constitute an unnecessarily high risk and waste of resources under the circumstances. Therefore cardiac surgery centres in developing regions often place more emphasis on palliative and closed heart procedures especially when just beginning (Rao, 2007; Mocumbi et al., 2011). Even so, in many of the least developed countries, the number of centres that have the capability to undertake these procedures may be very few and far between, so that the few families that can afford them do still have to travel long distances within or even outside their own country. Eventually, only a minority of children that might have benefitted from such procedures are able to do so.

3.5 Transportation of patients to other countries for treatment

Apart from the expense, comparatively few children can benefit from this option of treatment compared with the large number affected. It has been described as the worst option because it does not create human and organizational expertise for the country (Stolf, 2007). Also, several challenges have been associated with this alternative. Sometimes in an attempt to help the "neediest" there may be poor patient selection, especially when an inexperienced physician is involved. Very sick, advanced or complicated cases may be selected leading to such problems as:

3.5.1 Acute complications while airborne

Acute complications while airborne - such as hypercyanotic attacks. These may necessitate emergency landings. If there is no one on board knowledgeable enough to give the appropriate emergency management, death is a real possibility. Thus some airlines require mandatory medical escorts for such patients – which further increase costs.

3.5.2 Pre-operative or early operative mortality in the host country

Pre-operative or early operative mortality in the host country. This creates additional problems such as the need for a distraught parent to decide whether and how to bury the child in a foreign country, or whether to cremate or to transport the corpse back home for burial. Apart from the additional burden on the host organizations/families, this creates immediate and later psycho-social problems for the parents and families of the affected child.

3.5.3 Multiple-stage surgeries

Multiple-stage surgeries - if the patient turns out to have a complex heart lesion that requires 2 or more stages of surgery, decisions will also have to be taken as to whether to send the child back home untreated, perform the first stage of surgery only or commit to bringing the patient back after a few years to perform the subsequent stage(s) of surgery. Whatever decision is taken is associated with great cost either of the treatment or the emotional cost to the family of having to send their child home back untreated.

3.6 Intermittent cardiac surgery missions

It has been argued that transporting children to other countries for treatment coupled with intermittent "missions" to existing non-specialist hospitals to carry out cardiac surgery can act as "enabling projects" that help bring the problem into focus while the creation of a sustainable unit is being planned (Yacoub, 2007). Some have however criticized this treatment alternative because only a limited number of patients can be assisted and the results are not consistently satisfactory - since the local hospital conditions are often far from ideal and the team may not be on ground long enough to observe and manage some of the post-operative complications (Stolf, 2007). It is nevertheless a better option than no surgery at all and offers the possibility of training local surgeons and hospital personnel, which should be a major focus (Stolf, 2007; Yacoub, 2007).

3.7 Establishing treatment centres in developing countries

The ideal option remains the development or establishment of treatment centres in the developing countries themselves. This is the most challenging option because of the huge investments required – in terms of technology, infrastructure and the training of personnel (cardiologists, surgeons, intensive care personnel and other cardiovascular specialists) . Some of the success stories notably in India and Brazil have been as a result of home-grown efforts coupled in some cases with the efforts of returning citizens trained in developed countries. Others have been spearheaded by humanitarian efforts of individuals and groups from developed countries – notably in China, Vietnam, Mozambique and Guatemala (Pezella, 2010; Yacoub, 2007). It is a daunting task that requires great commitment in view of the tremendous social and economic challenges often encountered. The biggest challenge here is that of sustainability. The presence of home-grown technology (as in India, Brazil), cost-saving measures such as re-sterilizing and re-using consumables, long-term commitment and support from donor organizations in developed countries and incorporating research into the programme appear to be factors that favour sustainability (Rao 2007, Yacoub 2007).

4. Challenges of congenital heart disease prevention in developing countries

The prevention of congenital heart disease, like that of any other disease condition hinges on a basic understanding of its causes. There is widespread ignorance and misconception in many developing countries about the aetiology of congenital heart disease and other birth defects. Even in the developed world, it was only in the 20th century that the causes of birth defects including congenital heart disease were clearly categorized into the three broad groups now widely recognized: those originating in the pre-conception period and due primarily to genetic (chromosomal and single gene defects) and partly genetic causes (multifactorial inheritance involving interaction of genes and the environment); those arising after conception but before birth (these are usually due to teratogens); and those of unknown cause (Christianson & Modell, 2004 as cited in March of Dimes 2006).

The majority of CHD are attributable to multi-factorial inheritance which is largely not preventable based on the current state of our knowledge. The risk of chromosomal anomalies however increases with advancing maternal age, so that developing countries have a higher incidence of chromosomal trisomies because of limited access to family planning and a high percentage of pregnant women of advanced maternal age (35 years or older). There is often also deficient or absent prenatal screening, diagnosis, and associated services (Modell et al as cited in March of Dimes 2006; WHO 1996). Down syndrome or trisomy 21, the most common chromosomal disorder is associated with congenital heart disease in about 50% of cases. Trisomies 18 and 13 are much less common and are each associated with congenital heart disease in over 90% of cases (Park, 2007).

Teratogen-induced heart defects, though more readily preventable, are more common in developing countries because of higher frequency of intrauterine infection, notably rubella, lack of environmental protection policies, and poorly regulated access to medication (Penchaszadeh, 2002 as cited in Howson et al, 2008). Between 5 and 10% of birth defects in high income countries are of post-conception origin compared with approximately 10 to 15 % for developing countries. In countries with successful rubella immunization programs, congenital rubella has been largely eliminated. In the remaining 50 percent of countries, more than 100,000 infants are born with CRS annually (WHO 2000 as cited in March of Dimes, 2006).

Other factors that contribute to the higher burden of congenital heart disease in developing countries include: poverty, which predisposes women to malnutrition before and during pregnancy, and to a greater risk of exposure to environmental teratogens, parental consanguinity - a common practice in some developing countries and inadequate access to health care which hinders the control of some of the risk factors for congenital heart disease (Bassili et al., 2000; Children's HeartLink, 2007).

5. Reducing the toll of congenital heart disease in developing countries

The huge toll of congenital heart disease in developing countries obviously calls for urgent action. Management of congenital heart disease in developing countries has hitherto however focused primarily on treatment. While treatment is very important, the huge capital investments necessary to treat affected children and those yet to be born, is clearly beyond the limited health budgets of many developing countries. The need for a paradigm shift in the management of cardiac diseases from treatment only, to prevention plus treatment and rehabilitation has been highlighted (Pezzella 2010). This has implications as well for congenital heart disease, at least those that are clearly preventable and presents the need for paediatric cardiologists to be more involved in efforts to eliminate or minimize the occurrence of congenital heart diseases of preventable cause. Furthermore, the prevention of congenital heart disease would be difficult to separate from that of other birth defects and therefore should be an integral part of prevention strategies for birth defects generally.

Even though religious and socio-cultural differences may not permit the wholesale adoption some of the methods used, there are many lessons to be learnt from the experiences of more developed countries, where the incidence of birth defects have been reduced by about 75%

over the last few decades. Some of the steps taken by those countries (Howson et al, 2008) included:

- Improved collection and use of data
- Improved prenatal and peri-natal services including promotion of family planning, rubella immunization before pregnancy and folic acid fortification of commonly consumed foods.
- Training of health care professionals in best practices in care and prevention
- Educating the public on steps to take to promote a healthy pregnancy outcome including avoidance of teratogens during gestation, etc.

The foregoing coupled with the realities on ground in many developing countries today, inform certain broad areas of emphasis, including the urgent need for research and accurate data, improved diagnosis and treatment and a greater emphasis on prevention than has hitherto been the case. Preventive measures in particular deserve high priority and should be integrated into primary health care. As has been suggested, achieving the millennium development goals will also help to reduce the toll of paediatric heart disease, including congenital heart disease in developing countries (Leblanc, 2009). The need for community-based studies to generate accurate statistics on incidence, mortality and survival and the improved collection of routine data cannot be over-emphasized as such data are vital for planning intervention programmes and to justify more resource allocation. Longer term measures include the provision of more treatment facilities and the training of more specialists - obstetricians, paediatricians, cardiologists, paediatric cardiologists, cardiac surgeons, and all other allied health care professionals. This requires more resource allocation and more judicious use of available resources.

6. Conclusion

There is a need to increase public awareness about congenital heart disease in developing countries so as to encourage early presentation and enhance early diagnosis. Equally important is the need to educate all categories of health workers on early detection and referral coupled with prevention measures, including incorporating such teaching into the training curricula of the various categories of health workers. The need for good quality data and the training of more specialists so as to enhance treatment of affected children cannot be over-emphasized. Even though capital intensive, the need to provide more treatment centres for affected children can also not be avoided indefinitely. These measures require that health policymakers be made aware of the extent of the problem so that more resources can be allocated for primary level care which includes prevention, early detection and referral; secondary level care including medical treatment of some complications and tertiary care which includes surgical repair and rehabilitation. All these measures need to be complemented by research into local incidence and risk factors, and support from international agencies.

7. References

[1] Adams, F. (1959). Congenital heart disease: comments regarding incidence and natural history. *California Medicine,* Vol. 90, No. 3, (March 1959), pp. 213-216

[2] Bannerman, C. and Mahalu, W. (1998). Congenital heart disease in Zimbabwean children. *Annals of Tropical Paediatrics,* Vol. 18, No. 1, (March 1998), pp. 5-12, ISSN 0272-4936

[3] Bassili, A., Moktar, S., Dabous, N., et al. (2000). Risk factors for congenital heart disease in Alexandria, Egypt. *European Journal of Epidemiology,* Vol. 16, No. 9, (2000), pp.805-14

[4] Bode-Thomas, F., Okolo, S., Ekedigwe, J., et al. (2003). Paediatric echocardiography in Jos University Teaching Hospital: problems, prospects and preliminary audit. *Nigerian Journal of Paediatrics,* Vol. 30, (2003), pp. 143-149

[5] Children's HeartLink. (2007). *Linked by a common purpose: global efforts for improving pediatric heart health,* A report by Children's HeartLink, Retrieved from http://www.childrensheartlink.org/docs/globalreport

[6] Hoffman, J & Kaplan, S. (2002). The incidence of congenital heart disease. *Journal of the American College of Cardiology,* Vol. 39, No. 12, Jun 2002, pp. 1890-1900, ISSN 0735-1097/02/S22.00

[7] Howson, C., Christianson, A and Modell, B. (2008). Controlling birth defects: reducing the hidden toll of dying and disabled children in low-income countries. In: *Disease Control Priorities Project,* Accessed 22nd July 2011, Available from: http://www.dcp2.org

[8] Ibadin, M., Sadoh, W., Osarogiagbon, W. (2005). Congenital heart diseases at the University of Benin Teaching Hospital. *Nigeria Journal of Paediatrics,* Vol. 2, (2005), pp. 6-9

[9] Khalil, A., Aggarwal, R., Thirupuram, S., Arora, R. (1994). Incidence of congenital heart disease among hospital live births in India. *Indian Pediatrics,* Vol. 31, No. 5, (May 1994), pp. 519-527

[10] Leblanc, J. Creating a global climate for pediatric cardiac care. *World Journal of Pediatrics,* Vol. 5, No. 2, (May 2009), pp. 89-92

[11] March of Dimes. (2006). *Global report on birth defects,* Accessed 22nd July, 2011, Available from: http://www.marchofdimes.com/globalprograms

[12] Mocumbi, A., Lameira, E., Yaksh, A., Fereira, M., Sidi, D. (2011). Challenges on the management of congenital heart disease in developing countries. *International Journal of Cardiology,* Vol. 148, (2011), pp.285-288

[13] Park, M. (2007). *Pediatric Cardiology for Practitioners,* (5th edition), Elsevier, ISBN: 978-81-312-1304-9, New Delhi

[14] Pezzella , A. (2010). Global aspects of cardiothoracic surgery with focus on developing countries. *Asian Cardiovascular & thoracic annals,* Vol. 18, No. 3, 2010, pp. 299-310

[15] Rao, S (2007). Pediatric cardiac surgery in developing countries. *Pediatric Cardiology,* Vol. 28, (2007) pp. 144-148

[16] Sadoh, W. (2011). The cost of out-patient management of chronic heart failure in children with congenital heart disease. *Nigerian Journal of Clinical Practice,* Vol.14, No. 1, (April 2011), pp. 65-69

[17] Saxena, A. (2005). Congenital heart disease in India: a status report. *Indian Journal of Pediatrics,* Vol. 72, No. 7, (July 2005) pp. 595-598.

[18] Stolf, N. (2007). Congenital heart surgery in a developing country: a few men for a great challenge. *Circulation,* Vol. 116, pp. 1874-1875, ISSN: 0009-7322

[19] Subramanyan, R., Joy, J., Venugopalan, P., Sapru, A & al Khusaiby SM. (2000). Incidence and spectrum of congenital heart disease in Oman. *Annals of Tropical Paediatrics,* Vol. 20, No 4, (Dec 2000), pp 337-341.

[20] World Bank (2011). World Bank list of economies, In: *Changes in country classifications*, Accessed 23rd July 2011, Available from: http://www.data.worldbank.org
[21] World Health Organization. (1996). *Control of Hereditary Diseases.* WHO Technical Report Series 865. WHO, Geneva, Switzerland.
[22] Yacoub, M. (2007). Establishing pediatric cardiovascular services in the developing world: a wake-up call. *Circulation,* Vol. 116, (2007) pp. 1876-1878, ISSN 0009-7322

Part 6

Miscellaneous Issues

12

Myocardial Self-Repair and Congenital Heart Disease

Fariba Chalajour, Xiaoyuan Ma and R. Kirk Riemer
Stanford University, Stanford, CA
USA

1. Introduction

In this chapter we will explore the current understanding about the dynamics of myocardial cell populations after birth and how they may contribute to homeostasis and response to injury. Recent investigations of myocardial cell biology have revealed that the heart is not the terminally differentiated organ it was once thought to be. We now know that myocardium contains limited populations of cardiac progenitor cells (CPC) that are capable of generating all myocardial cell types. The changes in myocardial cell populations with time and the role these changes play in neonatal myocardial tissue expansion will be discussed. The contribution of CPC to heart growth and therapeutic strategies for congenital cardiac diseases will be explored.

2. Stem cells and heart development

2.1 Stem cells: The perspective has evolved

Pluripotent embryonic stem cells (ESC) are derived from the inner cell mass of an embryonic blastocyst (primitive ectoderm). The *pluri*potency of ESC defines that they are capable of differentiation into one of the three germ layers: ectoderm, mesoderm, or endoderm; reviewed in (Rossant, 2008; Bolli & Chaudhry, 2010). Embryonic mesoderm cells (identified by the expression of Brachyury T) in the developing primary heart field undergo committed differentiation into a pre-cardiac lineage (expressing Mesp-1) and have the potential to form committed cardiac progenitor cells (CPC, expressing Nkx2.5), which are capable of differentiation into cardiomyocytes, vascular smooth muscle cells, and endothelial cells; reviewed in (Sturzu & Wu, 2011). A cardiac progenitor cell is thus defined as a *multi*potent progenitor cell of the pre-cardiac lineage.

Originally it was thought that only ESC are pluripotent, and they could only be obtained from living embryos. Consequently, studies of human ESC have been impeded by ethical concerns. However, continued research has led to the realization that pluripotency is in fact a plastic multidirectional state. It has now been clearly demonstrated that a pluripotent state can be induced in adult somatic cells from humans, and other species; reviewed in Yamanaka (Yamanaka & Blau, 2010). The biochemical methods through which so-called induced pluripotent cells (iPSC) may be derived from adult cells are numerous and still expanding. Several recent reviews (Rossant, 2008; Yamanaka & Blau, 2010) of both the technology and the biology of iPSC may be consulted for the interested reader; the topic will not be further discussed here.

A variety of techniques have been used to induce the differentiation of ESC into a specific cell type of interest. The directed differentiation of ESC into cardiomyocytes has been achieved by several methods and has enabled the use of this approach to produce a large enough number of cells for repairing the injured heart to restore myocardial function (Gonzales & Pedrazzini, 2009; Laflamme & Murry, 2011). A large number of studies have been conducted and are still being conducted with the goal of restoring the function of infarcted myocardium using stem cell therapy with ESC-derived cardiomyocytes and also other cell types, with the expectation that they would continue to differentiate into cardiomyocytes after being delivered to the injured heart tissue (Murry et al., 2005). As this therapy is less relevant to *congenital* heart disease, it will not be further discussed here.

2.2 How cardiac progenitor cells form the developing heart

A brief review of cardiac development illustrates how cardiac stem cells are identified and how multiple distinct populations of pre-cardiac cells coalesce to form the distinct subregions of the heart.

2.2.1 Heart fields and cardiac progenitor cells

The development of the multi-chambered heart is complex and requires a precise regulation of cell migration, proliferation, and differentiation in a highly organized positional and temporal order. Several distinct CPC populations contribute to the formation of different heart fields. The first heart field (FHF) of cardiac progenitor cells is localized in the primitive streak and mostly contributes to formation of the left ventricle and part of the atria (Garcia-Martinez & Schoenwolf, 1993; Tam et al., 1997). A second heart field (SHF) of CPC from the pharyngeal mesoderm migrates into the arterial pole of the heart and is a major source of the cardiac progenitors that form the outflow tract (OFT), the right ventricle and the atria (Abu-Issa & Kirby, 2007). Continued development of the OFT and heart valves is achieved by migration of a population of non-mesodermal neural crest cells (NCC) from the neural fold into the arterial pole and endocardial cushion (Kirby & Waldo, 1995; Hutson & Kirby, 2007). Another population of mesenchymal CPC, the proepicardium, has been demonstrated to be an additional cell source contributing to the formation of coronary arteries and cardiac fibroblasts (Dettman et al., 1998). CPC from both FHF and SHF act in a close collaboration during the formation of the embryonic heart. During heart morphogenesis, CPC directed by different signaling pathways differentiate to mature cardiac cells. However, CPC of the postnatal heart have been shown to express markers common to both FHF and SHF. Whether these postnatal resident CPC contribute to remodeling and growth of the heart is considered likely but is still unsettled.

2.2.2 Second heart field and congenital heart disease

Studies of heart development in mice have shown that mutation of genes expressed by cells of the SHF causes congenital heart disease (CHD). Mutations in Nkx2.5 cause a spectrum of congenital heart defects including cardiac conduction abnormalities and ventricular- and atrial- septal defects (VSD, ASD) (Basson et al., 1997). Deletion of Tbx1 results in malformations of the cardiac outflow tract and VSDs due to failure in the migration of NCC to the heart (Jerome & Papaioannou, 2001; Merscher et al., 2001). Mutations in GATA4, some of which disrupt its interaction with Tbx5, cause ASDs and VSDs (Garg et al., 2003). Hand2 is essential for survival of second heart field progenitors and loss of Hand2 function in this cardiac progenitor population can cause a spectrum of congenital heart malformations

(Tsuchihashi et al., 2011). Cai (Cai et al., 2003) reported that Isl1+ cells are mostly localized in the SHF and give rise to the outflow tract. They demonstrated that disruption of Isl1 results in a complete failure to form the outflow tract in the mutant mice. The role of Fgf8 in early and late heart development has also been studied (Sun et al., 1999; Abu-Issa et al., 2002). Fgf8 is required for migration of mesoderm out of the primitive streak (Sun et al., 1999). In addition Fgf8 plays an important role in development of all the pharyngeal arches and in NCC survival (Abu-Issa et al., 2002). Cardiac NCC are multipotent and after migration to the SHF contribute to cardiovascular patterning (Kirby & Waldo, 1995). Ablation of the pre-migratory cardiac NCC causes numerous outflow tract septation defects: persistent truncus arteriosus, double-outlet right ventricle, tetralogy of Fallot, double-inlet left ventricle, tricuspid atresia, straddling tricuspid valve, and the absence of a varying combination of aortic arch arteries derived from pharyngeal arches 3, 4 and 6 (Nishibatake et al., 1987; Hutson & Kirby, 2007). Studies of interactions between cells of SHF origin with NCC in the pharyngeal region of mice (Vitelli et al., 2002; Moraes et al., 2005) have shown that mutation in Tbx1 disrupts formation of the pharyngeal arch arteries and causes septation defects due to failure in NCC migration. Bradshaw (Bradshaw et al., 2009) showed that abnormal distribution of Isl1-expressing cells in a neural crest-deficient mutant mouse causes instability of posterior arch arteries and outflow tract septation defects, leading to a double outlet right ventricle. Discovery of the presence and role of CPC in the normal and abnormal development of heart fields and their possible role in postnatal life suggests that targeting these cells is a valuable approach for both understanding the ontology of CHD and developing therapeutic approaches.

The implications of resident CPC expressing neural markers in the heart are manifold for congenital heart disease repair. First, the secondary heart field of cells creates the structures most affected by congenital disease: the outflow tracts and pulmonary and aortic trunks (Dyer & Kirby, 2009; Jain et al., 2010). Second, the resident CPC-derived from this field (i.e. Isl1+ or Nestin+ CPC) may form the primary cardiac stem cell pool that would potentially be mobilized to participate in the repair (cell replacement) of structures derived from the anterior/secondary heart field such as the OFT. Thirdly, therapeutics aimed at CPC mobilization may act more effectively on the right heart if they target NCC-derived CPC.

2.2.3 Postnatal distribution of CPC in the heart

Resident CPC have been localized in small groups or clusters in a unique microenvironment known as a "stem cell niche" which provides conditions for stem cells to maintain their multipotency and renewal capacity (Morrison & Spradling, 2008). Niches comprise a specific arrangement of stem cells, supporting cells, and extracellular matrix. The niche environment provides a paracrine signaling influence that maintains stem cells in their quiescent state and also responds to conditions outside the niche to initiate activation of stem cell replication and/or differentiation, for example in response to tissue injury (Morrison & Spradling, 2008). Classically, three well-characterized stem cell niches have been identified: germline, hematopoietic, and epithelial (Lemischka, 1997; Xie & Spradling, 2000; Spradling et al., 2001). However in the past decade, identification of resident stem cells in most mammalian organs suggests local tissue-specific niches are a general rule. Discovery of CPC niches in the adult mouse heart strengthens the growing appreciation that the heart is not a terminally differentiated organ and resident CPC might play a role in the postnatal remodeling and repair of cardiac tissue (Urbanek et al., 2006). The early study of Messina (Messina et al., 2004) demonstrated that cardiac stem cells are present in both atrial and ventricular human samples and in a wide range of ages (1 to 80 years old). According to this

study and mouse studies by Beltrami (Beltrami et al., 2003) and Oh (Oh et al., 2003), cardiac stem cells can be isolated from adult myocardium and differentiated into different cardiac cell lineages. Our own studies (Amir et al., 2008) have investigated the number and characteristics of CPC in human neonatal myocardium from patients with congenital heart disease. We demonstrated that CPC comprise a high percentage relative to cardiomyocytes in the human neonate and that their fractional representation declines as the heart grows in size, suggesting a dilutional effect. In other words, an apparently fixed population of CPC resides in the heart postnatally. Pouly (Pouly et al., 2008) reported that CPC concentration in the right atrium is greater than that of the septum of transplanted hearts. Other myocardial niches have been reported. Schenke-Layland (Schenke-Layland et al., 2011) reported that in human and mouse heart endogenous, multipotent $Isl1^{+}/Flk1^{+}$ CPC reside within niche clusters in the right ventricular free wall, the atria and outflow tracts. They were tightly circumscribed by the basement membrane proteins collagen V and laminin. However, systematic mapping of the complete heart to localize major niches and determine the distribution of these regions of high CPC density has not been reported. A general concept is that cardiac regions protected from greatest mechanical stress (atria, septum, apex) appear to contain the highest density of CPC. A more useful perspective may be consideration of the cardiac developmental sequence in which fields of CPC undergo migration and strategically controlled distribution, since the niches may constitute remnants of specific precursor fields in the primordial heart anlagen.
The role of niche-associated cells in regulating the stability and activation of resident stem cells is still poorly understood, especially in the heart. Recently, it has been shown that Notch-1 of murine CPC interacts with surrounding cells via the Jagged ligand. Through a Jagged-mediated activation signaling process induced in vitro, notch signaling, down regulation of c-Kit and upregulation of Nkx2.5 were found to be associated with increased myocyte proliferation (Boni et al., 2008). These data support the concept that interaction of CPC with supporting cells and matrix regulates their commitment to the myocyte lineage.

2.2.4 Postnatal Characterization of CPC fates

2.2.4.1 Prenatal formation of the heart from different fields

During heart development CPC express field-specific markers **(Figure 1.)** for FHF, SHF, and neural crest (Vincent & Buckingham, 2010). Mesp1 is one of the earliest markers for cardiac primordial cells (Saga et al., 1999). Depending on the stage of cell differentiation, genetic markers will be upregulated or down regulated in the CPC, which complicates clear classification of CPC originating from FHF and SHF based on markers. Nkx2.5 is a critical cardiac transcription factor in the first lineage, and Isl1 along with Foxh1, GATA factors, and Hand2 are key regulators in the second heart progenitor field (Moretti et al., 2006). The earliest differentiated cells in the cardiac crescent express GATA4 and Nkx2.5 (Vincent & Buckingham, 2010). The final differentiation to cardiomyocytes is controlled by Tbx (Takeuchi & Bruneau, 2009). Known markers for SHF CPC are Isl1, Tbx1 and Fgf10 (Kelly et al., 2001; Cai et al., 2003; Xu et al., 2004). Pax3 is recognized as a major regulatory gene for NCC, having an important role in their migration (Bradshaw et al., 2009). There is considerable overlap between the heart field-specific genetic markers. This issue is more evident in the case of the proepicardial organ, which gives rise to coronary arteries and epicardium. Both Isl1 and Nkx2.5 are expressed in the CPC from the proepicardial organ (Dettman et al., 1998), the cells of which also express Tbx18 and Wt1 (Martinez-Estrada et al., 2010).

2.2.4.2 Markers of CPC in the postnatal heart

In the postnatal heart, identification of CPC is based primarily on the cardiac lineage markers Nkx2.5, Mef2c, and Isl1. Identification of c-Kit$^+$ cells in adult mammalian heart suggests another postnatal source of CPC, however, the origin of these cells is unsettled. Although expression of the key CPC markers is preserved both in rodents and humans, species-specific markers limit translation of animal studies to human studies. Our studies of human infant RVOFT myocardium showed a mixed population of c-Kit$^+$, Isl1$^+$, and Nkx2.5$^+$ CPC (Amir et al., 2008). The neonatal human heart is a rich source of CPC bearing markers such as SSEA4, Isl1, Nkx2.5, and c-Kit. In addition to our report of myocardial SSEA4 localization(Amir et al., 2008), SSEA4 expression has been previously only reported in adult human kidney (Ward et al., 2011). Isl1$^+$ CPC have also been localized to the atrium (Laugwitz et al., 2005). Stem cell antigen-1 (Sca-1) is a marker for mouse resident CPC. In the mouse and human studies performed by Messina (Messina et al., 2004) and Beltrami (Beltrami et al., 2003) c-Kit$^+$ cells are considered to be CPC, whereas Oh (Oh et al., 2003) used c-Kit$^-$, Sca-1$^+$ cells as a marker for CPC. This apparent controversy may be explained by the existence of heterogeneous pools of cardiac stem cells in different stages of differentiation rather than multiple populations of distinct resident CPC. In addition, the anatomical location (i.e., heart field of origin) of the heart regions studied may determine the markers expressed by postnatal CPC.

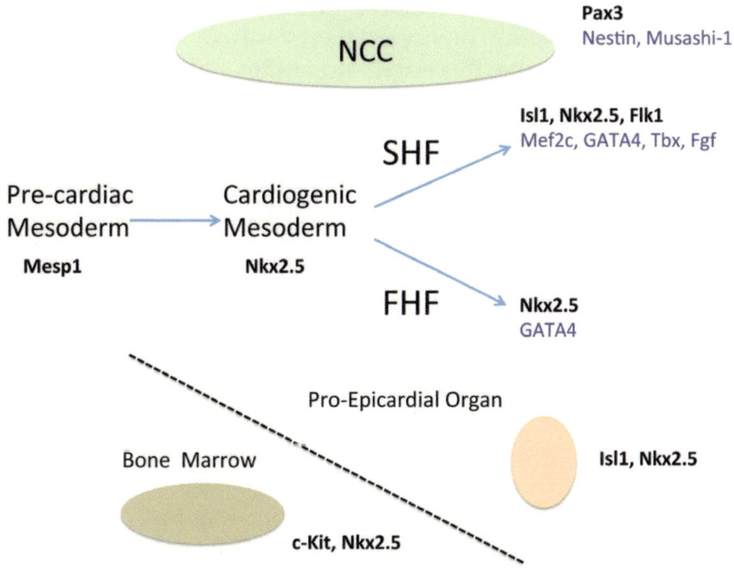

Fig. 1. Overview of myocardial CPC Markers in relation to their ontology.
Pre-cardiac mesoderm cells express Mesp1 until differentiation to cardiogenic mesoderm, marked by the expression of Nkx2.5. The cardiogenic mesoderm differentiates to form two heart fields. Cells in the first heart field (FHF) express GATA4 in addition to Nkx2.5. Cells of the secondary heart field (SHF) express Isl1 and Nkx2.5. The SHF also becomes populated by neural crest cells (NCC) expressing Pax3. Markers associated with the heart field cells but showing greater variation in their expression are indicated in blue type. In addition to cardiogenic mesoderm, cells from the pro-epicardial organ and also of hematopoietic lineage have been identified in the myocardium. Abbreviations: NCC, Neural crest cells; SHF, Second heart field; FHF, First heart field.

Mouse studies have demonstrated homing of bone marrow-derived stem cells into the infarcted myocardium, suggesting a hematopoietic origin for c-Kit+ CPC. However, transdifferentiation of these cells into cardiomyocytes is controversial (Orlic et al., 2001; Murry et al., 2004; Bearzi et al., 2007). On the other hand, Tallini (Tallini et al., 2009) reported that c-Kit is expressed by immature cardiomyocytes as well as endothelial cells during development of mouse heart and that the populations rapidly expanded during the first 2 days of postnatal life. Their study compared the difference between the multipotency potential of CPC derived from the neonatal heart and the adult injured heart. They concluded that the neonatal c-Kit+ cells showed an ability to differentiate into cardiomyocytes, smooth muscle cells, and endothelial cells. In contrast, they found that c-Kit+ cells in the adult injured mouse heart had no myogenic capacity. The co-expression of c-Kit and neuronal marker Nestin in neonatal CPC (Tallini et al., 2009) suggests a transitional status of NCC in postnatal life and the potential for NCC contributing to cardiac repair and remodeling (Drapeau et al., 2005).

2.3 Postnatal heart growth

The infant heart grows rapidly after birth. The pulmonary valve annular diameter doubles in the first 7 years of life and plateaus by age 14 (Sairanen & Louhimo, 1992) while left ventricular volume doubles over approximately the first 10 years of life (Nielsen et al., 2010). Although cardiomyocytes increase in volume (hypertrophic growth), in part by cellular fusion into very large multinucleate myocytes, there is also an overall increase in cellularity (cell number) in the heart during this rapid expansion phase of heart growth. That the number of myocytes continues to increase after birth has only recently been demonstrated. For decades, it was taken as fact that cardiomyocytes were incapable of dividing postnatally, if only because mitosis of a multinucleated cell is considered impossible.

One of the earliest reports of new cardiomyocytes appearing in the postnatal human heart was provided by studies of adult aortic stenosis patients, in which cells co-expressing cardiac and stem cell markers could be localized (Urbanek et al., 2003). Additionally, studies of transplanted adult donor hearts revealed the appearance of new cardiomyocytes in the donor heart by the presence of sex chromosomes opposite to that of the recipient host (Bayes-Genis et al., 2007). Highly compelling further evidence that new myocytes are added to the heart over time arises from carbon isotope data (Bergmann et al., 2009) showing that nearly 50% of myocytes are replaced over a lifetime. Studies of the hearts of dogs with advanced dilated cardiomyopathy performed by Leri (Leri et al., 2001) showed postnatal proliferation of cardiomyocytes, documented by the expression of cell proliferation marker Ki67 and telomerase. Telomerase activity is not only required for cardiac growth and survival but it also suppresses cardiomyocyte apoptosis (Oh & Schneider, 2002). We (Amir et al., 2008) also demonstrated that the neonatal human heart contains cardiomyocytes expressing Ki67. We also determined that the number of these proliferating myocytes declines nearly 6-fold in the first two months of life.

2.4 Summary: CPC in the postnatal myocardium

Work by a number of investigators has demonstrated that a population of multipotent cardiac lineage-determined cells (i.e., CPC) capable of further differentiation to all cardiac cell types is present in all hearts. Hence, continued cardiomyocyte renewal has slowly been gaining acceptance as both an important aspect of normal myocardial biology and a potential strategy to assist with repair of a diseased heart. The ability to expand the population of cardiomyocytes presents a potentially vast opportunity for therapeutic intervention for congenital heart diseases.

3. CPC and Therapy for CHD

3.1 Cardiac repair using CPC

3.1.1 Role of CPC in homeostatic repair and postsurgical healing

If the heart can add new cells, then the question arises regarding why it doesn't always heal itself? The generally offered explanation for the fact that resident CPC are unable to naturally rescue a moderately infarcted adult heart is that the region of damaged tissue is too great for this mechanism to work rapidly enough to restore function. Although not widely recognized, "silent "repair by CPC has been observed (see section 3.2.1). It is probable that small lesions in the myocardium are actually self-repaired silently through expansion of the resident CPC population. Large ischemic lesions would be expected to also result in the loss of resident CPC in the infarcted region, further impairing self-repair. However, progress has recently been reported. Intra-myocardial injection of autologous bone marrow derived stem cells has been used in adults with chronic ischemic heart disease (i.e. not infarcted) to achieve functional recovery and reverse ventricular remodeling (Williams et al., 2011). Such reports of success strengthen the concept that endogenous stem cells can provide clinically significant benefits to heart disease patients of all ages.

3.1.2 Therapies using CPC for tissue engineering

3.1.2.1 Tissue engineered myocardial grafts

Presently, many investigators are attempting to use cardiac stem cells to produce engineered myocardial sheet grafts for myoplasty of larger regions of infarct-damaged adult myocardium. Success has been limited to moderate. Major limiting factors to this approach remain. For example, integration of the graft into the existing myocardium so that it provides clinically significant augmented force development has been problematic. Additionally, achieving sufficient revascularization of the grafts to sustain viability has been difficult; see review by Sui (Sui et al., 2011). Although the potential utility of such grafts in congenital heart disease is not expectedly large, marked progress in this approach could conceivably provide alternative therapies for patients with failing Fontan circulations or possibly for those with cardiomyopathies.

3.1.2.2 Tissue engineered myocardial vascular and valve grafts

One area of potentially beneficial therapy that has previously received little attention in *congenital* heart disease patients is the engineering of vascular and valve grafts that are capable of meeting the rapid growth rate typical of the neonatal heart and great vessels during the first decade of life. The availability of graft materials with the ability to grow along with the young patient is highly desirable, but thus far not available. This is an area of recently increasing research interest, and one in which further research could provide enormous benefit to CHD patients.

3.1.3 Mobilizing resident CPC

3.1.3.1 Alternatives to cell delivery: "Activation" of resident CPC

Given the apparent difficulty in achieving clinically valuable augmentation of cardiac performance through the delivery of cardiomyocytes to a damaged heart, therapeutic approaches that are designed to mobilize resident CPC to expand the population of cardiomyocytes in situ are being given much more consideration. Therapeutic exploitation of the paracrine environments of the CPC niche and enhancing homing to sites of repair is a very attractive alternative approach to cell-based therapies. In concept, it is a matter of using biomolecules to mimic or enhance endogenous CPC "awakening" mechanisms to obtain greater quantities of cells to differentiate into functional cardiomyocytes. Recent reports reveal that this general approach has a high potential for success and is quite worthy of further investigation. High mobility group box protein 1 (HMGB1), an endogenous chromatin-associated protein, and Thymosine Beta4, a G-actin monomer binding protein, have been identified as paracrine factors potentially able to promote regeneration of myocardium. HMGB1 is released from necrotic cells and has been shown to stimulate the homing of fibroblasts and smooth muscle cells. It has been identified as a potential mediator of resident stem cell activation/mobilization (Palumbo & Bianchi, 2004). Limana (Limana et al., 2005) demonstrated that injection of HMGB1 into the infarcted region of mice induced the appearance of new myocytes and an increase in ventricular performance, leading these investigators to conclude that HMGB1 is a "potent inducer of myocardial regeneration." They demonstrated that c-kit+ CPC express the receptor for HMGB1 and that treatment increased the number of c-kit+ cells in mouse heart. Thymosine Beta4 has been shown to stimulate epicardial-derived cells (EPDC) to migrate and potentially promote neovascularization in the infarcted mouse heart (Smart et al., 2010); see review by (Bollini et al., 2011). Although there was no proof that EPDC were a source of the new cardiomyocytes, they may facilitate collateral vessel growth and thereby support the cardiomyocyte regeneration process. Damaged myocardium has a different paracrine environment, which if properly understood and exploited, may provide unique approaches for therapy via resident CPC activation.

Growth factor treatment has also been used to activate resident CPC populations for myocardial repair. Linke (Linke et al., 2005) used a canine MI model to show that IGF-1 and HGF treatment (intra-myocardial injection) could increase the density of proliferating ($Ki67^{+}$) CPC following MI. These same investigators recently extended their observations, showing that CPC aging is related to a decline in signaling through IGF-1 and HGF, which in turn reduces their effect to antagonize the aging effect that the local renin-angiotensin system induces on CPC. They found that IGF-1 and HGF were able to partially reverse age-related decline in cardiac function in rats (Gonzalez et al., 2008). Consistent with these reports of IGF-1 stimulation of CPC proliferation, D'Amario (D'Amario et al., 2011) has proposed that CPC senescence is regulated by paracrine and autocrine signaling: positive through IGF-1 & -2, and balanced by an opposing signal mediated primarily by angiotensin II, all acting via their cognate receptors. Accordingly, they propose that IGF-1 promotes CPC proliferation and survival via IGF-1 receptor signaling, CPC differentiation via action on both IGF-1 and -2 receptors, and increasing angiotensin signaling and reduced IGF-1 receptor signaling with aging promotes CPC and cardiomyocyte apoptosis.

CPC from the secondary/anterior heart field (i.e., $Nestin^{+}$) are resident in the secondary heart field regions of the rat heart (Drapeau et al., 2005). The recent review by Di Felice (Di Felice & Zummo, 2009) surveyed the many mutations of secondary heart field cells that are associated with human Tetralogy of Fallot. They concluded that potentially improved approaches to therapy would be better informed by a clearer understanding of the behavior and patterns of migration of CPC of the secondary heart field. That neural stem cells (CPC from the secondary heart field) may participate in recovery from myocardial injury in a region-specific manner has also been shown. These cells apparently migrate and home to infarcted region of rat hearts, although they differentiate into neuronal, not myocardial cells (Beguin et al., 2011). Tamura (Tamura et al., 2011) used a mouse transgenic approach to tag neural crest cells and show that these cells migrated to the ischemic border zone of an infarct and transdifferentiated into cardiomyocytes. Although evidence for Nestin$^+$ cells in the human heart is lacking, it is worth considering the different heart field lineages in the context of devising strategies for therapeutic targeting of human CPC. The targeting of neural crest-derived CPC to correct late ventricular arrhythmias occurring in patients after surgical repair operations for TOF is a potential therapeutic strategy(Di Felice & Zummo, 2009).

3.2 Potential roles of CPC in therapy for CHD
3.2.1 CPC silently contribute to therapy
3.2.1.1 (Pre-) Failing Fontan rescue via activation-RV strengthening

In the setting of failing Fontan physiology the potential for boosting cardiac performance through manipulation of cell number represents a new horizon. Ventricular assist devices (VAD) are presently used as a bridge to transplant in pediatric Fontan patients (Fynn-Thompson & Almond, 2007). VAD are also used to reduce ventricular load with the objective of enhancing the ability of the ventricle to support a greater load, i.e., to "rest" or re-train the ventricle of patients with dilated cardiomyopathy (CMP), even restoring function to the point of enabling pump removal (Birks et al., 2011). It is conceivable that the use of VAD may increase cardiomyocyte number, and evidence of this comes from recent prospective studies of myocardial biopsies showing an increased number of diploid myocytes in end stage congestive heart failure patients supported as a bridge to transplant with LVAD (Wohlschlaeger et al., 2010). Manginas (Manginas et al., 2009) has shown that endothelial progenitor cells are also mobilized by VAD use in patients. EPC may be stimulated to home into myocardium supported by VAD and improve myocardial function. As reviewed by Tsiavou (Tsiavou & Manginas, 2010), rescue of myocardial function during cardiac support by VAD may be mediated by CD45$^+$ EPC promoting neovascularization and transdifferentiating into or fusing with cardiomyocytes. However, the possible involvement of CPC fusion with existing myocytes as repair mechanism is not widely accepted. The implications of the above observations are that progenitor cells may at least be participating in, if not be a primary mechanism mediating these physiological changes observed with VAD therapy.

What physiological mechanisms might underlie the expansion of the myocardial cell population during VAD support? Current thinking is that paracrine mechanisms are involved. For example, mechanical stimulation by the VAD may induce the production of cytokines such as growth factors (see section 3.1.3.1), which then stimulate mitotic expansion of CPC. Additionally, the production of chemokines under the influence of the same mechanical stimulation may promote the homing of bone marrow-derived progenitor cells. Indeed, much of the success of cell delivery-based therapies, although still rather modest, are thought to be largely due to paracrine effects mediated through the injected cells, the carrier media or in some cases the physical-mechanical changes induced by injection of liquid boluses into the muscle wall.

3.2.2 Augmenting current therapy with CPC targeting

3.2.2.1 CPC activation as an adjuvant to VAD "resting" of ventricle

It has been reported that pharmacological therapy in conjunction with VAD support may enhance myocyte population expansion. Recent studies by Soppa used therapy with the beta-2 agonist clenbuterol (Soppa et al., 2008) in a murine heterotopic abdominal transplant of failing hearts. Testing the effects of clenbuterol on mechanical unloading, they were able to show that it improves LV function. Bhavsar demonstrated that clenbuterol positively affects cardiac physiology through myocyte hypertrophy, concluding that the effect was mediated by a paracrine action of fibroblast-derived IGF-1 (Bhavsar et al., 2010). At the present time, we can find no reports of an effect of clenbuterol on CPC recruitment/activation. It is conceivable that such combined pharmacological plus mechanical therapy approaches could provide a markedly re-strengthened ventricle capable of many more years of function if not for the rest of the patient's life. CPC recruitment could be combined with VAD-mediated myocardial unloading to augment myocardial tissue while "resting" the ventricle, whether left or right sided. Another possible use of therapies designed to expand the population of CPC is in the area of "ventricular training" a potential approach to prepare the LV of, e.g., delayed repair TGA patients for greater force production once the arterial switch operation has been performed. If VAD use can augment cardiomyocyte populations in otherwise normal ventricles, this could potentially help prepare the TGA patient for the switch operation by enhancing ventricular adaptation to increased loads.

3.2.2.2 Cardiomyopathy

Is it realistic to expect the manipulation of resident CPC populations to achieve a reversal in the decline in myocardial function in the setting of cardiomyopathy? Given the genetic nature of known lesions in sarcomeric proteins in this disease (Frazier et al., 2011), one may anticipate that the progenitor cell population may also harbor the same mutant alleles and therefore the expansion of that population may provide no benefit. However, for cardiomyopathy induced by chemical injury such as doxorubicin/adriamycin therapy (Shi et al., 2011), strategies to promote expansion of the resident CPC population could be considered an adjuvant or co-therapy used to mitigate cardiotoxicity. It is important to consider that, although the resident CPC may have an advantage in already being present within the muscular wall of the heart, therapies designed to help recruit bone marrow-derived CPC (and EPC) (see section 3.1.3.1) are certainly worthy of exploration while investigators try to understand the possibly different significance of resident versus bone marrow-derived CPC. Indeed, given the mismatch between patients in need of transplantation and the availability of transplantable hearts there would seem to be little reason not to emphasize the exploration of multiple approaches designed to utilize endogenous progenitor cells whether they be resident in the tissue or delivered to the tissue from sites such as the bone marrow.

3.2.2.3 Summary: Potential therapeutic opportunities

At present, investigators have only begun to exploit the potentials of using small molecule (drugs, growth factors) based therapies to expand desirable cell populations. We know of no examples of demonstrated CPC-based therapies for congenital cardiac disease at this time. Since CPC likely undergo senescence and their number as a percentage of total cells declines with expansion of the myocardial cell population, conceivably the benefits of such therapy may be far greater for the pediatric population than the adult.

4. Conclusions

The presence of resident CPC in myocardium is well supported through multiple studies. There is still much independent confirmation to be completed to clarify the promise of cardiac progenitor cell-mediated repair. Importantly, the major novel discoveries in the field of CPC biology have been made by only a small group of investigators and interpretation of some data is impaired by the lack of independent corroborating studies. Controversies also continue regarding the origin of CPC: during cardiac development, e.g., Isl1$^+$ CPC, or from bone marrow, e.g., c-Kit$^+$ CPC. Most likely, both sources are important but their therapeutic utilization may need to be approached with different strategies. Methods for activating resident CPC to realize their potential for effecting endogenous cardiac repair are still in the early discovery period. The fundamental question of CPC role in homeostatic maintenance of the myocardium throughout life has yet to be fully clarified, although an understanding of this highly significant role appears to be limited only by a lack of detection. Nonetheless, the potential applications of CPC-focused therapies in congenital heart disease treatments are likely manifold, awaiting only further investigation and implementation.

5. Acknowledgement

We thank Olaf Reinhartz, MD for reviewing this manuscript, and Laura Piechura for editorial assistance.

6. References

Abu-Issa, R. & Kirby, M. L. (2007). Heart Field: From Mesoderm to Heart Tube. *Annual review of cell and developmental biology* Vol.23, 2007) pp. 45-68, ISBN 1081-0706 (Print) 1081-0706 (Linking)

Abu-Issa, R., Smyth, G., Smoak, I., Yamamura, K. & Meyers, E. N. (2002). Fgf8 Is Required for Pharyngeal Arch and Cardiovascular Development in the Mouse. *Development* Vol.129, No.19, (Oct, 2002) pp. 4613-4625, ISBN 0950-1991 (Print) 0950-1991 (Linking)

Amir, G., Ma, X., Reddy, V. M., Hanley, F. L., Reinhartz, O., Ramamoorthy, C. & Riemer, R. K. (2008). Dynamics of Human Myocardial Progenitor Cell Populations in the Neonatal Period. *The Annals of thoracic surgery* Vol.86, No.4, 2008) pp. 1311-1319, ISBN 1552-6259

Basson, C. T., Bachinsky, D. R., Lin, R. C., Levi, T., Elkins, J. A., Soults, J., Grayzel, D., Kroumpouzou, E., Traill, T. A., Leblanc-Straceski, J., Renault, B., Kucherlapati, R., Seidman, J. G. & Seidman, C. E. (1997). Mutations in Human Tbx5 [Corrected] Cause Limb and Cardiac Malformation in Holt-Oram Syndrome. *Nature genetics* Vol.15, No.1, (Jan, 1997) pp. 30-35, ISBN 1061-4036 (Print) 1061-4036 (Linking)

Bayes-Genis, A., Roura, S., Prat-Vidal, C., Farre, J., Soler-Botija, C., de Luna, A. B. & Cinca, J. (2007). Chimerism and Microchimerism of the Human Heart: Evidence for Cardiac Regeneration. *Nature clinical practice. Cardiovascular medicine* Vol.4 Suppl 1, (Feb, 2007) pp. S40-45, ISBN 1743-4300 (Electronic) 1743-4297 (Linking)

Bearzi, C., Rota, M., Hosoda, T., Tillmanns, J., Nascimbene, A., De Angelis, A., Yasuzawa-Amano, S., Trofimova, I., Siggins, R. W., Lecapitaine, N., Cascapera, S., Beltrami, A. P., D'Alessandro, D. A., Zias, E., Quaini, F., Urbanek, K., Michler, R. E., Bolli, R., Kajstura, J., Leri, A. & Anversa, P. (2007). Human Cardiac Stem Cells. *Proc Natl Acad Sci U S A* Vol.104, No.35, (Aug 28, 2007) pp. 14068-14073, ISBN 0027-8424 (Print) 0027-8424 (Linking)

Beguin, P. C., El-Helou, V., Gillis, M. A., Duquette, N., Gosselin, H., Brugada, R., Villeneuve, L., Lauzier, D., Tanguay, J. F., Ribuot, C. & Calderone, A. (2011). Nestin (+) Stem Cells Independently Contribute to Neural Remodelling of the Ischemic Heart. *Journal of cellular physiology* Vol.226, No.5, (May, 2011) pp. 1157-1165, ISBN 1097-4652 (Electronic) 0021-9541 (Linking)

Beltrami, A. P., Barlucchi, L., Torella, D., Baker, M., Limana, F., Chimenti, S., Kasahara, H., Rota, M., Musso, E., Urbanek, K., Leri, A., Kajstura, J., Nadal-Ginard, B. & Anversa, P. (2003). Adult Cardiac Stem Cells Are Multipotent and Support Myocardial Regeneration. *Cell* Vol.114, No.6, (Sep 19, 2003) pp. 763-776, ISBN 0092-8674 (Print) 0092-8674 (Linking)

Bergmann, O., Bhardwaj, R. D., Bernard, S., Zdunek, S., Barnabe-Heider, F., Walsh, S., Zupicich, J., Alkass, K., Buchholz, B. A., Druid, H., Jovinge, S. & Frisen, J. (2009). Evidence for Cardiomyocyte Renewal in Humans. *Science* Vol.324, No.5923, (Apr 3, 2009) pp. 98-102, ISBN 1095-9203 (Electronic) 0036-8075 (Linking)

Bhavsar, P. K., Brand, N. J., Felkin, L. E., Luther, P. K., Cullen, M. E., Yacoub, M. H. & Barton, P. J. (2010). Clenbuterol Induces Cardiac Myocyte Hypertrophy Via Paracrine Signalling and Fibroblast-Derived Igf-1. *Journal of cardiovascular translational research* Vol.3, No.6, (Dec, 2010) pp. 688-695, ISBN 1937-5395 (Electronic)

Birks, E. J., George, R. S., Hedger, M., Bahrami, T., Wilton, P., Bowles, C. T., Webb, C., Bougard, R., Amrani, M., Yacoub, M. H., Dreyfus, G. & Khaghani, A. (2011). Reversal of Severe Heart Failure with a Continuous-Flow Left Ventricular Assist Device and Pharmacological Therapy: A Prospective Study. *Circulation* Vol.123, No.4, (Feb 1, 2011) pp. 381-390, ISBN 1524-4539 (Electronic) 0009-7322 (Linking)

Bolli, P. & Chaudhry, H. W. (2010). Molecular Physiology of Cardiac Regeneration. *Annals of the New York Academy of Sciences* Vol.1211, (Nov, 2010) pp. 113-126, ISBN 1749-6632 (Electronic) 0077-8923 (Linking)

Bollini, S., Smart, N. & Riley, P. R. (2011). Resident Cardiac Progenitor Cells: At the Heart of Regeneration. *Journal of molecular and cellular cardiology* Vol.50, No.2, (Feb, 2011) pp. 296-303, ISBN 1095-8584 (Electronic) 0022-2828 (Linking)

Boni, A., Urbanek, K., Nascimbene, A., Hosoda, T., Zheng, H., Delucchi, F., Amano, K., Gonzalez, A., Vitale, S., Ojaimi, C., Rizzi, R., Bolli, R., Yutzey, K. E., Rota, M., Kajstura, J., Anversa, P. & Leri, A. (2008). Notch1 Regulates the Fate of Cardiac Progenitor Cells. *Proc Natl Acad Sci U S A* Vol.105, No.40, (Oct 7, 2008) pp. 15529-15534, ISBN 1091-6490 (Electronic) 0027-8424 (Linking)

Bradshaw, L., Chaudhry, B., Hildreth, V., Webb, S. & Henderson, D. J. (2009). Dual Role for Neural Crest Cells During Outflow Tract Septation in the Neural Crest-Deficient Mutant Splotch(2h). *Journal of anatomy* Vol.214, No.2, (Feb, 2009) pp. 245-257, ISBN 1469-7580 (Electronic) 0021-8782 (Linking)

Cai, C. L., Liang, X., Shi, Y., Chu, P. H., Pfaff, S. L., Chen, J. & Evans, S. (2003). Isl1 Identifies a Cardiac Progenitor Population That Proliferates Prior to Differentiation and

Contributes a Majority of Cells to the Heart. *Dev Cell* Vol.5, No.6, (Dec, 2003) pp. 877-889, ISBN 1534-5807 (Print) 1534-5807 (Linking)

D'Amario, D., Cabral-Da-Silva, M. C., Zheng, H., Fiorini, C., Goichberg, P., Steadman, E., Ferreira-Martins, J., Sanada, F., Piccoli, M., Cappetta, D., D'Alessandro, D. A., Michler, R. E., Hosoda, T., Anastasia, L., Rota, M., Leri, A., Anversa, P. & Kajstura, J. (2011). Insulin-Like Growth Factor-1 Receptor Identifies a Pool of Human Cardiac Stem Cells with Superior Therapeutic Potential for Myocardial Regeneration. *Circulation research* Vol.108, No.12, (Jun 10, 2011) pp. 1467-1481, ISBN 1524-4571 (Electronic) 0009-7330 (Linking)

Dettman, R. W., Denetclaw, W., Jr., Ordahl, C. P. & Bristow, J. (1998). Common Epicardial Origin of Coronary Vascular Smooth Muscle, Perivascular Fibroblasts, and Intermyocardial Fibroblasts in the Avian Heart. *Developmental biology* Vol.193, No.2, (Jan 15, 1998) pp. 169-181, ISBN 0012-1606 (Print) 0012-1606 (Linking)

Di Felice, V. & Zummo, G. (2009). Tetralogy of Fallot as a Model to Study Cardiac Progenitor Cell Migration and Differentiation During Heart Development. *Trends Cardiovasc Med* Vol.19, No.4, (May, 2009) pp. 130-135, ISBN 1873-2615 (Electronic) 1050-1738 (Linking)

Drapeau, J., El-Helou, V., Clement, R., Bel-Hadj, S., Gosselin, H., Trudeau, L. E., Villeneuve, L. & Calderone, A. (2005). Nestin-Expressing Neural Stem Cells Identified in the Scar Following Myocardial Infarction. *Journal of cellular physiology* Vol.204, No.1, (Jul, 2005) pp. 51-62, ISBN 0021-9541 (Print) 0021-9541 (Linking)

Dyer, L. A. & Kirby, M. L. (2009). The Role of Secondary Heart Field in Cardiac Development. *Developmental biology* Vol.336, No.2, (Dec 15, 2009) pp. 137-144, ISBN 1095-564X (Electronic) 0012-1606 (Linking)

Frazier, A. H., Ramirez-Correa, G. A. & Murphy, A. M. (2011). Molecular Mechanisms of Sarcomere Dysfunction in Dilated and Hypertrophic Cardiomyopathy. *Progress in pediatric cardiology* Vol.31, No.1, (Jan 1, 2011) pp. 29-33, ISBN 1058-9813 (Print) 1058-9813 (Linking)

Fynn-Thompson, F. & Almond, C. (2007). Pediatric Ventricular Assist Devices. *Pediatric cardiology* Vol.28, No.2, (Mar-Apr, 2007) pp. 149-155, ISBN 0172-0643 (Print) 0172-0643 (Linking)

Garcia-Martinez, V. & Schoenwolf, G. C. (1993). Primitive-Streak Origin of the Cardiovascular System in Avian Embryos.Pdf. *Developmental Biology* Vol 159, 1993) pp. 706-719, ISBN

Garg, V., Kathiriya, I. S., Barnes, R., Schluterman, M. K., King, I. N., Butler, C. A., Rothrock, C. R., Eapen, R. S., Hirayama-Yamada, K., Joo, K., Matsuoka, R., Cohen, J. C. & Srivastava, D. (2003). Gata4 Mutations Cause Human Congenital Heart Defects and Reveal an Interaction with Tbx5. *Nature* Vol.424, No.6947, (Jul 24, 2003) pp. 443-447, ISBN 1476-4687 (Electronic) 0028-0836 (Linking)

Gonzales, C. & Pedrazzini, T. (2009). Progenitor Cell Therapy for Heart Disease. *Exp Cell Res* Vol.315, No.18, (Nov 1, 2009) pp. 3077-3085, ISBN 1090-2422 (Electronic) 0014-4827 (Linking)

Gonzalez, A., Rota, M., Nurzynska, D., Misao, Y., Tillmanns, J., Ojaimi, C., Padin-Iruegas, M. E., Muller, P., Esposito, G., Bearzi, C., Vitale, S., Dawn, B., Sanganalmath, S. K., Baker, M., Hintze, T. H., Bolli, R., Urbanek, K., Hosoda, T., Anversa, P., Kajstura, J. & Leri, A. (2008). Activation of Cardiac Progenitor Cells Reverses the Failing Heart

Senescent Phenotype and Prolongs Lifespan. *Circ Res* Vol.102, No.5, (Mar 14, 2008) pp. 597-606, ISBN

Hutson, M. R. & Kirby, M. L. (2007). Model Systems for the Study of Heart Development and Disease. Cardiac Neural Crest and Conotruncal Malformations. *Seminars in cell & developmental biology* Vol.18, No.1, (Feb, 2007) pp. 101-110, ISBN 1084-9521 (Print) 1084-9521 (Linking)

Jain, R., Rentschler, S. & Epstein, J. A. (2010). Notch and Cardiac Outflow Tract Development. *Annals of the New York Academy of Sciences* Vol.1188, (Feb, 2010) pp. 184-190, ISBN 1749-6632 (Electronic) 0077-8923 (Linking)

Jerome, L. A. & Papaioannou, V. E. (2001). Digeorge Syndrome Phenotype in Mice Mutant for the T-Box Gene, Tbx1. *Nature genetics* Vol.27, No.3, (Mar, 2001) pp. 286-291, ISBN 1061-4036 (Print) 1061-4036 (Linking)

Kelly, R. G., Brown, N. A. & Buckingham, M. E. (2001). The Arterial Pole of the Mouse Heart Forms from Fgf10-Expressing Cells in Pharyngeal Mesoderm. *Developmental cell* Vol.1, No.3, (Sep, 2001) pp. 435-440, ISBN 1534-5807 (Print) 1534-5807 (Linking)

Kirby, M. L. & Waldo, K. L. (1995). Neural Crest and Cardiovascular Patterning. *Circulation research* Vol.77, No.2, (Aug, 1995) pp. 211-215, ISBN 0009-7330 (Print) 0009-7330 (Linking)

Laflamme, M. A. & Murry, C. E. (2011). Heart Regeneration. *Nature* Vol.473, No.7347, (May 19, 2011) pp. 326-335, ISBN 1476-4687 (Electronic) 0028-0836 (Linking)

Laugwitz, K. L., Moretti, A., Lam, J., Gruber, P., Chen, Y., Woodard, S., Lin, L. Z., Cai, C. L., Lu, M. M., Reth, M., Platoshyn, O., Yuan, J. X., Evans, S. & Chien, K. R. (2005). Postnatal Isl1+ Cardioblasts Enter Fully Differentiated Cardiomyocyte Lineages. *Nature* Vol.433, No.7026, (Feb 10, 2005) pp. 647-653, ISBN 1476-4687 (Electronic) 0028-0836 (Linking)

Lemischka, I. R. (1997). Microenvironmental Regulation of Hematopoietic Stem Cells. *Stem cells* Vol.15 Suppl 1, 1997) pp. 63-68, ISBN 1066-5099 (Print) 1066-5099 (Linking)

Leri, A., Barlucchi, L., Limana, F., Deptala, A., Darzynkiewicz, Z., Hintze, T. H., Kajstura, J., Nadal-Ginard, B. & Anversa, P. (2001). Telomerase Expression and Activity Are Coupled with Myocyte Proliferation and Preservation of Telomeric Length in the Failing Heart. *Proceedings of the National Academy of Sciences of the United States of America* Vol.98, No.15, (Jul 17, 2001) pp. 8626-8631, ISBN 0027-8424 (Print) 0027-8424 (Linking)

Limana, F., Germani, A., Zacheo, A., Kajstura, J., Di Carlo, A., Borsellino, G., Leoni, O., Palumbo, R., Battistini, L., Rastaldo, R., Muller, S., Pompilio, G., Anversa, P., Bianchi, M. E. & Capogrossi, M. C. (2005). Exogenous High-Mobility Group Box 1 Protein Induces Myocardial Regeneration after Infarction Via Enhanced Cardiac C-Kit+ Cell Proliferation and Differentiation. *Circ Res* Vol.97, No.8, (Oct 14, 2005) pp. e73-83, ISBN 1524-4571 (Electronic) 0009-7330 (Linking)

Linke, A., Muller, P., Nurzynska, D., Casarsa, C., Torella, D., Nascimbene, A., Castaldo, C., Cascapera, S., Bohm, M., Quaini, F., Urbanek, K., Leri, A., Hintze, T. H., Kajstura, J. & Anversa, P. (2005). Stem Cells in the Dog Heart Are Self-Renewing, Clonogenic, and Multipotent and Regenerate Infarcted Myocardium, Improving Cardiac Function. *Proc Natl Acad Sci U S A* Vol.102, No.25, (Jun 21, 2005) pp. 8966-8971, ISBN 0027-8424 (Print) 0027-8424 (Linking)

Manginas, A., Tsiavou, A., Sfyrakis, P., Giamouzis, G., Tsourelis, L., Leontiadis, E., Degiannis, D., Cokkinos, D. V. & Alivizatos, P. A. (2009). Increased Number of Circulating Progenitor Cells after Implantation of Ventricular Assist Devices. *The Journal of heart and lung transplantation : the official publication of the International Society for Heart Transplantation* Vol.28, No.7, (Jul, 2009) pp. 710-717, ISBN 1557-3117 (Electronic) 1053-2498 (Linking)

Martinez-Estrada, O. M., Lettice, L. A., Essafi, A., Guadix, J. A., Slight, J., Velecela, V., Hall, E., Reichmann, J., Devenney, P. S., Hohenstein, P., Hosen, N., Hill, R. E., Munoz-Chapuli, R. & Hastie, N. D. (2010). Wt1 Is Required for Cardiovascular Progenitor Cell Formation through Transcriptional Control of Snail and E-Cadherin. *Nat Genet* Vol.42, No.1, (Jan, 2010) pp. 89-93, ISBN 1546-1718 (Electronic) 1061-4036 (Linking)

Merscher, S., Funke, B., Epstein, J. A., Heyer, J., Puech, A., Lu, M. M., Xavier, R. J., Demay, M. B., Russell, R. G., Factor, S., Tokooya, K., Jore, B. S., Lopez, M., Pandita, R. K., Lia, M., Carrion, D., Xu, H., Schorle, H., Kobler, J. B., Scambler, P., Wynshaw-Boris, A., Skoultchi, A. I., Morrow, B. E. & Kucherlapati, R. (2001). Tbx1 Is Responsible for Cardiovascular Defects in Velo-Cardio-Facial/Digeorge Syndrome. *Cell* Vol.104, No.4, (Feb 23, 2001) pp. 619-629, ISBN 0092-8674 (Print) 0092-8674 (Linking)

Messina, E., De Angelis, L., Frati, G., Morrone, S., Chimenti, S., Fiordaliso, F., Salio, M., Battaglia, M., Latronico, M. V., Coletta, M., Vivarelli, E., Frati, L., Cossu, G. & Giacomello, A. (2004). Isolation and Expansion of Adult Cardiac Stem Cells from Human and Murine Heart. *Circulation research* Vol.95, No.9, (Oct 29, 2004) pp. 911-921, ISBN 1524-4571 (Electronic) 0009-7330 (Linking)

Moraes, F., Novoa, A., Jerome-Majewska, L. A., Papaioannou, V. E. & Mallo, M. (2005). Tbx1 Is Required for Proper Neural Crest Migration and to Stabilize Spatial Patterns During Middle and Inner Ear Development. *Mechanisms of development* Vol.122, No.2, (Feb, 2005) pp. 199-212, ISBN 0925-4773 (Print) 0925-4773 (Linking)

Moretti, A., Caron, L., Nakano, A., Lam, J. T., Bernshausen, A., Chen, Y., Qyang, Y., Bu, L., Sasaki, M., Martin-Puig, S., Sun, Y., Evans, S. M., Laugwitz, K. L. & Chien, K. R. (2006). Multipotent Embryonic Isl1+ Progenitor Cells Lead to Cardiac, Smooth Muscle, and Endothelial Cell Diversification. *Cell* Vol.127, No.6, (Dec 15, 2006) pp. 1151-1165, ISBN 0092-8674 (Print) 0092-8674 (Linking)

Morrison, S. J. & Spradling, A. C. (2008). Stem Cells and Niches: Mechanisms That Promote Stem Cell Maintenance Throughout Life. *Cell* Vol.132, No.4, (Feb 22, 2008) pp. 598-611, ISBN 1097-4172 (Electronic) 0092-8674 (Linking)

Murry, C. E., Field, L. J. & Menasche, P. (2005). Cell-Based Cardiac Repair: Reflections at the 10-Year Point. *Circulation* Vol.112, No.20, 2005) pp. 3174-3183, ISBN 1524-4539

Murry, C. E., Soonpaa, M. H., Reinecke, H., Nakajima, H., Nakajima, H. O., Rubart, M., Pasumarthi, K. B. S., Virag, J. I., Bartelmez, S. H., Poppa, V., Bradford, G., Dowell, J. D., Williams, D. A. & Field, L. J. (2004). Haematopoietic Stem Cells Do Not Transdifferentiate into Cardiac Myocytes in Myocardial Infarcts. *Nature* Vol.428, No.6983, 2004) pp. 664-668, ISBN 1476-4687

Nielsen, J. C., Lytrivi, I. D., Ko, H. H., Yau, J., Bhatla, P., Parness, I. A. & Srivastava, S. (2010). The Accuracy of Echocardiographic Assessment of Left Ventricular Size in Children by the 5/6 Area X Length (Bullet) Method. *Echocardiography* Vol.27, No.6, (Jul, 2010) pp. 691-695, ISBN 1540-8175 (Electronic) 0742-2822 (Linking)

Nishibatake, M., Kirby, M. L. & Van Mierop, L. H. (1987). Pathogenesis of Persistent Truncus Arteriosus and Dextroposed Aorta in the Chick Embryo after Neural Crest Ablation. *Circulation* Vol.75, No.1, (Jan, 1987) pp. 255-264, ISBN 0009-7322 (Print) 0009-7322 (Linking)

Oh, H., Bradfute, S. B., Gallardo, T. D., Nakamura, T., Gaussin, V., Mishina, Y., Pocius, J., Michael, L. H., Behringer, R. R., Garry, D. J., Entman, M. L. & Schneider, M. D. (2003). Cardiac Progenitor Cells from Adult Myocardium: Homing, Differentiation, and Fusion after Infarction. *Proc Natl Acad Sci U S A* Vol.100, No.21, (Oct 14, 2003) pp. 12313-12318, ISBN 0027-8424 (Print) 0027-8424 (Linking)

Oh, H. & Schneider, M. D. (2002). The Emerging Role of Telomerase in Cardiac Muscle Cell Growth and Survival. *Journal of molecular and cellular cardiology* Vol.34, No.7, (Jul, 2002) pp. 717-724, ISBN 0022-2828 (Print) 0022-2828 (Linking)

Orlic, D., Kajstura, J., Chimenti, S., Jakoniuk, I., Anderson, S. M., Li, B., Pickel, J., McKay, R., Nadal-Ginard, B., Bodine, D. M., Leri, A. & Anversa, P. (2001). Bone Marrow Cells Regenerate Infarcted Myocardium. *Nature* Vol.410, No.6829, (Apr 5, 2001) pp. 701-705, ISBN 0028-0836 (Print) 0028-0836 (Linking)

Palumbo, R. & Bianchi, M. E. (2004). High Mobility Group Box 1 Protein, a Cue for Stem Cell Recruitment. *Biochemical pharmacology* Vol.68, No.6, (Sep 15, 2004) pp. 1165-1170, ISBN 0006-2952 (Print) 0006-2952 (Linking)

Pouly, J., Bruneval, P., Mandet, C., Proksch, S., Peyrard, S., Amrein, C., Bousseaux, V., Guillemain, R., Deloche, A., Fabiani, J. N. & Menasche, P. (2008). Cardiac Stem Cells in the Real World. *J Thorac Cardiovasc Surg* Vol.135, No.3, (Mar, 2008) pp. 673-678, ISBN 1097-685X (Electronic) 0022-5223 (Linking)

Rossant, J. (2008). Stem Cells and Early Lineage Development. *Cell* Vol.132, No.4, (Feb 22, 2008) pp. 527-531, ISBN 1097-4172 (Electronic) 0092-8674 (Linking)

Saga, Y., Miyagawa-Tomita, S., Takagi, A., Kitajima, S., Miyazaki, J. & Inoue, T. (1999). Mesp1 Is Expressed in the Heart Precursor Cells and Required for the Formation of a Single Heart Tube. *Development* Vol.126, No.15, (Aug, 1999) pp. 3437-3447, ISBN 0950-1991 (Print) 0950-1991 (Linking)

Sairanen, H. & Louhimo, I. (1992). Dimensions of the Heart and Great Vessels in Normal Children. A Postmortem Study of Cardiac Ventricles, Valves and Great Vessels. *Scandinavian journal of thoracic and cardiovascular surgery* Vol.26, No.2, 1992) pp. 83-92, ISBN 0036-5580 (Print) 0036-5580 (Linking)

Schenke-Layland, K., Nsair, A., Van Handel, B., Angelis, E., Gluck, J. M., Votteler, M., Goldhaber, J. I., Mikkola, H. K., Kahn, M. & Maclellan, W. R. (2011). Recapitulation of the Embryonic Cardiovascular Progenitor Cell Niche. *Biomaterials* Vol.32, No.11, (Apr, 2011) pp. 2748-2756, ISBN 1878-5905 (Electronic) 0142-9612 (Linking)

Shi, Y., Moon, M., Dawood, S., McManus, B. & Liu, P. P. (2011). Mechanisms and Management of Doxorubicin Cardiotoxicity. *Herz*(Jun 9, 2011) pp. ISBN 1615-6692 (Electronic) 0340-9937 (Linking)

Smart, N., Risebro, C. A., Clark, J. E., Ehler, E., Miquerol, L., Rossdeutsch, A., Marber, M. S. & Riley, P. R. (2010). Thymosin Beta4 Facilitates Epicardial Neovascularization of the Injured Adult Heart. *Annals of the New York Academy of Sciences* Vol.1194, (Apr, 2010) pp. 97-104, ISBN 1749-6632 (Electronic) 0077-8923 (Linking)

Soppa, G. K., Lee, J., Stagg, M. A., Felkin, L. E., Barton, P. J., Siedlecka, U., Youssef, S., Yacoub, M. H. & Terracciano, C. M. (2008). Role and Possible Mechanisms of

Clenbuterol in Enhancing Reverse Remodelling During Mechanical Unloading in Murine Heart Failure. *Cardiovascular research* Vol.77, No.4, (Mar 1, 2008) pp. 695-706, ISBN 0008-6363 (Print) 0008-6363 (Linking)

Spradling, A., Drummond-Barbosa, D. & Kai, T. (2001). Stem Cells Find Their Niche. *Nature* Vol.414, No.6859, (Nov 1, 2001) pp. 98-104, ISBN 0028-0836 (Print) 0028-0836 (Linking)

Sturzu, A. C. & Wu, S. M. (2011). Developmental and Regenerative Biology of Multipotent Cardiovascular Progenitor Cells. *Circ Res* Vol.108, No.3, (Feb 4, 2011) pp. 353-364, ISBN 1524-4571 (Electronic) 0009-7330 (Linking)

Sui, R., Liao, X., Zhou, X. & Tan, Q. (2011). The Current Status of Engineering Myocardial Tissue. *Stem cell reviews* Vol.7, No.1, (Mar, 2011) pp. 172-180, ISBN 1558-6804 (Electronic) 1550-8943 (Linking)

Sun, X., Meyers, E. N., Lewandoski, M. & Martin, G. R. (1999). Targeted Disruption of Fgf8 Causes Failure of Cell Migration in the Gastrulating Mouse Embryo. *Genes & development* Vol.13, No.14, (Jul 15, 1999) pp. 1834-1846, ISBN 0890-9369 (Print) 0890-9369 (Linking)

Takeuchi, J. K. & Bruneau, B. G. (2009). Directed Transdifferentiation of Mouse Mesoderm to Heart Tissue by Defined Factors. *Nature* Vol.459, No.7247, (Jun 4, 2009) pp. 708-711, ISBN 1476-4687 (Electronic) 0028-0836 (Linking)

Tallini, Y. N., Greene, K. S., Craven, M., Spealman, A., Breitbach, M., Smith, J., Fisher, P. J., Steffey, M., Hesse, M., Doran, R. M., Woods, A., Singh, B., Yen, A., Fleischmann, B. K. & Kotlikoff, M. I. (2009). C-Kit Expression Identifies Cardiovascular Precursors in the Neonatal Heart. *Proceedings of the National Academy of Sciences of the United States of America* Vol.106, No.6, (Feb 10, 2009) pp. 1808-1813, ISBN 1091-6490 (Electronic) 0027-8424 (Linking)

Tam, P. P., Parameswaran, M., Kinder, S. J. & Weinberger, R. P. (1997). The Allocation of Epiblast Cells to the Embryonic Heart and Other Mesodermal Lineages: The Role of Ingression and Tissue Movement During Gastrulation. *Development* Vol.124, No.9, (May, 1997) pp. 1631-1642, ISBN 0950-1991 (Print) 0950-1991 (Linking)

Tamura, Y., Matsumura, K., Sano, M., Tabata, H., Kimura, K., Ieda, M., Arai, T., Ohno, Y., Kanazawa, H., Yuasa, S., Kaneda, R., Makino, S., Nakajima, K., Okano, H. & Fukuda, K. (2011). Neural Crest-Derived Stem Cells Migrate and Differentiate into Cardiomyocytes after Myocardial Infarction. *Arterioscler Thromb Vasc Biol* Vol.31, No.3, (Mar, 2011) pp. 582-589, ISBN 1524-4636 (Electronic) 1079-5642 (Linking)

Tsiavou, A. & Manginas, A. (2010). Dynamics of Progenitor Cells and Ventricular Assist Device Intervention. *Journal of cardiovascular translational research* Vol.3, No.2, (Apr, 2010) pp. 147-152, ISBN 1937-5395 (Electronic)

Tsuchihashi, T., Maeda, J., Shin, C. H., Ivey, K. N., Black, B. L., Olson, E. N., Yamagishi, H. & Srivastava, D. (2011). Hand2 Function in Second Heart Field Progenitors Is Essential for Cardiogenesis. *Developmental biology* Vol.351, No.1, (Mar 1, 2011) pp. 62-69, ISBN 1095-564X (Electronic) 0012-1606 (Linking)

Urbanek, K., Cesselli, D., Rota, M., Nascimbene, A., De Angelis, A., Hosoda, T., Bearzi, C., Boni, A., Bolli, R., Kajstura, J., Anversa, P. & Leri, A. (2006). Stem Cell Niches in the Adult Mouse Heart. *Proc Natl Acad Sci U S A* Vol.103, No.24, (Jun 13, 2006) pp. 9226-9231, ISBN 0027-8424 (Print) 0027-8424 (Linking)

Urbanek, K., Quaini, F., Tasca, G., Torella, D., Castaldo, C., Nadal-Ginard, B., Leri, A., Kajstura, J., Quaini, E. & Anversa, P. (2003). Intense Myocyte Formation from Cardiac Stem Cells in Human Cardiac Hypertrophy. *Proc Natl Acad Sci U S A* Vol.100, No.18, (Sep 2, 2003) pp. 10440-10445, ISBN 0027-8424 (Print) 0027-8424 (Linking)

Vincent, S. D. & Buckingham, M. E. (2010). How to Make a Heart: The Origin and Regulation of Cardiac Progenitor Cells. *Curr Top Dev Biol* Vol.90, 2010) pp. 1-41, ISBN 1557-8933 (Electronic) 0070-2153 (Linking)

Vitelli, F., Morishima, M., Taddei, I., Lindsay, E. A. & Baldini, A. (2002). Tbx1 Mutation Causes Multiple Cardiovascular Defects and Disrupts Neural Crest and Cranial Nerve Migratory Pathways. *Human molecular genetics* Vol.11, No.8, (Apr 15, 2002) pp. 915-922, ISBN 0964-6906 (Print) 0964-6906 (Linking)

Ward, H. H., Romero, E., Welford, A., Pickett, G., Bacallao, R., Gattone, V. H., 2nd, Ness, S. A., Wandinger-Ness, A. & Roitbak, T. (2011). Adult Human Cd133/1(+) Kidney Cells Isolated from Papilla Integrate into Developing Kidney Tubules. *Biochimica et biophysica acta*(Jan 19, 2011) pp. ISBN 0006-3002 (Print) 0006-3002 (Linking)

Williams, A. R., Trachtenberg, B., Velazquez, D. L., McNiece, I., Altman, P., Rouy, D., Mendizabal, A. M., Pattany, P. M., Lopera, G. A., Fishman, J., Zambrano, J. P., Heldman, A. W. & Hare, J. M. (2011). Intramyocardial Stem Cell Injection in Patients with Ischemic Cardiomyopathy: Functional Recovery and Reverse Remodeling. *Circulation research* Vol.108, No.7, (Apr 1, 2011) pp. 792-796, ISBN 1524-4571 (Electronic) 0009-7330 (Linking)

Wohlschlaeger, J., Levkau, B., Brockhoff, G., Schmitz, K. J., von Winterfeld, M., Takeda, A., Takeda, N., Stypmann, J., Vahlhaus, C., Schmid, C., Pomjanski, N., Bocking, A. & Baba, H. A. (2010). Hemodynamic Support by Left Ventricular Assist Devices Reduces Cardiomyocyte DNA Content in the Failing Human Heart. *Circulation* Vol.121, No.8, (Mar 2, 2010) pp. 989-996, ISBN 1524-4539 (Electronic) 0009-7322 (Linking)

Xie, T. & Spradling, A. C. (2000). A Niche Maintaining Germ Line Stem Cells in the Drosophila Ovary. *Science* Vol.290, No.5490, (Oct 13, 2000) pp. 328-330, ISBN 0036-8075 (Print) 0036-8075 (Linking)

Xu, H., Morishima, M., Wylie, J. N., Schwartz, R. J., Bruneau, B. G., Lindsay, E. A. & Baldini, A. (2004). Tbx1 Has a Dual Role in the Morphogenesis of the Cardiac Outflow Tract. *Development* Vol.131, No.13, (Jul, 2004) pp. 3217-3227, ISBN 0950-1991 (Print) 0950-1991 (Linking)

Yamanaka, S. & Blau, H. M. (2010). Nuclear Reprogramming to a Pluripotent State by Three Approaches. *Nature* Vol.465, No.7299, (Jun 10, 2010) pp. 704-712, ISBN 1476-4687 (Electronic) 0028-0836 (Linking)

13

Accurate Measurement of Systemic Oxygen Consumption in Ventilated Children with Congenital Heart Disease

Jia Li
University of Alberta
Canada

1. Introduction

Measuring systemic oxygen consumption (VO_2) is a fundamental part of hemodynamic and oxygen transport assessment when using the Fick principle. This measure is pivotal for children with congenital heart disease, at cardiac catheterization and in the Intensive Care Unit (ICU) after cardiopulmonary bypass surgery (CPB). According to the direct Fick principle (Fick, 1870), VO_2 may be combined with the difference between arterial and venous oxygen content, and the pressure gradient, to allow the calculation of each parameter of systemic hemodynamics and oxygen transport. Parameters that may be calculated include systemic and pulmonary blood flows (Qs and Qp) and resistances (SVR and PVR), systemic oxygen delivery (DO_2), and oxygen extraction ratio (ERO_2). Importantly, these parameters can be derived in a variety of simple or complex circulations in congenital heart defects before and after surgical repair or palliation, including *1)* biventricular circulation with or without left to right or right to left shunt (Li, Hoschtitzky et al. 2004; Li, Schulze-Neick et al. 2000; Schulze-Neick, Li et al. 2001; Schulze-Neick, Li et al. 2002), *2)* functionally single ventricular circulation such as hypoplastic left heart syndrome before and after the Norwood procedure (Li, Zhang et al. 2006; Li, Zhang et al. 2006; Li, Zhang et al. 2007; Li, Zhang et al. 2007; Li, Zhang et al. 2008), and *3)* one-and-a-half ventricular circulation such as after the bidirectional cavopulmonary shunt operation (Hoskote, Li et al. 2004; Li, Hoskote et al. 2005).

If VO_2 needs to be measured, then accuracy of the measurement cannot be overemphasized (Kendrick, West et al. 1988; Laitinen and Rasanen 1998; Shanahan, Wilson et al. 2003). Any error in VO_2 measurement will translate directly into an equivalent magnitude of under-estimation or over-estimation of hemodynamics and oxygen transport parameters, which may misdirect surgical and clinical treatment strategies. Prognostic cardiac catheterization is often used for evaluation of systemic and pulmonary blood flows and vascular resistances, particularly pulmonary vascular resistance, in patients with primary or secondary pulmonary hypertension, and in patients with functionally single ventricular abnormalities undergoing staged surgical palliations. In this latter group, elevated pulmonary vascular resistance is a risk factor for poor outcome (Gentles, Gauvreau et al. 1997; Gentles, Mayer et al. 1997; Mair, Hagler et al. 1990), emphasizing the need for accurate hemodynamic assessment before staged palliations.

In ICU patients, the importance of the accurate measurement of VO_2 has been increasingly realized in the past decade or two. Significant alterations in systemic oxygen transport and the contribution of VO_2 in the impaired balance of oxygen transport during the early postoperative period after CPB are now better understood (Chiara, Giomarelli et al. 1987; Li, Hoschtitzky et al. 2004; Li, Schulze-Neick et al. 2000; Li, Zhang et al. 2007; Li, Zhang et al. 2007; Oudemans-van Straaten, Jansen et al. 1996). VO_2 has its own meaning in the balance of oxygen transport, which has been largely ignored. A hypermetabolic response with increased VO_2 occurs in patients after CPB, due mainly to *1)* a systemic inflammatory response (Li, Hoschtitzky et al. 2004; Oudemans-van Straaten, Jansen et al. 1996), *2)* rewarming from hypothermic CPB and fever (Li, Hoschtitzky et al. 2004; Li, Schulze-Neick et al. 2000), and *3)* the use of inotropes (Li, Zhang et al. 2006). The increase in VO_2 is an important contributor to the imbalance of oxygen transport in the early postoperative period, when cardiac function and oxygen delivery are depressed due to myocardial injury by surgery and ischemia-reperfusion (Li, Zhang et al. 2006; Li, Zhang et al. 2007; Wernovsky, Wypij et al. 1995). VO_2 varies greatly between patients and within individual patients over time. Variation in VO_2 results from varied circulatory, metabolic, and hormonal responses to CPB (Li, Hoschtitzky et al. 2004; Oudemans-van Straaten, Jansen et al. 1996), from patient body temperature (Li, Hoschtitzky et al. 2004; Li, Schulze-Neick et al. 2000;), and from pharmacological (Li, Zhang et al. 2006) and ventilator manipulations (Li, Hoskote et al. 2005; Li, Zhang et al. 2008) (please see section 4 for details). In this dynamic milieu, continuous or repeated monitoring of VO_2 is necessary to reflect changes over time.

Accurate measurement of VO_2 allows precise assessment of systemic hemodynamics and oxygen transport parameters in varied circulations after complete repair or palliations (Li, Hoschtitzky et al. 2004; Li, Hoskote et al. 2005; Li, Schulze-Neick et al. 2000; Li, Zhang et al. 2006; Li, Zhang et al. 2006; Li, Zhang et al. 2007; Li, Zhang et al. 2007; Li, Zhang et al. 2008; Schulze-Neick, Li et al. 2001; Schulze-Neick, Li et al. 2002). Actual measurements are superior to the indirect indicators, such as blood pressure and arterial and venous oxygen saturations that are most commonly used in postoperative management. Superiority of actual measurements is seen particularly clearly after the Norwood procedure, when profound hemodynamic instability and oxygen transport imbalance occurs. Furthermore, actual measurements of hemodynamics and oxygen transport parameters are fundamental to bedside physiological research on factors affecting the imbalance of oxygen transport, research aimed at improving the management of critically ill children. With direct and continuous measurement of VO_2 using state-of-the-art technique respiratory mass spectrometry, we have conducted extensive studies in neonates after the Norwood procedure (Li, Zhang et al. 2006; Li, Zhang et al. 2006; Li, Zhang et al. 2007; Li, Zhang et al. 2007; Li, Zhang et al. 2008; Li, Zhang et al. 2008; Li, Zhang et al. 2008; Li, Zhang et al. 2008). We use the Norwood circulation and physiology in this Chapter as a model to understand oxygen transport and the factors affecting oxygen kinetics in children after CPB.

The objectives of this chapter are two-fold. 1) To review the currently available techniques of VO_2 measurement, including published predictive equations and indirect Fick principle using themodilution, their advantages and disadvantages, with special emphasis on respiratory mass spectrometry to assess VO_2 in children undergoing cardiac cauterization and after CPB in the ICU. 2) Using the Norwood physiology as the model to introduce the concept of oxygen transport and further emphasize the importance of direct and continuous measurement of VO_2 in both clinical care and research in children with congenital heart disease before and after CPB.

2. The inaccurate techniques for measurement of VO_2

2.1 The inaccuracies of predictive equations

Although techniques for metabolic monitoring using indirect calorimetry or respiratory mass spectrometry are available for the direct measurement of VO_2, it is still common practice to estimate VO_2 values from tables or published predictive equations (LaFarge and Miettinen 1970; Lindahl 1989; Lundell, Casas et al. 1996; Wessel, Rorem et al. 1969). Despite attempts to improve the accuracy of estimated VO_2 values, large discrepancies are still observed between measured and estimated values (Laitinen and Rasanen 1998; Shanahan, Wilson et al. 2003; Wolf, Pollman et al. 1998). Such discrepancies present challenges in the clinical application of predictive equations e.g., in the catheterization laboratory setting, because subsequent hemodynamic calculations will be impaired. In ICU patients during the early postoperative period after CPB, estimation of VO_2 is even further exposed to inaccuracies due to significant variability of VO_2 between and within patients over time (Li, Zhang et al. 2006; Li, Zhang et al. 2006; Li, Zhang et al. 2007; Li, Zhang et al. 2008). Furthermore, estimating VO_2 by predictive equations gives a single value for a given patient and makes no provision for the dynamic patient milieu that is inevitable in the early post-operative period (Li, Zhang et al. 2006; Li, Zhang et al. 2006; Li, Zhang et al. 2007; Li, Zhang et al. 2008).

We have compared results from four commonly used equations for estimating VO_2 (LaFarge and Miettinen 1970; Lindahl 1989; Lundell, Casas et al. 1996; Wessel, Rorem et al. 1969) against VO_2 measured directly by respiratory mass spectrometry. Both the equations and the direct measurements were applied to children with congenital heart defects, during cardiac catherization and in the ICU after CPB. We found poor agreement between the direct measurements and all estimated values, especially in children younger than 3 years of age and in the ICU patients (Li, Bush et al. 2003; Rutledge, Bush et al. 2010).

2.1.1 VO_2 values during cardiac catheterization versus in the ICU after CPB

In patients undergoing cardiac catheterization, there is a general *over-estimation* of VO_2 introduced by the equations (Figure 1) (Li, Bush et al. 2003). The conditions of conscious sedation with spontaneous ventilation were used to generate the predictive equations decades ago. In contrast in current practice, general anesthesia and mechanical ventilation are used in most children undergoing cardiac catheterization. General anesthesia and muscle relaxants with mechanical ventilation may decrease the cardiopulmonary work and metabolic rate, resulting in a reduction in VO_2 of up to 20 to 30%.(Nisbet, Dobbinson et al. 1973; Westenskow, Jordan et al. 1978)

In the ICU patients, a general *under-estimation* of VO_2 is introduced by the equations, with very poor agreement to actual measurements, as the equations were generated in preoperative patients undergoing cardiac catheterization (Li, Bush et al. 2003). After CPB, VO_2 is significantly increased and highly variable between patients and within each patient (Figure 2) (Li, Zhang et al. 2006; Li, Zhang et al. 2007; Li, Zhang et al. 2008). Thus, the direct measurement of VO_2 is essential for these patients; continuous or repeated measurements are also essential to reflect the dynamic changes in these patients that occur over time.

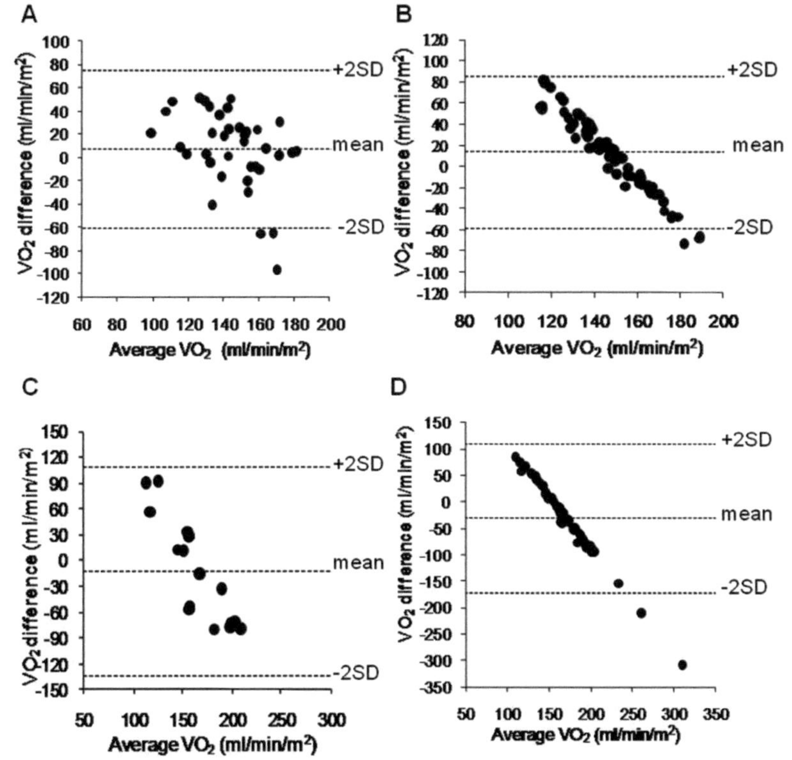

Fig. 1. Agreement of measured and estimated VO_2. Measured VO_2 minus estimated VO_2 is plotted against average VO_2; in patients undergoing cardiac catheterization, (A) using the LaFarge equation and (B) the Wessel equation; and after cardiac surgery in the ICU, (C) using the LaFarge equation and (D) the Wessel equation .

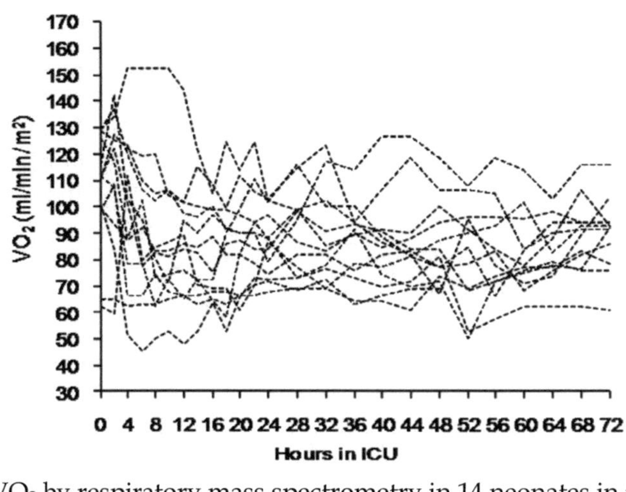

Fig. 2. Measured VO_2 by respiratory mass spectrometry in 14 neonates in the first 72 hours after the Norwood procedure

2.1.2 VO_2 values in patients > 3 years old versus ≤ 3 years old

Of the equations we tested initially, the LaFarge equation is the most commonly used and gives the closest estimation to measured results with the lowest bias and limits of agreement (Li, Bush et al. 2003). However, despite the fact that the LaFarge equation was generated and intended for use in patients between 3 and 40 years of age, it is applied in patients of all ages. With advances in surgical techniques and perioperative management, increasing numbers of younger patients with complex congenital heart defects, such as functionally single ventricular abnormalities, undergo cardiac surgery. This in turn increases the need for diagnostic cardiac catheterization in children younger than 3 years, often with the single goal of accurately evaluating pulmonary vascular resistance.

Our initial study, comparing measured and estimated VO_2, excluded patients whose ages fell outside the range used in the derivation of LaFarge equation, that is, younger than 3 years. We revisited the data to compare estimates of VO_2 in patients younger than 3 years to the earlier data from patients older than 3 years of age. Estimations were significantly poorer in the group younger than 3 years, with a bias of 55 mL/min/m^2, compared to a bias of 11 mL/min/m^2 in the older group. The limits of agreements were -42 to +153 mL/min/m^2 for children < 3 years versus -39 to +61 mL/kg/m^2 for those ≥ 3 years (Figure 3) (Rutledge, Bush et al. 2010)

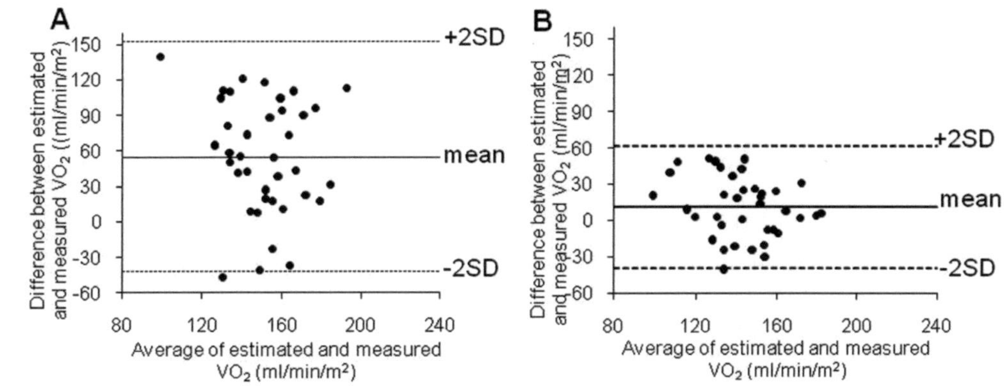

Fig. 3. Agreement of measured and estimated VO_2 during cardiac catheterization in patients (A) < 3 years old and (B) > 3 years old.

The LaFarge equation (LaFarge and Miettinen 1970) includes a logarithmic transformation of age for male patients (equation 1) and for female patients (equation 2).

$$VO_2\ (mL/min/m^2) = 138.1-(11.49 \times \log_e age) + (0.378 \times \text{heart rate}) \quad (1)$$

$$VO_2\ (mL/min/m^2) = 138.1- (17.04 \times \log_e age)+(0.378 \times \text{heart rate}) \quad (2)$$

The logarithmic transformation of age intrinsically results in a faster increase in estimated VO_2 as age decreases, particularly within the first 3 years of life (Figure 4A). Interestingly, the directly measured VO_2 has almost exactly the opposite trend, being lowest in the youngest patients and quickly increasing in the first 3 to 4 years (Figure 4B). As a result, the errors of estimated VO_2 are dramatically related to age (Figure 4C). The reasons for lower VO_2 in younger children remain unclear, but body composition may be a factor. In particular, 'fat mass' is relatively higher in younger children (Fomon, Haschke et al. 1982; Moukarzel, Salas et al. 2003) and VO_2 in fat mass is about 20 times lower than in muscular mass (Moukarzel, Salas et al. 2003).

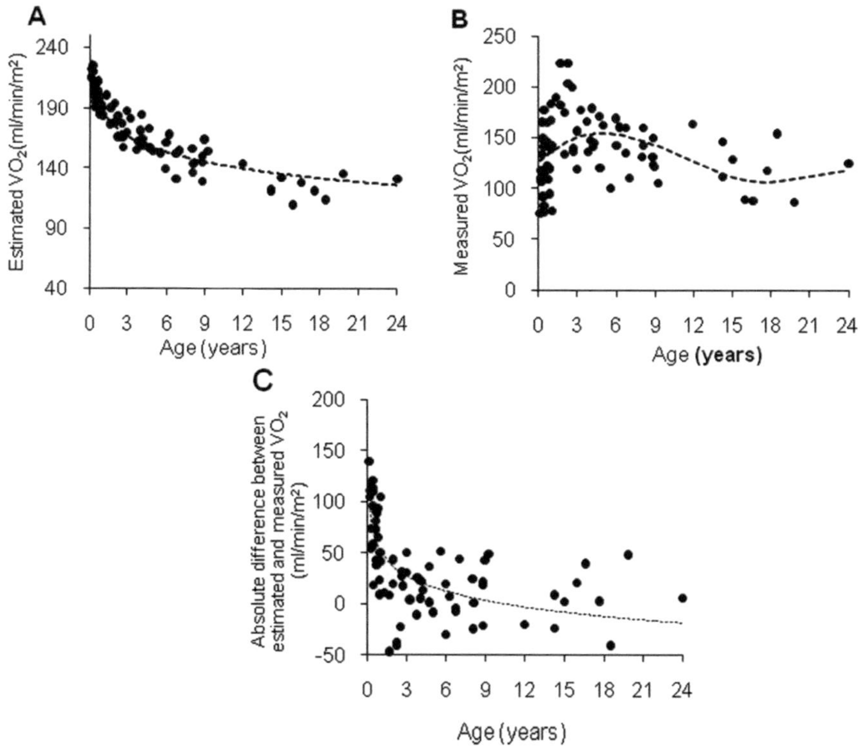

Fig. 4. The trends in relation to age of (A) estimated VO_2, (B) measured VO_2, and (C) their difference, in 75 patients undergoing cardiac catheterization.

We conclude that estimation of VO_2 is unacceptably inaccurate for clinical decision-making and research. Direct measurement of VO_2 is appropriate for young children with congenital heart defects undergoing cardiac catheterization and in the ICU after CPB. Direct and continuous measurement of VO_2 is essential, particularly in those younger than 3 years and in the early postoperative period after CPB.

2.2 Inadequacy of the reverse Fick method

VO_2 can also be calculated by the reverse Fick method from the cardiac output, directly measured by the thermodilution technique, for example. This method has obvious limitations for clinical application in patients with congenital heart defects. First, the calculation is clearly intermittent. Second, the presence of intracardiac shunting and tricuspid regurgitation can significantly affect the accuracy of the calculation. Most important, certain complex circulations preclude the use of the thermodilution technique (e.g., after the Norwood procedure, bidrectional caval pulmonary shunt, or the Fontan operation), because of anatomical (e.g., parallel systemic and pulmonary circulations) and methodological (e.g., inadequate mixing) limitations.

3. Direct measurement of VO_2 using respiratory mass spectrometry

The concept of mass spectrometry (measuring fractional proportions of substances in a mixture, according to their molecular mass-charge ratios) was first introduced at the end of the 19th century. The recruitment of mass spectrometry into respiratory physiology in the 1940s, and its subsequent refinement over the decades, has established a 'state-of-the-art' method for measuring VO_2 using highly accurate and rapid multiple gas analysis. The mixed expirate method (Davies and Denison 1979) enabled use of the mass spectrometer alone to measure metabolic gas exchange and ventilation volume. This technique has been used widely to measure VO_2 in a broad spectrum of clinical and experimental conditions. We have adapted the method to continuously measure VO_2 with a variety of pediatric ventilators and anesthesia ventilators before, during, and after CPB, using the AMIS 2000 Medical Respiratory Mass Spectrometer System (Innovision A/C Odense, Denmark). Our combination of techniques and equipment makes respiratory mass spectrometry a unique and powerful tool in multiple settings: in the cardiac catheterization laboratory (Schulze-Neick, Li et al. 2002 ; Shekerdemian, Bush et al. 1997; Shekerdemian, Bush et al. 1997), in the operating room (Li, Stokoe et al. 2004), and in the ICU (Li, Hoschtitzky et al. 2004; Li, Schulze-Neick et al. 2000; Li, Zhang et al. 2006; Li, Zhang et al. 2006; Li, Zhang et al. 2007; Li, Zhang et al. 2007; Li, Zhang et al. 2008; Schulze-Neick, Li et al. 2001).

3.1 Principles of mass spectrometry

Mass spectrometers analyze substances in the gas phase by performing a sequence of five operations: *1)* accept and vaporize a minute controlled quantity of sample; *2)* reduce the sample vapor to a very low pressure; *3)* ionize a representative part of the vapor; *4)* separate the ionized particles produced, according to their mass-to-charge ratio; and *5)* read the abundance of particles at specific values of the mass-to-charge ratio.

3.2 Hardware design

Features of a mass spectrometer are outlined in Figure 5.

A Teflon capillary tubing (A) with an internal diameter 0.3 mm and a length of 3 to 6 m provides the gas transport from the sampling site (B) to the vacuum system. There are three sample inlets, one for the on-line continuous monitoring of O_2 and CO_2 fractional concentrations, the other two for the inspiratory and expiratory gas sampling. The gas sample at atmospheric pressure is drawn at a sampling rate of 10 to 20 mL/min down the tubing (A), passing through the three static electro-magnetic valves (C), which are selected in turn as appropriate to the sequence of gas analysis needed for the metabolic calculations. The sample is drawn by the inlet rotary vacuum pump (D) into the sample chamber (E), and all but a small fraction of it is pumped away continuously at the low-pressure end of the inlet tubing. The turbo molecular pump (F), supported by a second backing rotary pump (G), provides a very high vacuum environment of around 5×10^{-7} mBar in the dispersion chamber (H), housing ionization chamber (I), mass filter (J), and ion detector (K). Thus, the high vacuum provided by the turbo molecular pump draws the remaining gas sample through the molecular leak (L) into the ionization chamber, where the gas molecules are ionized. The ions are focused into a tight beam, enter the aperture of the quadrupole mass filter, and are separated by the quadrupole mass filter (J). The use of appropriate voltages in this field allows only ions of a definite mass interval to pass and reach the ion detector (K), suppressing the inevitable 'noise' which would otherwise be created by the contaminants that cross the mass filter as a result of scatter. The ions are then collected and pre-amplified in a current-voltage pre-amplifier prior to signal processing. The resulting signal is therefore made as pure as possible before being amplified by the secondary electron multiplier (SEM). Amplification enables a higher sensitivity and faster operation. The resulting output of the detection unit is proportional to the ion current, which in turn is proportional to the partial pressure of the gas species. (Pressures indicated are at normal operating conditions).

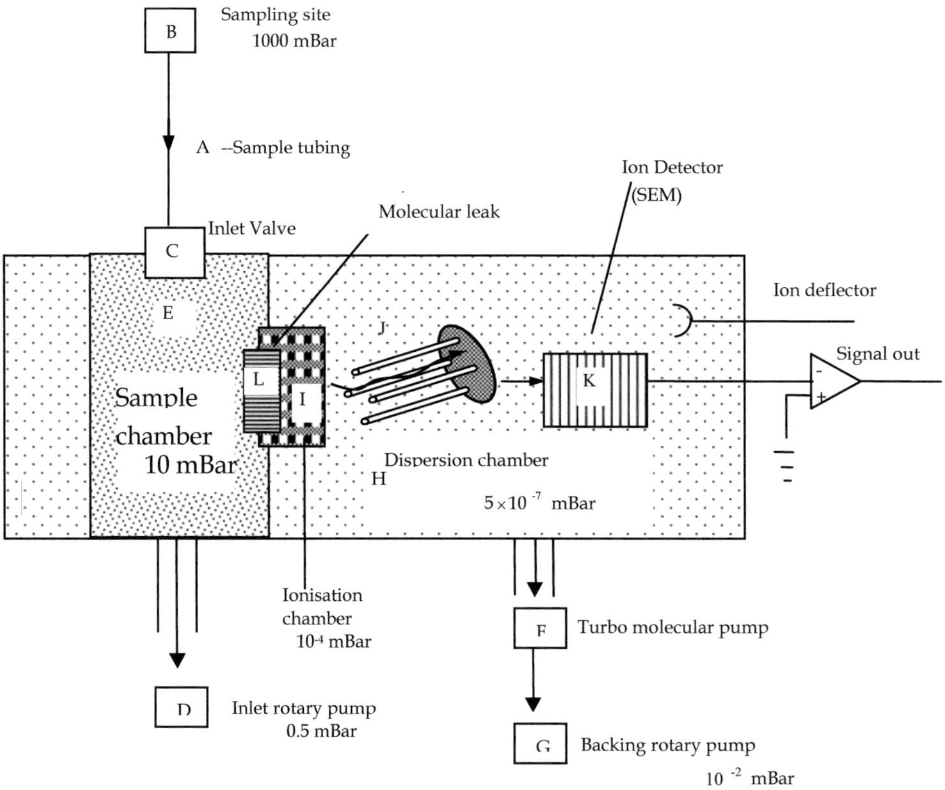

Fig. 5. Design of AMIS 2000 respiratory mass spectrometer.

3.3 The measurement of VO_2

The mass spectrometer measures metabolic gas exchange by the 'inert gas dilution method'. 'A known mass flow of a marker gas is injected into expired gas upstream of a mixing box, and the resulting gas composition downstream used to deduce the mass flows of all its components' (Davies and Denison 1979). VO_2 is then calculated every 30 seconds as:

$$VO_2\,(STPD) = V_{Tr}\,(STPD) \bullet [F_{IO2} \bullet (1\text{-}F_{MCO2}\text{-}F_{MTr})\text{-}F_{MO2} \bullet (1\text{-}F_{ICO2}\text{-}F_{ITr})] \,/\, D \qquad (3)$$

$D = F_{MTr} \bullet (1\text{-}\ F_{IO2}\text{-}\ F_{ICO2})\ \text{-}\ F_{Itr} \bullet (1\text{-}\ F_{MO2}\text{-}\ F_{MCO2})$

V_{Tr} = added flow of indicator gas (tracer, Argon)

F_{IO2}, F_{ICO2}, F_{Itr} = constant fractional concentrations of O_2, CO_2 and tracer gas in inspired air

F_{MO2}, F_{MCO2}, F_{MTr}: = measured fractional concentrations of O_2, CO_2 and tracer gas at the outlet of the mixing chamber
STPD = Standard temperature and pressure dry.

3.4 Setup of respiratory mass spectrometer in the cardiac catheterization laboratory with anesthesia ventilators

Accurate measurement of minute ventilation relies on the complete collection of expired gas and therefore a leak-free circuit. Ideally, patients are intubated with cuffed endotracheal tubes. Precise VO_2 measurement requires a steady-state period, thus patients are sedated and paralyzed to obviate the confounding effects of movement, agitation, and pain on VO_2. We have adapted the AMIS2000 respiratory mass spectrometer in the cardiac catheterization laboratory to anesthesia ventilators with a partial rebreathing system (Figure 6).

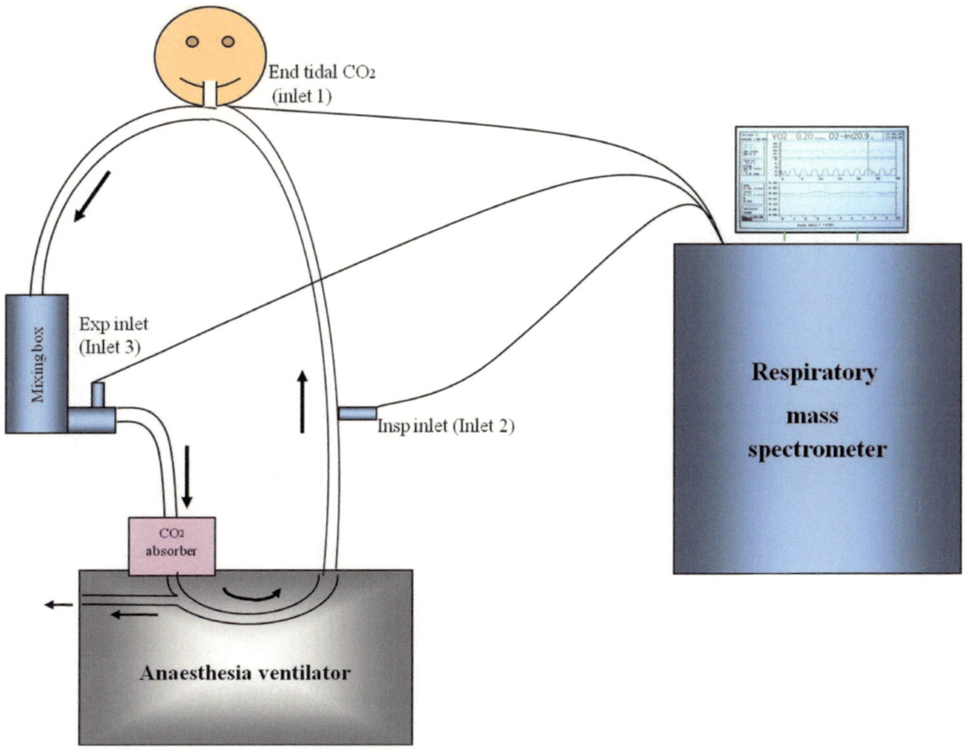

Fig. 6. The setup of the AMIS2000 respiratory mass spectrometer sampling inlets, mixing box, and the circuit of the anesthesia ventilator in the cardiac catheterization laboratory.

Most children undergoing cardiac catheterization are paralyzed and mechanically ventilated by an anesthesia ventilator with a partial rebreathing system, whereby the exhaled gas is re-circulated via a CO_2 absorber and fresh gas mixture is continuously supplied. The mixing box is inserted in the expiratory limb of the ventilator circuit to collect the expired gas. Inlet 1 is placed at the mouth piece close to the endotracheal tube, for continuous on-line monitoring of breath-to-breath oxygen and carbon dioxide fractional concentrations. This checks that the steady state had not been perturbed. Another two inlets are used for the measurement of VO_2. Inlet 2, which is placed in the inspiratory limb of the ventilator circuit, samples inspiratory gas; Inlet 3 samples the 'effluent' mixed expirate from the distal end of the mixing box.

3.5 Setup of respiratory mass spectrometer in the ICU with pediatric ventilators

We have also adapted the AMIS2000 respiratory mass spectrometer in the ICU to various pediatric ventilators with continuous flow (Figure 7). Pediatric ventilators in the ICU use continuous flow to supply fresh gas throughout the breathing cycle. This avoids increasing the amount of work required to trigger spontaneous breathing. In a setup different from the anesthesia ventilator, the mixing box is connected to the exit port of the pediatric ventilator to collect the expired gas, and is also connected to an 'expiratory' inlet (Inlet 3). The expiratory inlet allows sampling of the 'effluent' mixed expirate from the distal end of the mixing box. Inlets 1 and 2 are placed at the mouth piece and in the inspiratory limb respectively, in the same way as in the anesthesia ventilator.

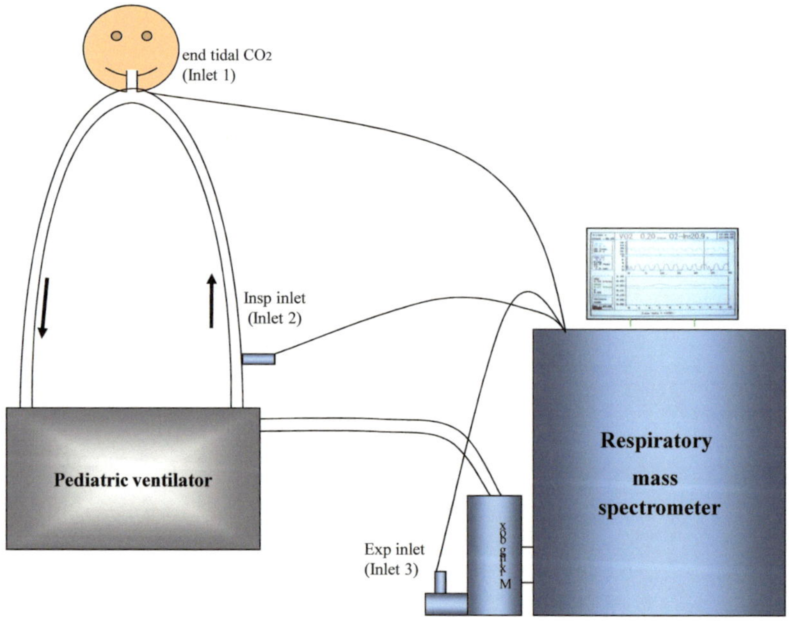

Fig. 7. The setup of the AMIS2000 respiratory mass spectrometer sampling inlets, mixing box, and the circuit of the pediatric ventilator in the ICU.

3.6 Clinical applications of respiratory mass spectrometry in the ICU

Respiratory mass spectrometers were first produced for commercial applications in the late 1980s. The reported precision of the mass spectrometer was as low as 5% in spontaneous breathing at rest or during exercise. The precision increases in paralyzed and ventilated patients. Precision was further improved by avoiding the use of flow sensors. Versatility of the respiratory mass spectrometer is greatly increased by the use of long sampling probes up to 30 meters(Davies and Denison 1979). Long probes allow the study of subjects who otherwise might be inaccessible due to the size of the equipment, such as patients undergoing cardiac catheterization, intensive care, or surgery, where space at the bedside is severely limited. Long probes also enable simultaneous events to be examined sequentially, and permit a single mass spectrometer to be shared between several patients or laboratories. Respiratory mass spectrometers have become valuable clinical research tools. Our adaptation of the respiratory mass spectrometer to pediatric ventilators has allowed us to extensively study systemic hemodynamics and oxygen transport, and the factors affecting them, before and after cardiac surgery in children with congenital heart defects (Li, Hoschtitzky et al. 2004; Li, Hoskote et al. 2005; Li, Schulze-Neick et al. 2000; Li, Zhang et al. 2006; Li, Zhang et al. 2006; Li, Zhang et al. 2007; Li, Zhang et al. 2007; Li, Zhang et al. 2008; Zhang 2008; Zhang, Holtby et al. 2008).

The importance of oxygen transport is increasingly appreciated in the care of critically ill patients, particularly after CPB (Gilbert, Haupt et al. 1986; Haupt, Gilbert et al. 1985; Hoffman, Ghanayem et al. 2000; Li, Hoschtitzky et al. 2004; Li, Hoskote et al. 2005; Li, Schulze-Neick et al. 2000; Li, Zhang et al. 2006; Li, Zhang et al. 2006; Li, Zhang et al. 2007; Li, Zhang et al. 2007; Li, Zhang et al. 2008; Oudemans-van Straaten, Jansen et al. 1996; Powers, Mannal et al. 1973; Tweddell, Hoffman et al. 1999; Zhang 2008; Zhang, Holtby et al. 2008). The fundamental requirement of ICU management is to match systemic oxygen delivery (DO_2) to VO_2, to sustain cellular metabolism and end-organ function. Many patients requiring ICU support have reduced DO_2, usually as a result of decreased myocardial function. However, in many patients the reduced cardiac output and DO_2 are further compounded by secondary abnormalities of VO_2 that amplify the deficiency of DO_2 and contribute to the overall imbalance of oxygen transport. This combination is seen in many situations such as sepsis and trauma (Gilbert, Haupt et al. 1986; Haupt, Gilbert et al. 1985; Powers, Mannal et al. 1973), but is a consistent feature of cardiac surgery (Hoffman, Ghanayem et al. 2000; Li, Hoschtitzky et al. 2004; Li, Schulze-Neick et al. 2000; Li, Zhang et al. 2007).

Most children experience a phase of reduced cardiac output during the first few hours after CPB (Hoffman, Ghanayem et al. 2000; Li, Zhang et al. 2007; Wernovsky, Wypij et al. 1995). At the same time, VO_2 is increased and highly dynamic in relation to central body temperature (Li, Hoschtitzky et al. 2004; Li, Schulze-Neick et al. 2000), the systemic inflammatory response (Li, Hoschtitzky et al. 2004; Oudemans-van Straaten, Jansen et al. 1996), pharmacological manipulations (Hayes, Timmins et al. 1994; Li, Zhang et al. 2006), and ventilatory manipulations (Li, Hoskote et al. 2005; Li, Zhang et al. 2008). VO_2 is an important constituent in the balance of oxygen transport, but has been largely ignored in ICU management. Traditional management of these patients has focused on augmenting myocardial performance through the use of inotropes, for example, to enhance cardiac output and DO_2. However, inotropic agents may not effectively enhance cardiac output in the presence of myocardial injury, and may paradoxically stimulate systemic and myocardial oxygen consumption, offsetting any gains in DO_2 (Fowler, Alderman et al. 1984; Hayes, Timmins et al. 1994; Li, Zhang et al. 2006). An alternative (and in some ways more rational) approach to improving the balance of oxygen transport may be to decrease VO_2. For example, the use of skeletal muscle paralysis and assisted ventilation is a standard therapy directed at reducing metabolic demands. These simple maneuvers may reduce VO_2 by up to 20 to 30% (Nisbet, Dobbinson et al. 1973; Westenskow, Jordan et al. 1978). Similarly, profound reductions in VO_2 may be achieved simply by controlling central body temperature. We have shown in infants after cardiac surgery, for example, that central pyrexia increases VO_2 by approximately 11% per degree Celsius (Li, Schulze-Neick et al. 2000). Therefore, in the current conceptualization of oxygen transport, emphasis should shift beyond cardiac output and oxygen delivery to the balance between DO_2 and VO_2.

4. Calculation of oxygen transport parameters using directly measured VO_2

4.1 The Fick principle

The Fick principle states that 'The total uptake or release of any substance by an organ is the product of blood flow to the organ and the arteriovenous concentration difference of the substance.' (Fick 1870).

The Fick principle implies that if the flow in a system cannot be measured directly, then it can be measured using an indicator, provided that the indicator is removed at a known rate. Fick described the theory of a method to calculate cardiac output but never actually measured it himself. He argued: 'It is astonishing that no one has arrived at the following obvious method by which the amount of blood ejected by the ventricle of the heart with each systole may be determined directly, at least in animals. One measures how much oxygen an animal absorbs from the air in a given time. During the experiment one obtains a sample of arterial and venous blood; in both the oxygen content is measured. The difference in oxygen content tells how much oxygen each cubic centimeter of blood takes up in its passage through the lungs. As one knows the total quantity of oxygen absorbed in a given time one can calculate how many cubic centimeters of blood passed through the lungs in this time.' (Vandam and Fox 1998).

Verification of the Fick principle in humans was initially accomplished in 1930, through the daring exploits of Baumann and Grollman at a time when cardiac catheterization had yet to be established as a clinical tool. They obtained samples of mixed venous blood by inserting a spinal tap needle just to the right of the sternum; the needle entered the right ventricular chamber by puncturing its wall (Grollman 1932).

The direct Fick principle using VO_2 is one of the oldest methods of measuring systemic and pulmonary blood flows, but nonetheless remains the gold standard. It can be used in simple biventricular and varied complex circulations in congenital heart defects, before or after surgical repair palliations. Relevant equations are provided in the following sections.

4.2 In normal circulation

The direct Fick method measures cardiac output (CO, which is systemic blood flow, Qs, and is equal to pulmonary blood flow, Qp) with VO_2 according to the following equation:

$$CO = VO_2 / (CaO_2 - CvO_2) \tag{4}$$

where CaO_2 and CvO_2 are arterial and the mixed venous oxygen contents, respectively. Then:

$$SVR = (MaP - MsvcP)/CO \tag{5}$$

$$PVR = (MpaP - MpvP)/CO \tag{6}$$

$$DO_2 = CO \times CaO_2 \tag{7}$$

$$ERO_2 = VO_2 / DO_2 \tag{8}$$

where MaP, MsvcP, MpaP, and MpvP are mean systemic arterial, superior vena cava, pulmonary arterial, and pulmonary venous pressures; CaO_2 is systemic arterial oxygen content.

4.3 In biventricular circulation with shunt

In a biventricular circulation, the left to right, right to left, or bidirectional shunt may be present at the atrial, ventricular, or great vessel levels, such as in atrial septal defect, ventricular septal defect, patent arterial duct, or tetrology of Fallot.

$$Qs = VO_2 / (CaO_2\text{-}CvO_2) \tag{9}$$

$$Qp = VO_2 / (CpvO_2\text{-}CpaO_2) \tag{10}$$

$$SVR = (MaP - MsvcP)/Qs \tag{11}$$

$$PVR = (MpaP - MpvP)/Qp \tag{12}$$

$$DO_2 = CO \times CaO_2 \tag{13}$$

where CaO_2, CvO_2, and $CpvO_2$ are systemic arterial and venous, and pulmonary venous oxygen contents; and MaP, MvP, and MpvP are mean systemic arterial, venous, and pulmonary venous pressures. ERO_2 is calculated as in the normal circulation (Equation 8).

4.4 In one-and-a-half ventricular circulation: Bidirectional cavopulmonary shunt

In bidirectional cavopulmonary shunt circulation, the blood from the superior vena cava is directed to the pulmonary arteries, passing through the pulmonary circulation (Qp) and becomes oxygenated before it reaches the systemic circulation. Once in the systemic circulation, the blood from the superior vena cava mixes with systemic venous blood from the inferior vena cava (Qivc) to form total cardiac output (CO). Therefore, as stated by Salim, Case et al. (1995):

$$Qsvc = Qp \tag{14}$$

$$CO = Qp + Qivc \tag{15}$$

$$Qp = VO_2 / (CpvO_2 - CsvcO_2) \tag{16}$$

$$CO = VO_2 \times (CpvO_2 - CivcO_2) / [(CpvO_2 - CsvcO_2) \times (CaO_2 - CivcO_2)] \tag{17}$$

$$Qivc = CO - Qp \tag{18}$$

$$SVR = (MaP - MivcP)/Qs \tag{19}$$

$$PVR = (MsvcP - MpvP)/Qp \tag{20}$$

where CaO_2, $CivcO_2$, $CsvcO_2$, and $CpvO_2$ are arterial, inferior and superior vena cava and pulmonary venous oxygen contents; MaP, MivcP, MsvcP, and MpvP are mean systemic arterial, inferior and superior vena cava, and pulmonary venous pressures. DO_2 and ERO_2 are calculated as in the normal circulation (Equations 7 & 8).

4.5 In single ventricular circulation: Hypoplastic left heart syndrome and the Norwood circulation

In functionally single ventricular circulation, a single outlet from the heart provides both systemic and pulmonary circulations via an interposed B-T shunt or right ventricle to pulmonary artery shunt. Therefore:

$$CO = Qs + Qp \tag{21}$$

$$Qs = VO_2 / (CaO_2 - CvO_2) \tag{22}$$

$$Qp = VO_2 / (CpvO_2 - CaO_2) \tag{23}$$

$$SVR = (MaP - MsvcP)/Qs \tag{24}$$

$$'PVR' = (MaP - MpvP)/Qp \tag{25}$$
(including the shunt)

$$DO_2 = Qs \times CaO_2 \tag{26}$$

Where CaO_2, CvO_2 and $CpvO_2$ are systemic arterial, superior vena caval and pulmonary venous oxygen contents; MaP, MsvcP, and MpvP are mean systemic arterial, superior vena cava, and pulmonary venous pressures; 'PVR' is pulmonary vascular resistance including the shunt in the classic Norwood procedure (Li, Zhang et al. 2006; Li, Zhang et al. 2007). ERO_2 is calculated as in the normal circulation (Equation 8).

In this Chapter, the Norwood circulation is used as the model to understand the balance of oxygen transport and the factors affecting it. This is an ideal model to understand the concept of oxygen transport, since the Norwood physiology is characterized by profound hemodynamic instability and oxygen transport imbalance, and represents the most challenging group of children for postoperative management after CPB. Data presented in this chapter were obtained in neonates after the classic Norwood procedure with the Blalock-Taussig shunt, but the basic physiology of the classic Norwood procedure is largely the same as the modified procedure with the right ventricle to pulmonary artery conduit, i.e., a single neonatal ventricle provides the parallel pulmonary and systemic circulations.

5. Improved understanding of the Norwood physiology and postoperative management using direct measurement of VO_2

The Norwood procedure for hypoplastic left heart syndrome, and similar anatomic variants, continues to have significant morbidity, and a mortality rate that ranges from 6% to 25% (Azakie, Merklinger et al. 2001; Gaynor, Mahle et al. 2002; Ohye, Sleeper et al. 2010; Sano, Huang et al. 2009). Despite advances in surgical and postoperative management, these infants have little hemodynamic reserve. Instability following repair is inherent in the neonatal single ventricle supplying parallel pulmonary and systemic circulations, and is compounded by the variable effects of CPB and ischemia and reperfusion injury. Our understanding of the Norwood physiology has been based on theoretical studies using computational models (Barnea, Austin et al. 1994; Migliavacca, Pennati et al. 2001), and on animal models (Kitaichi, Chikugo et al. 2003). Necessarily, these models do not reflect the true functionally single ventricular physiology. In previous studies in humans, arterial superior vena caval oxygen saturations, and their derivations were most commonly used as surrogates of DO_2 (Charpie, Dekeon et al. 2001; Hoffman, Ghanayem et al. 2000; Maher, Pizarro et al. 2003; Tweddell, Hoffman et al. 1999). In some human studies, derived values of pulmonary and systemic blood flows have been obtained, but are based on the key assumption of a fixed VO_2 of 160 or 180 $mL/min/m^2$ (Charpie, Dekeon et al. 2001; Hoffman, Ghanayem et al. 2000; Maher, Pizarro et al. 2003; Tweddell, Hoffman et al. 1999). However, as demonstrated above in section 2.1.1 (Figure 2), postoperative VO_2 has wide inter- and intra-patient variability in children (Li, Schulze-Neick et al. 2000; Li, Zhang et al. 2006; Li, Zhang et al. 2007; Li, Zhang et al. 2008). Thus, significant errors may be introduced in the calculation of hemodynamic and oxygen transport indices incorporating fixed values of VO_2. The introduction of such errors has greatly limited our understanding of postoperative hemodynamics and oxygen transport in these patients.

The adaptation of the respiratory mass spectrometer (AMIS2000, Innovision A/S, Demark) to continuously measure VO_2 allows the measurement of actual values for each element of systemic hemodynamics and oxygen transport. Use of actual values has significantly improved our understanding of the Norwood physiology and its postoperative management.

5.1 Profiles of hemodynamics and oxygen transport after the Norwood procedure

The Norwood physiology is an ideal model for understanding oxygen transport, since it is characterized by profound hemodynamic instability and oxygen transport imbalance (Li, Zhang et al. 2007). Wide, unstable, inter-individual and intra-individual variations in all the elements of hemodynamics and oxygen transport are observed, particularly on the systemic side (including systemic vascular resistant and blood flow). Pulmonary vascular resistance and blood flow are less variable, due to the mechanical limitation of the Blalock-Taussig shunt in the classic Norwood procedure or to the right ventricle to pulmonary artery shunt in the modified Norwood procedure.

5.2 VO_2 and its contribution to the balance of oxygen transport

Previous studies used assumptions for VO_2 of 160 or 180 mL/min/m² to calculate hemodynamics (Charpie, Dekeon et al. 2001; Hoffman, Ghanayem et al. 2000; Maher, Pizarro et al. 2003; Tweddell, Hoffman et al. 1999). Those values are much higher than the directly measured VO_2 in our patients, which ranged from 45 to 152 mL/min/m² (Figure 8).

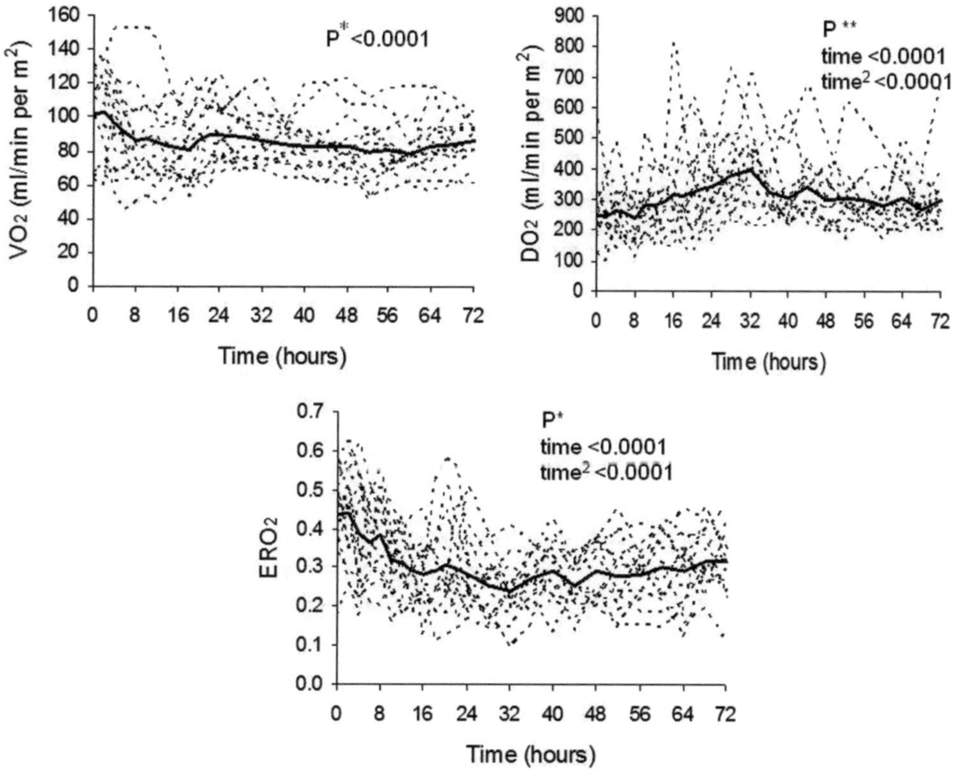

Fig. 8. The changes in oxygen consumption (VO_2), oxygen delivery (DO_2) and oxygen extraction ration (ERO_2) in neonates in the first 72 hours after the Norwood procedure. Dotted lines indicate individual patients; solid line indicates the mean.

An overestimation of VO_2 leads to a direct proportional change in the estimates for the calculated variables. For example, an assumed VO_2 of 170 mL/min/m^2, compared with the measured mean VO_2 on arrival in ICU of 101 mL/min/m^2, leads to a 68% overestimation of total CO, Qp, and Qs, and a 68% underestimation of PVR and SVR. Even more important, VO_2 is highly variable both between and within individual patients over time. Using a single assumed VO_2 makes no provision for the highly dynamic patient milieu that is inherent in the Norwood physiology.

VO_2 increases immediately after the Norwood procedure, mainly due to the systemic inflammatory response (Li, Hoschtitzky et al. 2004; Oudemans-van Straaten, Jansen et al. 1996), re-warming from hypothermic CPB and fever (Li, Hoschtitzky et al. 2004; Li, Schulze-Neick et al. 2000), and the use of inotropes (Li, Zhang et al. 2006). After arrival of the patient in the ICU, VO_2 decreases rapidly in the first 24 hours, followed by a slower decrease over the following 48 hours. In the first 24 hours, CO, Qs, and DO_2 are the variables most decreased. However, during the critical first 24-hour period, the balance of VO_2 and DO_2 improves significantly, as indicated by the rapid decrease in ERO_2 (Figure 8). The observed improvement in balance results primarily from a decrease in VO_2, rather than DO_2 as previously reported. After 24 hours, DO_2 became the primary contributor to the balance of oxygen transport.

5.3 Optimizing oxygen delivery

Historically, the postoperative management strategy for patients after the Norwood procedure was directed at diminishing Qp by increasing PVR, in order to increase Qs and DO_2. Analysis of our data reveals that SVR is far more important in determining Qs and DO_2 than is PVR. This indicates that both the systemic and pulmonary vascular compartments have variable resistance, but the systemic circulation has a more profound effect on DO_2, whereas the pulmonary compartment is relatively fixed with the mechanical limitation of the shunt. Interestingly, increases in SaO_2 and PaO_2 have only a weak positive correlation with Qp, implying that relative hypoxia to increase PVR and reduce Qp yields little benefit to DO_2. Our data also show that hemoglobin is an important contributor to DO_2, with a tight correlation between DO_2 and hemoglobin values. Therefore, treatment strategies should be designed to improve DO_2 and its balance with VO_2. Specifically, management strategies to maintain a high hemoglobin value, a low VO_2, and a relatively low and stable SVR appear to be rational.

5.4 Factors that affect the balance of oxygen transport

Direct measurements of VO_2 have allowed us to study the complex effects of some routine treatments on oxygen transport. Some routine treatments used in an effort to improve the balance of oxygen transport in fact have adverse effects.

5.4.1 Catecholamines

Catecholamines, such as dopamine, epinephrine, and norepiphrine, are commonly used in patients after CPB to augment cardiac contractility and DO_2 (Kawamura, Minamikawa et al. 1980; Merin, Bitran et al. 1977; Rosenblum and Frieden 1972). Catecholamines also stimulate VO_2 through their effects on myocardial work and metabolic rate (Cori and Buchwald 1930; Ensinger, Weichel et al. 1993; Maxwell, Crompton et al. 1985). If the increase in DO_2 is greater than the increase in VO_2, catecholamines will improve the overall balance of oxygen transport and tissue oxygenation. Some reports indicate favorable responses to catecholamine treatment in adults and older children after cardiac surgery (Kawamura, Minamikawa et al. 1980; Merin, Bitran et al. 1977; Rosenblum and Frieden 1972). In neonates, however, catecholamines have additional thermogenic actions through their effects on brown adipose tissue, resulting in an exaggerated increase in VO_2 (Maxwell, Crompton et al. 1985; Penny, Sano et al. 2001; Sell, Deshaies et al. 2004). Furthermore, neonatal hearts are known to have limited reserves to increase cardiac contractility. The reserves might become marginal in a Norwood circulation, with the injured single right ventricle providing parallel pulmonary and systemic circulations. In these patients, efforts to improve DO_2 by catecholamines are more likely to be associated with predominately adverse effects. As we have reported, terminating a moderate dose of dopamine (5 μg/kg/min) was not associated with any significant changes in CO or DO_2, but with a significant decrease in heart rate and rate-pressure product, an indirect indicator of myocardial oxygen consumption (Li, Zhang et al. 2006). VO_2 also decreased by 16±14 mL/min/m^2, representing a change of 20±11%. Terminating dopamine resulted overall in an improvement of the balance of oxygen transport, as indicated by the significant decrease in ERO_2 (Figure 10). Therefore, a moderate dose of dopamine induces predominantly an increase in VO_2, adversely affecting the VO_2–DO_2 relationship. Figure 11 shows examples of on-line VO_2 monitoring before and after dopamine termination.

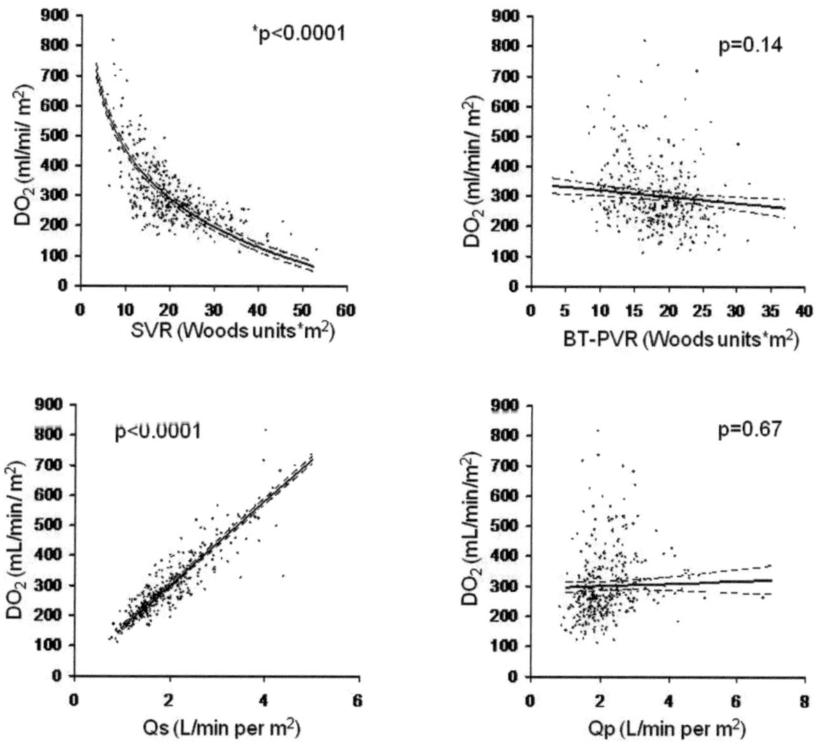

Fig. 9. Correlations between oxygen delivery (DO_2) and systemic vascular resistance (SVR), systemic blood flow (Qs), total pulmonary vascular resistance including the B-T shunt (BT-PVR), and pulmonary blood flow (Qp).

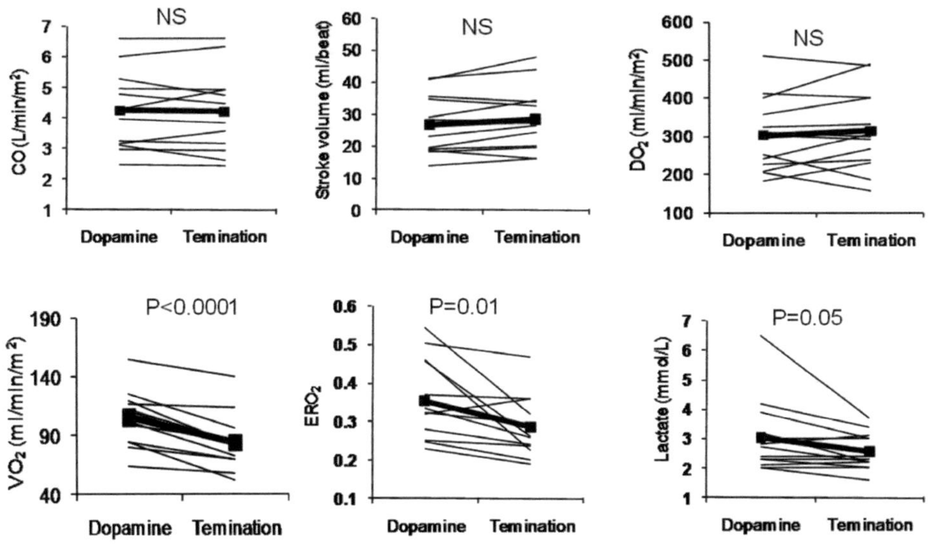

Fig. 10. The individual (thin line) and mean (bold line) changes in systemic hemodynamics and oxygen transport before and after termination of dopamine following the Norwood procedure.

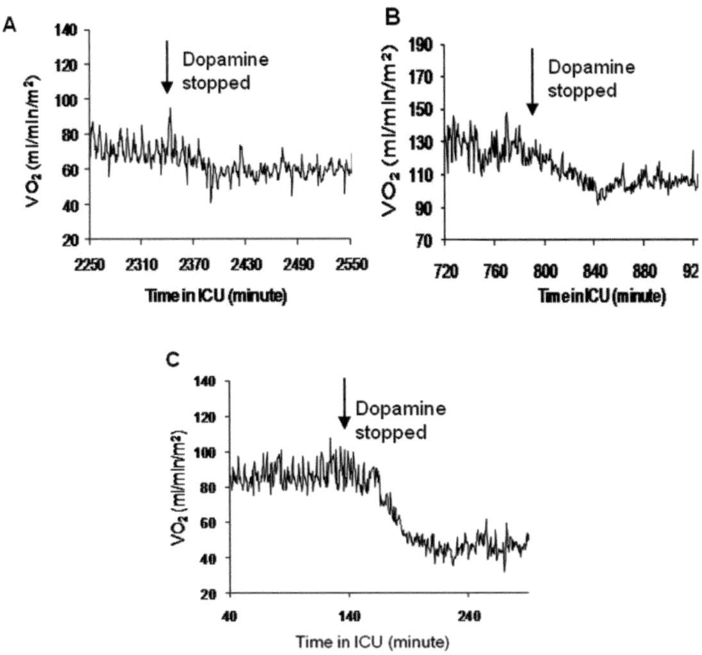

Fig. 11. Examples of the on-line measurement of oxygen consumption (VO_2) in three patients showing rapid and (A) small, (B) moderate, and (C) large decreases in VO_2 after terminating dopamine.

5.4.2 CO_2

CO_2 has been suggested as a factor increasing DO_2 in neonates both before and after the Norwood procedure (Bradley, Simsic et al. 2001; Mora, Pizarro et al. 1994). Consequently, it is a common practice to maintain a relatively high arterial CO_2 tension ($PaCO_2$), primarily by hypoventilation. The potent pulmonary vasoconstrictive effect of CO_2 was believed to decrease pulmonary blood flow (Qp), thereby increasing Qs (Mora, Pizarro et al. 1994). We studied the effect of stepwise increases in $PaCO_2$ from 40 to 50 to 60 mmHg, and found complex effects of CO_2 on systemic and regional oxygen transport (Li, Zhang et al. 2008). Moderate hypercapnia increases Qs as a result of its effect on SVR, rather than via PVR as previously proposed. The increase in systemic blood flow is primarily a consequence of increased cerebral blood flow that compromises splanchnic circulation. Moderate hypercapnia also decreases VO_2 and stimulates the release of catecholamines. The decrease in VO_2 improves the balance of oxygen transport, but the increase in catecholamines may be undesirable (Figures 12). Clinically, CO_2 should be used with caution when the aim is to improve oxygen delivery.

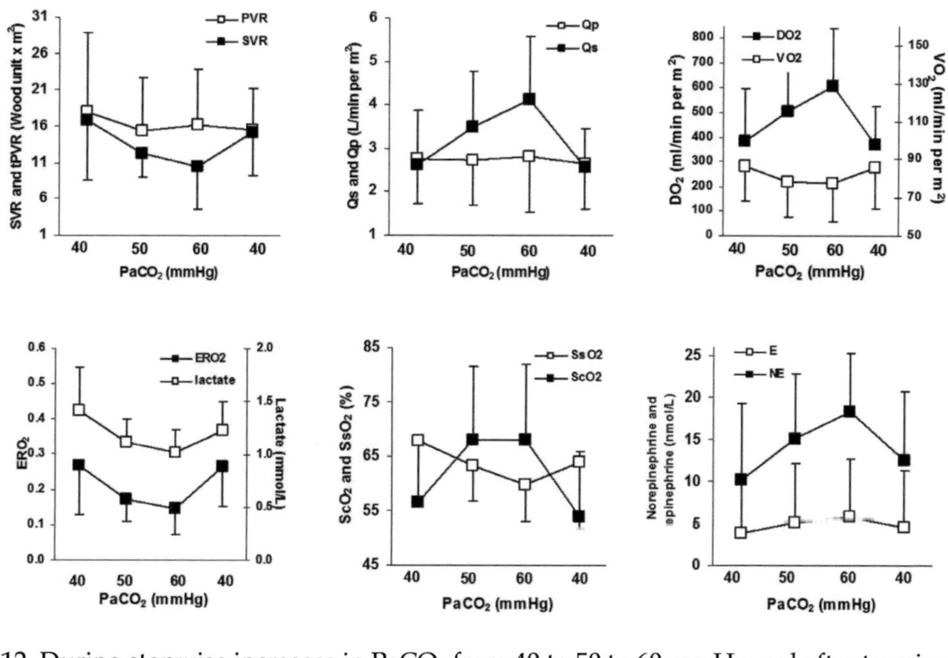

Fig. 12. During stepwise increases in $PaCO_2$ from 40 to 50 to 60 mmHg and after termination of CO_2, changes in systemic and total pulmonary vascular resistances (SVR and PVR), systemic and pulmonary blood flow (Qp and Qs), oxygen consumption and delivery (VO_2 and DO_2), oxygen extraction ration (ERO_2), and lactate, cerebral and splanchnic oxygen saturations (ScO_2 and SsO_2) and in epinephrine and norepinephrine.

5.4.3 Hyperglycemia

Hyperglycemia has been identified as a risk factor for adverse outcomes in critically ill patients, including those after CPB. Tight glucose control with insulin therapy has been shown to improve outcomes, but is not common practice for children following CPB. In our data, elevated glucose level showed negative correlations with CO and DO_2, and positive correlations with SVR and ERO_2 (Figure 13) (Zhang 2008). Therefore, hyperglycemia is

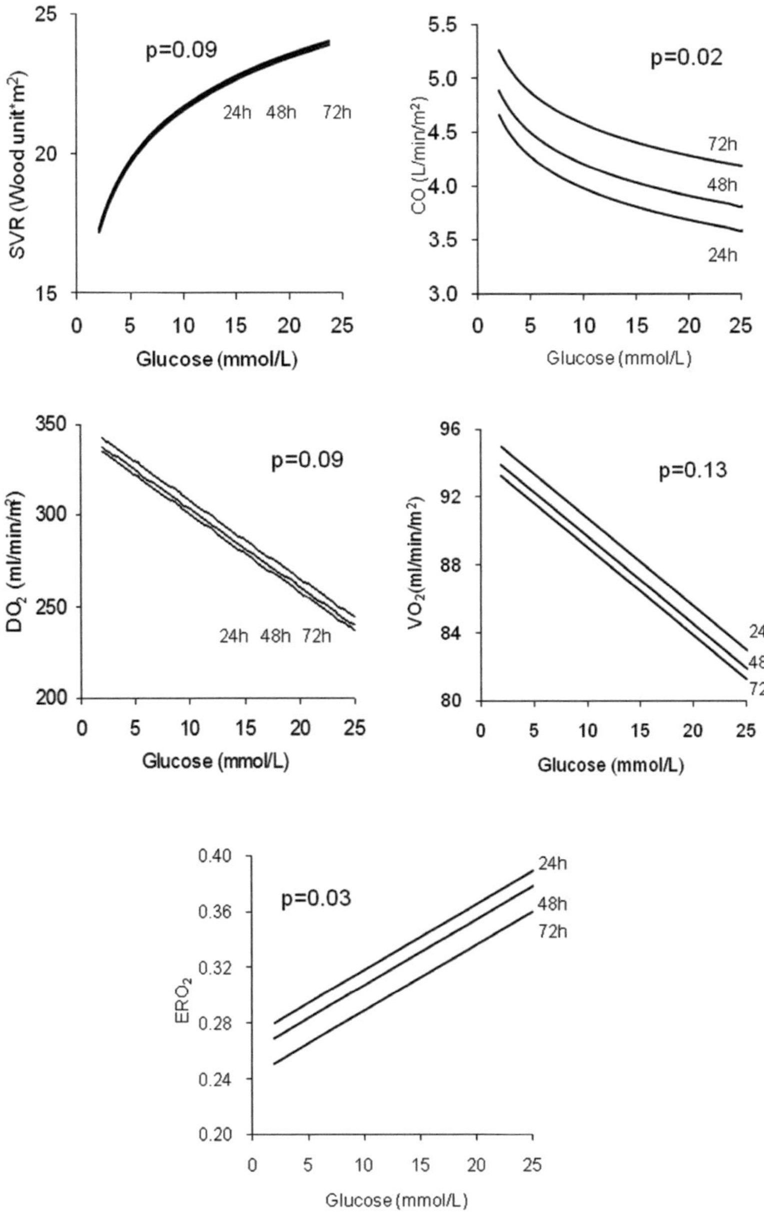

Fig. 13. Representative regression lines for the model predicting correlations between blood glucose and systemic vascular resistance (SVR), cardiac output (CO), systemic oxygen delivery (DO_2), oxygen consumption (VO_2), and oxygen extraction (ERO_2), at 24, 48, and 72 hours after the Norwood procedure for 17 neonates in the ICU.

negatively associated with systemic hemodynamics and oxygen transport status. Randomized clinical trials of glucose control with insulin therapy are warranted to identify the cause-and-effect relationship and to provide important information regarding appropriate glucose management strategies for children following CPB.

5.4.4 Other factors

To date, we have found a few factors in current routine postoperative management that have varied effects on oxygen transport. Further investigations are required to identify other factors in clinical management with favourable or adverse effects, and to design new treatment strategies to improve postoperative oxygen transport and clinical outcomes.

6. Conclusion

The predictive equations currently in use are unacceptable to measure VO_2 in ventilated children with congenital heart disease, particularly in those younger than 3 years of age, and in the early postoperative period after CPB. Direct, continuous, and precise measurement of VO_2 is fundamental for accurate assessments of hemodynamics and oxygen transport in children undergoing cardiac catheterization and in the ICU after cardiac surgery. Respiratory mass spectrometry is the 'state-of-the-art' method, allowing highly sensitive and precise measurement of VO_2. Measured VO_2 and the Fick principle allow the calculation of each parameter of systemic hemodynamic and oxygen transport, in varied circulations in congenital heart defects, both before and after complete surgical repair or palliation. These actual measurements are not only useful in clinical management, but important for bedside physiological studies on the balance of systemic oxygen transport in children after CPB. Some routine treatments in current use are intended to improve the balance of oxygen transport, but may actually worsen it. When considering clinical management of unbalanced oxygen transport, clinicians should choose therapies that address both decreased DO_2 and increased VO_2. ICU management strategies need to be refined to optimize the balance of systemic oxygen transport in children with congenital heart defects undergoing cardiac surgery. The resultant improved clinical outcomes in the early postoperative period and at long term follow-up will improve the quality of life for these vulnerable children.

7. References

Azakie, T., S. L. Merklinger, et al. (2001). "Evolving strategies and improving outcomes of the modified norwood procedure: a 10-year single-institution experience." Ann Thorac Surg 72(4): 1349-1353.

Barnea, O., E. H. Austin, et al. (1994). "Balancing the circulation: theoretic optimization of pulmonary/systemic flow ratio in hypoplastic left heart syndrome." J Am Coll Cardiol 24(5): 1376-1381.

Bradley, S. M., J. M. Simsic, et al. (2001). "Hemodynamic effects of inspired carbon dioxide after the Norwood procedure." Ann Thorac Surg 72(6): 2088-2093; discussion 2093-2084.

Charpie, J. R., M. K. Dekeon, et al. (2001). "Postoperative hemodynamics after Norwood palliation for hypoplastic left heart syndrome." Am J Cardiol 87(2): 198-202.

Chiara, O., P. P. Giomarelli, et al. (1987). "Hypermetabolic response after hypothermic cardiopulmonary bypass." Crit Care Med 15(11): 995-1000.

Cori, C. F. and K. W. Buchwald (1930). "Effect of continuous injection epinephrine on the carbohydrate metabolism, basal metabolism and vascular system of normal man." Am J Physiol(95).

Davies, N. J. and D. M. Denison (1979). "The measurement of metabolic gas exchange and minute volume by mass spectrometry alone." Respir Physiol 36(2): 261-267.

Davies, N. J. and D. M. Denison (1979). "The uses of long sampling probes in respiratory mass spectrometry." Respir Physiol 37(3): 335-346.

Ensinger, H., T. Weichel, et al. (1993). "Effects of norepinephrine, epinephrine, and dopamine infusions on oxygen consumption in volunteers." Crit Care Med 21(10): 1502-1508.

Fick, A. (1870). "U ¨ ber die Messung des Blutquantums in der Herzventrikeln." Sitzungsberichte der physikalisch-medicinischen Gesellschaftzu Wurtzberg: XVI–XVII.

Fomon, S. J., F. Haschke, et al. (1982). "Body composition of reference children from birth to age 10 years." Am J Clin Nutr 35(5 Suppl): 1169-1175.

Fowler, M. B., E. L. Alderman, et al. (1984). "Dobutamine and dopamine after cardiac surgery: greater augmentation of myocardial blood flow with dobutamine." Circulation 70(3 Pt 2): I103-111.

Gaynor, J. W., W. T. Mahle, et al. (2002). "Risk factors for mortality after the Norwood procedure." Eur J Cardiothorac Surg 22(1): 82-89.

Gentles, T. L., K. Gauvreau, et al. (1997). "Functional outcome after the Fontan operation: factors influencing late morbidity." J Thorac Cardiovasc Surg 114(3): 392-403; discussion 404-395.

Gentles, T. L., J. E. Mayer, Jr., et al. (1997). "Fontan operation in five hundred consecutive patients: factors influencing early and late outcome." J Thorac Cardiovasc Surg 114(3): 376-391.

Gilbert, E. M., M. T. Haupt, et al. (1986). "The effect of fluid loading, blood transfusion, and catecholamine infusion on oxygen delivery and consumption in patients with sepsis." Am Rev Respir Dis 134(5): 873-878.

Grollman, A. (1932). The Cardiac Output in Man in Health and Disease. Springfield, Illinois, Charles C Thomas.

Haupt, M. T., E. M. Gilbert, et al. (1985). "Fluid loading increases oxygen consumption in septic patients with lactic acidosis." Am Rev Respir Dis 131(6): 912-916.

Hayes, M. A., A. C. Timmins, et al. (1994). "Elevation of systemic oxygen delivery in the treatment of critically ill patients." N Engl J Med 330(24): 1717-1722.

Hoffman, G. M., N. S. Ghanayem, et al. (2000). "Venous saturation and the anaerobic threshold in neonates after the Norwood procedure for hypoplastic left heart syndrome." Ann Thorac Surg 70(5): 1515-1520; discussion 1521.

Hoskote, A., J. Li, et al. (2004). "The effects of carbon dioxide on oxygenation and systemic, cerebral, and pulmonary vascular hemodynamics after the bidirectional superior cavopulmonary anastomosis." J Am Coll Cardiol 44(7): 1501-1509.

Kawamura, M., O. Minamikawa, et al. (1980). "Combined use of phenoxybenzamine and dopamine for low cardiac output syndrome in children at withdrawal from cardiopulmonary bypass." Br Heart J 43(4): 388-392.

Kendrick, A. H., J. West, et al. (1988). "Direct Fick cardiac output: are assumed values of oxygen consumption acceptable?" Eur Heart J 9(3): 337-342.

Kitaichi, T., F. Chikugo, et al. (2003). "Suitable shunt size for regulation of pulmonary blood flow in a canine model of univentricular parallel circulations." J Thorac Cardiovasc Surg 125(1): 71-78.

LaFarge, C. G. and O. S. Miettinen (1970). "The estimation of oxygen consumption." Cardiovasc Res 4(1): 23-30.

Laitinen, P. O. and J. Rasanen (1998). "Measured versus predicted oxygen consumption in children with congenital heart disease." Heart 80(6): 601-605.

Li, J., A. Bush, et al. (2003). "Measured versus estimated oxygen consumption in ventilated patients with congenital heart disease: the validity of predictive equations." Crit Care Med 31(4): 1235-1240.

Li, J., A. Hoschtitzky, et al. (2004). "An analysis of oxygen consumption and oxygen delivery in euthermic infants after cardiopulmonary bypass with modified ultrafiltration." Ann Thorac Surg 78(4): 1389-1396.

Li, J., A. Hoskote, et al. (2005). "Effect of carbon dioxide on systemic oxygenation, oxygen consumption, and blood lactate levels after bidirectional superior cavopulmonary anastomosis." Crit Care Med 33(5): 984-989.

Li, J., I. Schulze-Neick, et al. (2000). "Oxygen consumption after cardiopulmonary bypass surgery in children: determinants and implications." J Thorac Cardiovasc Surg 119(3): 525-533.

Li, J., J. Stokoe, et al. (2004). "Continuous measurement of oxygen consumption during cardiopulmonary bypass: description of the method and in vivo observations." Ann Thorac Surg 77(5): 1671-1677.

Li, J., G. Zhang, et al. (2007). "Comparison of the profiles of postoperative systemic hemodynamics and oxygen transport in neonates after the hybrid or the Norwood procedure: a pilot study." Circulation 116(11 Suppl): I179-187.

Li, J., G. Zhang, et al. (2008). "Energy expenditure and caloric and protein intake in infants following the Norwood procedure." Pediatr Crit Care Med 9(1): 55-61.

Li, J., G. Zhang, et al. (2008). "Carbon dioxide--a complex gas in a complex circulation: its effects on systemic hemodynamics and oxygen transport, cerebral, and splanchnic circulation in neonates after the Norwood procedure." J Thorac Cardiovasc Surg 136(5): 1207-1214.

Li, J., G. Zhang, et al. (2008). "Significant correlation of comprehensive Aristotle score with total cardiac output during the early postoperative period after the Norwood procedure." J Thorac Cardiovasc Surg 136(1): 123-128.

Li, J., G. Zhang, et al. (2008). "The influence of systemic hemodynamics and oxygen transport on cerebral oxygen saturation in neonates after the Norwood procedure." J Thorac Cardiovasc Surg 135(1): 83-90, 90 e81-82.

Li, J., G. Zhang, et al. (2006). "Adverse effects of dopamine on systemic hemodynamic status and oxygen transport in neonates after the Norwood procedure." J Am Coll Cardiol 48(9): 1859-1864.

Li, J., G. Zhang, et al. (2006). "Inclusion of oxygen consumption improves the accuracy of arterial and venous oxygen saturation interpretation after the Norwood procedure." J Thorac Cardiovasc Surg 131(5): 1099-1107.

Li, J., G. Zhang, et al. (2007). "Profiles of hemodynamics and oxygen transport derived by using continuous measured oxygen consumption after the Norwood procedure." J Thorac Cardiovasc Surg 133(2): 441-448.

Lindahl, S. G. (1989). "Oxygen consumption and carbon dioxide elimination in infants and children during anaesthesia and surgery." Br J Anaesth 62(1): 70-76.

Lundell, B. P., M. L. Casas, et al. (1996). "Oxygen consumption in infants and children during heart catheterization." Pediatr Cardiol 17(4): 207-213.

Maher, K. O., C. Pizarro, et al. (2003). "Hemodynamic profile after the Norwood procedure with right ventricle to pulmonary artery conduit." Circulation 108(7): 782-784.

Mair, D. D., D. J. Hagler, et al. (1990). "Fontan operation in 176 patients with tricuspid atresia. Results and a proposed new index for patient selection." Circulation 82(5 Suppl): IV164-169.

Maxwell, G., S. Crompton, et al. (1985). "The effect of dopamine upon oxidative metabolism of brown fat adipocytes." Eur J Pharmacol 116(3): 293-297.

Merin, G., D. Bitran, et al. (1977). "The hemodynamic effects of dopamine following cardiopulmonary bypass." Ann Thorac Surg 23(4): 361-363.

Migliavacca, F., G. Pennati, et al. (2001). "Modeling of the Norwood circulation: effects of shunt size, vascular resistances, and heart rate." Am J Physiol Heart Circ Physiol 280(5): H2076-2086.

Mora, G. A., C. Pizarro, et al. (1994). "Experimental model of single ventricle. Influence of carbon dioxide on pulmonary vascular dynamics." Circulation 90(5 Pt 2): II43-46.

Moukarzel, A. A., J. S. Salas, et al. (2003). "Estimate of specific energy expenditure of fat-free mass and fat mass in children receiving total parenteral nutrition." J Med Liban 51(4): 206-210.

Nisbet, H. I., T. L. Dobbinson, et al. (1973). "Oxygen uptake in ventilated children during methoxyflurane anaesthesia." Can Anaesth Soc J 20(3): 334-346.

Ohye, R. G., L. A. Sleeper, et al. (2010). "Comparison of shunt types in the Norwood procedure for single-ventricle lesions." N Engl J Med 362(21): 1980-1992.

Oudemans-van Straaten, H. M., P. G. Jansen, et al. (1996). "Increased oxygen consumption after cardiac surgery is associated with the inflammatory response to endotoxemia." Intensive Care Med 22(4): 294-300.

Penny, D. J., T. Sano, et al. (2001). "Increased systemic oxygen consumption offsets improved oxygen delivery during dobutamine infusion in newborn lambs." Intensive Care Med 27(9): 1518-1525.

Powers, S. R., Jr., R. Mannal, et al. (1973). "Physiologic consequences of positive end-expiratory pressure (PEEP) ventilation." Ann Surg 178(3): 265-272.

Rosenblum, R. and J. Frieden (1972). "Intravenous dopamine in the treatment of myocardial dysfunction after open-heart surgery." Am Heart J 83(6): 743-748.

Rutledge, J., A. Bush, et al. (2010). "Validity of the LaFarge equation for estimation of oxygen consumption in ventilated children with congenital heart disease younger than 3 years--A revisit." American Heart Journal 160(1): 109-114.

Salim, M. A., C. L. Case, et al. (1995). "Pulmonary/systemic flow ratio in children after cavopulmonary anastomosis." J Am Coll Cardiol 25(3): 735-738.

Sano, S., S. C. Huang, et al. (2009). "Risk factors for mortality after the Norwood procedure using right ventricle to pulmonary artery shunt." Ann Thorac Surg 87(1): 178-185; discussion 185-176.

Schulze-Neick, I., J. Li, et al. (2001). "Pulmonary vascular resistance after cardiopulmonary bypass in infants: effect on postoperative recovery." J Thorac Cardiovasc Surg 121(6): 1033-1039.

Schulze-Neick, I., J. Li, et al. (2002). "The endothelin antagonist BQ123 reduces pulmonary vascular resistance after surgical intervention for congenital heart disease." J Thorac Cardiovasc Surg 124(3): 435-441.

Sell, H., Y. Deshaies, et al. (2004). "The brown adipocyte: update on its metabolic role." Int J Biochem Cell Biol 36(11): 2098-2104.

Shanahan, C. L., N. J. Wilson, et al. (2003). "The influence of measured versus assumed uptake of oxygen in assessing pulmonary vascular resistance in patients with a bidirectional Glenn anastomosis." Cardiol Young 13(2): 137-142.

Shekerdemian, L. S., A. Bush, et al. (1997). "Cardiopulmonary interactions in healthy children and children after simple cardiac surgery: the effects of positive and negative pressure ventilation." Heart 78(6): 587-593.

Shekerdemian, L. S., A. Bush, et al. (1997). "Cardiopulmonary interactions after Fontan operations: augmentation of cardiac output using negative pressure ventilation." Circulation 96(11): 3934-3942.

Tweddell, J. S., G. M. Hoffman, et al. (1999). "Phenoxybenzamine improves systemic oxygen delivery after the Norwood procedure." Ann Thorac Surg 67(1): 161-167; discussion 167-168.

Vandam, L. D. and J. A. Fox (1998). "Adolf Fick (1829-1901), physiologist: a heritage for anesthesiology and critical care medicine." Anesthesiology 88(2): 514-518.

Wernovsky, G., D. Wypij, et al. (1995). "Postoperative course and hemodynamic profile after the arterial switch operation in neonates and infants. A comparison of low-flow cardiopulmonary bypass and circulatory arrest." Circulation 92(8): 2226-2235.

Wessel, H. U., D. Rorem, et al. (1969). "Continuous determination of oxygen uptake in sedated infants and children during cardiac catheterization." Am J Cardiol 24(3): 376-385.

Westenskow, D. R., W. S. Jordan, et al. (1978). "Correlation of oxygen uptake and cardiovascular dynamics during N2O-fentanyl and N2O-thiopental anesthesia in the dog." Anesth Analg 57(1): 37-41.

Wolf, A., M. J. Pollman, et al. (1998). "Use of assumed versus measured oxygen consumption for the determination of cardiac output using the Fick principle." Cathet Cardiovasc Diagn 43(4): 372-380.

Zhang, G., H. Holtby, et al. (2008). "Aortic atresia is associated with an inferior postoperative systemic, cerebral and splanchnic oxygen transport status in neonates with hypoplastic left heart syndrome after the Norwood procedure. ." Circulation 118(Suppl).

Zhang, G. M., M; Holtby, H; Cai,S; Van Arsdell,G; Li,J (2008). "Blood Glucose Negatively Correlates with Systemic Hemodynamics and Oxygen Transport and Cerebral Oxygenation in Neonates after the Norwood Procedure." Circulation 118(Suppl.): 913.

14

Myocardial Lactate Metabolism in Children with Non-Cyanotic Congenital Heart Disease

Toshiyuki Itoi
Department of Pediatric Cardiology and Nephrology,
Graduate School of Medical Science,
Kyoto Prefectural University of Medicine
Japan

1. Introduction

It is well recognized that main energy source for myocardium is fatty acids (Wisneski et al.,1987, Lopaschuk et al.,2010). However, in failing heart or in hypertrophied heart, fatty acid oxidation ability was reported to be impaired and, on the contrary, carbohydrates were preferred to use for provision of energy demand (Stanle et al.,2005,Lopaschuk et al.,1992). The fetal heart is exposed to relatively high lactate concentrations. Immediately after birth, plasma lactate concentrations decrease. In the immature heart, *lactate dehydrogenase (LDH) is* predominated by the M type isozyme, as higher activity, resulting in greater lactate production from pyruvate (Brooks et al., 1985). This requires greater NADH levels than seen in the adult heart. The dominance of glycolytic flux in immature hearts leads to accumulation of lactate to a greater extent than is seen in adult hearts during profoundly hypoxic states (Brooks et al., 1985).

It has been shown that, in the isolated perfused rat heart, lactate significantly contributes to acetyl-CoA formation more than glucose. When fatty acid oxidation is activated, pyruvate dehydrogenase (PDH) activity is suppressed by increase of the NADH/NAD+ ratio followed by an enhancement of lactate production from accumulated pyruvate. As a result, lactate is released from myocardium even under aerobic status (Brooks et al., 1985). Immediately after birth, fatty acids are not the major energy substrate in newborn hearts, although the capacity of the heart for oxidization of fatty acids rapidly increases. Of interest, lactate is also important ATP provider in newborn heart (Lopaschuk et al. 1991).

Patho-physiology of congenital heart defects (CHD) is very wide ranging from the right ventricular (RV) volume overload and/or pressure overload to the left ventricular (LV) volume overload and/or pressure overload. CHD with left-to-right shunt is basically a non-cyanotic status. However, the myocardial cells may be in the milieu of relatively low oxygen because of relative decreased of coronary circulation from hypertrophy. Despite the evidence that lactate may be an important fuel for myocardial energy metabolism, there is remarkably little information on the lactate utilization in immature hearts especially in CHD. Lactate plays the other important role as a regulator of cellular redox state. *The redox state described in this chapter is defined as the balance of* $NADH/NAD^+$ *in the myocardium.* The cytosolic $NADH/NAD^+$ ratio in most tissues is enhanced by activation of glycolysis. If lactate dehydrogenase (LDH) activity is high such as in heart, the lactate/pyruvate (L/P)

ratio of a given cell is regarded to reflect the cytosolic $NADH/NAD^+$ ratio. The lactate and pyruvate are thought to provide for a redox coupling between organs through blood since plasma level of these metabolites equilibrate with cytosolic concentrations of cells. In view of "lactate shuttle theory" by Brooks (Brooks, 2002), lactate released into the coronary venous circulation and taken up by distal tissue that is to say myocardium via coronary artery circulation may affect redox state in the myocardial cells .
The energy substrates use in CHD had been focused on cyanotic disease (Scheuer et al.,1970, 1972, Rudolph et al.,1971, Fridli et al.,1977). As such, the studies of myocardial metabolism have long history but are very limited (Scheuer et al.,1970, 1972, Fridli et al.,1977, Åmark et al., 2007). In recent years, advancement of intensive care before and after surgical treatment, and carrying out of the long-term care of the circulation are getting to require precise *understanding* of myocardial metabolism in CHD.
In this article, we focused on myocardial use of energy substrates, especially lactate, in young patients with RV volume overload (*represented in the atrial septal defect, ASD*) or with both RV pressrure load and LV volume load (represented in the ventricular septal defect, VSD). The author will also consider the myocardial redox state of non-cyanotic CHD in young patients with reviewing of myocardial substrate use.

2. Patients and methods

Twenty one patients were enrolled into this study. Their ages range from ten-month to 11 years: patient details are summarized in Table 1. The patients were divided into three groups; Seven patients of Kawasaki disease without coronary lesions over 6 months after healing (KD group), seven patients of ASD as a representative of RV volume overload (ASD group), *(ASD group),* seven patients of VSD or patent ductus arteriosus (PDA) as a representative of RV pressure overload in addition to LV volume overload (PH group). *(PH group). All the patients in the PH group were received diuretics.*
All patients were not fed for at least four hours. Conbination of *ketamine-HCl and diazepan were used for general anesthesia with spontaneous respiration.* Heparin (100U/kg) was administered *after insertion of* arterial sheath. Intravenous infusion including 4.3% glucose and 20 mEq/l lactate maintained during the protocol. A coronary sinus catheter was inserted into the mid-to-anterior region of the coronary sinus via the inferior vena cava under fluoroscopy (Hamaoka et al., 1989). Blood sample collection was done at least 10 min after the end of all catheterization and angiography for the diagnosis because the influence of contrast medium to myocardial metabolism was reported to maintain 10-20 minutes by Wisneski et al (Wisneski et al., 1982). The verification of appropriate catheter position was determined by measuring oxygen saturation.
Oxygen saturation was measured by Oxygen Saturation Monitor system (Erma). Blood samples were obtained simultaneously from coronary sinus and femoral artery for the chemical analysis of concentrations of glucose, lactate and free fatty acids and oxygen concentration. Blood samples for glucose were mixed with titrate and, for lactate and pyruvate with 6% perchloric acid. This protocol was performed by the guideline of the Committee on Research of Kyoto Prefectural University of Medicine and informed consents were obtained from parents.

Calculations on energy substrate metabolism:

Pulmonary blood flow to systemic blood flow ratio (Qp/Qs) was calculated by means of Fick's method. Blood oxygen concentration was calculated as the product of Hb

concentration, oxygen saturation, and an oxygen-binding capacity of 1.34 ml/g. The oxygen extraction rate (OER) for each substrate was calculated using the following formula:
- OER = (AVDsubstrate/AVDoxygen) x substrate factor
- AVD; arteriovenous concentration difference

The substrate factor for glucose or lactate is 0.75 and 5.7 for free fatty acids (FFA). FFA concentration of whole blood was calculated by multiplying plasma concentration with (100-hematocrit)/100.

Redox potential (Eh) = -204+30.7x log([pyruvate]/[lactate]) (Gudbjarnason & Bing, 1962).

$\Delta Eh = Eh_{cv} - Eh_{ao}$ (Eh_{cv} and Eh_{ao} represent Eh of coronary venous blood and of aortic blood, respectivelty)

Statistical analysis

Values are expressed as mean ± standard deviation. All statistical tests were performed using JMP (ver.6, SAS Institute Japan, Co). We used Kruskal-Wallis one way analysis of variance on ranks to compare overall differences among three groups. We compared median value of all groups using two tailed Mann-Whitney U tests. Because three pairwise planed comparisons were made we considered $P<0.016$ as significant. In case of comparison of paired samples, Wilcoxon signed-rank test was applied and $P<0.05$ was considered as significant.

3. Results

3.1 Patients profiles (Table 1)

There was no significant difference among the groups on age. Heart rates (HR) and left ventricular systolic pressure (LVSP) were similar among groups, so the double products (LVSP x HR) of the left ventricle in PH group was same to those in ASD group. The ratio of the right ventricular systolic pressure (RVSP) to the LVSP was higher in PH group than in ASD group (0.35 ± 0.13 mmHg vs 0.79 ± 0.17 mmHg) . Qp/Qs of 1.7 ± 0.5 in PH group was also the same level in comparison with that of 1.8 ± 0.2 in ASD group.

3.2 Oxygen uptake

The arterial-coronary vein oxygen concentration differences were similar among three groups; 11.1 ± 0.7 Vol% for KD, 11.1 ± 2.3 Vol% for ASD group, and 10.9 ± 0.9 for PH group. However, this does not mean that the myocardial oxygen consumption of each group was similar, because we could not measure coronary flow in each group. Among three groups, however, the similar LV double products value may suggest the same levels of the LV oxygen consumption. On the other hand, the RV double products of the PH group were the highest level. These results suggested that the myocardial oxygen consumption in PH group may be the highest level among the groups.

3.3 Myocardial substrate uptake

The concentrations of glucose, lactate, and FFA in the artery were same levels among the groups (Table 2). Plasma FFA concentrations were thought to be higher levels in all groups than normal values due to heparinization, although blood FFA was not measured before heparin injection. Concerning substrate concentrations in the coronary vein, lactate levels of PH group was significantly higher than other groups. Pyruvate concentrations of PH group showed no significant difference in comparison with values of other groups. Continuous

infusion of low dose lactate and glucose did not influence the concentrations of both lactate and glucose since blood levels of those substrates were within the normal values.
We calculated myocardial OER of each substrate since, in this study, coronary sinus blood flow could not be measured. Figure 1 shows OER of each substrate in each group. Glucose OER in each patient was quite variable so that there was no significant difference on the mean value; 2.0±13.0% for KD group, 8.4±11.0% for ASD group, and 15.5±20.4% for PH group. Mean arterio-venous difference of lactate in PH group was negative resulting in -5.3±11.2% of calculated lactate OER. This value was significantly lower than both of KD group (7.8±9.2 %, p=0.013) and of ASD group (19.7±9.5, p=0.004). On the other hand, the lactate OER of ASD group showed higher trend than both KD group and PH group. There were no significant difference on FFA OER in each group; 62.8±28.2% for KD group, 63.6±9.8% for ASD group, and 62.8±28.0% for PH group. Sum of each glucose, lactate, and FFA OER was calculated as a total OER of heart.

3.4 Myocardial redox state or anaerobic metabolism (Table 3)

The lactate/pyruvate (L/P) ratios in coronary vein were similar among the groups. However, the L/P ratios of both ASD group and PH group were relatively higher values than those of KD group. Each values of redox potential (Eh) calculated from blood lactate and pyruvate showed no significant difference among groups. The ΔEh also showed no significant difference among the groups but the ΔEh of PH group was relatively lower value than other groups.

3.5 The effects of oxygen inhalation

As some patients in PH group were supposed myocardial relative ischemia or hypoxic state, we measured the major energy substrates under administration of oxygen for CHD patients. Figure 2 demonstrates the change of lactate OER both from ASD group and PH group. Lactate OER of ASD group did not change with oxygen inhalation. On the other hand, its PH group increased from -6.3±10.9% to 3.0±9.9%. However, of interest, both the CS L/P ratio and ΔEh of each group showed no remarkable changes even after inhale of oxygen (Table 3).

4. Discussion

4.1 Characteristics of methodology on myocardial energy metabolism study

In humans, the coronary sinus, which empties into the right atrium, receives blood from 96% of veins from the left ventricular free wall and septum (Sethna et al., 1986). The coronary sinus system drains approximately three fourths of the blood entering the left coronary artery and only 10 to 20 % of the inflow of the right coronary artery. The rate of tissue metabolism (uptake or release) can only be measured by multiplying the artery-coronary vein difference by the blood flow if the flow, the arterial concentration, and the rate of tissue metabolism are all constant. We did not measure coronary sinus blood flow in this study because of technical difficulties for infants. Then, we calculated oxygen extraction ratio for standardizing and comparing the substrate use in the heart.
This kind of studies to adult patients carried without heparinization but with frequent wash of catheter for prevention of thrombus formation, since it is well known that heparin induces the production of free fatty acids from lipoprotein by activation of lipoprotein lipase. We used, in this study, heparin for anti-coagulation and obtained blood samples

under heprinized state because of two reasons; 1) for preservation of veins and arteries from obstruction in younger children and 2) for our aim of studying myocardial metabolism in patients under critical states as in pediatric intensive care unit or in surgical intervention where many patients were heparinized.
In spite of these limitation, this method we applied here is still useful for clinical study on myocardial metabolism (Vánky et al. 2006) because data obtained are supposed not far from animal model study (Lopaschuk et al., 1992), computer simulation study and isotopical study in human.

4.2 Myocardial use of lactate and other substrates in non-cyanotic CHD

It is very important to know the myocardial energy substrate use *during the management of heart failure* or cardiac surgery of children with CHD. However, myocardial metabolism even in the normal immature heart has not been fully elucidated. Although data we can refer on myocardial energy substrate use in normal children are limited, myocardial fatty acids uptake of KD group *resembles the results that Rudolph demonstrated* (Rudorph et al., 1971). For this reason, we considered that results from KD group represented normal myocardial substrate use in children. Table 4 shows the comparison among some previous reports on the substrates use in hearts in young including cyanotic CHD. Myocardial FFA uptake in children shows very similar levels among the reports. The very variable glucose uptake shown in other reports including adults suggested that glucose may not play an important role for myocardial energy supply for children at rest. (Vánky et al. 2006,Lopaschuk et al., 1992).
It has been demonstrated that adult hypertrophied hearts prefer to oxidize glucose. Increase of glucose oxidation may be beneficial for hypertrophied heart on production of ATP with less myocardial oxygen consumption than fatty acid oxidation. Allard *et al* reported that the steady-state palmitate oxidation rates were decreased in the hypertrophied hearts compared with control hearts (Allard et al., 1994). Although the uptake of glucose of CHD hearts, in our study, was quite variable, both hearts with the volume overloaded RV (ASD group) and with the pressure overloaded RV (PH group) showed tendency of increase of glucose uptake. (Figure 1, Table 4). These suggest that a myocardial potential of glucose use in children with CHD may not be an inferior level in comparison with adult hearts against overload. However, *one should note in our results that* FFA use was high levels even in PH group and that lactate was dominant energy supplier more than glucose in ASD group.
Gertz *et al* have reported that in subjects with high blood free fatty acids, myocardial lactate extraction may be low (Gertz et al., 1980). However, this is not the case at least in children with CHD (Table 4). The lactate use including of cyanotic CHD is relatively high even under the high levels of fatty acid use. From another point of view, it is speculated that fatty acid use in children with CHD *have reached to* near maximum levels and, as a result, lactate regulated the energy supply against additional loads on the heart. Some studies have clarified that fatty acids oxidation increased with elevation of ventricular workload in immature hearts (Itoi et al., 1993a,Ascuitto et al., 1999). The lactate oxidation rates of the immature hearts were also increased by the addition of preload to the RV without significant change of glucose oxidation (Itoi et al., 1993b). The ASD group in our study showed the very same result of this experimental model on change of the lactate oxidation (Figure 1). Recently, Vánky *et al* revealed that no significant uptake of glucose was detected before or after surgery for aortic stenosis but the uptake of lactate was significant before surgery (Vánky et al. 2006).

The blood lactate levels in the resting state are low, in the range of 0.5-1 mM, in human adults. Results of our study showed that, even in children with CHD, arterial lactate levels were the same as in adults (Table 2). Then, the lactate use changes in hearts of children with non-cyanotic CHD might not be influenced by blood lactate levels. Lactate oxidation occurs because the lactate dehydrogenase (LDH) isozyme found in heart has a low affinity for pyruvate, although the equilibrium constant for the LDH is in the direction of lactate formation. In addition, the hydrogen ion, pyruvate, and NADH formed by the LDH reaction are rapidly removed in the aerobic heart, forcing the reaction in the direction of the formation of pyruvate (Drake-Holland, 1983). Furthermore, in the setting of a fully activated FFA oxidation, glycolysis flux and the pyruvate dehydrogenase complex (PDC) activity are supressed with increased NADH from β-oxidation. This phenomenon may result in not only deceleration of glucose oxidation but also acceleration of lactate oxidation (Figure 3). This scenario may happen in mildly overloaded hearts as in ASD group.

The very characteristic finding in our study was the efflux of lactate under the stable fatty acids use in PH group (Figure 1). In RVH, there is a mitochondrial metabolic switch from glucose oxidation to glycolysis due to myocardial ischemia (Pio et al., 2010, Gomez et al., 2001). Positron emission tomography studies in patients with RVH suggested that there is increased RV glucose uptake, which is thought to reflect enhanced glycolysis. The less efficient production of ATP by glycolysis in RVH meant the formation of lactate, rather than pyruvate (Oikawa et al., 2005). In the immature heart, lactate dehydrogenase (LDH), which is predominated by the M type isozyme, as higher activity, resulting in greater lactate production from pyruvate (Brooks et al., 2002). This requires greater NADH levels than seen in the adult heart. The dominance of glycolytic flux in immature hearts leads to accumulation of lactate to a greater extent than is seen in adult hearts during profoundly hypoxic states (Brooks et al., 2002). Now, does the spillover of lactate from hearts of PH group indicate the existence of profound myocardial ischemia of the right ventricle?

4.3 Redox-potential of the lactate-pyruvate system in CHD

The redox-potential of the coronary sinus blood approaches that of cardiac tissues, and the redox-potential of the coronary venous blood becomes more negative than that of arterial blood. When ΔEh is positive there is active cellular oxidation and the energy required is supplied by oxidative phosphorylation. When ΔEh is negative there is glycolysis and anaerobic phosphorylation becomes an important energy source (Gudbjarnason & Bing, 1962). The RV overloaded heart, especially PH group, showed a tendency of decrease of ΔEh (Table 3). Since some hearts of CHD were supposed to be under hypoxic state, we administered oxygen to patients. The results that oxygen inhalation increased influx of lactate (Figure 2) without changes of both the L/P ratio and ΔEh (Table 3) suggested that myocardial hypoxic state may not be only one cause of the lactate efflux from hearts of the PH group.

Kobayashi *et al* demonstrated that, in isolated perfused heart, both the intracellular and the perfusate L/P ratio increases at higher cardiac workloads (Kobayashi & Neely, 1979). The L/P ratio of a given cell is thought to reflect the cytosolic NADH/NAD ratio (Rassmussen et al., 2009). Since the coronary venous L/P ratio at rest has been reported around 10 (Friedli 1977), our results suggested that the cytosolic NADH/NAD ratio may be higher in the CHD groups, although statistically not significant, than in KD group at rest (Table 3).

Our results suggested that, under the high potential of fatty acids oxidation, 1) the low level of acceleration of oxidative metabolism as in ASD group resulted in increasing of lactate oxidation for filling NADH because of limitation of glycolysis activity by fatty acids oxidation, 2) the higher level of cardiac work as in PH group results in the faster rates of glycolysis by cellular hypoxia and/or adrenaline (Brooks et al., 2002, Massie et al., 1995), which were also accompanied by increased conversion of pyruvate to lactate by over-production of NADH (Figure 3).

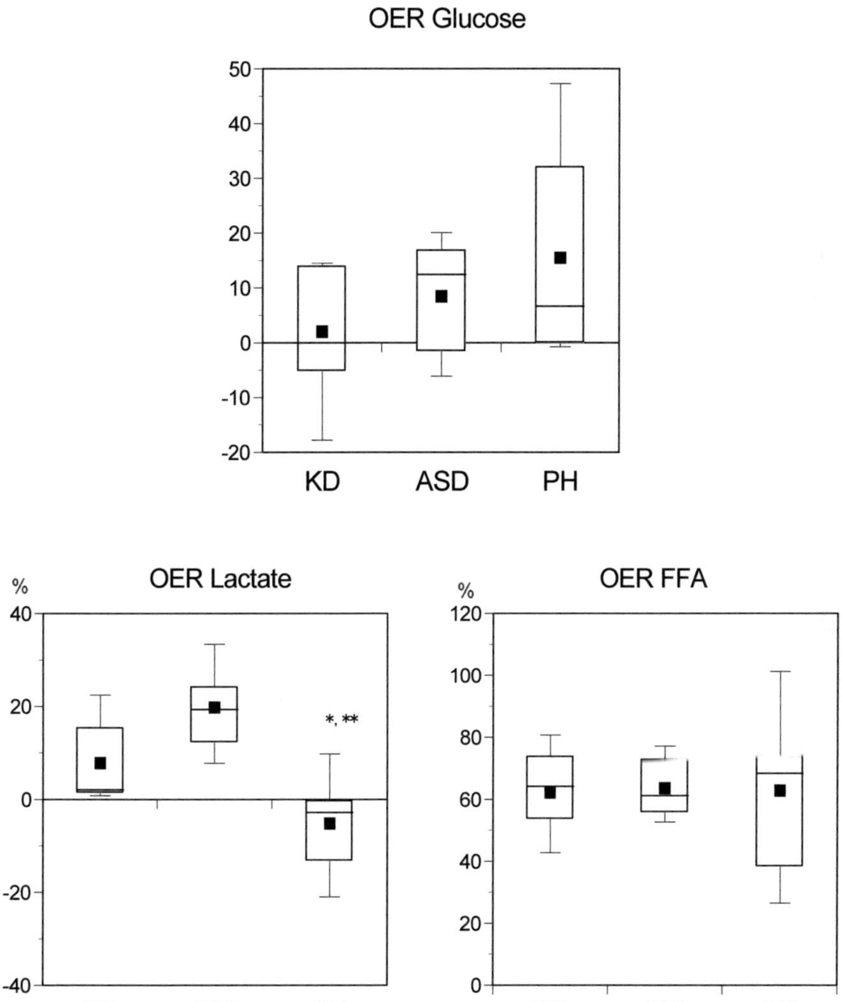

KD, Kawasaki disease; ASD, atrial septal defect; PH, pulmonary hypertension;
*, significantly different from KD; **, significantly different from ASD.

Fig. 1. Myocardial oxygen extraction rate (OER) of glucose, lactate, and fatty acids

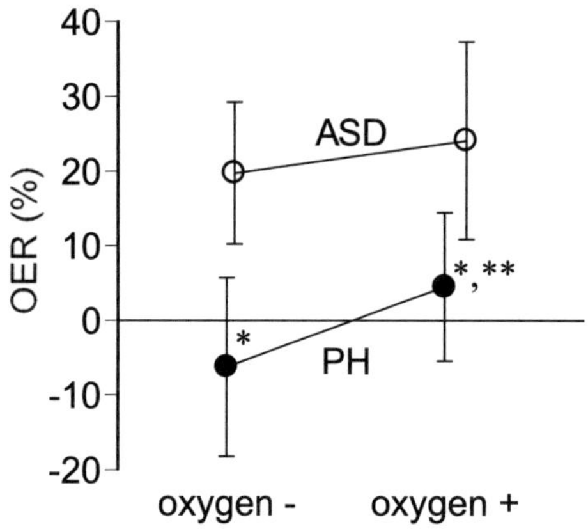

ASD, atrial septal defect; PH, pulmonary hypertension.
*, significantly different from ASD; **, significantly different from oxygen -

Fig. 2. Effects of oxygen administration of myocardial lactate use

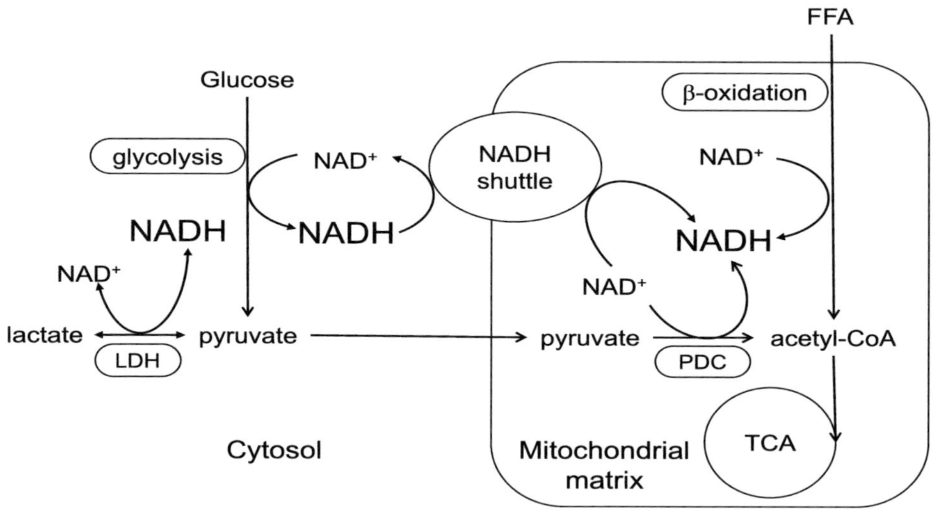

LDH, lactate dehydrogenase; PDC, pyruvate dehydrogenase complex.
NADH produced by glycolysis or conversion of lactate to pyruvate is carried into the mitochondrial matrix via NADH shuttle. In mitochondrial matrix, NADH is produced from conversion of pyruvate to acetyl-CoA catalyzed by PDC.

Fig. 3. Relationship between myocardial energy substrate use and pathways for oxidation of NADH

	KD	ASD	PH	ANOVA *P*
Age (year)	3.5±2.3	6.9±3.0	2.1±0.8†	0.005
HR (bpm)	123±24	118±1	129±27	NS
RVPsys (mmHg)	24±4	40±12*	80±22**, †	<0.001
LVPsys (mmHg)	112±15	116±9	100±10	NS
RVP/LVP	0.22±0.05	0.35±0.13	0.79±0.17**,†	<0.001
LV DP (x1000)	13.63±2.06	13.61±1.7	12.95±2.82	NS
RV DP (x1000)	2.94±0.65	4.80±1.94	10.32±3.28**,†	0.001
Qp/Qs	1	1.8±0.2	1.7±0.5	-
Hb(g/dl)	12.5±0.7	13.3±0.7	12.9±0.9	NS

HR, heart rate; RVPsys, systolic right ventricular pressure; LVPsys, systolic left ventricular pressure; DP, double products (=ventricular systolic pressure x heart rate); Qp/Qs, pulmonary-sysytolic flow ratio; Hb, hemoglobin
*, significantly different between KD vs ASD; **, significantly different between KD vs VSD; †, significantly different between ASD vs VSD

Table 1. Patients profiles

	KD	ASD	PH	ANOVA *p*
Aorta				
O2 sat (%)	97.7±0.5	97.1±0.8	95.1±3.3	NS
Glucose (mmol/L)	4.95±1.07	5.48±0.33	5.17±0.88	NS
lactate (mmol/L)	0.72±0.19	0.83±0.44	0.86±0.36	NS
pyruvate (mmol/L)	0.045±0.023	0.048±0.015	0.092±0.093	NS
FFA (mmol/L)	1.28±0.33	1.41±0.44	1.34±0.3	NS
Coronary sinus				
O2 sat (%)	31.5±4.3	35.2±12.5	32.2±5.6	NS
Glucose (mmol/L)	4.93±1.07	5.46±0.28	5.18±0.95	NS
lactate (mmol/L)	0.53±0.16	0.53±0.3	0.95±0.47**,†	0.033
pyruvate (mmol/L)	0.052±0.027	0.037±0.01	0.1±0.081	NS
FFA (mmol/L)	1.08±0.34	1.2±0.46	1.15±0.3	NS

**, significantly different from ASD group; †, significantly different from ASD group

Table 2. Myocardial substrate uptake

	O2	KD	ASD	PH	ANOVA *p*
CV L/P	-	11.8±3.3	15.1±8.7	15.6±13.0	NS
	+	11.6±4.3	15.8±6.0	14.0±8.8	NS
Redox potential					
Eh_{cv} (mV)	-	-236.2±4.7	-238.3±7.7	-237.7±8.8	NS
	+	-235.6±6.7	-239.9±5.4	-237.2±7.5	NS
Eh_{ao} (mV)	-	-241.9±7.2	-241.6±5.4	-238.9±9.7	NS
	+	-240.5±6.8	-245.6±4.8	-239.6±6.4	NS
ΔEh (mV)	-	5.7±4.7	3.3±5.9	1.2±4.7	NS
	+	5.0±3.7	5.7±2.7	2.3±4.9	NS

CV, coronary vein; Eh, redox potential, ΔEh, difference of redox potential between artery and coronary vein

Table 3. Anaerobic Metabolism

5. Conclusion

Myocardial energy metabolism in non-cyanotic CHD was basically sustained by fatty acids oxidation whether or not with increasing workloads. The glucose use was accelerated with overload with cellular hypoxia although very variable. Lactate seemed to play an important role to maintain lactate-pyruvate redox potential. When myocardial workloads were mild as in ASD group, the NADH demand was complemented by lactate oxidation. On the other hand, when workloads were as strong as producing a myocardial hypoxic state as in PH group, lactate production was accelerated to maintain the cellular redox state.

6. Acknowledgements

The author would like to thank all colleagues who collaborated in catheter examination.

7. References

Allard MF, Schönekess BO, Henning SL, English DR, & Lopaschuk GD. (1994). Contribution of oxidative metabolism and glycolysis to ATP production in hypertrophied hearts. *Am J Physiol.*, 267 (Heart Circ. Physiol. 36), H742-H750. ISSN: 0363-6135

Åmark K, Ekroth R, Nilsson K, Sunnegårdh J, & Söderberg B. (2007). Myocardial substrates in children with congenital heart disease: relationship to substrate supply, age, growth and desaturation.*Act Pediatr*, 96, 1677-1680 ISSN: 0803-5253

Ascuitto RJ, Joyce JJ, & Ross-Ascuitto NT. (1999). Mechanical function and substrate oxidation in the neonatal pig heart subjected to pacing-induced tachycardia. *Mol Genet Metab*, 66, 212-223. ISNN: 1096-7192

Brooks W, Ekblom B, & Bing OHL.(1985) . Comparative response to a 2-week and 6-month old rat myocardium to hypoxia.*J Dev Physio*, 7, 229-40. ISSN: 0141-9846

Brooks GA. (2002). Lactate shuttle in nature. *Biochem Soc Trans.*,30(2), 258-264. ISSN: 0300-5127

Drake-Holland AJ. (1993). Substrate utilization. Cardiac Metabolism Ed. Drake-Holland AJ and Noble MIM, pp.195-213..John Willey & Sons LTd, ISBN 0-471-10249-0, Northern Ireland.

Fridli B, Haenni B, Moret P, & Opie LH. (1977). Myocardial metabolism in syanotic congenital heart disease studied by arteriovenous differences of lactate, phosphate, and potassium at rest and during atrial pacing. *Circulation*, 55, 647-652. ISSN: 0009-7322

Gertz EW, Wisneski JA, Neese R, Houser A, Korte R, & Bristow JD. (1980). Myocardial lactate extraction: multi-determined metabolic function. *Circulation*, 61, 256-261. ISSN: 0009-7322

Gomez A, Bialostozky D, Zajarias A, Santos E, Palomar A, Martinez ML, & Sandoval J. (2001). Right ventricular ischemia in patients with primary pulmonary hypertension. J Am Coll Cardiol; 38:1137–1142. ISSN: 0735-1097

Gudbjarnason S & Bing RJ. (1962). The redox potential of the lactate-pyruvate system in blood as an indicator of the functional state of cellular oxidation. *Biochim Biophys Acta*, 60, 158-162. ISSN: 0005-2736

Hamaoka K, Itoi T, Nakagawa M, Kamiya Y, & Sawada T. (1989). Coronary sinus cannulation via the femoral vein. *Pediatr Cardiol.*, 10, 91-92. ISSN: 0172-0643

Itoi T, Huang L, & Lopaschuk GD. (1993a). Glucose use in neonatal rabbit hearts reperfused after global ischemia. *Am J Physiol.*, 265 (Heart Circ. Physiol. 34), H427-H433. ISSN: 0363-6135

Itoi T, & Lopaschuk GD. (1993b). The contribution of glycolysis, glucose oxidation, lactate oxidation to ATP production in isolated bibentricular working hearts from 2-week-old rabbits. *Pediatr Res.*, 34, 735-741.ISSN: 0031-3998.

Kobayashi K & Neely JR. (1979). Control of maximum rates of glycolysis in rat cardiac muscle. *Circ Res.*, 44, 166-175. ISSN: 0009-7300

Lopaschuk GD, Spafford MA, & Marsh DR. (1991). Glycolysis is predominant source of myocardial ATP production immediately after birth. *Am J Physiol.*,261 (Heart Circ. Physiol. 30) ,H1698-H1705. ISSN: 0363-6135

Lopaschuk GD, Collins-Nakai RL, & Itoi T. (1992). Developmental changes in energy substrate use by the heart. *Cardiovasc Res.*, 26, 1172–1180. ISSN: 1755-3245

Lopaschuk GD, Ussher JR, Folmes DL, Jaswal JS, & Stanley WC.(2010). Myocardial fatty acid metabolism in health and disease. *Physiol Rev.*, 90, 207-258. ISSN: 0031-9333

Massie BM, Schaefer S, Garcia J, McKirnan MD, Schwartz GG, Wisneski JA, Weiner MW, & White FC. (1995).

Myocardial high-energy phosphate and substrate metabolism in swine with moderate left ventricular hypertrophy. *Circulation.*, 91, 1814-1823. ISSN 0009-7322

Oikawa M, Kagaya Y, Otani H, Sakuma M, Demachi J, Suzuki J, Takahashi T, Nawata J, Ido T, Watanabe J, & Shirato K. (2005). Increased [18F]fluorodeoxyglucose accumulation in right ventricular free wall in patients with pulmonary hypertension and the effect of epoprostenol. *J Am Coll Cardio.*, 45, 1849–1855. ISSN: 0375-1097

Piao L, Marsboom G, & Archer SL. (2010). Mitochondrial metabolic adaptation in right ventricular hypertrophy and failure. *J Mol Med.*, 88, 1011–1020. ISSN: 0946-2716

Rassmussen P, Madsen CA, Nielsen HB, Zaar M, Gjedde A, Secher NH, & Quistorff B. (2009), Coupling between the blood lactate-to-pyruvate ratio and MCA *Vmean* at the onset of exercise in humans. *J Appl Physiol* 107, 1799–1805. ISSN: 0021-8987

Rudolph W. (1971/72). Myocardial metabolism in cyanotic congenital heart disease. *Cardiol,* 56, 209-215. ISSN: 0008-6312

Scheuer J, Shaver JA, Kroetz FW, & Leonard JJ. (1970). Myocardial metabolism in cyanotic congenital heart disease. *Cardiol*, 55, 193-210. ISSN: 0008-6312

Scheuer J, Corpus M, Lamarre R, Yuan S-H, Kypson J, & Cheng G. (1972). Alteration of glucose and insulin metabolism in congenital heart disease. *Circulation*, 46, 333-346. ISSN 0009-7322

Sethna DH & Moffitt EA. (1986). An appreciation of the coronary circulation. *Anesth Analg.* 65, 294-305

Stanley WC, Recchia FA, & Lopaschuk GD. (2005). Myocardial Substrate Metabolism in the Normal and Failing Heart. *Physiol Rev*, 85, 1093–1129. ISSN: 0031-933

Vánky FB, Håkanson E, Szabó Z, Jorfeldt L, & Svedjeholm R. (2006). Myocardial metabolism before and after valve replacement for aortic stenosis. *J Cardiovasc Surg.*, 47, 305-313. ISSN: 0021-9509

Wisneski JA, Gertz EW, Neese RA, Soo W-J, Bristow JD, Adams JR, & Beaurdry J-P. (1982). Myocardial metabolic alteration after contrast angiograpy. *Am J Cardiol.*, 50, 239-245. ISSN 0002-9149

Wisneski JA, Gertz EW, Neese RA, & Mayr M. (1987) Myocardial metabolism of free fatty acids. *J Clin Invest.*, 79, 359-366. ISSN: 0021-9738

15

Chemical Elements and Structural/Molecular Properties of Myocardium in Infants with Transposition of Great Arteries

Okuneva G.N.[1], Karaskov A.M.[1], Trunova V.A.[2], Zvereva V.V.[2]
Kliever Ye.E.[1], Volkov A.M.[1] and Vlasov Yu.A.[1]
[1]*E.N. Meshalkin Research Institute of Circulation Pathology,*
[2]*A.V. Nikolayev Institute of Inorganic Chemistry*
Russian Federation

1. Introduction

The imbalance of chemical elements (CE) during the prenatal development of a foetus might cause foetal heart abnormalities and even miscarriages (Skalny, 1999; Kudriyn, 2000), while the deficit of many vital CE during the gestation period could lead to congenital heart diseases. The deficiency of Cu in the course of this period might provoke the development of aortic aneurysms and impairment of vessel elasticity (Panchenko, 2004), while the lack of Zn could bring about transposition of the great arteries (TGA) (Shankar & Prasad, 1998; Beerli et al., 2000). The content of Fe, Cu, Zn, Se and Mn in optimal quantities is indispensable for adequate support of the cellular cycle, growth and differentiation of cells, including cardiomyocytes (Ruff, 1999). TGA comprises a special group of congenital heart diseases (CHD) with concordant atrioventricular and discordant ventricular-arterial junctions (Fozzard et al., 1986; Hoffman, 2006). This complicated disease occurs in newborns with CHD in an excess of 10 % of cases, with significant mortality and morbidity (Bokeria & Gorbachevsky, 1996). This is because it is yet unclear why this disease occurs, how this pathology progresses during the growth and development of newborns and, most importantly, which metabolic processes get impaired in cardiomyocytes that lead to the death of myocardium. Nowadays, a high level of immunofluorescent methods allows for identifying the cardiomyocytes that are involved in DNA replication (Re, 1987; Bolli, 2002). The main difficulty encountered in treating this disease is to correctly evaluate the ventricular function providing an adequate cardiac output (Castaneda, 1993, 1998). Age is also an important factor in determining the speed and functional reaction of the myocardium to pressure overload (Isoyama et al., 1987; Re, 1987; Scholzen & Gerders, 2000). Further research is needed to answer the following questions: 1. How is CE distribution disrupted in different parts of the heart and how is this disruption related to pathomorphological abnormalities? 2. How are morphology and the molecular structure of cardiomyocytes changed in the course of growth and development of infants with TGA, from newborns to 1-year-old babies? 3. What pathomorphological distinctions are typical for 2 anatomical types of TGA: with intact ventricular septum (IVS) and with ventricular septum defect (VSD)?

The purpose of this research is to study the content of chemical elements and the morphological structure of the myocardium in infants with different TGA types. Three tasks were set to achieve this goal: 1. To investigate some features of the content of CE and the structure of cardiomyocytes in 3 age groups: newborns aged 1 to 6 months and babies aged 6 to 12 months. 2. To study the concentration of CE in different parts of the heart in infants with TGA and in patients whose death was not caused by cardiac problems (control group). 3. To compare the features of CE and pathomorphological structure of 2 anatomic types of TGA: with atrial septal defect (ASD) and intact ventricular septum (IVS) and with atrial septal defects (ASD) and (VSD).

2. Methods

A pathomorphological study was carried out using autopsy material of 68 infants aged under 1 who died during the follow-up period, as well as 10 infants of the same age whose death was not caused by cardiac problems. All TGA patients were broken down in 2 groups according to patients' anatomical type: the first group included patients with a simple form of TGA - TGA with atrial septum defect (ASD) and intact ventricular septum (IVS) - 37 patients (19 aged under 1 month and 18 aged 1 to 6 months), while 31 patients having TGA with ASD and VSD (7 aged under 1 month, 13 aged 1 to 6 months and 11 patients aged 6 to12 months) were assigned to the second group.

Biopsy samples were preserved in 4 % phosphate-buffered formalin and then washed off in a distilled water solution followed by processing in cryoprotectans (solutions of saccharose: 5 % for 2 hours, 10 % for 2 hours, 15 % for 12 hours). Fluorometry of histologic specimens was carried out by using an Axioskop 40FL microscope and an AxioCamHRc camera. To get a good computerized image of each histologic specimen, a Zeiss Plan-Neofluar x 40 lens was used for 20 s at a +24 °C room temperature. The images obtained were processed by AxioVision 3.1 software (Carl Zeiss).

Fluorescent probes containing ethidium bromide and chlortetracycline were used to perform fluorometry of the myocardium. Staining myocardium slices with ethidium bromide was done in a phosphate buffer pH=7.4 that contained 5.0 * 10 3 g/l of ethidium bromide for 5 minutes at a temperature of 25 °C, while chlortetracycline, also done in a phosphate buffer pH=7.4 containing 2.6 * 10 2 g/l of chlortetracycline, was applied for 1 minute at a temperature of 25 °C. Fluorometry of histological preparations was then carried out. In the case of ethidium bromide, uptake was equal to 510-523 nm, emission - to 595-605 nm, while in the case of chlortetracycline, those parameters came to 400 nm and 520 nm respectively. In addition, myocardium samples were stained with antibodies for Monoclonal Anti Skeletal Myosin (FAST) Clone MY-32 skeletal myosin. FITS-conjugated secondary antibodies were used as a secondary marker.

The following properties were measured: muscle fibre diameter, relative area of muscle tissue, its apparent density, number of nuclei, mean area of a nucleus, nucleus-cytological relations and number of intramyocardial vessels.

Microsoft Excel 2000 was used to perform statistical processing of the results. T-tests were employed to provide the reliability of differences of mean quantities and correlation relationships. Differences $p<0.05$ were considered as reliable.

The concentrations of CE were determined by X-ray fluorescence analysis with synchronous radiation (SRXRF). All measurements were carried out at the station of X-ray fluorescent elemental analysis in the Siberian Centre of Synchrotron and Terahertz Radiation (Budker Institute of Nuclear Physics SB RAS). The parameters of the storage ring VEPP-3 and experimental station are as follows: E_{ex} = 2 GeV, B = 2 T, I_e = 100 mA; chamber for the analysis is made from elconait; maximum diameter of the sample is 30 mm; the spot size is 1 ÷ 30 mm^2; exposure time is 10 ÷ 1000 c; the excitation energy is from 12 to 45 keV; elements determined: from S to U; X-ray fluorescence from the sample is registered by 10mm^2 Si(Li) detector (OXFORF, Oxford Instruments Inc., USA) with energy resolution 150 eV at 5.9 keV, respectively (Trounova et al., 1998).

The advantages of the application of SR as a primary source of excitation are as follows: the high intensity → the better peak/background ratio → analysis of samples with low masses (down to 0.5 mg, dry weigh); linear polarization → lower background → lower detection limits (down to 0.02 ppm for organic matrices); the wide spectrum of radiation → optimization of excitation energy, the possibility to measure samples, as well as varying the excitation energy.

The concentrations of CE in the samples of heart muscle and vessels were calculated by the external standard method (different certified reference materials [CRM]) were used). The corresponding approaches were elaborated upon, using different certified reference materials with similar matrices: the applicability of different standards and the absorption characteristics of their matrices were investigated (Trunova et al., 2008). All spectra obtained were processed by the AXIL programme (Canberra Packard, Benelux). The samples investigated are the fragments of myocardium tissue with masses from 2 to 10 mg (dry weigh). At one of the steps of the sample procedure they are dried for 48 hours and longer to obtain a dry sample with a flat surface.

The content of CE was measured in 40 samples of myocardium of TGA infants aging from 1 to 4.5 months (mean age 3.0+0.7 months, heart's mass 54.0+5.0 g, body mass 4.2+0.3 kg). The concentrations of the following 14 CE were studied: S, Cl, K, Ca, Cr, Mn, Fe, Ni, Cu, Zn, Se, Br, Rb, Sr by SRXRF (Okuneva et al., 2010). By using X-ray fluorescence analysis with synchronous radiation (XFA SR), concentrations of the following 14 CE were studied: S, Cl, K, Ca, Cr, Mn, Fe, Ni, Cu, Zn, Se, Br, Rb, Sr (Okuneva et al., 2010). Myocardium samples were taken from ventricles and atria not later than 24 hours after death. Overall, more than 270 X-ray fluorescence spectra of CE were obtained. The content of CE was determined on the basis of 1 μg per 1 g of tissue.

3. The clinical examination of infants with TGA

All patients with TGA were broken down in 2 groups: the first group included patients with intact ventricular septum (IVS), while the second one incorporated those with ventricular septum defects (VSD). Two tasks were set; firstly, to study the clinical characteristics of patients depending on their age, for which purpose all of them were classified into 3 age groups: newborns aged 1 to 6 months and babies aged 6 to12 months. The second task was to compare the clinical characteristics of the deceased patients (subgroup I) and patients with favourable outcomes after surgical repair of the disease (subgroup II). Anthropometric measurements of patients with IVS depending on their age in the first and second group are given in Table 1.

Group	Sub group	At birth		By the time of surgery			
		Weight, kg	Height, cm	Weight, kg	Norm	Height, cm	Norm
Newborns	I (n=19)	3.2±0.6	50.4±3.2	3.1±0.1*	4.1±0.2	53.5±0.5	52.8±0.2
	II (n=5)	3.2±0.1	52.0±1.3	3.2±0.1*	4.1±0.2	52.4±1.1	
1-6 months old	I (n=18)	3.2±0.6	51.2±0.2	4.7±0.1	4.9±0.2	57.3±0.4	55.8±0.2
	II (n=5)	3.1±0.2	51.0±1.3	5.3±0.9	4.9±0.2	58.8±3.1	
6 to 12 months old	II (n=5)	3.1±0.1	50.0±0.8	7.4± 0.7	9.5±0.2	70.2±3.0	70.5±0.2

** P < 0.05*

Table. 1. Anthropometric measurements of TGA patients with IVS

As can be seen from Table 1, the weight of patients in all groups was close to the norm. However, by the moment of surgery the delay in body weight gain as compared to the norm in newborns in both subgroups amounted to 1000 g, in infants - 200 g, while in those who survived in the third group it came to 1500 g. Dynamics of height measurements slightly exceeded the benchmark indicators. Similar anthropometric data were also obtained for the VSD group (Table 2).

Group	Sub group	At birth		By the moment of surgery			
		Weight, kg	Height, cm	Weight, kg	Norm	Height, cm	Norm
Newborns	I	3,2±0,2	52,0±1,0	3,3±0,3	3,8±0,2	53,5±1,3	52,8±0,2
	II	3,0±0,1	51,2±0,6	3,5±0,1	3,8±0,2	51,7±1,0	
1 to 6 months old	I	2,8±0,5	51,1±0,8	4,1±0,6*	5,0±0,2	58,1±2,5	55,8±0,2
	II	3,2±0,1	50,8±0,2	4,0±0,1*	5,0±0,2	56,8±0,7	
6 to12 months old	I	3,4±0,4	50,6±1,2	6,0±0,8*	9,8±0,2	63,3±3,0	70,5±0,2
	II	3,0±0,1	50,6±0,3	7,0±0,5*	9,4±0,2	70,5±2,1	

** P < 0.05*

Table 2. Anthropometric measurements of TGA patients with VSD

By the moment of surgery, the delay in body weight gain as compared with the norm in newborns was on average 400 g, in the 1 to 6 months old - 900 g, in 6 to 12 months old infants in the deceased subgroup this difference came to 3800 g, while in those who survived - 2400 g. Dynamics of height measurements slightly exceeded the benchmark indicators in both groups. Based on the data obtained, one might conclude that disruption of metabolic processes in TGA infants evidently manifests itself only by a decrease in body weight, with the height parameters remaining the same. Table 3 looks at echocardiographic (ECHO) measurement data in patients with IVS depending on their age.

Group	Newborns		1 to 6 months old		6 to 12 months old
Subgroup	I	II	I	II	II
End-systolic dimension, cm	1.3±0.7	0.8±0.1	1.1±0.2	0.8±0.1	1.3±0.1
End-systolic volume, ml	1.4±0.7	1.4±0.7	3.8±1.5	1.7±0.5	5.8±1.0
Systolic output, ml	6.0±2.1	4.6±1.0	20.4±13.6	7.3±1.9	16.9±1.7
Shortening fraction, %	44.1±4.9	51.2±2.1	40.7±6.6	47.2±2.2	48.0±5.1
Ejection fraction, %	79.1±4.4	82.4±1.7	77.8±6.8	83.0±1.5	75.6±4.1
LV thickness, cm	0.5±0.1	0.5±0.1	0.6±0.1	0.5±0.1	0.6± 0.1
End-diastolic dimension, cm	1.6±0.2	1.5±0.1	2.0±0.3	1.7±01	2.5± 0.1
End-diastolic volume, ml	8.6±3.0	5.6±1.8	19.1±8.7	6.5± 2.5*	22.7±3.6

Table 3. Echocardiographic measurement data for TGA patients with IVS

As the table shows, the age does not influence the following values of ECHO: RV end-systolic dimension, LV shortening fraction and LV ejection fraction. There was a slight age-related increase in ASD, as well as a decrease in the unclosed ductus arteriosus size. As compared with the newborns, the following ECHO values tended to increase: RV size, end-systolic volume, systolic output, end-diastolic dimension, LV end-diastolic volume and LV thickness, thus indicating a reduction of myocardial contractility. ECHO data on TGA patients with VSD are given in Table 4.

Group	Newborns		1 to 6 months old		6 to 12 months old	
Subgroup	I	II	I	II	I	II
RV size, cm	1.2± 0.2	0.8± 0.1	1.0± 0.2	0.9± 0.2	1.5±0.4	1.4± 0.2
End-systolic dimension, cm	1.1± 0.3	1.2± 0.1	1.5± 0.4	1.3± 0.2	1.4±0.3	1.4± 0.2
End-systolic volume, cm	2.7±0.5	3.5± 0.9	9.4± 5.0	4.8±1.8	6.4± 2.3	6.4± 1.9
Systolic output, ml	10.1±3.5	9.3± 3.1	19.7±9.2	15.7±3.4	18.9±2.0	17.9±1.9
Shortening fraction,%	45.0±4.5	38.5±5.0	35.1±3.0	42.1±15.4	42.3±4.2	48.2±7.2
Ejection fraction, %	69.7±3.4	72.0±5.7	66.5±5.6	75.0±4.6	73.5±4.6	75.6±6.2
LV thickness, Cm	0.51±0.1	0.3± 0.1	0.54±0.1	0.5± 0.1	0.6±0.1	0.7± 0.1
End-diastolic dimension, cm	1.3± 0.3	1.9± 0.2	4.6± 3.3	2.4± 0.2	2.5±0.3	2.5± 0.2
End-diastolic volume, cm	11.6±1.5	13.3±4.6	25.8±11.9	20.6±5.0	24.2±5.9	22.7±4.8

Table 4. Echocardiographic measurement data for TGA patients with VSD

In the 1 to 6 and 6 to 12 months old groups, as compared with the newborn group, the following ECHO values were found to increase considerably: RV size, end-systolic volume, systolic output, end-systolic dimension, end-diastolic volume and end-systolic dimension. In addition, there was a trend toward an increase in the size of ASD, VSD and LV thickness. However, the size of unclosed ductus arteriosus tended to decrease. The shortening fraction (SF) and ejection fraction (EF) values matched the age-related indices. The pressure in the pulmonary artery was elevated in all groups, but it was particularly high in the 6 to 12 months old group.
Clinical/functional examination of TGA patients demonstrated that in terms of basic clinical indicators there were no statistically significant differences between the deceased and surviving infants with TGA. Moreover, average indicators of all 3 age subgroups (newborns, 1 to 6 months old and 6 to 12 months old) in both groups are identical within a time period. From this it follows that negative factors causing the death of infants with TGA are related to molecular disorders of metabolic processes in cardiomyocytes that, in turn, brought us to start studying the content of CE and structural/molecular characteristics of TGA infants' myocardium.

4. Distribution of chemical elements in different parts of the heart and their impact on the development of pathologies in TGA patients

The following mechanisms were identified when analyzing the content of CE in the deceased infants' myocardium (Table 5A,B).

		Intact myocardium		TGA patients' myocardium	
Parts of the heart		Left ventricle (n=5)	Right ventricle (n=5)	Left ventricle (n=15)	Right ventricle (n=20)
Content of CE, μg/g	S	3380±631	3260±335	3268±424	3547±331
	Cl	842±311	624±142	405±45*	435±56
	K	792±257	630±133	508±60	560±55
	Ca	1352±218	1264±94	1256±89	1224±99
	Cr	1.0±0.22	0.9±0.12	0.4±0.15*	0.6±0.23
	Mn	2.4±0.2	2.4±0.2	2.6±0.8	5.1±2.0
	Fe	344±30	422±83	321±42	342±33
	Ni	0.4±0.05	0.6±0.09	0.2±0.03*	0.2±0.05*
	Cu	8.9±0.68	10.1±0.87	14.6±2.99	16.1±2.58
	Zn	360±39	392±43	240±22*	307±42
	Se	0.7±0.1	0.8±0.1	0.2±0.05*	0.1±0.04*
	Br	12±1.6	13±1.6	6±0.7*	8±0.8*
	Rb	1.4±0.23	1.4±0.18	0.8±0.20	0.6±0.08*
	Sr	6.1±0.7	6.3±0.6	3.7±0.7	3.8±0.5*

* $P < 0.05$

Table 5A. Distribution of CE in infants' ventricle with intact myocardium and TGA infants

It follows from Tables 5A and 5B that in 65 % of TGA patients, as compared to those with intact myocardium, the content of CE was reduced: K was lower, down to 78 %, concentration of Cl, Cr, Sr, Zn decreased to 50 % and the concentration of Br, Ni, Rb was also low. The content of Se equalled to just 25 % of the benchmark value. Three CE: S, Ca and Fe had an appropriate concentration. It was found out that only 2 CE had an increased concentration: Cu – 160 % and Mn – 170 to 200 %. According to the distribution of CE in the heart parts, the lowest concentrations of CE were found in LV and RA myocardium.

		Intact myocardium		TGA patients' myocardium	
Parts of the heart		Left atrium (n=5)	Right atrium (n=5)	Left atrium (n=21)	Right atrium (n=20)
Content of CE, μg/g	S	2560±180	2575±370	2398±300	2505±260
	Cl	504±83	615±158	348±43	290±42*
	K	494±71	580±165	444±58	421±38
	Ca	990±54	1112±96	1148±105	1109±86
	Cr	0.8±0.11	1.1±0.44	0.6±0.25	0.7±0.18
	Mn	2.0±0.2	2.0±0.2	3.1±1.1	4.2±1.4
	Fe	404±101	340±23	338±53	375±38
	Ni	0.3±0.06	0.4±0.09	0.2±0.04	0.2±0.04
	Cu	9.0±0.49	8.9±1.14	13.0±2.18	14.3±2.70
	Zn	344±38	298±57	183±21*	192±27
	Se	0.7±0.1	0.7±0.2	0.2±0.06*	0.2±0.05*
	Br	12±1.2	11±2.2	6±0.7*	6±0.6*
	Rb	1.2±0.17	1.1±0.24	0.5±0.10*	0.5±0.07*
	Sr	5.7±0.6	5.1±0.9	3.2±0.3*	3.5±0.4

* $P < 0.05$

Table 5B. Distribution of CE in infants' atrium with intact myocardium and TGA infants

Hence, irreversible hemodynamic disorders of the myocardial function and development of cardiac insufficiency might be connected with a low concentration of Cl, Cr, Sr, Zn, Br, Rb, Ni and specifically Se, which in this case drops to 25 % and even beyond the measurement limit. An increased content of Mn and Cu mostly in the right parts of the heart could be explained by an elevated functional load and plays a compensatory role. The content of S, Fe and Ca matches the benchmark values and does not affect the changes in the myocardium. On the basis of the results obtained it may be concluded that in order to maintain normal functional activity of the myocardium in TGA infants, the content of Cl, Zn, Sr, Cr, Ni, Rb, Br and especially Se that protects cardiomyocytes from lipid peroxidation should be optimal. The following relationships were revealed while comparing CE impoverishment in the myocardium of TGA infants in different heart parts (Table 6).

CE	LV		CE	RV		CE	LA		CE	RA	
	Mean	±m		Mean	±m		Mean	±m		M	±m
S	3268	424	S	3547	331	S	2398	330	S	2505	260
Ca	1256	89	Ca	1224	99	Ca	1148	105	Ca	1109	86
K	508	60	K	560	55	K	444	58	K	421	38
Cl	405	45	Cl	435	56	Cl	348	43	Fe	375	38
Fe	321	42	Fe	342	33	Fe	338	53	Cl	290	42
Zn	240	22	Zn	307	42	Zn	183	21	Zn	192	27
Cu	14.6	2.99	Cu	16	2.58	Cu	13	2.18	Cu	14.3	2.7
Br	6	0.7	Br	8	0.8	Br	6	0.7	Br	6	0.6
Sr	3.7	0.7	Mn	5.1	5	Sr	3.2	0.3	Mn	4.2	1.4
Mn	2.6	0.8	Sr	3.8	0.5	Mn	3.1	1.1	Sr	3.5	0.4
Rb	0.8	0.2	Rb	0.6	0.08	Cr	0.6	0.25	Cr	0.7	0.18
Cr	0.4	0.15	Cr	0.6	0.23	Rb	0.5	0.1	Rb	0.5	0.07
Ni	0.2	0.03	Ni	0.2	0.05	Se	0.2	0.06	Se	0.2	0.05
Se	0.2	0.05	Se	0.1	0.04	Ni	0.2	0.04	Ni	0.2	0.04

Table 6. CE impoverishment in the heart parts of TGA infants

It was found that in the hypertrophied myocardium of LV (and RV) there was a decreased content of K, Cl, Zn, while the content of S, Fe and Ca remained at an adequate level (see Fig. 1).

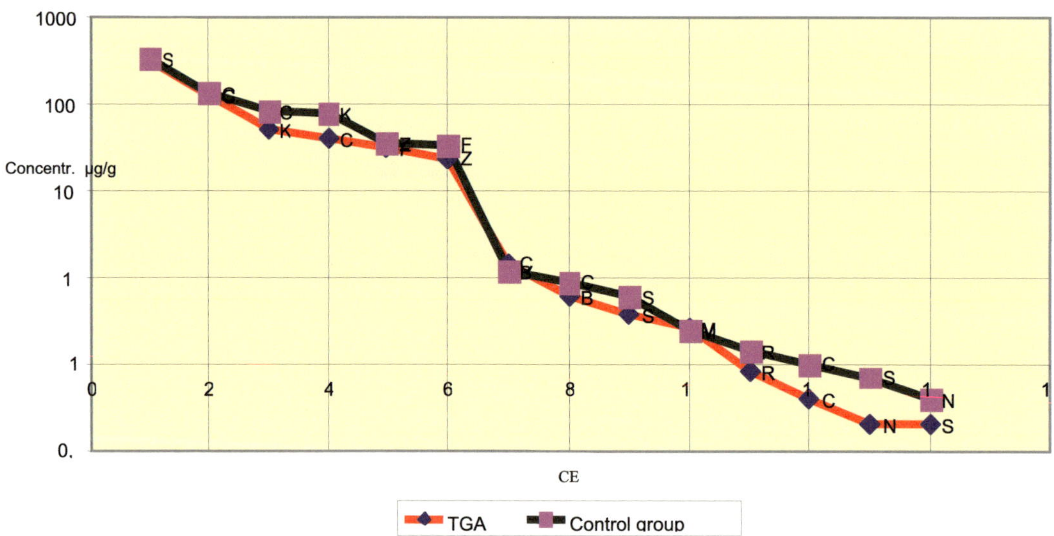

Fig. 1. Distribution of CE in LV of TGA infants, CE are arranged by concentration decrease.

The concentration of microelements Cr, Rb, Ni, Se was notably lowered, while the remaining CE had values that were close to the benchmark ones. The data obtained led us to conclude that the hypertrophied myocardial function in TGA infants was impaired due to a decreased concentration of microelements. These changes were more pronounced in the left parts of the heart. These results were also confirmed by the morphological examination data. Hypertrophic changes in the heart make rapid strides over age, exceeding the benchmark age values by 2 times at the age of up to 1 month and by 3.5 - 4.5 - at the age of 6 to 12 months. At the same time, the linear dimensions of LV and RV in patients with IVS (first group) were practically identical, while in the VSD group (second group) the thickness of RV exceeded that of LV by 133 % (Table 7).

Group	Heart's mass, g*	Wall thickness, cm		Muscle fibre diameter, μm		Inflow, cm		Outflow, cm	
		RV	LV	RV	LV	RV	LV	RV	LV
1st group	52.6 ±8.31	0.60 ±0.15	0.61 ±0.17	11.65 ±2.12	11.85 ±1.95	2.5 ±0.41	2.6 ±0.24	3.6 ±0.61	3.7 ±0.47
2nd group	48.7 ±9.33	0.60 ±0.12	0.55 ±0.14	11.90 ±3.11	11.60 ±2.55	2.5 ±0.21	2.8 ±0.36	3.6 ±0.52	4.0 ±0.54

* The norm is 24±0.15 g

Table 7. Cardiometric parameters of TGA newborns (first and second groups)

Heart part	Anatomic group	S	K	Fe	Cu	Sr	Zn
RV	1st group	0.15	0.09	0.58*	-0.26	-0.19	0.12
	2nd group	0.31	0.15	-0.29	-0.60*	0.13	0.08
LV	1st group	0.92**	0.75**	0.82**	-0.92**	0.67**	-0.18
	2nd group	0.46	0.47	0.50	-0.33	0.30	-0.25

* - Reliability of correlation relationship ($p<0.05$)
** – Reliability of correlation relationship ($p<0.01$)

Table 8. Correlation relationships (r) between myocardium thickness and content of some chemical elements

A statistically reliable relationship between LV myocardium thickness and the content of S, K, Fe, Sr and a negative correlation relationship with Cu were revealed for the first group with IVS (Table 8).

According to our data, an impaired myocardial function in TGA infants resulting in death might be related to a considerable reduction of metabolism, the markers of which appeared to be a lowered content of Br, Ni, Rb (down to 50 %), Cr, Sr, Zn, Cl (down to 60 %) and particularly Se (down to 25 %). What role do these CE play in myocardium metabolism in TGA infants? Some of these CE are mostly of an endonuclear nature (Cr, Mr, Ni), while others are found outside the nucleus and accumulated in microsomes, mitochondria, lysosomes and Golgi's complex (Cu, Zn, Se, Br, Sr) (Kudrin et al., 2000). Of great importance is Zn, which activates more than 300 enzymes and is part of over 200 metalloproteins (Skalny, 1999; Beerli, 2000). Zinc deficiency results in the development of congenital heart diseases (Panchenko, 2004), Br plays an important role in the development of a foetus and its shortage leads to a greater number of miscarriages. Ni might be a co-factor of many enzymes: urease, hydrogenase, a number of dehydrogenases and methyl-coenzyme M-reductase, while its deficiency affects metabolic processes in the cells. It was found out that the activity of b-DNA-polymerase directly depends on the content of Cr, a vital chemical element (Panchenko, 2004). Cr deficiency is observed in premature infants, whose mothers do not get enough of it in their diet. Chlorous channels can be found in mitochondrial membranes and muscle tissue. Also, chloride ions regulate the liquid volume and stabilize pH of the cells (Sing & Snow, 1998). Rb is an analogue of K and together with Cl they are very active in redoxreactions. A considerable deficiency of Se, which protects cardiomyocytes from detrimental effects of free radicals, has the greatest impact on cardiomyocyte metabolism. A decrease in muscle mass and a developmental lag were observed in newborns whose mothers were short of Se during pregnancy (Panchenko et al., 2004). In the case of Se deficiency, the cells start dying both in the form of apoptosis and necrosis, which might result in the sudden death of newborns (Azoicai et al., 1997; Bolli, 2002). On the strength of these data, we suggest that a very low content of CE, and Se in particular, in the myocardium could lead to structural disorders in the development of heart parts and, consequently, to deaths among TGA infants.

5. Pathomorphological measurements of myocardium in TGA infants

Data on morphological measurements of myocardium samples of TGA infants and infants of the same age but with intact myocardium are given in Table 9. As is seen from Table 9, the myocardium mass increased by 2.0 - 2.5 times and it tended to increase over age, i.e. in TGA infants the increase in the heart's mass considerably exceeded the normal age-related values for the heart's mass. Morphometric measurement data show that, in comparison with the intact myocardium, the TGA infants' myocardium had a reduced diameter of muscle fibres and a reduced mean area of nucleus and lowered nucleus-cytoplasma ratios in RV. However, the volumetric density and relative area of muscle tissue surface tended to increase.

Morphometric parameters	Heart part	Infants	TGA infants
Muscle tissue diameter, μm	LV	14.6±0.79	12.0±1.47
	RV	13.1±1.13	11.4±1.35
Relative area of muscle tissue surface, μm^2	LV	265±22.8	287±27.3
	RV	274±27.3	286±37.6
Volumetric density of muscle tissue	LV	0.78±0.067	0.85±0.08
	RV	0.81±0.081	0.84±0.11
Number of nuclei per field of vision	LV	41±2.5	45±7.1
	RV	53±1.5	34±7.7
Mean area of nucleus, μm^2	LV	2358±211.8	2073±107.1
	RV	2534±289.1	2063±355.8
Nucleus-cytoplasmic ratio	LV	0.37	0.33
	RV	0.49	0.26

Table 9. Morphometric parameters of TGA infants' myocardium

Depending on the anatomic type, 2 groups of TGA patients prevail: the first group, the so-called simple TGA form, TGA with atrial septal defect (ASD) and intact ventricular septum (IVS), and the second group, which includes TGA patients with ASD and VSD.

From the point of view of hemodynamics, the first group of TGA patients with IVS features a two-directional shunt, the volume of which, when performing isolated shunting on the level of atria, will depend on compliance of atria, a pressure differential in them during different phases of the cardiac cycle, size of atrial defect and a difference in resistance of the systemic and pulmonary circulation. Since the systemic circulation and pulmonary circulation are separated, the main compensation strategy is to increase the volume of circulating blood, which leads to overflow of the pulmonary circulation system (Adkin et al., 2002). In this anatomic type of TGA, the functional load on the ventricles is practically the same, which is confirmed by the results obtained while staining the myocardium with ethidium bromide. These results indicate that the peak of active synthesis of genetic material uptake in both ventricles in this group, as compared to that in the control group (see Fig. 2A), occurs during the neonatal period and manifests itself as a dramatic drop in colour intensity in fluorescence (see Fig. 2B).

The second group of TGA patients with VSD is hemodynamically characterized by the presence of 2 defects, on the level of atrial and ventricular septa, which improves blood mixing on the ventricular level due to crossed shunting. With VSD size being small, the pressure in pulmonary circulation grows slightly, when the size of VSD is large, the pressure in both circulation systems is levelled out which results in high pulmonary hypertension (HPHT) and augmentation of hypoxemia (Bokeria, 1996; Isoyama et al., 1987). In this anatomic type of TGA, due to an increase in the blood volume, both ventricles are subject to a large functional load as compared with the first group of patients, which makes itself evident in a reduced level of fluorescence in infancy (1 to 6 months old). From our point of view, this phenomenon can be defined as the start of the heart remodelling processes, which at the age of older than 6 months also include hyperplastic processes. These processes are related to polyploidization of nuclear material and subsequent hypertrophic phenomena determined by appropriate hemodynamic conditions developed during the postnatal period.

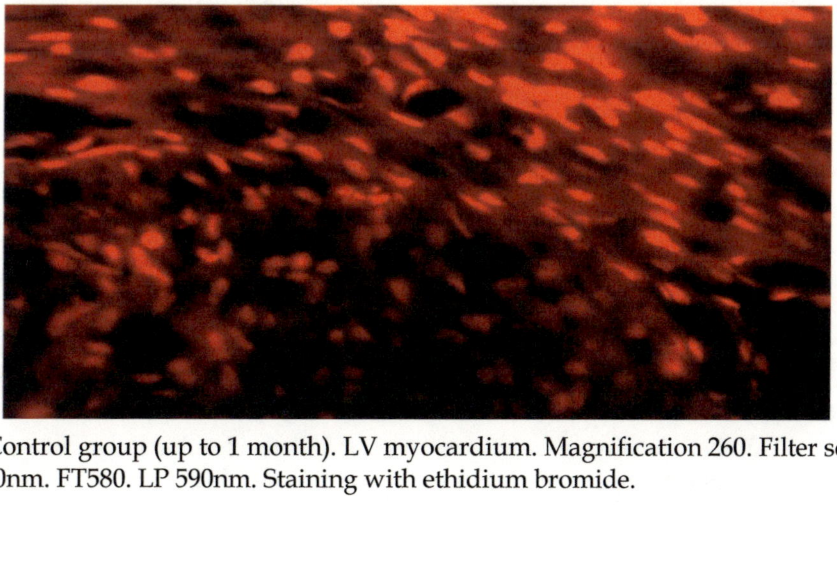

Fig. 2A. Control group (up to 1 month). LV myocardium. Magnification 260. Filter set 14. BP510-560nm. FT580. LP 590nm. Staining with ethidium bromide.

Fig. 2B. TGA with IVS. Lowered fluorescence level. LV myocardium (1 to 6 months). Magnification 260. Filter set 14. BP510-560nm. FT580. LP 590nm. Staining with ethidium bromide.

Clinical examination of TGA patients classified as belonging to the first anatomic type, i.e. with IVS, revealed an increase with age in cardiac insufficiency, respiration rate, liver dimensions, as well as a reduction in blood oxygen saturation on average, down to 60.9+13.5%. Arterial pressure and cardiac rate were within the normal age limits.

All TGA patients from the VSD group had pronounced cardiac insufficiency, increased respiration rate and liver dimensions, and decreased blood oxygen saturation, down to 32. 5+12.5% ($p<0.05$). Arterial pressure and cardiac rate were within the normal age limits. According to echocardiographic data, TGA patients from both groups, as compared with newborns, tended to show with age an increase in the following indicators: RV size (end-systolic dimension, stroke output, end-diastolic volume) and LV thickness. These changes imply a tendency towards a decrease in the contractile potential of the myocardium. The senior group of patients with VSD demonstrated a higher pressure in the pulmonary artery, up to 76.5+2.1 mm Hg.

LV muscle mass was growing faster by 6 to 12 months in the patients with VSD, with this value remaining stable in the IVS group. The mean quantity of nuclei was initially lower than in the control group, while the average area of nuclei was, to the contrary, higher but tended to decrease with age as well. The total area of nuclei in the control group tended to decrease. In the first group with IVS, this process took place faster, while in the second group there was an increase of this value, which is indicative of a compensatory reaction of LV. With age the surface density of cardiomyocytes smoothly grew in all the groups. The nucleus-cytoplasmic ratio in LV gradually decreased with age in infants of all groups. More pronounced was this tendency in RV of TGA patients with IVS. Conversely, a slight increase in this ratio was noted in TGA patients with VSD.

Studying the number density of capillaries revealed their simultaneous changes in both groups, with the highest point occurring at the age of 1 month in LV and RV in patients with

IVS. Measuring the content of CE in groups with IVS and VSD resulted in the following findings. The content of Cu, Zn and Mn in the group with VSD is 1.3 - 1.5 times higher than in the group with IVS. The content of CE in LV and RV of patients with IVS was about the same, except for an increased content of Mn in LV. At the same time, the content of CE in RV of patients with VSD increased, compared with that in LV, notably higher were concentrations of Zn, Mn and, to a lesser extent, Cu, Cr, Br, Rb. These findings are also confirmed by the cardiometric data (see the Table). In the case of the type with IVS, hypertrophic processes in LV and RV develop uniformly, and CE concentrations in LV and RV do not differ essentially. In the second type of TGA with VSD, the right ventricle has to bear a large functional load, therefore, CE concentration in RV is higher than in LV. It agrees with more pronounced structural changes in coronary arteries in the functionally overloaded RV in patients with VSD. However, despite intensive cardiac work in the cases of ASD and VSD, oxygen delivery in this group of patients is worse because of lower blood oxygen saturation down to 32 %.

The reduction of the numeric content of total ions Ca^{2+} is caused by the development of hypertrophic phenomena in the myocardium of patients with congenital heart diseases (see Fig. 3A and 3B). Most probably, these hypertrophic phenomena result from a decrease in the number of myofibrils, which aggravates cardiac insufficiency.

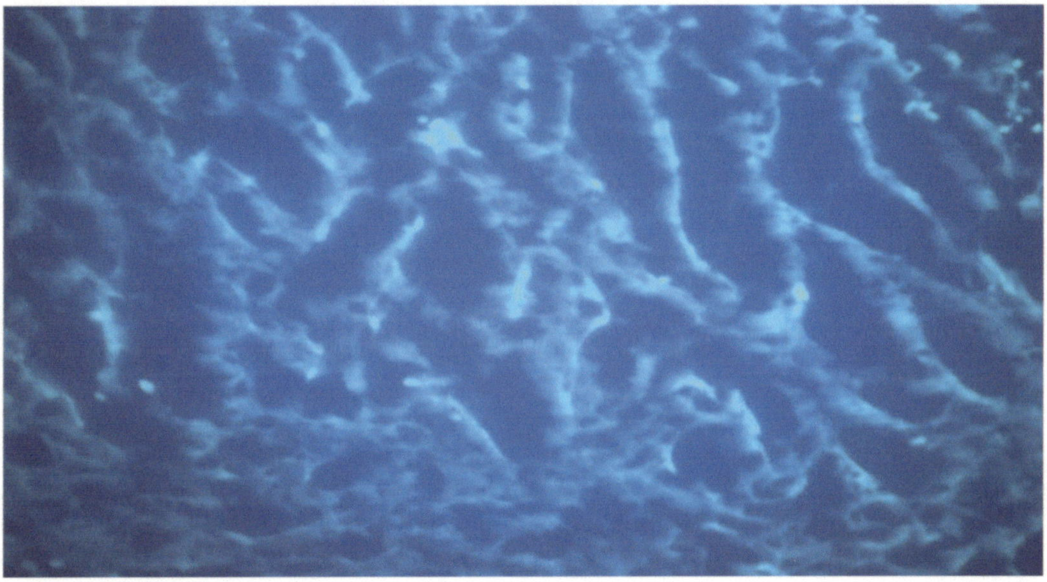

Fig. 3A. Control group. Native sample of LV wall. A high level of fluorescence. Filter set 05. BP395-440nm. FT460. LP 470nm. Magnification 260. Staining with chlortetracycline.

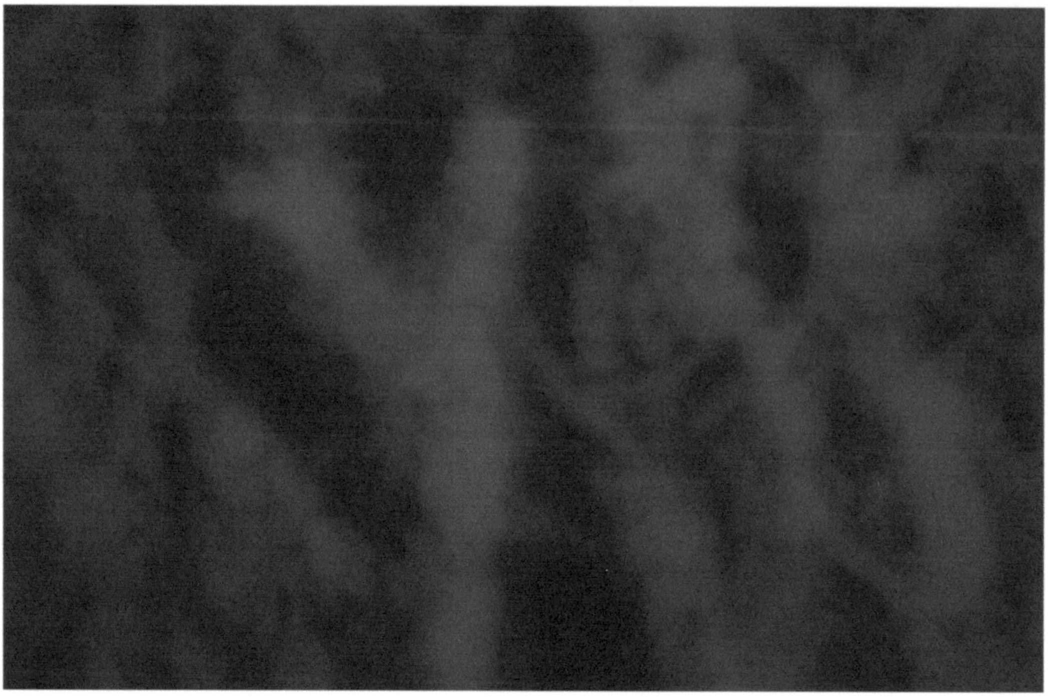

Fig. 3B. TGA with IVS (6 to 12 months). Native sample of LV wall. A lowered level of fluorophore fluorescence. Filter set 05. BP395-440nm. FT460. LP 470nm. Magnification 260. Staining with chlortetracycline.

In the case of hypertrophy not only is the volume (size) of muscle cells changed, but their phenotype as well. In the conditions of overload the contractile proteins in these cells are replaced by protein forms typical for foetuses and newborns. For example, the ß- myosin (ß-MHC) heavy chain is activated and, simultaneously with the suppression of α-MHC gene, the activity is changed over from the genes of the cardial α-actin to the genes of the skeletal one. This results in a reduction of the contractility speed of hypertrophied fibres. As hypertrophy proceeds, a few other genes are activated, including some early growth regulators, genes responding to thermal shock and growth factors, as well as a gene of the atrial natriuretic factor. The latter represents a peptide hormone that facilitates a decrease in hemodynamic overload by regulating blood pressure and salt discharge by the kidneys. Taking into account the preceding, we stained the myocardium samples with antibodies for Monoclonal Anti-Skeletal Myosin (FAST) Clone MY-32 skeletal myosin. As a secondary marker, we made use of FITS-conjugated secondary antibodies. As a result of the technique used, skeletal myosin was found in the myocardium of TGA patients (Fig. 4).

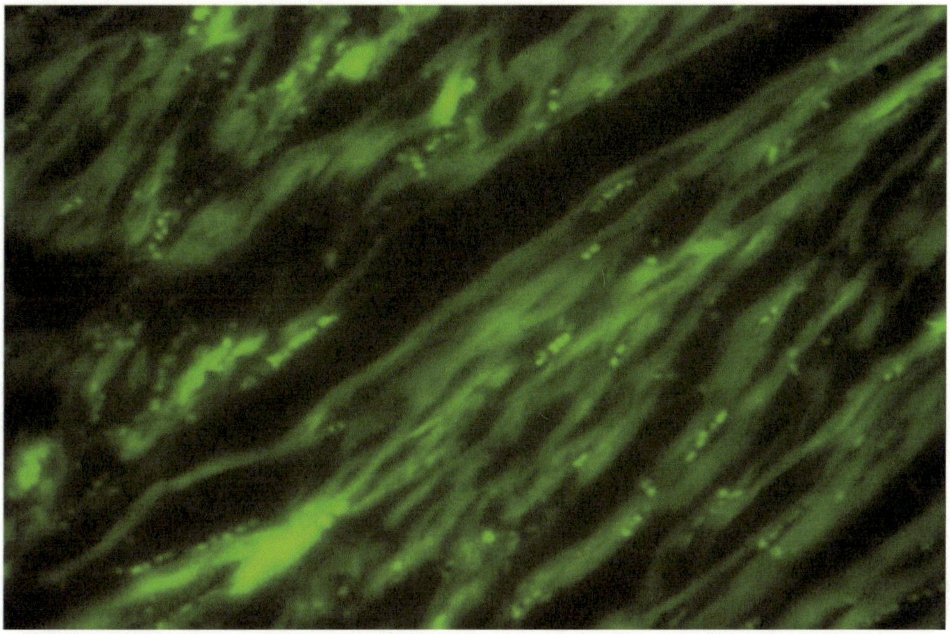

Fig. 4. TGA with IVS (1 to 6 months). Sample of LV wall. Appearance of skeletal myosin granules in the myocardial structure. Filter set 09. BP395-440nm. FT460. LP 470nm. Magnification 260. Monoclonal Anti-Skeletal Myosin (FAST) Clone MY-32, secondary antibody FITS-conjugated.

Thus, considering the dynamics of intensity of the above morphological processes taking place in the myocardium of TGA infants not older than 1 year, it should be noted that hypertrophic changes in TGA patients' myocardium make progress with age. Hyperplastic processes associated with intensive polyploidization of the genetic material and an increase in the quantity of desoxyribonucleic acid play an important role in the remodelling of the heart in patients older than 6 months. On the basis of fluorometric measurement data, the decrease in the level of total calcium ions in cardiomyocytes of TGA patients is dependent on the occurrence of cardiosclerosis zones when hypertrophy of the myocardium is progressing. While adapting to these processes and to chronic hypoxia typical for congenital heart diseases and due to a less energy-consuming mechanism of skeletal muscle contractility, the synthesis changes over from cardiac myosin to a skeletal one, which, in turn, enhances clinical presentations of cardiac insufficiency because of a lowered speed of hypertrophied fibre contractility. In the case of hypertrophy of cardiomyocytes, not only is their volume (size) changed, but their phenotype as well. The synthesis of the ß-myosin (ß-MHC) heavy chain is activated and, simultaneously with suppression of α-MHC, the synthesis of cardio-specific proteins is changed over to proteins specific for skeletal muscles, for example, skeletal a-actin is expressed. This results in a reduction of the contractility speed of hypertrophied fibres. As hypertrophy proceeds, a few other genes are activated including some early growth regulators, genes responding to thermal shock and growth factors, as well as a gene of the atrial natriuretic factor, which facilitates a reduction in hemodynamic overload by regulating blood pressure and discharge of salt by the kidneys. Immunohistochemical examinations of the samples of TGA infants' myocardium made it possible to observe the appearance of skeletal myosin in the cardiomyocytes. This testifies that, during hypertrophy development, the synthesis changes over from cardiac myosin to a skeletal one. Plain fluorescent microscopy of preparations stained with ethidium bromide revealed a drastic decrease in intensity of the fluorescent marker in infants aged under 6 months, as compared to the control group, and a rapid growth of ethidium bromide incorporation in infants aged 6 months and upward. It indicates a prevalence of the population of cardiomyocytes with diploid nuclei in the hearts of infants aged up to 6 months. In patients aged above 6 months, the heart remodelling process proceeds, with the processes associated with polyploidization of nuclear material and subsequent development of cell hypertrophy dominating. It should be emphasized that the level of polyploidization in LV cardiomyocytes is essentially higher than that in RV. Hence, the hyperplastic processes associated with intensive polyploidization of the genetic material and an increase in the quantity of desoxyribonucleic acid play an important role in the remodelling of the heart in patients aged above 6 months.

6. Conclusion

This study enabled us to come to the following conclusion on the development of a pathological mechanism causing the deaths of TGA patients at an early age. As a result of aorta and pulmonary artery transposition, low-oxygen venous blood flows into the systemic circulation system, limits the growth of newborns. The need for a sufficient volume of oxygen can be met only by increased load on the myocardium, with the development of heart hypertrophy uniform for LV and RV in patients with IVS and more pronounced in RV in patients with VSD. In this case the growth of TGA infants conforms to the age norm and even slightly exceeds it, while the body mass falls far short of the norm by 25-30 %. For hypertrophy and hyperplasia to develop dramatically, there should be an increased supply of nutritional and caloric substances, including CE. As the delivery of CE turns out to be insufficient, or their consumption increases, a 50 % deficiency of such microelements as Cl, Cr, Sr, Zn, Br, Rb and especially Se, which, as an active antioxidant, protects cardiomyocytes from lipid peroxidation, can be seen. As a consequence, structural disorders of the myocardium occur on the morphological/molecular level. Also observed are the following abnormalities: a decrease in the diameter of muscle fibres and the average area of nuclei, a drop in the level of the total calcium ions against the background of intensive polyploidization of genetic material, an increase in the content of the quantity of desoxyribonucleic acid, and change from the cardiac myosin synthesis over to a skeletal one. All these changes lead to alteration of the myocardium, occurrence of cardiosclerosis, development of cardiac insufficiency and reduction of arterial blood saturation down to 32 % and below, which is fatal, and results in death of the organism. This is a picture of TGA development pathogenesis of infants from neonatal age up to 1 year old. In this case, only definitive repair of the disease can break the pathogenetic chain of TGA in an early period, and the best time when effective cardiac surgery could be performed for TGA infants is in the neonatal period.

We suppose, that to prevent the development of congenital heart diseases including TGA, pregnant women and nursing mothers should get the optimum quantity of microelements Cr, Zn, Sr, Ni, Rb, Br and most of all Se, protecting the myocardium from lipid peroxidation.

7. References

Adkin, D.V.; Gnusayev, S.F. & Ilyin, V.N. (2002). Criteria of early detection and tactics of early preoperative treatment of TGA. *Pediatry*, No.3, (2002), pp. 88-91

Azoicai, D.; Ivan, A. & Bredatean, M. et al. (1997). The importance of use of selenium in the role of an antioxidant in preventing cardiovascular disease. *Rev Med Chir Soc Med Nat Lasi.*, Vol. 101, No. 2, (1997) , pp. 109-115

Beerli, R.R.; Schopfer, U. & Dreier, B. et al. (2000). Chemically regulated zinc finger transcription factors. *J Biol Chem.*, Vol. 275, No. 42, (2000), pp. 2617-2627

Bokeria, L.A. & Gorbachevsky, S.V. (1996). Congenital heart diseases: state-of-the-art in Russia. *Proceedings of Thoracic and cardiovascular surgery*, Moscow, Russia, No. 3, (1996), pp. 31-34

Bolli, R. (2002). Regeneration of the human heart-no chimera? *N. Engl. J. Med*, Vol 346, No. 1, (2002), pp. 55-56

Castaneda, A.R. (1993). Surgical management of transposition of the great arteries. *Acta Chir. Austriaca*, Vol 25, No 2, (1993) , pp. 80-82

Castaneda, A.R.; Trusier, G.A. & Paul, M. H. et al. (1998). The early results of treatment of simple transposition in the current era. *J. Thorac. Cardiovasc. Surg*, Vol. 95, No 1, (1998), pp 14-28

Fozzard, H.A.; Haber, E. & Jennings, R.B. et al. (1986). *The Heart and Cardiovascular System.* New York: Raven Press, ISBN 0881671266, pp. 1491-1495, USA

Hoffman, J. (2006). *Pediatric cardiology*. ISBN 5-89816-071-X, Moscow, Russia

Isoyama, S.; Wei, JY. & lzumo, S. et al. (1987). Effect of age on the development of cardiac hypertrophy produced by aortic constriction in the rat. *J Clin invest*, Vol. 81, No. 6 (1988), pp. 1850-1857

Kudrin, A.V.; Skalny, A.A. & Zhavoronkov, A.A. (2000). *Immunopharmacology of microelements*. ISBN 5-87317-077-0, KMK Publishing House, Moscow, Russia

Okuneva, G.N. et al. (2010). *Chemical elements in the cardiovascular system of cardiac patients.* GEO Publishing House, ISBN 978-5-904682-22-4, Novosibirsk, Russia

Panchenko, L.F.; Mayev, I.V. & Gurevich, K.G. (2004). *Clinical biochemistry of microelements.* GOU VUNMC Publishing House, ISBN 5-89004-077-4, Moscow, Russia

Re, R.M. (1987). Cellular mechanisms of growth in cardiovascular tissue. *Am.J.Cardiol.*, No. 60, (1987), pp. 100-104

Reiss, K.; Cheng, W. & Ferber, A. et al. (1996). Overexpression of insulin-like growth factor-1 in the heart is coupled with myocyte proliferation in transgenic mice, *Proc. Natl. Acad. Sci.* USA. Vol. 93, No. 16, (1996), pp. 8630-8635.

Ruff, H.A. (1999). Population-based data and development of individual children: case of low to moderate lead levels and intelligence. *J. Dev. Behev. Pediatr.*, Vol. 20, No 1, pp. 42-79

Scholzen, T. & Gerders, J. (2000). The Ki-67 protein: from the known and the unknown. *J. Cell. Physiol.* Vol. 182, (2000), pp. 311-313

Shankar, A.H. & Prasad, A.S. (1998). Zinc and immune function: the biological basis of altered resistance to infection. *Am. J. Clin. Nutr.* Vol. 68 (Suppl.), (1998), pp. 447-463

Singh, J. & Snow, E.T. (1998). Chromium (III) decreases the fidelity of human DNA polymerase beta. *Biochemistry*, Vol. 37, No. 26, (1998), pp. 9371-9378

Skalny, A.V. & Rudakov I.A. (2004). *Bioelements in medicine.* Moscow, Mir Publishing House, ISBN 5-03-003645-8, Moscow, Russia

Trounova, V.A.; Zolotarev, K.V. & Baryshev, V.B. et al. (1998). Analytical possibilities of SRXRF station at VEPP-3 SR source. *Nuclear Instruments and Methods A*, Vol. 405, (1998), pp. 532-536

Trunova, V. A. & Zvereva, V. V. (2008). Investigation of the distribution macro - and traceelements in human myocardium and vessels by SRXRF. *Journal of Structural Chemistry*, Vol. 49, (2008), pp. 211-216